Complementary
& Alternative Therapies
in Nursing

Tai Chi (17)
Relaxation
Breathing (18)

Ruth Lindquist, PhD, RN, FAAN, is a professor at the University of Minnesota School of Nursing, and a faculty member of the Center for Spirituality and Healing in the Academic Health Center. She also is a member of the Academy of Distinguished Teachers at the University of Minnesota. Her past research has focused on critical care nurses' attitudes toward and use of complementary and alternative therapies. Currently, her research focuses on the use of complementary and alternative therapies (exercise, mindfulness meditation, problem-solving therapy) to improve the health of patients with peripheral arterial disease, heart disease, and stroke. She has also incorporated the use of complementary and alternative therapies in her work with the women's cardiac patient support group, and in research to promote self-care among nurses.

Mariah Snyder, PhD, is professor emerita at the University of Minnesota School of Nursing. Her professional career included teaching courses on complementary therapies, conducting research on the use of these therapies in people with dementia, and in managing stress in individuals with chronic illnesses. She also worked with international nurses to further the use of complementary therapies across the globe. Dr. Snyder was a founding member of the Center for Spirituality and Healing at the University of Minnesota and promoted the establishment of the center's graduate interdisciplinary minor. In her retirement, Dr. Snyder devotes time to assisting women recovering from addiction and homelessness and in developing the library at Cristo Rey Jesuit High School in Minneapolis.

Mary Fran Tracy, PhD, RN, CCNS, FAAN, is a critical care clinical nurse specialist at the University of Minnesota Medical Center, Fairview. She is an adjunct clinical professor at the University of Minnesota School of Nursing and adjunct assistant professor at the University of Minnesota School of Medicine. Dr. Tracy has been the principal investigator or coinvestigator on a number of major funded research projects, including several focused on nurses' use of alternative therapy interventions in critical care, and reduction of reliance on traditional medicine therapies in critical care settings. Dr. Tracy has published numerous papers and book chapters, including several in the current and past editions of the Snyder/Lindquist, *Complementary & Alternative Therapies in Nursing*. Additional authored chapters appear in other well-regarded critical care, progressive care, and advanced practice nursing textbooks. Dr. Tracy has been the journal editor for *AACN Advanced Critical Care* since 2008.

Complementary
& Alternative Therapies
in Nursing

SEVENTH EDITION

Ruth Lindquist, PhD, RN, FAAN
Mariah Snyder, PhD
Mary Fran Tracy, PhD, RN, CCNS, FAAN

SPRINGER PUBLISHING COMPANY
NEW YORK

Springer Publishing Company, LLC
11 West 42nd Street
New York, NY 10036
www.springerpub.com

Acquisitions Editor: Margaret Zuccarini
Composition: Amnet Systems Pvt. Ltd.

ISBN: 978-0-8261-9612-5
e-book ISBN: 978-0-8261-9762-7

14 15 / 5 4 3 2

The author and the publisher of this Work have made every effort to use sources believed to be reliable to provide information that is accurate and compatible with the standards generally accepted at the time of publication. The author and publisher shall not be liable for any special, consequential, or exemplary damages resulting, in whole or in part, from the readers' use of, or reliance on, the information contained in this book. The publisher has no responsibility for the persistence or accuracy of URLs for external or third-party Internet websites referred to in this publication and does not guarantee that any content on such websites is, or will remain, accurate or appropriate.

Library of Congress Cataloging-in-Publication Data

Complementary & alternative therapies in nursing / [edited by] Ruth Lindquist, Mariah Snyder, Mary Fran Tracy. — Seventh edition.
      p. ; cm.
  Complementary and alternative therapies in nursing
  Includes bibliographical references and index.
  ISBN 978-0-8261-9612-5 (print edition : alk. paper) — ISBN 978-0-8261-9762-7 (e-book)
  I. Lindquist, Ruth (Professor of nursing), editor of compilation. II. Snyder, Mariah, editor of compilation. III. Tracy, Mary Fran, editor of compilation. IV. Title: Complementary and alternative therapies in nursing.
  [DNLM: 1. Complementary Therapies—nursing. 2. Holistic Nursing. WY 86.5]
  RT41
  610.73—dc23

                                                                              2013024628

Printed in the United States of America by McNaughton & Gunn.

To providers around the world who strive to care for and comfort those seeking health and healing, through the offering of complementary and alternative therapies.

Contents

Contributors

Susan M. Bee, MS, RN, PMHCNS-BC
Clinical Nurse Specialist
Pediatric Pain Rehabilitation Center
Mayo Clinic
Rochester, Minnesota

Carie A. Braun, PhD, RN
Professor
Chair, Department of Nursing and Chair Joint Faculty Senate
College of Saint Benedict/Saint John's University
Saint Joseph, Minnesota

Ulf G. Bronäs, PhD, ATC, ATR, FSVM, FAHA
Assistant Professor
School of Nursing
University of Minnesota
Minneapolis, Minnesota

Miriam E. Cameron, PhD, MS, MA, RN
Graduate Faculty and Lead Faculty, Tibetan Healing Initiative
Center for Spirituality and Healing
Academic Health Center
University of Minnesota
Minneapolis, Minnesota

Kuei-Min Chen, PhD, RN
Professor, College of Nursing
Director, Master Degree Program of Aging and Long-Term Care
Kaohsiung Medical University
Director, Kaohsiung Elderly Research and Development Center, Kaohsiung City
  Government
Kaohsiung, Taiwan

Corjena K. Cheung, PhD, RN
Assistant Professor
School of Nursing
University of Minnesota
Minneapolis, Minnesota

Linda L. Chlan, PhD, RN, FAAN
Distinguished Professor of Symptom Management Research
College of Nursing
Ohio State University
Columbus, Ohio

Michael S. Christopher, PhD
Associate Professor
School of Professional Psychology
Pacific University
Forest Grove, Oregon

Susanne M. Cutshall, DNP, RN, ACNS-BC, HWNC-BC
Assistant Professor and Integrative Health Specialist
Mayo Clinic
Rochester, Minnesota

Michele M. Evans, MS, RN, PMHCNS-BC, APNG
Clinical Nurse Specialist
Pain Rehabilitation Center
Mayo Clinic
Rochester, Minnesota

Maura Fitzgerald, RN, MS, MA, CNS
Clinical Nurse Specialist
Children's Hospitals and Clinics of Minnesota
Pain Medicine, Palliative Care, and Integrative Medicine Program
Minneapolis/St. Paul, Minnesota

Melissa H. Frisvold, PhD, RN, CNM
Assistant Professor
School of Nursing & Health Sciences
Georgetown University
Washington, DC

Marion Good, PhD, RN, FAAN
Professor Emerita
Frances Payne Bolton School of Nursing
Case Western Reserve University
Cleveland, Ohio

Cynthia R. Gross, PhD
Professor
School of Nursing and College of Pharmacy
University of Minnesota
Minneapolis, Minnesota

Thora Jenny Gunnarsdottir, PhD, RN
Associate Professor
Faculty of Nursing
University of Iceland
Reykjavik, Iceland

Niloufar Niakosari Hadidi, PhD, RN, ACNS-BC, FAHA
Assistant Professor
School of Nursing
University of Minnesota
Minneapolis, Minnesota

Linda L. Halcón, PhD, MPH, RN
Associate Professor and Cooperative Head
School of Nursing
University of Minnesota
Minneapolis, Minnesota

Melodee Harris, PhD, APN, GNP-BC, FNGNA
Clinical Assistant Professor
University of Arkansas for Medical Sciences
College of Nursing
Little Rock, Arkansas

Annie Heiderscheit, PhD, MT-BC, LMFT
Center for Spirituality and Healing
Academic Health Center
University of Minnesota
Minneapolis, Minnesota

Mary Jo Kreitzer, PhD, RN, FAAN
Director, Center for Spirituality and Healing
Professor, School of Nursing
University of Minnesota
Minneapolis, Minnesota

Mary Langevin, RN, MSN, NP-C, CPON, HBN-BC
Family Nurse Practitioner
APRN-Hematology/Oncology
Children's Hospitals and Clinics of Minnesota
Minneapolis, Minnesota

Laura Lathrop RN, DNP, CNP
Advanced Certified Hospice and Palliative Care Nurse
Palliative Consult Service, Allina Health
St. Paul, Minnesota

Barbara Leonard, PhD, RN, FAAN
Professor Emerita
School of Nursing
University of Minnesota
Minneapolis, Minnesota

Ruth Lindquist, PhD, RN, FAAN
Professor
School of Nursing
University of Minnesota
Minneapolis, Minnesota

Margaret P. Moss, PhD, JD, RN, FAAN
Associate Professor
School of Nursing
Yale University
New Haven, Connecticut

Kathleen Niska, PhD, RN
Associate Professor
Graduate Department of Nursing
College of St. Scholastica
Duluth, Minnesota

Susan O'Conner-Von, PhD, RN
Associate Professor
School of Nursing
University of Minnesota
Minneapolis, Minnesota

Sue Penque, PhD, RN, NE-BC
Senior Vice President
South Nassau Communities Hospital
Oceanside, New York

Elizabeth L. Pestka, MS, RN, PMHCNS-BC, APNG
Assistant Professor and Clinical Nurse Specialist
Pain Rehabilitation Center
Mayo Clinic
Rochester, Minnesota

Gregory A. Plotnikoff, MD
Medical Director, Institute for Health and Healing
Abbott Northwestern Hospital
Minneapolis, Minnesota

Maryanne Reilly-Spong, PhD
Research Associate
College of Pharmacy
University of Minnesota
Minneapolis, Minnesota

Debbie Ringdahl, DNP, RN, CNM, Reiki Master
Clinical Assistant Professor
School of Nursing and Center for Spirituality and Healing
University of Minnesota
Minneapolis, Minnesota

Dereck Salisbury, MS
Doctoral Candidate
Department of Kinesiology
University of Minnesota
Minneapolis, Minnesota

Yeoungsuk Song, PhD, RN, ACNP-BC
Assistant Professor
College of Nursing
Kyungpook National University
Daegu, South Korea

Mariah Snyder, PhD
Professor Emerita
School of Nursing
University of Minnesota
Minneapolis, Minnesota

Mary Fran Tracy, PhD, RN, CCNS, FAAN
Critical Care Clinical Nurse Specialist
University of Minnesota Medical Center, Fairview
Minneapolis, Minnesota

Diane Treat-Jacobson, PhD, RN
Associate Professor and Cooperative Head
School of Nursing
University of Minnesota
Minneapolis, Minnesota

Shirley K. Trout, PhD, Med
Pedagogy of Engagement (pedENG)
Faculty Development Consultant
Owner, Teachable Moments
Lincoln, Nebraska

Alexa W. Umbreit, MS, RN-BC, CHTP, CCP
Independent Practitioner
St. Paul, Minnesota

Shigeaki Watanuki, PhD, RN
Professor of Gerontological Nursing
National College of Nursing
Tokyo, Japan

Pamela Weiss-Farnan, PhD, MPH, RN, Dip.Ac., L.Ac
Integrative Therapist
Institute for Health and Healing
Abbott Northwestern Hospital
Minneapolis, Minnesota

Jaclene A. Zauszniewski, PhD, RN-BC, FAAN
Kate Hanna Harvey Professor in Community Health Nursing
Frances Payne Bolton School of Nursing
Case Western Reserve University
Cleveland, Ohio

Terri Zborowsky, PhD, EDAC
Center for Spirituality and Healing
University of Minnesota
Minneapolis, Minnesota

International Sidebar Contributors

AUSTRALIA
Trisha Dunning, PhD, AM, RN, CDE, MEd
Professor and Chair in Nursing (Barwon Health)
School of Nursing and Midwifery
Deakin University
Victoria, Australia

Alison Short, PhD, MT-BC, RMT
Australian Institute of Health Innovation
University of New South Wales
Sydney, Australia

BRAZIL
Milena Flória-Santos, PhD, MS, RN
Assistant Professor
University of São Paulo at Ribeirão Preto College of Nursing
WHO Collaboration Centre for Nursing Research Development
Ribeirão Preto, São Paulo, Brazil

CAMBODIA
Sivchhun Hun
Nursing Student
Carr College of Nursing
Harding University
Searcy, Arkansas

CANADA
Linda Lindeke, PhD, RN, CNP
Director of Graduate Studies
Associate Professor
School of Nursing
University of Minnesota
Minneapolis, Minnesota

Kelly Penz, PhD, RN
Assistant Professor
College of Nursing
University of Saskatchewan
Regina, Canada

Larissa Pinczuk
Nursing Student
Carr College of Nursing
Harding University
Searcy, Arkansas

CHINA
Fang Yu, PhD, RN, GNP
Associate Professor
School of Nursing
University of Minnesota
Minneapolis, Minnesota

GAZA
Jehad Adwan, PhD, RN
Clinical Assistant Professor
School of Nursing
University of Minnesota
Minneapolis, Minnesota

GHANA
Esi Fosua Yeboah
Nursing Student
Carr College of Nursing
Harding University
Searcy, Arkansas

ICELAND
Thora Jenny Gunnarsdottir, PhD, RN
Associate Professor
Faculty of Nursing
University of Iceland
Reykjavik, Iceland

IRAN
Mansour Hadidi, MA
Architect
Shoreview, Minnesota

JAPAN
Ikuko Ebihara, MBA
3rd-degree Reiki Practitioner
NPO Reiki Association, Japan Reiki Association
St. Paul, Minnesota

Konomi Nakashima, PhD, RN
Associate Professor
Department of Nursing
School of Health Sciences
Bukkyo University
Kyoto Prefecture, Japan

Kenji Watanabe, MD, PhD, FACP
Associate Professor
School of Medicine
Director, Center for Kampo Medicine
Keio University
Shinjuku-ku, Japan

Shigeaki Watanuki, PhD, RN
Professor of Gerontological Nursing
National College of Nursing
Tokyo, Japan

KENYA
Eunice M. Areba, PhD candidate, RN, PHN
School of Nursing
University of Minnesota
Minneapolis, Minnesota

NEPAL
Deb Gauldin, RN, PMS
Deb Gauldin Productions
Raleigh, North Carolina

PERÚ
Margaret Kehoe, Dip.Ed-CHTP/1
Lima, Perú

Sasha Orange
Nursing Student
School of Nursing
University of Minnesota
Minneapolis, Minnesota

PHILIPPINES
Zapora Burillo, MSN, RN, CNN
South Nassau Communities Hospital
Oceanside, New York

Azel Peralta
Nursing Student
Carr College of Nursing
Harding University
Searcy, Arkansas

REPUBLIC OF SINGAPORE
Siok-Bee Tan, PhD, MN, RN
Advanced Practice Nurse and Assistant Director of Nursing
Singapore Nursing Division
Singapore General Hospital
Republic of Singapore

RUSSIA AND UKRAINE
Olga Formogey, MN, RN
Doctoral Student
School of Nursing
University of Minnesota
Minneapolis, Minnesota

SOUTH AFRICA
Karin Gerber, M. Cur (c), B. Cur, Dipl N Edu
Associate Lecturer and Level Coordinator for B.Cur 2
Nursing Science Department
School of Clinical Care Sciences
Nelson Mandela Metropolitan University (NMMU) North Campus
Port Elizabeth, South Africa

SOUTH KOREA
Sohye Lee, BSN
Doctoral Student
School of Nursing
University of Minnesota
Minneapolis, Minnesota

SWEDEN
Ulf G. Bronäs, PhD, ATC, ATR, FSVM, FAHA
Assistant Professor
School of Nursing
University of Minnesota
Minneapolis, Minnesota

TAIWAN
Jing-Jy Sellin Wang, PhD, RN
Professor
Department of Nursing & Institute of Gerontology
College of Medicine
National Cheng Kung University
Tainan City, Taiwan

Miaofen Yen, PhD, RN, FAAN
Professor
Department of Nursing & Institute of Allied Health Sciences
College of Medicine
National Cheng Kung University
Tainan City, Taiwan

THAILAND
Kesanee Boonyawatanangkool, APN
Nursing Care Management Center (NCMC)
Nursing Division
Srinagarind Hospital, Faculty of Medicine
Khon Kaen University
Khon Kaen, Thailand

Nutchanart Bunthumporn, PhD, RN
Lecturer, Faculty of Nursing
Thammasat University
Klong Luang, Pathum Thani
Thailand

Sukjai Charoensuk, PhD, RN
Boromarajonani College of Nursing
Chon Buri
Thailand

TIBET AND INDIA
Tashi Lhamo, RN, BTMS
Staff Nurse
Unity Hospital
Minneapolis, Minnesota

UNITED KINGDOM
Graeme D. Smith, PhD, RN, BA, FEANS
Senior Lecturer
School of Health in Social Science
University of Edinburgh
Edinburgh, United Kingdom

WEST AFRICA
Maria Keita, MSN, RN, CNS
Clinical Nurse Specialist
Regions Hospital
St. Paul, Minnesota

Preface

Welcome to the new seventh edition of *Complementary & Alternative Therapies in Nursing*. Widespread popularity of complementary and alternative therapies continues, compelling us to update the evidence underlying the therapies and to incorporate new information related to their use. We took this opportunity to also refresh the look and feel of book and chapter content, especially by adding views and perspectives of international colleagues in each chapter. You are sure to enjoy these international perspectives! However, even as we embrace change, we deliberately carry forward all of the book's well-recognized strengths into this edition. We kept the chapter format, organization, practice applications, examples, and evidence-based approach of the book. We believe that the up-to-date, easy-to-retrieve, authoritative information on commonly used complementary and alternative therapies have contributed to the book's success and use by nurses in the United States and around the world. The book is unique in its field, and is relied upon for accurate and useful information from scholars and practitioners in varied fields. Attesting to this is the fact that the book has been translated into three languages—Chinese, Japanese, and Spanish. The volume will continue to be a valued asset for busy professionals, popular among nursing faculty, nursing students, and practicing nurses. A majority of the general population is using these therapies; never have our patients and the public desired complementary and alternative therapies more. This new edition is timely, and it offers the latest information and evidence to arm nurses with the knowledge and application guides for use of these high-in-demand therapies.

This work is an essential resource for nurses, and provides current information on many of the most commonly used complementary and alternative therapies. Having such a resource at hand is needed to keep us up to date regarding evidence supporting use of the various procedures. It also enables us to provide our patients with basic information about selected complementary therapies, including the ability to better answer questions about their use—especially questions regarding safety and efficacy. As providers, nurses need to be informed about potential contraindications for procedures, as well as their possible interactions with concurrently prescribed conventional medical solutions. We also need to be knowledgeable about these therapies so that we may offer them to our patients as safe and effective options for comfort, relief of symptoms, or for health and healing. We believe that this book meets these essential needs for information. The usefulness of the volume is enhanced by the inclusion of links to various websites, where further details and current and updated information may be found.

We are eager to share our excitement about what is "new" about this edition. The first thing you might notice on the binding and cover of the book is the inclusion of a new editor, Dr. Mary Fran Tracy. Dr. Tracy is a clinical nurse specialist with experience in the field, particularly as a member of a collaborative interdisciplinary team that researches use of complementary therapies. She brings visionary viewpoints and evidence she has gained through her past national complementary and alternative therapy survey of practicing critical care nurses. She brings editorial skills from her years of experience as chief editor of the journal *AACN Advanced Critical Care.*

Also, in this edition, new authors with fresh viewpoints join more senior authors who have a wealth of experience and expertise, resulting in a rich blend of vigor and wisdom. We have worked diligently to provide cutting-edge information from the available evidence base, as well as from the experience of the numerous experts who have authored the chapters of this book. Many of the authors regularly use these therapies in practice, in their research, or in their own self-care. The wisdom of seasoned authors, many of whom are at the peak of their research or practice careers, is obvious in the writing. The contributor lists in the front of the text contain a roster of authors who have distinguished positions, roles, credentials, and achievements that attest to their authority in the area of their therapeutic specialty. These contributors have acquired expertise from the work they do across a broad array of practice settings of various sizes and structures—encompassing large and small health care institutions, schools, academic health centers, public health settings, and private practice.

All of the chapters describing therapies have sections that include background, definitions, scientific basis, intervention(s), and one or more techniques that can be used to implement a therapy. There are precautions to be aware of in applications, conditions, and patient populations in which these therapies have been used, as well as cultural applications and suggestions for research. The uniform format is a structure that provides a clear way to organize knowledge and educate patients.

The chapter on "Creating Optimal Healing Environments" has found a new home in the "Foundations" section of the text in recognition of the primary, essential role that the environment plays in the administration or practice of healing therapies. The material on education, practice, and research continues to be housed in separate chapters, with even greater depth and concentration of focus in those areas. New references provide current and relevant cutting-edge information for today's practicing nurse or nurse scholar. These references also point out new avenues for science and discovery to pursue in the exploration of the science and art underlying the procedures. The information provided is practical. The holistic and caring aspects of these therapies have been and continue to be valued both by nurses and by those to whom care is provided in the United States and worldwide. Nursing roles continue to evolve; however, within all of these varied roles and settings in which nurses practice, concern for the comfort and healing of patients remains uppermost in their minds.

In this edition, as in the past, we continue to draw upon the expertise of authors from around the world, including South Korea, Sweden, Iceland, Iran, Taiwan, and Japan. However, in this seventh edition, we have expanded the perspectives within each chapter to specifically include viewpoints from outside the United States. Within each chapter is the "voice" of those giving or receiving effective healing therapies and practices from countries and cultures around the globe. The world is becoming increasingly smaller; hence, we need to understand the use of complementary and alternative therapies and practices indigenous to various cultures and populations. Thus, besides the expanded emphasis on culture in Chapter 1, the most exciting addition to this new volume is the international sidebars found throughout the book in each chapter. Contributors of these sidebars come from more than 20 countries on six continents. They provide tremendous perceptions that broaden, enrich, and deepen our understanding of the basis for and use of complementary therapies.

Complementary therapies play a key role in the promotion of healing, comfort, and care worldwide. Many therapies used by nurses have been used over the past centuries. Now, an increasing number of these procedures that have long been a part of systems of care across the globe are receiving attention in the United States. The increasing mobility of society, whether through immigration, travel, or attendance at international conferences, requires that nurses be knowledgeable about ancient therapies that are still used by many people around the world. Throughout this work, attention is paid to health care practices of other cultures, so that nurses may acquire knowledge about and respect for these practices and therapies and, if possible, incorporate them into the plan of care. Thus, this book is needed more than ever to help prepare students and practitioners for the broad range of complementary and alternative therapies that they will encounter in their practice.

This actively developing frontier of science is generating important and much-needed evidence to support our informed use of complementary and alternative therapies. Various groups, including the National Academy of Science, have proposed goals to expand research on complementary therapies. There is a concomitant increase in the number of journals focusing on these therapies. We trust that we have captured the most current evidence for the therapies in the seventh edition of this text. Conducting and disseminating the research-based evidence for the use of complementary therapies is an endeavor in which nurses can be integrally involved. Many nurses have provided leadership in research, education, and practice applications of these practices.

As consumer demand for and use of complementary therapies continue to increase, it is critical that nurses gain knowledge about complementary therapies, so that they can select and include them in their practice; provide patients with information about them; be informed about research and practice guidelines related to complementary therapies; alert patients to possible contraindications; and even incorporate some of these procedures into their own self-care. The recognized benefits experienced in personal use of the therapies in self-care fuel the enthusiasm for their application and use in practice.

Finally, we want to thank the countless nurses and nursing students who across the years have used our text and who have encouraged us to continue updating the information. The interest they have shown in the use of complementary therapies for practice and self-care has prompted us to continue our quest to obtain new information about complementary therapies that can be used by nurses. We thank the authors—some new, many returning—who have spent countless hours in writing or revising the chapters to bring you the most useful and updated information. We also thank the many international contributors who have enriched the chapters, and in their writing helped us to see the therapies through fresh eyes and help us to develop new possibilities for their use. Their stories will "stick" with us as we ponder the use of these therapies with other individuals we encounter requiring our care. We thank our colleagues at the School of Nursing and the Center for Spirituality and Healing at the University of Minnesota for their ongoing efforts to develop the knowledge base for complementary therapies through research, and to educate students about these therapies for their future practice, to the benefit of countless patients whom they have yet to encounter.

Ruth Lindquist, PhD, RN, FAAN
Mariah Snyder, PhD
Mary Fran Tracy, PhD, RN, CCNS, FAAN

Part I: Foundations for Practice

Complementary therapies have become widely known and used in Western health care. However, the therapies included in many of the surveys that have been done about the use of complementary therapies are sometimes limited in scope. Expanding the perspectives on complementary therapies' medicine so that nurses become more knowledgeable about therapies that are practiced by people in multiple cultures across the globe is critical to competent health care. In Chapter 1 and in subsequent chapters throughout this book, the authors have taken a new tack: to examine the use of complementary therapies from a global perspective. Nurses from across the globe discuss how a specific therapy is or is not used in their countries. This approach conveys the growing use of complementary therapies not only in the United States but worldwide.

Modeling the holistic, caring philosophy that underlies many of the complementary therapies typically used is an important aspect of care. Taking care of oneself is even more important in the increasingly pressure-filled health care settings in which nurses and other health professionals practice today. In Chapter 2, therapies and practices are discussed that nurses can use to lessen stress and thereby better focus on the patient and the patient's family.

Two therapies—presence and communication—are critical elements in the implementation of any of the complementary therapies. Many patients and families comment about a nurse who was "really present when providing care." Presence is difficult to define; however, as an old adage goes, "You know it when you see it." The multiple facets of communication, both verbal and nonverbal, are likewise important keys to providing the holistic care that is part of the philosophy underlying the use of complementary therapies. Nonverbal communication becomes more important when interacting with people who are not from Western cultures. The increasing cultural diversity found in many countries requires that all health professionals be attuned to health practices that patients may be using. The knowledge of customs—as basic as whether it is acceptable to shake the hands of the patient and family, or touch someone of another gender—is foundational in establishing the kind of therapeutic relationship that is integral to the success of complementary therapies. Discussions in Chapters 3 and 4 seek to heighten the nurse's awareness of the importance of presence and communication skills in building such relationships.

Chapter 5 describes the final foundation for healing—creating an optimal healing environment. The physical or "built" environment is a main focus of this chapter. However, in the international sidebar of this chapter, we are reminded of the importance of the roles of food, family, and spirituality in the creation of a healing environment.

Chapter 1: Evolution and Use of Complementary and Alternative Therapies

Mariah Snyder, Kathleen Niska, and Ruth Lindquist

Complementary and alternative therapies have become an integral part of health care in the United States and other countries. Although the term *complementary therapies* is used in this book, numerous other designations have been used for such remedies that are not a part of the Western system of medical care. The word *complementary* is preferred by some because it conveys that a procedure is used as an adjunct to Western or conventional therapies, whereas *alternative* indicates a therapy that is used in place of a Western approach to health care. Both terms are in the title of the National Institutes of Health (NIH) agency responsible for these aids: the National Center for Complementary and Alternative Medicine (NCCAM). More recently, the term *integrative medicine* has been used to convey that care provided in a health care facility is a blend of Western medicine, complementary therapies, and possibly procedures from other systems of health care. A growing body of research to support use of complementary therapies is emerging.

DEFINITION AND CLASSIFICATION

Numerous definitions of complementary therapies exist. Nursing and other health professions frequently call the area complementary *therapies*, whereas NCCAM refers to them as complementary *medicine*. The broad scope of these remedies and the many health professionals and therapists who are involved in delivering them create challenges for finding a definition that captures the breadth of this field.

As defined by the NCCAM, "Complementary and alternative medicine is a group of diverse medical and health care systems, practices, and products that are not presently considered to be part of conventional medicine" (NCCAM, 2012, p. 1). In this context, *conventional* refers to Western biomedicine. The NCCAM definition acknowledges that other systems of health care exist and are used. According to the World Health Organization, 80% of health care in developing countries is comprised of indigenous traditional health practices rather than Western biomedicine (World Health Organization, 2012).

The lack of precision in the meaning of complementary therapies poses challenges when comparing findings across surveys that have been conducted on use of complementary procedures. Some surveys have included a large number of practices, whereas others have been limited in scope. For example, in the NCCAM/National Center for Health Statistics Survey (NCCAM, 2008a), adding prayer for health reasons to the analyses increased the percentage of use of complementary therapies from 36% to 62%.

The field of complementary therapies is constantly changing as new remedies are identified—a number of which are from other systems of care or used in a variety of native cultures. NCCAM now classifies these multiple therapies and systems of care into three categories, although acknowledging the existence of many other practices and systems of care. One large category of therapies that is used in nursing is not included as a specific group in the recent NCCAM classification: energy therapies. The NCCAM categories and examples of the types of therapies in each classification plus other major categories are shown in Exhibit 1.1. Some of these procedures have been widely used and researched, whereas others are relatively unknown in the United States. A number of the therapies noted in Exhibit 1.1 have been a part of nursing for many years.

Other methods for classifying complementary therapies are provider-based and nonprovider-based administration. Remedies that are provider based require a professional/therapist to administer them, whereas therapies that are nonprovider based do not require the presence of a professional. For example, a therapist is required for acupuncture but one is not required for acupressure. Herbal preparations and food supplements—the most used groups of complementary therapies—are self-administered. For many procedures, once the technique has been taught, a therapist is not needed. Meditation is an example of this type of self-administered therapy. Nonprovider therapies are usually much less costly than the provider-administered therapies.

Globally, as people migrate for economic reasons, wars, drought, or political factors, health professionals are becoming increasingly aware

Exhibit 1.1. *NCCAM Classification for Complementary Therapies and Examples of Therapies*

Natural Products

Therapies use substances found in nature. Examples: herbal medicine (botanicals), vitamins, minerals, dietary supplements, probiotics.

Mind–Body Therapies

Interventions use a variety of techniques to enhance the mind's ability to affect body functions and symptoms. Examples: imagery, meditation, yoga, music therapy, prayer, journaling, biofeedback, humor, Tai Chi, art therapy, acupuncture.

Manipulative and Body-Based Therapies

Therapies are based on manipulation or movement of one or more parts of the body. Examples: chiropractic medicine, massage, bodywork such as rolfing.

***Energy Therapies**

Therapies focus on the use of energy fields such as magnetic and bio-fields that are believed to surround and permeate the body. Examples: healing touch, therapeutic touch, Reiki, external Qi gong, magnets.

***Systems of Care**

Whole systems of care are built on theory and practice and often evolved apart from and earlier than Western medicine. Each has its own therapies and practices. Examples include traditional Chinese medicine, Ayurvedic, naturopathy, and homeopathy.

***Traditional Healers**

Healers use methods from indigenous theories, beliefs, and experiences handed down from one generation to the next. An example is the Native American healer or shaman.

*Categorized by the NCCAM as *Other Practices* and not as a distinct category.
Source: NCAAM (2012).

of culture-specific health practices used in other countries. These remedies may be ones carried out by shamans, healers, family members, or the patient. Knowledge about common practices in various ethnic groups assists nurses in providing culturally sensitive care to promote health. A danger health professionals face is assuming that all people from a culture, a country, or an area of the world engage in the same health practices. For example, assuming that all Native Americans use sage as part of their healing services is erroneous. Health practices vary across the many Native American tribes/nations found in the Americas. Likewise, health practices differ among those from the huge African continent. Thus, individual assessments are needed to determine the healing practices a given person might be using, and acceptable therapies that might be employed.

USE OF COMPLEMENTARY THERAPIES

Interest in, and use of, complementary/alternative therapies has increased exponentially in recent years. Many individuals often used these therapies (e.g., prayer, meditation, herbal preparations); however, they were not called complementary therapy. Surveys have addressed use within English-speaking and largely Caucasian groups (Barnes, Powell-Griner, McFann, & Nahin, 2004; Sharafi, 2011; Su & Li, 2011). Recently, surveys have explored complementary therapy use within minority groups in the United States: African Americans (Barner, Bohman, Brown, & Richards, 2010); Hispanic adolescents (Feldman, Wiemann, Sever, & Hergenroeder, 2008); Whites, Mexican Americans, and Chinese Americans (Chao & Wade, 2008); and Asian Americans (Mirsa, Balagopal, Klatt, & Geraghty, 2010).

Interest in the use of complementary therapies is a phenomenon found not only in the United States but in many other countries as well. Research on the use of these therapies has been conducted in various countries, including Saudi Arabia (Al-Faris et al., 2008), Germany (Ernst, 2008), Japan (Hori, Mihaylov, Vasconcelos, & McCoubrie, 2008), Scotland (Thomson, Jones, Evans, & Leslie, 2012), and Turkey (Erci, 2007). The number of people using complementary therapies varied in these survey reports, but percentage of use was near 50% in all of the countries reporting.

Numerous studies have explored the use of complementary therapies in specific health conditions, including obesity (Bertisch, Wee, & McCarthy, 2008), asthma (Fattah & Hamdy, 2011), cancer (Wyatt, Silorskii, Wills, & Su, 2010), stroke (Shah, Englehardt, & Ovbiagele, 2009), and arthritis (Hoerster, Butler, Mayer, Finlayson, & Gallo, 2011). The Cochrane Database of Systematic Reviews contains reviews of the efficacy of numerous complementary therapies in the treatment of specific conditions (Cochrane Database of Systematic Reviews, 2012). In addition to the use of complementary therapies for health conditions, complementary therapies are often used to promote a healthy lifestyle. An example would be the use of Tai Chi to promote flexibility and prevent falls in older adults.

Some researchers have attempted to identify characteristics of users of complementary therapies. Nguyen and colleagues (2011) found that more women than men use these therapies. They also noted that a higher percentage of individuals using complementary therapies have academic degrees as compared with a nonuser group. These findings were further validated in the national survey conducted by the NCCAM and the National Center for Health Statistics (NCCAM, 2008a). Struthers and Nichols (2004) reviewed studies on the use of complementary therapies in racial and ethnic minority populations. They found that the use of complementary therapies was not greater in minority groups. However, it is not known how many therapies not listed on surveys were used by immigrants or those in minority groups.

What has prompted this rapidly growing interest in complementary therapies? First, the holistic philosophy underlying complementary therapies differs significantly from the dualistic or Cartesian philosophy that for several centuries has permeated Western medicine. In the administration of complementary therapies, the total person is considered—physical, emotional, mental, and spiritual. The goal of CAM (complementary/alternative medicine) is to bring harmony or balance within the person. People are seeking complementary therapists or care from facilities that offer complementary therapies because they want to be treated as a whole person—not as a heart attack or a fractured hip.

A second reason suggested for the popularity of CAM is that individuals want to be involved in the decision making in matters related to their health. The increasing pressure of cost containment in health care has reduced the amount of time physicians and nurses spend with their patients. A goal of health care related to reducing the cost of health care is to have people assume more responsibility for their well-being, which may explain the increase in using complementary therapies in addition to conventional care.

A third reason cited for seeking care from complementary therapists relates to quality of life. Patients have reported they do not want the treatment for a health problem to be worse than the initial problem itself. The focus of Western medicine largely has been on curing problems, whereas the philosophy underlying the use of complementary therapies is focused on harmony within the person and promotion of health. As noted earlier, this has many ramifications with the growing number of those with chronic illnesses.

The personal qualities of the complementary guide (whether a nurse, physician, or other therapist) are key in the healing process. Caring, which has been integral to the nursing profession through the years, is also a key component in the administration of complementary therapies. Two aspects of administration of CAM therapies—presence and active listening—are covered in subsequent chapters. Both convey caring. Remen (2000), a physician who is involved in cancer care, has stated:

> I know that if I listen attentively to someone, to their essential self, their soul, as it were, I often find that at the deepest, most unconscious level, they can sense the direction of their own healing and wholeness. If I can

remain open to that, without expectations of what the someone is supposed to do, how they are supposed to change in order to be better, or even what their wholeness looks like, what can happen is magical. By that I mean that it has a certain coherency or integrity about it, far beyond any way of fixing their situation or easing their pain that I can devise on my own. (p. 90)

The heightened interest in complementary therapies prompted the NIH to establish the Office of Alternative Medicine in 1992, which was elevated to the NCAAM in 1998 (NCCAM, 2012). What was significant about the establishment of this NIH office was that it was lobbied for by consumers rather than health professionals. The purposes of the NCCAM are fourfold:

- To define through rigorous research the usefulness and safety of complementary therapies and their role in improving health
- To promote translational research on the use of these therapies
- To train researchers to carry out studies on CAM therapies, and
- To facilitate education and outreach related to CAM

The NCAAM has funded research for individual investigators and for centers that explore the efficacy of a number of specific complementary therapies such as acupuncture and St. John's wort. Other centers explore the use of complementary procedures in the treatment of specific conditions such as addictive disorders, arthritis, cardiovascular disease, and neurological disorders. Additionally, the NCAAM has funded educational centers in the health professions to prepare practitioners and researchers.

REIMBURSEMENT AND COSTS

Currently, third-party payers such as insurance companies pay for a limited number of complementary therapies. The therapies most frequently covered are chiropractic medicine, acupuncture, and biofeedback. In most instances, physician referral is required for reimbursement. According to Nahin and colleagues (2009), Americans spent $33.9 billion on complementary remedies in 2007 with nearly two thirds being paid out of pocket by the consumer. Interestingly, $22 billion was for nonprovider-related expenses with only $11.9 billion being paid to practitioners. Obviously, people must feel that complementary techniques produce positive results if they continue to personally pay for these aids.

Some states, such as Washington, require the inclusion of complementary therapists in private, commercial insurance products (Lafferty et al., 2004). Other states have instituted legislation that provides protection for persons using complementary procedures. For example, legislation in Minnesota, titled the Complementary and Alternative

Health Care Freedom of Access bill, allows unlicensed complementary health care providers (non–health care professionals) to administer the therapies for which they have been trained. These therapists must provide their clients with a patient bill of rights and also supply them with proof of their education and practice.

Are complementary therapies cost-effective in terms of outcomes of care? Lind, Lafferty, Tyree, and Diehr (2010) examined differences in costs of health care for patients with back pain, fibromyalgia, and menopause symptoms who used CAM and those who did not. They found that CAM users had overall lower health care costs than those who did not use CAM: $1,420 less. Other researchers reported that individuals with chronic illnesses who used CAM were more likely to report feeling healthier (Nguyen et al., 2011).

The recently enacted Patient Protection and Affordable Care Act (PPACA) notes that health insurance providers are forbidden to discriminate against health care professionals who are acting within the scope of their license or certification (Thompson & Nichter, 2011). This opens the possibility for greater use of complementary therapists. How this provision may be challenged and/or implemented should be interesting—particularly in the care of the currently uninsured who seek insurance coverage.

CULTURE-RELATED ASPECTS OF COMPLEMENTARY THERAPIES

Human cultures pervade the globe. One's culture lends structure to a shared way of life in health and illness. McElroy and Townsend (2004) specified, "the culture of a group is an information system transmitted from one generation to another through nongenetic mechanisms" (p. 110). Culture is basically the shared way of life of a group of people. Culture theory and anthropology underscore the need for the inclusion of both complementary therapies and biomedical solutions into quality health care systems. All cultures have either systems of health care or numerous health care practices/therapies that are used by the members of that culture. Many of these remedies remain unknown to Western health care providers.

Singer and Baer (2012) noted that medical anthropology "builds a theoretical based understanding of what health is, how culture and health interact, the role of social realities in shaping disease, the importance of health/environmental interface, and a range of other issues" (p. vii). Emerging infections are occurring from human intrusion into ecosystems, with people encountering pathogens such as the Hanta virus found in wildlife within dried, aerosolized urine of rodents. These pathogens, foreign to humans, are spread as refugees move from one area to another due to war or natural occurrences such as drought. Thus, constant vigilance is needed to detect health problems in immigrants, refugees, and migrants.

Migration of people brings not only diseases but also their health care practices. Traditional healers traveling in populations of refugees include midwives, herbalists, shamans, priests or priestesses, bonesetters, and surgeons. There is a great need for healers because 47% of global morbidity is attributable to chronic conditions, with 60% mortality arising from such conditions (Manderson & Smith-Morris, 2010). Quinlan (2011) stated that 85% of traditional remedies are herbal, and more than 70% of the world's population depends on common herbal medicine for their primary care (p. 394). Beliefs about the cause of a number of chronic conditions point to the type of therapy used to "cure" the illness. Some individuals may seek care from a sorcerer. Humoral balance is a focus in some cultural systems of care such as traditional Chinese medicine (yin/yang) and Latin American medicine (hot/cold). Therapies to promote this balance such as Qi in traditional Chinese medicine and other systems in Latin American medicine may be used by immigrants from these areas.

Entire systems of health care have survived for thousands of years in various regions of the world. With the increasing movement of people either for short periods of time such as for study, business, or vacation or for permanent immigration, aspects of diverse systems of care will be encountered both by those in transit and by health care providers. The impact of Western medicine in most areas of the world is growing. However, individuals will continue to use all or portions of their traditional system of health care. These different ways of healing can work well together; however, it is imperative for Western care providers to assess for therapies or practices that may be used so that the patient is receiving safe care. Because minimal information is known about the outcomes of many of these therapies, close observations are needed to ensure that the therapy is enhancing, not interfering, with the biomedical treatment.

Although nurses may not know minute details of healing traditions in other cultures, it is helpful for them to gain some knowledge about the specific heritage of a patient. With today's technology, key points about the health practices of the culture can be obtained from web sources. When nurses are familiar with the patient's worldview, they can ask subjects and family members about specific needs and preferences that are natural parts of the individual's or the family's healing traditions.

An example of the importance of knowledge about cultural health practices in caring for Native Americans can be found in their traditional health care practices. As noted previously, the health professional must not make generalizations about health practices of Native Americans because great variations exist among the more than 500 Native American nations. In a number of instances the healing practices or rituals are kept secret and passed on from healer to healer (American Cancer Society, 2012).

Purifying the body is a foundational healing component of health rituals in a number of Native American nations. The basis for cleansing is to rid the person of bad feelings, negative energy, or bad spirits.

The individual is cleansed both physically and spiritually (Borden & Coyote, 2012). Cleansing can take a variety of forms such as smudging or sweat lodges. Sage and sweetgrass are commonly used by Plain Native Americans for their smudging ceremonies. Borden and Coyote describe a smudging ceremony:

> [B]urn the clippings of the herbs [dried], rub your hands in the smoke, and then gather the smoke and bring it into your body—or rub it onto yourself; especially onto any area you feel needs spiritual healing. Keep praying all the while that the unseen powers of the plant will cleanse your spirit. Sometimes, one person will smudge another, or a group of people using hands—or more often a feather—to lightly brush the smoke over the other person(s). (p. 3)

Native American families may wish to use smudging for family members who are hospitalized. This will require creativity on the part of nurses and others to make this possible.

Each complementary therapy chapter details how the specific therapy is implemented in countries other than the United States. Although similarities across nations and cultures in administration of the therapies are noted, cultural differences are recognized in the handling of the therapies globally. Sidebars that highlight both cross-cultural similarities and differences are included in most chapters.

Sidebar 1.1 relates the use of therapies in Palestine and their importance to health. The author also notes the transmission of these practices from generation to generation.

Sidebar 1.1. *International Perspective—Palestine*

Jehad Adwan, Gaza, Palestine

Growing up in a refugee camp in Rafah, on the Gaza Strip, I heard stories from my parents and grandparents about how they treated their sick. My paternal grandfather, Hassan, died long before I was born, but my grandmother, Aisha, lived until I was 15 years old. Hassan was perceived by his village as man of God (*Darwish*). He once predicted, according to the story my father told us many times, that my father (his son, Zaki) would fall and hurt himself or even die while sleeping one hot summer night on the roof—as many people did during summer. He asked his wife, Aisha, to remove the large pottery jars (used to cool water off in the shade) from under the assumed spot where my father would fall. Sure enough, my father fell that night and landed on soft sand rather than on a pottery jar. He was unscathed.

(continued)

Sidebar 1.1. *International Perspective—Palestine (continued)*

My grandmother inherited the skill of massage from her mother. Massaging the sick has been practiced in Palestine for many generations. My great-grandmother specialized in massage, which she learned from her mother. She incorporated hand skills and locally harvested olive and sesame seed oils with spiritual recitation of healing verses from the Qur'an. This skill is usually kept in families and handed down from mother to daughter, or father to son. I still feel her warm hands on my neck and chest as a child whenever I had a cold or sore throat. The warm oil in her hands touching my neck and chest with her firm yet gentle pressure on the troubled spot—combined with her reassuring whisper of the Qur'an verses—were hypnotizing. In a calming voice she would whisper:

> Say, I seek refuge in the Lord of daybreak from the evil of that which He created; from the evil of darkness when it settles; from the evil of the blowers in knots [witchcraft]; and from the evil of an envier when he envies. (Qur'an 113, 1–5)

Envy was often perceived as a cause of illness and misfortune in Palestine. However, as people become more accustomed to Western-style health care practices, less believe today that envy alone is the source of illness; and it's becoming more accepted that physical and environmental factors cause illness. Traditional healing, however, still exists to a large extent in rural communities that modern clinics and hospitals often cannot reach. You can find traditional healers delivering babies, fixing bones, and prescribing herbal and natural remedies for a variety of minor ailments and diseases. Some of these remedies include hibiscus teas, honey, vinegar, and numerous local herbs such as sage, thyme, and anise.

My older brother, Ra'ed, a superintendent for our hometown school district, is a strong believer in herbal medicine. We used to argue about the efficacy of these herbal remedies—he defending them, whereas I took the side of the Western-style approach of pharmacology. In retrospect, I see where he was coming from. I believe that although not all traditional Palestinian remedies do what they claim, there are elements that I do miss about them. I miss my grandmother's gentle, healing touch on my tiny neck and body as a sick little boy. I miss her comforting voice. If her touch wasn't comforting and healing to me, I don't know what else was.

IMPLICATIONS FOR NURSING

Although the term *complementary therapies* was not used, numerous therapies and their underlying philosophy have been a part of the nursing profession since its beginnings. In *Notes on Nursing* (1935/1992), Florence

Nightingale stressed the importance of creating an environment in which healing could occur and the significance of therapies such as music in the healing process. Complementary therapies today simply provide yet another opportunity for nurses to demonstrate caring for patients.

As noted in the chapters on self-care, education, practice, and research, nursing has embraced complementary practices. Although it is indeed gratifying to see that medicine and other health professions are recognizing the importance of listening and presence in the healing process, nurses need to assert that many of these therapies have been taught in nursing programs and have been practiced by nurses for centuries. Procedures such as meditation, imagery, support groups, music therapy, humor, journaling, reminiscence, caring-based approaches, massage, touch, healing touch, active listening, and presence have been practiced by nurses throughout time.

Complementary therapies are receiving increasing attention within nursing. Journals such as the *Journal of Holistic Nursing* and *Complementary Therapies for Clinical Practice* are devoted almost exclusively to complementary solutions. Many journals have devoted entire issues to exploring the use of complementary remedies. Articles inform nurses about complementary therapies and how specific procedures can be used with various patient conditions, including promoting health.

Because of the increasing use of complementary therapies by patients to whom nurses provide care, it is critical that nurses possess knowledge about these therapies. Patients expect health professionals to know about complementary therapies; nurses need such knowledge so that they can:

- Assess appropriateness and safety of therapies used
- Answer basic questions about use of complementary techniques
- Refer patients to reliable sources of information
- Suggest therapies having evidence of benefit for condition
- Provide patients with guidelines for identifying competent therapists
- Assist in determining whether insurance will reimburse for a specific therapy
- Administer a selected number of complementary remedies

Obtaining a complete health history requires that questions about the use of complementary therapies be an integral part of the health history. Many patients may not volunteer information about using complementary procedures unless they are specifically asked; others may be reluctant to share this information unless the practitioner displays an acceptance of complementary techniques. Although facts are needed about all complementary therapies, getting feedback about use of herbal preparations is critical because interactions between certain prescription drugs and certain herbal preparations may pose a threat to health.

The vast number of complementary therapies makes it impossible for nurses to be knowledgeable about all of them, but familiarity with the more common therapies will assist health providers in answering basic questions. Many organizations, professional associations, individuals, and groups have excellent websites that provide information about specific therapies. Caution is needed, however, in accepting information from any website. The NCAAM (2008b) urges that the following questions be posed:

- What group/organization operates the site and funds it?
- What is the purpose of the site?
- Where does the information originate and what guides the content presented?
- Who, such as an editorial board, selects the data contained on the site?
- How often is the content updated?
- Do links to other sites exist?
- How is information about the user of the site collected and can the user contact someone if questions arise?

Websites for specific therapies are identified throughout this book.

Assisting patients to identify criteria to use in identifying competent therapists is another role for nurses—and this is not an easy task. Because many complementary therapists are not members of a health profession, licensure and regulations often do not apply to them, and rules vary greatly from state to state. Numerous websites related to specific remedies contain information about therapists and what consumers can expect, and may also help in identifying practitioners in one's geographical area.

CONCLUSION

More and more people not only know about complementary therapies but also are using them or considering using them. Thus, it is mandatory for nurses to increase their knowledge about these therapies, which are often used in conjunction with Western biomedical treatments. Patients desire the emphasis on holistic care that underlies many complementary techniques. Holistic practice has permeated nursing for centuries. Incorporating complementary procedures into nursing care carries on this tradition.

REFERENCES

Al-Faris, E. A., Al-Rowais, N., Mohamed, A. G., Al-Rukban, M. O., Al-Kurdi, A., Al-Noora, M. A., . . . Sheikh, A. (2008). Prevalence and pattern of alternative medicine use: The results of a household survey. *Annals of Saudi Medicine, 28,* 4–10.

American Cancer Society. (2012). *Native American healing.* Retrieved December 3, 2012, from http://www.cancer.org/treat/treatmentandsideeffects/complementary therapies

Barner, J. C., Bohman, T. M., Brown, C. M., & Richards, K. M. (2010). Use of complementary and alternative medicine (CAM) for treatment among African Americans: A multivariate analysis. *Research in Social and Administrative Pharmacy, 6*(3), 196–208.

Barnes, P. M., Powell-Griner, E., McFann, K., & Nahin, R. L. (2004). Complementary and alternative medicine use among adults: United States, 2002. *Advance Data, 343,* 1–19.

Bertisch, S. M., Wee, C. C., & McCarthy, E. P. (2008). Use of complementary and alternative therapies by overweight and obese adults. *Obesity, 16,* 1610–1615.

Borden, A., & Coyote, S. (2012). *The smudging ceremony.* Retrieved December 6, 2012, from http://www.asunam.com/smudge_ceremony.html

Chao, M. T., & Wade, C. M. (2008). Socioeconomic factors and women's use of complementary and alternative medicine in four racial/ethnic groups. *Ethnicity & Disease, 18,* 65–71.

Cochrane Database of Systematic Reviews. (2012). *Table of contents—Cochrane Database of Systematic reviews.* Retrieved December 13, 2012, from http://www.the cochranelibrary.com/view/0/13996979657.a.html

Erci, B. (2007). Attitudes towards holistic complementary and alternative medicine: A sample of healthy people in Turkey. *Journal of Clinical Nursing, 16,* 761–768.

Ernst, E. (2008). Complementary medicine in Germany. *Climacteric, 11,* 91–92.

Fattah, M. A., & Hamdy, B. (2011). Pulmonary functions of children with asthma improve following massage therapy. *Journal of Alternative and Complementary Medicine, 17*(11), 1065–1068.

Feldman, J. M., Wiemann, C. M., Sever, L., & Hergenroeder, A. C. (2008). Folk and traditional medicine use by a subset of Hispanic adolescents. *International Journal of Adolescent Medicine & Health, 20,* 41–51.

Hoerster, K. D., Butler, D. A., Mayer, J. A., Finlayson, T., & Gallo, L. C. (2011). Use of conventional care and complementary/alternative medicine among U.S. adults with arthritis. *Preventive Medicine, 54*(1), 13–17.

Hori, S., Mihaylov, I., Vasconcelos, J. C., & McCoubrie, M. (2008). Patterns of complementary and alternative medicine use amongst outpatients in Tokyo, Japan. *BMC Complementary & Alternative Medicine, 8,* 14.

Lafferty, W. E., Bellas, A., Corage Baden, A., Tyree, P. T., Standish, L. J., & Patterson, R. (2004). The use of complementary and alternative medical providers by insured cancer patients in Washington state. *Cancer, 100,* 1522–1530.

Lind, B. K., Lafferty, W. E., Tyree, P. T., & Diehr, P. K. (2010). Comparison of health care expenditures among insured users and nonusers of complementary and alternative medicine in Washington state: A cost minimization analysis. *Journal of Alternative and Complementary Medicine, 16*(4), 411–417.

Manderson, L., & Smith-Morris, C. (2010). *Chronic conditions, fluid states: Chronicity and the anthropology of illness.* New Brunswick, NJ: Rutgers University Press.

McElroy, A., & Townsend, P. (2004). *Medical anthropology in ecological perspective.* Boulder, CO: Westview Press.

Mirsa, R., Batagopal, P., Klatt, M., & Geraghty, M. (2010). Complementary and alternative medicine use among Asian Indians in the United States: A national study. *Journal of Alternative & Complementary Medicine, 16,* 843–852.

Nahin, R. L., Barnes, P. M., Stussman, B. J., & Bloom, B. (2009). Costs of complementary and alternative medicine (CAM) and frequency of visits to CAM practitioners:

United States, 2007. *National statistics reports; no 18.* Hyattsville, MD: National Center for Health Statistics.

National Center for Complementary and Alternative Medicine. (2012). *What is complementary and alternative medicine?* Retrieved from http://nccam.nih.gov/health/whatiscam

National Center for Complementary and Alternative Medicine. (2008a). *The uses of complementary and alternative medicine in the United States.* Retrieved November 17, 2008, from http://nccam.nih.gov/news/camsurvey_fs1.htm

National Center for Complementary and Alternative Medicine. (2008b). *What 10 things to know about evaluating medical resources on the web?* Retrieved from http://nccam.nih.-gov/health/webresrources

Nguyen, L. T., Davis, R. B., Kaptchuk, T. J., & Phillips, R. S. (2011). Use of complementary and alternative medicine and self-rated health status: Results from a national survey. *Journal of General Internal Medicine, 26*(4), 399–404.

Nightingale, F. (1992). *Notes on nursing.* Philadelphia, PA: Lippincott. (Original work published 1935).

Quinlan, M. (2011). Ethnomedicine. In M. Singer & P. Erickson (Eds.), *A companion to medical anthropology* (pp. 381–404). Ames, IA: Wiley-Blackwell.

Remen, R. N. (2000). *My grandfather's blessings.* New York, NY: Riverhead Books.

Shah, S. H., Englelhardt, R., & Ovbiagele, B. (2009). Patterns of complementary and alternative medicine use among United States stroke survivors. *Journal of Neurological Science, 27,* 180–185.

Sharafi, S. (2011). Complementary and alternative medicine (CAM) among hospitalized patients: Reported use of CAM and reasons for use, CAM preferred during hospitalization, and the socio-demographic determinants of CAM users. *Complementary Therapies in Clinical Practice, 17,* 199–205.

Singer, M., & Baer, H. (2012). *Introducing medical anthropology: A discipline in action.* Lanham, MD: Rowman & Littlefield.

Struthers, R., & Nichols, L. A. (2004). Utilization of complementary and alternative medicine among racial and ethnic minority populations. Implications for reducing health care disparities. In J. Fitzpatrick & A. Villarruel (Eds.), *Annual review of nursing research* (Vol. 22, pp. 285–313). New York, NY: Springer Publishing Company.

Su, D., & Li, L. (2011). Trends in the use of complementary and alternative medicine in the United States: 2002–2007. *Journal of Health Care for the Poor and Underserved, 22*(1), 296–310.

Thompson, J. J., & Nichter, M. (2011). *CAM & health reform.* Retrieved December 6, 2012, from http://www.medanthro.net/research/cagh/insurancestatements/Thompson%26Nichter(CAM).pdf

Thomson, P., Jones, J., Evans, J. M., & Leslie, S. L. (2012). Factors influencing the use of complementary and alternative medicine and whether patients inform their primary care physicians. *Complementary Therapies in Medicine, 20*(1/2), 45–53.

World Health Organization. (2012). *Health of indigenous peoples.* Retrieved November 21, 2012, from http://www.who.int/mediacentre/factsheets/fs326/en/index.html

Wyatt, G., Sikorski, A., Wills, C. E., & Su, H. (2010). Complementary and alternative medicine use, spending, and quality of life in early stages of breast cancer. *Nursing Research, 59*(1), 58–66.

Chapter 2: Complementary Therapies: Nurse's Self-Care

Barbara Leonard

Complementary therapies are becoming widely used by people around the world. Nurses need to know about these therapies. First, nurses must be able to answer patients' questions and perhaps integrate some of these procedures into their own health practices. Second, nurses often may find that selected interventions are helpful to them in leading healthful and less stressful lives.

This chapter focuses on the nurse's use of complementary therapies as a commitment to wholeness so that this health care provider can use "self" as an instrument of healing. Self-care is critical for nurses and patients alike. The need for holistic self-care is essential for one's body, mind, and spirit. Self-awareness is integral to reflective holistic nursing practice. The American Holistic Nurses Association (AHNA) notes that the nurse "has a responsibility to model health behaviors. Holistic nurses strive to achieve harmony in their own lives and assist others striving to do the same" (AHNA, 2009, p. 2). Self-care is especially important for nurses and other health professionals who encounter life-and-death issues in their daily lives at a much higher rate than most other individuals. Stress mastery, general well-being, how complementary therapies can be incorporated into one's life, and care of one's spirit are discussed in this chapter.

STRESS MASTERY

Since the mid-20th century, science has demonstrated the impact of stress on human health, especially on the immune system. Although stress is a fact of modern life, many health professionals experience it regularly in their work. Fosarelli states that "for the health professional, the experience of bad situations and events is almost constant, depending on the medical specialty in which he or she practices" (2012, p. 41). She further emphasizes that in order to protect themselves, some health professionals will:

- Develop a hard shell, a brusque demeanor that ensures that no patient will draw close
- Take on only those patients who are likely to survive and thrive
- Become addicted to something that makes them feel better
- Bottle up their issues, keeping up a façade

Nurses cannot avoid stressful situations because they are part of nursing practice. Stress mastery goes beyond stress management as an understanding of stress mechanisms, the effect of stress on the human body, and how to develop the knowledge and skill that are needed to master stress. These are part of everyday life for nurses and other health professionals in the 21st century.

Understanding the toll of constant stress on one's body/mind is essential to learning stress mastery. In the animal world, threatened animals have extremely high adrenaline levels; however, levels decline rapidly and return to normal as soon as the threat passes. The mechanism for recovery from stress is inherent in animals. Human beings, on the other hand, can remain stressed, so the body/mind is in a constant state of threat. When this happens, the body's cells go into a protective modality that prevents growth because the two are mutually exclusive (Lipton, 2005). Because emotions link our physical body and our consciousness, consciousness and cells are intimately connected. For example, if one engages in reviewing old traumas, the brain goes into the protective mode that inhibits growth. The brain treats the old hurt as though it were current. Lipton emphasizes that eliminating stressors only puts one at the neutral point; to thrive one must not only eliminate stressors but also actively seek joyful, loving, fulfilling lives that stimulate growth processes.

Similarly, Hanson's (2008) research revealed that the human brain evolved to accentuate negative experiences for survival purposes. Even fleeting negative experiences leave traces in the brain. Monitoring one's thinking and practicing mindfulness are helpful in reducing stress. Hanson recommends that human beings store positive experiences in the brain by highlighting them through conscious attention. He suggests that individuals should let a good experience register deeply in emotional memory. One method for doing this is to imagine a positive experience soaking into one's chest, back, and brainstem or imagining a treasure chest in the heart where positive images are stored. Warm, good experiences have important benefits because they promote optimism, a bulwark against depression. Over time positive experiences counteract the effects of trauma or other painful experiences. They help to increase resilience, promote optimism, and identify key states of mind so one can find one's way back to peace, contentment, strength, well-being, and loving kindness.

SELF-CARE PRACTICES

Aspects of self-care involve basic activities such as eating a balanced diet, exercising, getting adequate sleep and rest, praying and/or meditating, keeping a sense of humor, and learning stress mastery skills. These general areas of health are the *foundation* for holistic health; they are by no means trivial. Holistic nurses are aware of the interrelationship among the body's systems: body, mind, and spirit. Pert states that "awareness is the property of the whole organism; and in the psychosomatic network, we see the conscious and the unconscious mind infusing every aspect of the physical body" (2008, p. 18). The term *body/mind/spirit* suggests that the cells of the entire body are always interrelating. Unlike the Cartesian philosophy in which the mind and body are separated, in the philosophy underlying holistic care, all systems affect each other. For example, a person with a headache is less interested in interacting with others, the appetite is often decreased, the ability to concentrate is lessened, and the spirit is less drawn to prayer. Similarly, if one's spirit is deadened, social, physical, and mental realms are impacted.

One strategy suggested for improving health is for the person to set goals and to keep track of progress toward these goals. Helpful information for setting goals can be found at the website (takingcharge.csh.umn.edu/create-healthy-lifestyle/your-healthy-lifestyle-tools). This site contains scientifically based information to assess and implement lifestyle improvements in physical activity, emotions, diet and nutrition, self-care, stress mastery, life purpose, relationships, and environment. Self-tests allow the individual to assess and determine areas in which changes are needed and how to set realistic goals in particular spheres.

The work of nurses requires that they are intentional about living holistically. No one integrative health modality can substitute for the kinds of daily holistic behaviors needed to remain whole in body, mind, and spirit. Buettner (2010) studied four geographic areas around the world—in which a disproportionate number of centenarians were found—to discover factors contributing to their vitality and longevity. Factors differed across the four areas; however, based on their findings, the researchers found commonalities to arrive at the following recommendations:

- Walking is the best activity for achieving longevity.
- Become aware of your values, passions, and talents and share these with others.

- Find time each day to meditate, nap, pray, or enjoy a happy hour; this helps to reduce stress and ultimately inflammation.
- Eat a healthy diet and reduce calories by 20%; eat a big breakfast; offer premeal expressions of appreciation.
- Shift to a mostly plant-based diet heavy on beans, nuts, and green plants; eat meat once or twice weekly.
- Engage in a happy hour, drinking in moderation.
- Giving attention to family life adds years to one's life.
- Make spirituality a part of one's life; it does not matter if a person is Christian, Jewish, Muslim, Buddhist, or part of another religious group; participating in a religious group four times a month adds 4 to 14 years to life.
- Expand (or retain) friendships.

These can be found on (www.bluezones.com/live-longer/power-9). These findings provide a holistic approach to life and address physical, spiritual, mental, and social aspects of living. The nine recommendations complement the website (takingcharge.csh.umn.edu/create-healthy-lifestyle/your-healthy-lifestyle-tools) that discusses lifestyle changes.

It is important to remember that basic, daily, good health practices are the foundation for holistic health. The right amount of sleep, for example, is essential not only for physical health but for spiritual, emotional, and mental health as well. During deep sleep the brain stores into long-term memory in the hippocampus the preceding day's events. Without deep sleep, memory is affected negatively. Likewise, regular exercise is needed for memory just as it is for myriad other health benefits. Sleep is essential for emotional health as well. Glozier et al. (2010) demonstrated with almost 3,000 young adults that for each hour of sleep lost, levels of psychological stress rose by 5%. Those getting the least amount of sleep were 14 times more likely to report symptoms of psychological stress. The researchers found that if the subjects were not anxious to begin with, those who slept less than 5 hours per night tripled their odds of becoming psychologically stressed. Something as basic as loss of sleep can have an extraordinary impact on a person's health. Sleep is but one of the necessary components in achieving holistic health.

Some people may feel the need for social support or guidance as they embark on incorporating self-care practices into their lives. A personal life coach is an option that some may find helpful in this endeavor. Life coaches assist individuals in discovering the important things in their lives, designing a plan to help reach goals, and partnering with a person to eliminate obstacles. The coach partners with an individual and is available for support on the journey. Visits with the coach can be in person as well as by telephone or the Internet.

INTEGRATING COMPLEMENTARY THERAPIES

Many nurses may find numerous complementary therapies useful in living a more stress-free life and in personal growth. Not only may these procedures prove uniquely helpful, but subjective knowledge about them may assist the nurse in using them in practice. Personal experience with specific therapies provides information about a technique that is not found in articles and books.

Journaling (Chapter 13) is a therapy that may assist nurses in gaining personal insight about one's values, strengths, causes of stress, and areas in which one wishes to expand and grow. Taking a few minutes at the end of a day and letting what is within come out on paper can be helpful. Reviewing how one dealt with a difficult situation or challenge may provide understanding of how to approach a similar situation, should it arise. Sidebar 2.1 details how journaling is used by palliative care nurses in Canada.

Sidebar 2.1. *Use of Canadian Palliative Care Nurses' Reflective Journaling as Contributing to Nurses' Health and Well-Being*

Kelly Penz, Regina, Canada

Traditionally, journaling in nursing, worldwide and in Canada, has been used as an educative tool to facilitate reflective practice and to bridge the theory–practice gap for students involved in clinical nursing experiences. It is generally accepted that reflective writing activities, such as journaling, enable nursing students to develop their critical thinking and reasoning skills and, more important, facilitate a smooth transition to the role of competent and independent practitioner. Less information is available on the effectiveness of journaling as related to the health and well-being of practicing nurses.

As part of my doctoral research using a qualitative grounded-theory study on the experience of hope of RNs [registered nurses] who provide palliative and end-of-life care in community settings (Penz & Duggleby, 2012; Penz & Duggleby, 2011), I asked the registered nurse participants to keep a journal about their thoughts regarding their practice in palliative and end-of-life care over a 1- to 2-week period. Although the personal journaling activity was a form of data collection, I was pleasantly surprised to hear the positive reflections that were shared by the participants. In follow-up interviews, many RN participants shared that they felt that taking the time to reflect on their practice in a written format was very therapeutic and contributed to their overall well-being. The guided

(continued)

Sidebar 2.1. *Use of Canadian Palliative Care Nurses' Reflective Journaling as Contributing to Nurses' Health and Well-Being (continued)*

journaling activity allowed them to share their significant experiences, reflect on what kept them hopeful when dealing with death and dying, and disclose the aspects of their nursing experiences that were most difficult. Some participants also perceived that the journaling activity provided a safe avenue, and that this was one of the first times they felt they were given a voice.

Nurses are well versed in attending to the psychosocial needs of their patients and their patients' family members. Yet, as a professional group, they face significant occupational stressors and an increasing complexity of practice in most settings. Perhaps the Latin phrase attributed to Juvenal from his *Satires* captures the concern for nurses best, "Quis custodiet ipsos custodes?" Alternate translation: "Who cares for the caregivers?" Although personal journaling may not be of interest to every practicing nurse, the potential supportive benefit of such an intervention should be explored in more depth. Nurses have important stories to tell, and reflective practice for nurses begins with being able to articulate their most significant concerns and celebrate their outstanding contributions to ensuring high-quality care for their patients. Whether these personal journal reflections are shared with others or kept private, they offer nurses a tangible way to consider the meaning they find in their work, thereby enhancing their identity as expert practitioners who really do make a difference. Overall, the use of reflective journaling—individually or even in combination with group discussions of journal entries—may provide an important self-care strategy to support the psychosocial health and well-being of nurses in practice.

References

Penz, K., & Duggleby, W. (2012). "It's different in the home…" The contextual challenges and rewards of providing palliative nursing care in community settings. *Journal of Hospice and Palliative Nursing, 14*(5), 365–373. doi:10.1097/NJH.0b013e3182553abc

Penz, K., & Duggleby, W. (2011). Harmonizing hope: A grounded theory study of the experience of hope of registered nurses who provide palliative care in community settings. *Palliative and Supportive Care, 9*(3), 281–294. doi:10.1017/S147895151100023X

Numerous relaxation therapies exist (Chapter 18). Strategies as simple as pausing and using diaphragmatic breathing in a difficult situation may be enough to lower stress, clear the mind, and provide a new perspective. The nurse's calmness may transfer to the patient, family, and coworkers.

Becoming aware of the tenseness in one's muscles helps to make one conscious of the increasing tenseness and reducing the tension before it escalates to high levels. Considering yoga (Chapter 9) or Tai Chi (Chapter 17) may bring many personal benefits to a tired back or tense muscles. Just getting out for a 10-minute walk may revive the spirits and provide new energy.

Massage (Chapter 16) is a luxury many long for—and many nurses would enjoy. However, a simple hand massage can do much to not only relieve tension but provide enjoyment. Finding time in a busy day is difficult; however, taking 2 minutes to massage the hands of a coworker and having this reciprocated can be the uplift that sparks the rest of the day. Family members and volunteers may be taught how to provide hand massage to patients.

The number of therapies a nurse may choose for personal use is endless: music, prayer, imagery, healing touch, aromatherapy, or Reiki are just a few examples. The challenge faced is which one best fits with me? What is wonderful is that so many of the procedures do not require a therapist for implementation. They can be used personally after a brief introduction to the technique.

One practice that nurses may wish to consider is spiritual direction that addresses the spiritual component of one's life. Just as a personal life coach helps with aspects of one's life, a spiritual director walks with the individual. The following section is a description of spiritual direction and its holistic benefits.

SPIRITUAL DIRECTION

Spiritual direction is a time-honored tradition of accompanying other people as they seek to grow in their relationship with God or the sacred in their lives. Spiritual direction is not psychotherapy or pastoral counseling, even though it has similar professional boundaries, ethics, and listening skills in common with them. Spiritual direction does not try to fix problems; instead, it helps individuals find meaning and purpose in their life circumstances. Spiritual directors have completed specialized graduate education and undergo continual direction and supervision themselves.

Some form of spiritual direction is found in many of the major religions of the world. Among traditional Native Americans a medicine man/woman will guide a "vision quest" and interpret the dreams and visions of the seeker. A Zen master gives spiritual guidance to a seeker in the Buddhist tradition. In Christianity, spiritual direction has existed since the 4th century CE. Until recently, spiritual direction was exclusive to those in religious life; laypersons rarely sought direction (Moon, 2002). Today it is found in many Protestant denominations as well as in the Roman Catholic Church. Benner (2002) states that although large sectors within Christianity had never heard of spiritual direction until recently, seminaries and colleges of many denominations are now busy refashioning departments of Christian education into programs of spiritual formation. Clergy and laity alike are seeking opportunities to learn about spiritual direction. Susanka (2007) suggests it is often necessary to find a place of stillness within oneself and, through that stillness, an opening to the spiritual life.

The modern spiritual director has received education in the art and practice of spiritual direction and adheres to professional ethics such as those specified by SDI (Spiritual Directors International). SDI is a global organization of people from many faiths who share a common concern and passion for the practice of spiritual direction. Opportunities are available for sharing of resources and ideas online at www.sdiworld.org. A person seeking direction should inquire about a director's educational preparation, supervision, and practice. A spiritual director, with permission of the directee, may collaborate with other professionals working with a directee. When a directee is in crisis, working with both a counselor and a director may be very beneficial; for others, it may be best to work with a counselor first and then with a director.

Nurses who seek spiritual direction do so to reflect on how God or the sacred is present in their lived experience as a nurse and a person. The focus of spiritual direction is on the inward movement of the Spirit in the nurse's life. A health care provider may seek direction during a life transition or crisis, or during ordinary times, to gain a deeper relationship with God or the sacred. All of life's experiences can be brought to bear, but always at the discretion of the person seeking direction (Munger, 2009). In the course of receiving direction, some of the circumstances of one's life may appear unchanged; however, the inner transformation may be evident in one's professional work and personal relationships, even in one's environment. Problems may resolve as a side benefit of direction. A nurse, for example, working with a group of women in transition from prison to society, said of herself, "I no longer *say* prayers; I *am* prayer." She went on to describe how she had become less judgmental and more accepting, more patient, more peaceful, more relaxed, and more joyful. The work was still the same; the women's problems just as serious; but she was different and, as a result, has become much more present to the women she works with.

Spiritual direction is especially useful to nurses whose working lives are spent in high-stress health care environments, dealing with life-and-death questions on a regular basis. Spiritual direction is about reflection on one's life in all of its complexity. At the heart of direction is one's unique relationship with the sacred. Direction can help nurses become more sensitive to God's presence in their work and God's desire to "partner" with them. Developing an awareness of this partnership with God or the sacred provides a serenity that can prevent emotional and spiritual burnout so that relationships with patients, families, colleagues, and oneself become healthy and healing (Fosarelli, 2012). Spiritual directors typically suggest ways of prayer and meditation. They may also recommend reading materials, as well as different ways of listening to the sacred in their lives, for instance—through journal writing, art, music, and review of dreams and images from meditation (Steinhauser, 1999). Dreams serve many functions for the psyche in healing and maintenance of health. They give emotional compensation, reveal truths about life situations that the ego resists, provide warnings, and uncommonly provide what Jung called archetypal understanding (Sanford, 1989). *Archetype* is a term used to denote an idea or image that is part of the collective unconscious of humanity across time. Some spiritual directors work with their directees' dreams to help them see what the dream is suggesting.

Spiritual direction typically occurs monthly, or more frequently if the individual desires it. Spiritual directors may meet with individuals over several years or months, depending on the circumstances of the directee. Group spiritual direction is also available. The director and directee assess their work together periodically. For access to a spiritual director, individuals can contact their religious denomination or SDI. Directors are usually willing to see people from any religious tradition. Some directors will have expertise in areas such as addiction (Woodbridge, 2000), different ways of praying, dreamwork, or particular life circumstances.

FUTURE RESEARCH

Research in the following areas will contribute to knowledge about self-care and the nurse:

- Qualitative studies on the holistic lifestyle practices of nurses
- Studies about the health outcomes on nurses using complementary therapies, including spiritual direction
- Surveys of nurses to identify the therapies they use in self-care

REFERENCES

American Holistic Nurses Association. (2009). *Code of ethics for holistic nurses.* Retrieved February 15, 2009, from www.ahna.org/Resourses/Publications/PositionStatements/tabid/1926/default.aspx/ p. 2

Benner, D. G. (2002). Nurturing spiritual growth. *Journal of Religion and Theology, 30,* 355–361.

Buettner, D. (2010). *Blue zones: Lessons for living longer from people who've lived the longest.* New York, NY: National Geographic.

Fosarelli, P. (2012). Facilitating healing of the healers: Spiritual direction with physicians and other health professionals. *Presence, 18* (6), 41–53.

Glozier, N. A., Maratiniuk, G., Patton, R., Ivers, Q., Li, I., Hickie, T., ... Stevenson, M. (2010). Short sleep duration in prevalent and persistent psychological distress in young adults: The DRIVE study. *Sleep, 33* (9), 1139–1145.

Hanson, R. (2008). Seven facts about the brain that incline the mind to joy. In T. Simon (Ed.), *Measuring the immeasurable* (pp. 269–286). Boulder, CO: Sounds True.

Lipton, B. H. (2005). *The biology of belief: Unleashing the power of consciousness, mind matters.* New York, NY: Hay House.

Moon, G. W. (2002). Spiritual direction: Meaning, purpose, and implications for mental health professionals. *Journal of Religion and Theology, 30,* 264–275.

Munger, C. (2009). Field notes: Spiritual direction. *Listen: A Seeker's Resource for Spiritual Direction, 3*(1), 1.

Pert, C. (2008). The science of consciousness and emotions. In T. Simon (Ed.), *Measuring the immeasurable: The scientific case for spirituality* (pp. 15–34). Boulder, CO: Sounds True.

Sanford, J. (1989). *Dreams: God's forgotten language.* San Francisco, CA: Harper & Row.

Steinhauser, J. (1999). Art prayer: A dance with the holy. *Presence. The Journal of Spiritual Directors International, 5,* 8–17.

Susanka, S. (2007). *The not so big life: Making room for what really matters.* New York, NY: Random House.

Woodbridge, B. (2000). Spiritual direction with an addicted person. In N. Vest (Ed.), *Still listening: New horizons in spiritual direction* (pp. 37–47). Harrisburg, PA: Moorehouse.

Chapter 3: Presence

SUE PENQUE AND MARIAH SNYDER

Being, sharing ou authentic self (handwritten)

Presence is an intervention integral to the administration of all complementary therapies and may be used in conjunction with or independently of other procedures. It is closely related to the therapy of active listening, and the two share many similar characteristics. Although presence has been recognized for centuries within nursing, research has only recently been initiated on this subject. This research has largely been conducted in conjunction with the concept of caring.

DEFINITION

Philosophical views of existentialism assisted with the development of the concept of presence for nursing. Sartre (1943/1984) described awareness as a means toward knowing a person and a way of presence. Sartre coined the term *authentic self* as bringing self to "being with" a person. Heidegger (1962), in his philosophical teachings, introduced the term *Dasein* or "being there" for another. "Being" is the unique quality of a person and is experienced through sharing one's authentic self (Heidegger, 1962). According to nursing author T. P. Nelms (1996), being is presence and the heart of nursing practice. Thus, being there and being with are core definitions of presence. Preliminary to developing a presence scale, Kostovich (2012) had 10 registered nurses validate the following definition of presence: "Nursing presence is an intersubjective human connectedness shared between the nurse and patient" (p. 169).

The connection between philosophy and nursing regarding the concept of presence began to emerge in the 1960s. Vaillot (1962) used the phenomenon of presence to describe therapeutic relationships as crucial to patient care. Two other pioneers in this field, Paterson and Zderad (1976), described presence as the process of being available with the whole of oneself and open to the experience of another through a reciprocal interpersonal encounter. According to Paterson and Zderad (1976), presence is an intervention the nurse uses to establish a relationship with the patient.

Benner (1984) coined the verb *presencing* to denote the existential practice of being with a patient. "Presencing" is one of the eight competencies Benner identifies as constituting the helping role of the nurse. This view of presence in nursing was supported by Parse (1998), who characterized presence as "the primary mode of nursing practice" (p. 40). More recently, McMahon and Christopher (2011) have developed a midrange theory of nursing presence in which they identified five variables that characterize presence: individual client characteristics, the characteristics of the nurse, shared characteristics with the nurse–patient dyad, the environment, and the intentional decisions of the nurse related to practice. Kostovich (2012) developed a model for presence that includes antecedents and possible outcomes.

Presence may be reciprocal when both parties are connecting and may be meaningful to both the patient and the nurse. Melnechenko (2003) noted: "to be invited to share in another's unfolding health, to be asked to journey with another through the process of moving and choosing, is without doubt an honor and privilege" (p. 24). The transactional characteristic of presence was emphasized by McKivergin and Day (1998). Hessel (2009), in a concept analysis of presence, noted that presence involves a spiritual connection that is felt when the nurse and patient share the experience of being together. In presence, the nurse is available to the patient with the wholeness of his or her unique individual being. Presence can be characterized as an exchange in which meaningful awareness on the part of the nurse helps to bring integration and balance to the life of the patient (Snyder, Brandt, & Tseng, 2000) and perhaps satisfaction and meaning for the nurse.

Two classifications of presence have been developed (McKivergin & Daubenmire, 1994; Osterman & Schwartz-Barcott, 1996). The continuum in both classifications extends from merely being physically present with the patient to being available with the wholeness of self. Exhibit 3.1 describes the dimensions of presence and provides an example of each type of presence. It is only the transcendent (Osterman & Schwartz-Barcott, 1996) or therapeutic presence (McKivergin & Daubenmire, 1994) that constitutes the complementary therapy designated as presence.

Presence is an intervention used by nurses but takes practice if used as a complementary therapy. Nurses may increase their use of transcendent presence by practicing journaling, mindfulness, active listening, unitasking, holding silence with a partner, focus on the breath, and purposeful activities such as smiling and centering. These activities enable a person to experience presence and evoke it as an intervention when needed.

Exhibit 3.1. *Dimensions of Presence*

Dimensions of Presence	Example
Physical presence	Nurse is competent in carrying out patient care; has minimal interaction with patient and is seemingly unaware of nonverbal communication; exits room without noting future plan of care.
Full presence	Nurse enters room and greets patient by name; nurse carries out care while communicating with patient; senses patient's nonverbal communication; plans care in collaboration with patient.
Transcendent presence *uses touch*	Before entering patient's room, nurse centers self so entire focus will be on patient; greets patient by name and uses touch. During the time with the patient the nurse conveys complete interest and is responsive to patient's holistic needs. This is done while providing competent care.

The universality of presence and caring has been documented (Jonsdóttir, Litchfield, & Pharris, 2004). Presence transcends cultures and modes of communication. The Buddhist way of life through mindfulness implies one is attentive, aware, and fully present in the moment (Kabat-Zinn, 1990). Even if the nurse and patient are unable to communicate verbally, the patient perceives the presence of a caring nurse. The psychological evidence of presence is apparent. According to Paulson (2004), presence requires an emotional, subjective interaction in which the nurse conveys genuine concern for patients, not just as patients but as human beings.

SCIENTIFIC BASIS

Paterson and Zderad (1976) recognized presence as an integral component of their theory of humanistic nursing. Presence implies openness, receptivity, readiness, and availability on the part of the nurse. Many nursing situations require close proximity to another person; however, that in itself does not constitute presence. To experience the lived dialogue of nursing, the nurse responds with an openness to a "person-with-needs" and with an "availability-in-a-helping way" (Paterson & Zderad, 1976). Reciprocity often emerges through the dialogue.

Nurse scientists have described presence as a subconstruct of the broad concept of caring (Nelms, 1996; Watson, 1985), but Melnechenko (2003) contends that presence is more than caring and active listening. Presence involves the nurse as "co-participant" in the caring process (Watson, 1985). Caring requires the nurse to be keenly attentive to the needs of the patient, the meaning the patient attaches to the illness or problem, and how the patient wishes to proceed. The use of presence helps lead the patient to heal, discover others, and find meaning in life.

Research on the expert practice of critical care nurses has demonstrated the importance of presence. Minick (1995) found that connectedness with the patient was important not only as a caring behavior but also because it assisted the nurse in the early identification of postoperative problems. Therapeutic presence may help nurses to be more attentive and to detect subtle changes that may not be evident without it. Nurses lacking connectedness were perceived by their patients as detached. Wilkin and Slevin (2004) further validated the fact that the importance of the critical care nurse being present to the patient was as essential a part of nursing care as were the skills needed to reach unresponsive and intubated patients.

Kostovich (2012), in developing a presence scale, identified the following as attributes of presence: teaching, surveillance, concern, empathy, companionship, educated skillfulness, availability, responsive listening, coordination of care, spiritual enhancement, reassurance, and personalization of care (p. 169). Antecedents of presence found in studies include connection through personal stories, informal interactions, and empathic interactions (Evans, Coon, & Crogan, 2007). These factors are important in establishing real connection with a patient.

When presence is used as a complementary therapy, consequences or effects occur for the patient, family, and nurse. Easter (2000) reported a decrease in pain for the patient, an increase in satisfaction for the nurse, and improved mental well-being for the nurse through presence. According to Drick (2003), presence creates healing and changes the atmosphere in the nurse–patient relationship. Jonas and Crawford (2004) reported calcium flux at the cellular level and lower, more stable heart rates as a result of healing presence within minutes to hours of the intervention. Tavernier (2006) identified three consequences of presence: (a) relationship, (b) healing, and (c) reward. The importance of presence in care has been recognized and valued as a key nursing intervention. A midrange theory of nursing presence, developed by McMahon and Christopher (2011), identifies presence as integral to the nurse–patient relationship. The nurse must have the ability to recognize the need for presence and be open to the invitation to be present. Further investigation on why and how presence plays a positive and vital role in health outcomes needs to be encouraged.

INTERVENTION

The description of presence related by Mitch Albom (1997) in *Tuesdays with Morrie* succinctly captures its essential elements. Albom is reporting how Morrie, a man with advanced amyotrophic lateral sclerosis, views presence:

I believe in being fully present. That means you should be with the person you're with. When I'm talking with you now, Mitch, I try to keep focused only on what is going on between us. I am not thinking about something we said last week. I am not thinking about what's coming up this Friday. I am not thinking about doing another Koppel show, or about medications I'm taking. I am talking to you; I am thinking about you. (pp. 135–136)

Centering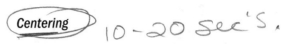

Presence entails conscious attention to the upcoming interaction with the patient. The nurse must be available with the whole self and be open to the personal and care needs of the patient. This process is called *centering*, a meditative state. The nurse takes a short time, sometimes only 10 or 20 seconds, to eliminate distractions, so that the focus can be on the patient. Some people find that taking a deep breath and closing the eyes helps in freeing them of distractions and becoming centered. This may be done outside the room (or other setting) in which the encounter will occur. Centering may also be as simple as the nurse pausing before contact with the patient and repeating the patient's name to help focus attention on that person.

Technique

Exhibit 3.2 lists the key component of presence and the skills necessary for practicing it. Sensitivity to others requires the nurse to be an excellent listener and observer. (Therapeutic listening is addressed in Chapter 4.) Good observation skills assist nurses in identifying nuances in expression and communication that may reveal the real concerns of the patient. Presence often means periods of silence in which subtle interchanges occur. Continuing attentiveness on the part of the nurse is a critical aspect of this therapy. Both the nurse and the client experience a sense of union or joining for a moment in time. Focusing on the moment—not the past or the future—is inherent in being present.

Exhibit 3.2. *Skills for Implementing Presence*

Key Component	Skills
Holistic attention to patient	Centering Active listening Openness to others Sensitivity Verbal communication that is at level of patient Use of touch when culturally appropriate Nonverbal demonstration of acceptance

Exhibit 3.3. *Possible Outcomes of Presence*

Patient feeling comforted and supported

Patient sensing that whole being is cared for

Patient level of stress decreased

Patient feeling less lonely

Patient has an increased sense of peace and hope

Patient feeling increased self-worth

Patient perceiving decreased pain

Patient feeling motivated and encouraged

Little is known about the length of a therapy session or when therapeutic presence should be used. Often the nurse identifies it intuitively: "It just seems like this patient truly needs me now." Because of the intense nature of the interaction, the length of time the nurse is present to the patient may seem greater even though only 30 seconds or a minute may have passed. Although presence is often used in conjunction with another therapy or treatment, identifying when a patient needs someone to just be present for a few minutes may be the most effective technique.

Measurement of Effectiveness

Measuring outcomes of presence interventions involve both the patient and the nurse because of their reciprocal interaction. Comments from the patient about feeling cared for, being able to express concerns, and perceiving understanding are some outcome measures derived from patient satisfaction tools. McMahon and Christopher (2011) reviewed literature on presence and identified potential client outcomes. These are shown in Exhibit 3.3. The correlation between high patient satisfaction and excellent nursing care is well documented. Incorporating the effects of presence in patient surveys should be considered among the important outcomes indicating a positive health experience and healing. Because of the intangibles that often occur with the use of presence, finding words or indices to measure presence may be challenging.

A tool developed by Kostovich (2012) may be used to measure patient's perceptions of nursing presence. The Presence of Nursing Scale is a 25-item scale measuring nursing presence. The internal consistency reliability using Cronbach's alpha was 0.95. This tool showed a high correlation with patient satisfaction.

Precautions

The major precaution in the use of presence is to take one's cue from the patient and not force an encounter. A true presence encounter considers the wants and needs of the patient and is not for the nurse's primary benefit. If the nurse is "available with the whole of oneself and open to the experience" of the client, as the definition states, the nurse will act in accordance with the wishes and needs of the patient.

A negative consequence of presence is that colleagues may be critical of the nurse who spends time "just being" with patients and/or families. Certainly this should not be a deterrent to the use of presence, but rather a concern that should be discussed and resolved by nursing staff. Finfgeld-Connett (2008) stated that a supportive work environment that starts at the highest administrative level of the facility helps promote the use of presence.

Professional maturity has been identified as a factor having an impact on the use of presence. McMahon and Christopher (2011) noted that a novice nurse may be so focused on the skill to be performed as to be unable to detect the subtle signs that the patient requires the intervention of presence.

USES

Presence can be used in any nursing situation. Persons struggling with a new diagnosis, an exacerbation of a condition, or a loss are especially in need of moments of presence. An and Jo (2009) found that a 30-minute nursing-presence intervention reduced stress in older adults in nursing homes. Use of presence is also important in patients in hospice settings.

Presence is needed with patients in critical care settings (Wilkin & Slevin, 2004) and emergency departments (Wiman & Wikblad, 2004). Patients and their families often feel lost in high-tech critical care settings. The use of presence helps prevent critical care nurses from being viewed by their patients as emotionally distant and focusing only on the machines and technology. Other patient populations in which use of presence has been documented include women with postpartum psychosis (Engqvist, Ferszt, & Nilsson, 2010) and in midwifery practice (Hunter, 2009).

As health care and nursing encompass more technology, including telemedicine, as part of the modes for delivery of care, explorations of virtual presence are needed. Educators using distance teaching have been investigating the impact of the emotional presence of the instructor on learners and the effect this has on learning outcomes. Sandelowski (2002) noted that people involved in designing technology and nurses are interested in creating environments for patients and nurses that produce feelings of interaction that are immediate, intimate, and *real*. The rapidly increasing use of telephones, home monitoring, and other forms of telemedicine challenge nurses to convey attentive care in these settings that includes presence. Nurses can ask themselves, "Am I truly listening; present to the patient who is invisible?"

CULTURAL APPLICATIONS

Culture is closely interlaced with nationality, race, ethnicity, social class, and even generations, and is important in considering the meaning of presence for the patient, family, and nurse. Presence may also hold a special interpretation for the individual based on past experience or family influence. The key is to identify and acknowledge the meaning of presence for the patient and all family members in the relationship. Mitchell (2006) provides an exemplar of presence among young, middle-aged, and older adults. The themes of attentive presence and "being with" in the exemplar are apparent in each of the generations. As described by Mitchell, cultural connection is necessary in bringing meaning to life experience and is emotional and healing.

In addition, each person has a preference for a communication style, and that may be influenced by his or her cultural background. In several cultures, gestures of respect and knowing the person hold high importance in establishing a relationship. In other cultures, too much eye contact may be seen as offensive. Communication and trust are shown to be the largest factors that create connection among Hispanic families (Evans et al., 2007). Conversational silence is important in some cultures as a mechanism to becoming present with another person or the environment. Buddhists use silence as a respectful technique to being present and are comfortable with long periods of silence, whereas other cultures may not be. Mindfulness, being in the present moment and aware of everything around you—is the Buddhist way of life.

A nurse who trained in the Philippines gives her expert opinion on the meaning of presence in the countries where nurses received nursing degrees (Sidebar 3.1).

Sidebar 3.1. *Use of Presence in the Philippines*

Zapora Burillo

Filipino's believe that "presence heals the spirit." In this culture, sickness and hospitalization of an individual is a family matter. Family members stay with the patient 24/7; they schedule coverage for 24-hour

---

(continued)

> ### Sidebar 3.1. *Use of Presence in the Philippines* *(continued)*
>
> vigils until the patient is discharged home or is fully recovered. The person who stays with the patient is called *bantay*, which translates as "watcher." The presence of a familiar face at the bedside alleviates the fear and anxiety of the patient; it promotes an environment of trust and confidence. The nurse works collaboratively with the family member to provide physical and emotional comfort to the patient during the healing process. The nurse's presence provides a sense of reassurance.
>
> Nurses need to make an assessment of the cultural needs of patients before therapeutic presence can be attained. Presence has special meaning to the individual, depending on culture and according to level of development. It is critical to understand how one connects with others and creates an intimate awareness.

FUTURE RESEARCH

Nurses document assessments made and treatments administered, but rarely do they document the use of presence and the outcomes of this therapy. Despite the challenges in identifying and documenting outcomes of presence, current interest in complementary therapies provides an opportunity for nurses to validate the positive outcomes of the use of presence. Areas in which research is needed include the following:

- Although every patient could benefit from presence, large case-loads often place restrictions on nurses' time. What are assessments that would alert nurses to patients who most need the therapy of presence?
- What are strategies that can be used to teach nursing students and other health professionals how to implement presence?
- With the advent of telemedicine, how can virtual presence be introduced into these contacts with patients? Is physical presence essential or is presence a nonlocal phenomenon, like prayer?
- What are the barriers to becoming present?
- What needs to occur in the work environment for presence to have meaning for both the patient and the nurse?
- What are the cultural differences in the meaning of presence, and how can a nurse identify those differences?
- Is there a relationship between the quantity and/or quality of presence and patient outcomes?

REFERENCES

Albom, M. (1997). *Tuesdays with Morrie*. New York, NY: Doubleday.

An, G., & Jo, K. (2009). The effect of a nursing presence program on reducing stress in older adults in two Korean nursing homes. *Australian Journal of Advanced Nursing, 26*, 79–85.

Benner, P. (1984). *From novice to expert: Excellence and power in clinical nursing practice*. Menlo Park, CA: Addison-Wesley.

Drick, C. A. (2003). Back to basics: The power of presence in nursing care. *Journal of Gynecologic Oncology Nursing, 13*(3), 13–18.

Easter, A. (2000). Construct analysis of four modes of being present. *Journal of Holistic Nursing, 18*, 362–377.

Engqvist, I., Ferszt, G., & Nilsson, K. (2010). Swedish registered nurses' description of presence when caring for women with post-partum psychosis: An interview study. *International Journal of Mental Health Nursing, 19*, 193–196.

Evans, B. C., Coon, D., & Crogan, N. L. (2007). Personalismo and breaking barriers: Accessing Hispanic populations for clinical services and research. *Geriatric Nursing, 28*(5), 289–296.

Finfgeld-Connett, D. (2006). Meta-synthesis of presence in nursing. *Journal of Advanced Nursing, 55*, 708–714.

Heidegger, M. (1962). *Being and time* (J. Macquarrie & E. Robinson, trans.). San Francisco, CA: HarperCollins.

Hessel, J. (2009). Presence in nursing practice: A concept analysis. *Holistic Nursing Practice, 23*, 276–281.

Hunter, L. (2009). A descriptive study of "being with women" during labor and birth. *Journal of Midwifery & Women's Health, 54*, 111–118.

Jonas, W. B., & Crawford, C. C. (2004). The healing presence: Can it be reliably measured? *Journal of Alternative and Complementary Medicine, 10*(5), 751–756.

Jonsdóttir, H., Litchfield, M., & Pharris, M. D. (2004). The relational core of nursing practice in partnership. *Journal of Advanced Nursing, 47*, 241–248.

Kabat-Zinn, J. (1990). *Full catastrophe living*. New York, NY: Delacorte Press.

Kostovich, C. T. (2012). Development and psychometric assessment of the Presence of Nursing Scale. *Nursing Science Quarterly, 25*(2), 167–175.

McKivergin, M., & Daubenmire, J. (1994). The essence of therapeutic presence. *Journal of Holistic Nursing, 12*(1), 65–81.

McKivergin, M., & Day, A. (1998). Presence: Creating order out of chaos. *Seminars in Perioperative Nursing, 7*, 96–100.

McMahon, M., & Christopher, K. (2011). Toward a mid-range theory of nursing presence. *Nursing Forum, 46*(2), 71–82.

Melnechenko, K. (2003). To make a difference: Nursing presence. *Nursing Forum, 38*, 18–24.

Minick, P. (1995). The power of human caring: Early recognition of patient problems. *Scholarly Inquiry for Nursing Practice: An International Journal, 9*, 303–317.

Mitchell, M. (2006). Understanding true presence with elders: A story of joy and sorrow. *Perspectives, 30*(3), 17–19.

Nelms, T. P. (1996). Living a caring presence in nursing: A Heideggerian hermeneutical analysis. *Journal of Advanced Nursing, 24*, 368–374.

Osterman, P., & Schwartz-Barcott, D. (1996). Presence: Four ways of being there. *Nursing Forum, 31*, 23–30.

Parse, R. (1998). *The human becoming school of thought: A perspective for nurses and other health professionals*. Thousand Oaks, CA: Sage.

Paterson, J. G., & Zderad, L. T. (1976). *Humanistic nursing.* New York, NY: Wiley.

Paulson, D. S. (2004). Taking care of patients and caring for patients are not the same. *AORN Online, 79,* 359–360, 362, 365–366.

Sandelowski, M. (2002). Visible humans, vanishing bodies, and virtual nursing: Complications of life, presence, place, and identity. *Advances in Nursing Science, 24,* 58–70.

Sartre, J. P. (1943/1984). *Being and nothingness.* New York, NY: Washington Square Press.

Snyder, M., Brandt, C. L., & Tseng, Y. (2000). Use of presence in the critical care unit. *AACN Clinical Issues, 11,* 27–33.

Tavernier, S. (2006). An evidence-based conceptual analysis of presence. *Holistic Nursing Practice, 20*(3), 152–156.

Vaillot, S. M. C. (1962). *Commitment to nursing: A philosophic investigation.* Philadelphia, PA: Lippincott.

Watson, J. (1985). *Nursing: Human science and human care: A theory of nursing.* Norwalk, CT: Appleton-Century-Crofts.

Wilkin, K., & Slevin, E. (2004). The meaning of caring to nurses: An investigation into the nature of caring work in an intensive care unit. *Journal of Clinical Nursing, 13,* 50–59.

Wiman, E., & Wikblad, K. (2004). Caring and uncaring encounters in nursing in an emergency department. *Journal of Clinical Nursing, 13,* 422–429.

Chapter 4: Therapeutic Listening

SHIGEAKI WATANUKI, MARY FRAN TRACY,
AND RUTH LINDQUIST

*L*istening is an active and dynamic process of interaction with a client that requires intentional effort to attend to a client's verbal and nonverbal cues. Listening is an integral part and foundation of nurse–client relationships, and one of the most effective therapeutic techniques available to nurses. The theoretical underpinnings of listening can be traced back to counseling psychology and psychotherapy. Rogers (1957) used counseling and listening to foster independence and promote growth and development of clients. Rogers also emphasized that empathy, warmth, and genuineness with clients were necessary and sufficient for therapeutic changes to occur. Listening has been identified as a significant component of therapeutic communication with patients and therefore fundamental to a therapeutic relationship between the nurse and patient (Foy & Timmins, 2004). Listening is also a key to improving health professionals' teamwork effectiveness and patient safety in complex clinical settings (Denham et al., 2008).

DEFINITION

Many modifiers are used with the word listening—*active, attentive, empathic, therapeutic,* and *holistic.* The choice of modifier seems to depend more on an author's paradigm than on differences in the descriptions of listening (Fredriksson, 1999). Unless active listening was explicitly used by researchers in the articles reviewed in this chapter, the term *therapeutic listening* is used here to focus on the formal, deliberate actions of listening for therapeutic purposes (Lekander, Lehmann, & Lindquist, 1993). Therapeutic listening is defined as "an interpersonal, confirmation process involving all the senses in which the therapist attends with empathy to the client's verbal and nonverbal messages to facilitate the understanding, synthesis, and interpretation of the client's situation" (Kemper, 1992, p. 22). Beyond the therapist, this empathetic attending pertains to nurses and to other care providers.

SCIENTIFIC BASIS

Therapeutic listening is a topic of interest and concern to a variety of disciplines. A number of qualitative and quantitative studies provide a scientific basis of intervention effects in relation to process—behavioral changes of providers that foster communication—and outcomes: client satisfaction, improved clinical indicators.

A systematic review of 20 intervention studies that aimed at improving patient–doctor communication revealed the effectiveness of interventions that typically increased patient participation and clarification (Harrington, Noble, & Newman, 2004). Although few improvements in patient satisfaction were found, significant improvements in perceptions of control over health, preferences for an active role in health care, adherence to recommendations, and clinical outcomes were achieved. Likewise, preferable client outcomes were found in another study in nursing. A survey of 195 parents of hospitalized pediatric patients demonstrated that health care providers' use of immediacy and perceived listening were positively associated with satisfaction, care, and communication (Wanzer, Booth-Butterfield, & Gruber, 2004).

Qualitative studies provide rich understanding of the nature of therapeutic listening and explore the meaning and experience of being listened to in the context of real-world settings. Self-expression opportunities that enable clients to be listened to and understood can promote clients' self-discovery—meaning reconstruction and healing (Sandelowski, 1994). A discourse analysis of 20 nurse–patient pairs at community hospitals, however, indicated insufficient active listening skills on the part of nurses (Barrere, 2007). The study results showed that nurses often missed cues that patients needed nurses to listen to their concerns, or overlooked potential opportunities for health teaching, especially in "asymmetrical" communication patterns (dominance of nurse or patient) as compared to "symmetrical" patterns (nurse–patient communication involving active listening).

Studies evaluating training of health care providers in therapeutic communication skills have shown that training can be effective in improving therapeutic communication skills. A randomized controlled study tested the efficacy of 25-hour training sessions in self-control techniques and communication skills with 61 nurse volunteers. The participating nurses were presented with simulated encounters with relatives of seriously ill patients and their role-plays were evaluated by blinded raters. The results showed significant improvements in the skills of listening, empathizing, not interrupting, and coping with emotions after controlling for baseline performance scores (Garcia de Lucio, Garcia Lopez, Marin Lopez, Mas Hesse, & Caamano Vaz, 2000).

A combination of learning sessions (cognitive interventions), administrative support, and coaching activities (affective and behavioral interventions) enables long-term improvement in communication styles of nurses. A quasiexperimental study was undertaken to test the effectiveness of an integrated communication skills training program for 129 oncology nurses at a hospital in China. Continued significant improvements in overall basic communication skills, self-efficacy, outcome expectancy beliefs, and perceived support in the training group were observed after 1 and 6 months of training intervention. No significant improvements were found in the control group (Liu, Mok, Wong, Xue, & Xu, 2007).

These studies attempted to identify complex relationships among multiple phenomena and variables, including the immediate and long-term effects of training interventions, clinical supervision and support, and cognitive and behavioral changes on the part of nurses. Further systematic studies are needed to enhance knowledge related to intervention effectiveness, especially the link between client characteristics, client satisfaction, and type of interventions. This is particularly important in light of today's health care emphasis and reimbursement aligned with patient satisfaction, patient engagement, and symptom management such as alleviation of pain.

INTERVENTION

Therapeutic listening enables clients to better understand their feelings and to experience being understood by another caring person. Effective engagement in therapeutic listening requires nurses to be aware of verbal and nonverbal communication that conveys explicit and implicit messages. When verbalized words contradict nonverbal messages, communicators rely more often on nonverbal cues; facial expression, tone of voice, and silence become as important as words in determining the meaning of a message (Kacperek, 1997). Nonverbal communication is inextricably linked to verbal communication and can change, emphasize, or distract from the words that are spoken (Bush, 2001).

Guidelines

Listening is an active process, incorporating explicit behaviors as well as attention to choice of words, quality of voice (pitch, timing, and volume), and full engagement in the process (Burnard, 1997). Therapeutic listening requires a listener to tune in to the client and to use all the senses in analyzing, inferring, and evaluating the stated and underlying meaning of the client's message. As providers feel increasing time pressures, it can be easy to attempt to guide or limit the conversation rather than allowing the patient to fully express concerns. However, to be fully heard without interruption can be viewed as supportive by the patient (Bryant, 2009), and may ultimately strengthen the therapeutic relationship. Therapeutic listening requires concentration and an ability to differentiate between what is actually being said and what one wants or expects to hear. It may be difficult to listen accurately and interpret messages that one finds difficult to relate to, or to listen to information that one may not want to hear. Therapeutic listening is both a cognitive and an emotional process (Arnold & Underman Boggs, 2007). When not fully engaged, it can be easy to become distracted or to start formulating a response rather than to stay focused on the message. Three components have been identified as being foundational to therapeutic listening:

1. Rephrasing the patient's words and thoughts to ensure clarity and accuracy
2. Conveying an understanding of the speaker's perceptions
3. Asking questions and prompting to clarify (De Vito, 2006)

These and other techniques for therapeutic listening intervention are presented in Exhibit 4.1.

Therapeutic listening with children can be even more complex because it frequently involves the presence or participation of more parties: the nurse, the child, parents, and/or other family members. This may take particular skill on the part of the nurse as he or she attends to both the spoken messages as well as the nonverbal communication/reactions of two, three, or more persons simultaneously. In addition, the nurse must be sensitive to the clarification of information and cues in front of either the child or the caregiver, depending on the child's age and developmental stage.

Adolescents especially may be willing to talk openly with an adult who is not a family member. However, they may respond quickly, abruptly, or defensively to any perceived indications of judgment, indifference, or disrespect on the part of the listener. It is extremely important with adolescents to be fully attentive, allow for complete expression of thoughts, and avoid statements or facial expressions that imply disapproval or that can be misinterpreted.

Exhibit 4.1. *Therapeutic Listening Techniques*

Active presence: Active presence involves focus on the client to interpret the message that he or she is trying to convey, recognition of themes, and hearing what is left unsaid. Short responses such as "yes" or "uh-huh" with appropriate timing and frequency may promote clients' willingness to talk. *My bodies w/ you*

Accepting attitude: Conveying an accepting attitude is assuring, and can help clients to feel more comfortable about expressing themselves. This can be demonstrated by short affirmative responses or gestures.

Clarifying statements: Clarifying statements and summarizing can help the listener verify message interpretation and create clarity. Encourage specificity rather than vague statements to facilitate communication. Rephrasing and reflection can assist the client in self-understanding. Using phrases such as "tell me more about that" or "what was that like?" may be helpful, rather than asking "why," which may elicit a defensive response from the client.

Use of silence: Use of silence can encourage the client to talk, facilitate the nurse's focus on listening rather than the formulation of responses, and reduce the use of leading questions. Sensitivity toward cultural and individual variations in the seconds of silence may be developed by paying detailed attention to the patterns of client communication.

Tone: Tone of voice can express more than the actual words through empathy, judgment, or acceptance. Match the intensity of the tone to the message received to avoid minimizing or overemphasizing.

Nonverbal behaviors: Clients relaying sensitive information may be very aware of the listener's body language and will be viewed as either accepting of the message or closed to it, judgmental, and/or disinterested. Eye contact, or a nodding head, are essential to conveying the listener's true interest and attention. Maintaining a conversational distance and judicious use of touch may increase the client's comfort. Cultural and social awareness are important so as to avoid undesired touch. *Crossed arms, fidgeting*

Environment: Distractions should be eliminated to encourage the therapeutic interchange. Therapeutic listening may require careful planning to provide time for undivided attention or may occur spontaneously. Some clients may feel very comfortable having family present; others may feel inhibited when others are present. *manage environment*

Because therapeutic listening involves both cognitive and emotional processes, it is important that nurses recognize the role of emotional intelligence in their therapeutic interactions. *Emotional intelligence* is defined as an ability to recognize emotions in self and other, and to understand and utilize these emotions in thinking processes and interactions with others (Vitello-Cicciu, 2002). Nursing requires a significant amount of emotional labor, resulting in expectations of expressions of caring, understanding, and empathy with patients and families. Strategies such as reflection, empathizing, and skilled therapeutic listening can promote a healing environment for patients and families (Molter, 2003).

A listening technique referred to as *change-oriented reflective listening* targets behavioral change of health care providers (Strang, McCambridge, Platts, & Groves, 2004) and has a strong potential for incorporation into the repertoire of nursing interventions. This technique has been adapted from the core principles of motivational interviewing (Rollnick et al., 2002). Change-oriented reflective listening is a brief motivational enhancement intervention that encourages providers' consideration of the quality of primary care, and then stimulates their intent to change behavior in the direction desired. This method takes the form of a brief telephone conversation (15–20 min), in which reflective listening statements are interspersed with open questions about the issue at hand. A menu of questions with the range of possible areas for discussion is constructed in advance. The technique has been successfully piloted with general practitioners to motivate them to intervene with opiate users and as part of alcohol intervention (McCambridge, Platts, Whooley, & Strang, 2004; Strang et al., 2004).

Communicating with a patient and family in difficult situations necessitates careful and considerate listening skills. Basic communication skills such as "ask-tell-ask" and "tell me more" principles have been introduced to oncology settings (Back, Arnold, Baile, Tulsky, & Fryer-Edwards, 2005) and end-of-life care in critical care settings (Shannon, Long-Sutehall, & Coombs, 2011). The first "ask" is used for the provider to assess perceptions and understanding of a patient or family regarding the current situation or issue at hand. This step would help the provider to obtain a basic idea about the patient's or family's level of knowledge or emotional state. The "tell" portion is used for the provider to convey the most pressing needed or desired information to the patient/family. The information should be provided in understandable, brief chunks, kept at no more than three pieces of information at a time. Then, the second "ask" is used to check understanding of the patient/family and their additional questions. The "ask-tell-ask" cycle would be repeated until a final "ask" is a summary of agreed-upon decisions or plans. "Tell me more" can be used to get back on track when the conversation appears diverted. It also can be used to allow patient/family to share more of their emotions, while letting the health provider get past his or her own initial reactions and respond in a less defensive or emotional mode (Back et al., 2005; Shannon et al., 2011).

Measurement of Outcomes

Inclusion of multiple measurements, such as self-report, behavioral observation, physiological indicators, and qualitative accounts, provides rich data for the study of therapeutic listening. For example, the Active Listening Observation Scale (ALOS-global) is a validated seven-item behavioral observational scale that measures the general practitioner's attentiveness and acknowledgment of suffering among patients presenting minor ailments (Fassaert, van Dulmen, Schellevis, & Bensing, 2007).

Challenges to outcome measurement may include the isolation of therapeutic listening as an independent variable from other confounding variables. Other challenges may be related to the complexity of the multifaceted phenomenon of therapeutic listening that may necessitate different study designs. Antecedents to interventions such as clients' characteristics have to be taken into consideration; likewise, the process-related components of interventions such as short- and long-term improvements in nurses' knowledge, skills, and attitudes after training and client outcomes need to be evaluated (Harrington et al., 2004; Kruijver, Kerkstra, Francke, Bensing, & van de Weil, 2000).

Positive changes in psychological variables such as anxiety, depression, hostility, or nursing care satisfaction are potential client outcomes of therapeutic listening. It may also be useful to examine physiological measures (e.g., heart rate, blood pressure, respiratory rate, immunological measures, electroencephalography results) as outcomes of therapeutic interchange. Outcomes may include clinical variables such as patients' response to illness, mood, adherence, disease control, morbidity, and health care cost. Boudreau and colleagues believe that therapeutic listening can result in multiple outcomes: listening gives patients opportunities to articulate concerns that provide insight into their "personhood"; it can generate data for providers to use in the provision of optimal care and it may actually assist in healing (Boudreau, Cassell, & Fuks, 2009).

Precautions

Therapeutic listening has at its heart the intent to be helpful; however, a few precautions are warranted. Questions that start with the word "why" may take clients out of the context of their experience or feelings and direct them into an intellectual thinking mode or cause defensive responses. Rather, phrases such as "tell me more about that," or "what was that like?" (Shattell & Hogan, 2005, p. 31) may be helpful.

The provider needs to be engaged fully when using therapeutic listening. If the provider is only half-listening, using selective listening, or is distracted, the patient may sense his or her concerns are being minimized or the provider may actually reach an inaccurate diagnosis. This weakens the therapeutic relationship between patient and provider (Boudreau et al., 2009).

The provider also needs to be aware of the potential negative self-consequences if the caregiver is involved in emotionally charged situations. Clinical supervision may be helpful for the provider in addressing such difficulties (Jones & Cutcliffe, 2009).

Practitioners and clinicians are cautioned to avoid use of active listening skills especially with patients presenting minor ailments. Active listening behavior of general practitioners was observed to correlate with nonadherence of medication regimens if patients felt good prior to the consultation. Rather, general practitioners' being sensitive to the emotional state of a patient, and providing a clear explanation of the condition and preferable prognosis were observed to correlate with patients' reduced anxiety and better overall health (Fassaert, van Dulmen, Schellevis, van der Jagt, & Bensing, 2008).

Maintaining professional boundaries during therapeutic listening is important; empathy is to be demonstrated, but within the professional relationship with clients. Referrals for professional counseling may be indicated in such cases as psychiatric crises. Ethical dilemmas may result if the principle of respecting clients' autonomy and confidentiality conflicts with the principle of maintaining professional responsibility and integrity, such as taking action based on sensitive information shared in the therapeutic exchange. Open discussion and negotiation of the use of such sensitive information, within the context of the nurse–client relationship, relies on the trust relationship that has been established such that the trust is retained or even deepened.

USES

Therapeutic listening is an intervention that is applicable to a virtually unlimited number of care situations. It is beneficial for practitioners to continue listening to a patient throughout the entire visit. Indeed, according to a study of audiotaped office visits, approximately 21% of patients disclosed new and vital information in the closing moments of an appointment (White, Levinson, & Roter, 1994). Selected patient population-based examples in which the use of listening is described are included in Exhibit 4.2. Managers in the health care field may also reap benefits from active listening (Kubota, Mishima, & Nagata, 2004). Exhibit 4.3 presents websites of national and international professional organizations where online resources for therapeutic listening can be found.

Technology is becoming increasingly important in assuring that patients have effective means to communicate and ways to be fully

Exhibit 4.2. *Selected Uses of Listening With Patient Populations or in Care Settings*

Adolescent mental health (Claveirole, 2004)

Cancer (Back et al., 2005; Liu et al., 2007)

Culturally diverse populations (Davidhizar, 2004)

Day surgery (Foy & Timmins, 2004)

Emergency care (O'Gara & Fairhurst, 2004; O'Hagan, Webb, & Moore, 2004)

End-of-life care in critical care settings (Shannon et al., 2011)

Heart failure: To improve self-care (Riegel et al., 2006)

Older adults (Williams, Kemper, & Hummert, 2004)

Perinatal care (Battersby & Deery, 2001)

Posttraumatic stress (Gidron et al., 2001)

Relatives of critically ill patients: Use of training simulation for providers (Garcia de Lucio et al., 2000)

Terminal care (Cherin, Enguidanos, & Brumley, 2001)

Traumatic stress/disasters (Liehr, Mehl, Summers, & Pennebaker, 2004)

Women with breast cancer (Harris & Templeton, 2001)

Young people in foster care (Murphy & Jenkinson, 2012)

heard and understood. Devices such as Passy-Muir tracheal valves that can allow mechanically ventilated patients to speak, computer programs that can "speak" the patient's electronic input, and laryngeal devices are now more frequently available and expected to promote communication. When alternative methods are being used, nonverbal communication is even more important to observe and monitor.

Exhibit 4.3. *Professional Organizations and Online Resources for Therapeutic Listening*

The International Communication Association (www.icahdq.org)

The International Listening Association (www.listen.org)

Communication Institute for Online Scholarship (www.cios.org)

CULTURAL APPLICATIONS

Sensitivity and awareness of cultural variations in communication styles are vital to intervention effectiveness. Cultural differences in meanings of certain words, styles, and approaches, or in certain nonverbal behaviors such as silence, touch, eye contact, or smile may adversely affect the effectiveness of therapeutic communication. For example, there may be tendencies for clients from certain cultures to talk loudly, to be direct in conversation, and to come to the point quickly. Clients from other cultures may tend to talk softly, be indirect in their communication, or "talk around" points while emphasizing attitudes and feelings. In some cultures, it is believed that open expression of emotions is unacceptable. Whether in the dominant culture or in nondominant cultures, however, persons may simply smile when they do not comprehend. The skills of therapeutic listening are particularly useful in ensuring that communication in such cases is effective. It is important that nurses explore and understand clients' cultural values and assumptions, as well as their patterns of behavior related to communication, while avoiding stereotyping (Seidel et al., 2011). Awareness of cultural differences is key to therapeutic communication. Sidebar 4.1 provides a look at the use of therapeutic listening in a Japanese population.

Sidebar 4.1. *Nurses' Therapeutic Listening Skills Used for Older Postesophagectomy Patients in Japan*

Shigeaki Watanuki, Tokyo, Japan

Many esophageal cancer patients in Japan undergo thoracoabdominal esophageal surgery. Such patients frequently experience multiple signs and symptoms after surgery for months and sometimes even years due to gastrointestinal (GI) conditions. Such conditions may include vocal cord paralysis, esophageal stenosis, or reflux, which may result in coughing, dysphagia, difficulty swallowing, vomiting, weight loss, or reduced physical activity.

Surgeons, due to their limited time and a large number of patients, have only a few minutes to listen to postsurgical patients in outpatient departments. Older Japanese patients usually hesitate to ask surgeons about their symptoms, changes in daily life, or their concerns. It is as though these elders think they have problems that are "too small" to ask their surgeons. Such problems, however, are often very important

(continued)

Sidebar 4.1. *Nurses' Therapeutic Listening Skills Used for Older Postesophagectomy Patients in Japan (continued)*

and may actually be an indication of major complications or GI conditions; reporting them may actually aid in diagnosis.

Nurses' therapeutic listening skills play a key role in detecting patients' problems. Nurses at this hospital are trained in the "ask-tell-ask" and "tell me more" educational programs. Designated nurses are assigned to the GI surgical outpatient department to see postsurgical patients and to listen to their stories. If the nurses "sense" patients' problems through therapeutic exchange, they continue to explore the type and degree of the patients' problems, and how the problems affect their daily lives. The nurses listen to the patients' entire experiences of living after esophagectomy.

One day, a nurse saw a patient who complained of nothing special, but had eaten sushi the previous evening as a celebration of his 80th birthday—3 months after his esophagectomy. The nurse kept exploring the client's story, and found that he had continuously experienced decline in food intake, due to increased difficulty in passing food through his esophagus. The nurse assessed that such a condition might be associated with esophageal stenosis, an indication of balloon or bougie for dilatation by his surgeon. The nurse immediately reported this to the surgeon. The surgeon examined his patient and, as expected, diagnosed that the client had severe esophageal stenosis. This patient's condition might otherwise have been overlooked by nurses and surgeons, if this nurse had not had an outstanding "sense" and effective therapeutic listening skills.

The nurses additionally provide the patients with assurance and positive feedback if the patients are on the right track and are trying to adhere to the expected "healthy behavior." Such behavior includes eating small amounts of food slowly, engaging in regular physical activity, and keeping the upper body elevated while asleep. If patients would benefit from behavioral changes in their daily lives, nurses work with them to find acceptable common ground.

After seeing patients, the nurses convey the clients' critical information or questions to the surgeon if indicated and desired. Otherwise, nurses encourage the patients to relate their concerns to the surgeons; or the nurse may ask surgeons questions on behalf of the patients. The patients and surgeons of this department have reported that the nurses are sensitive to the patients' needs, and have noted how helpful nurses are in working together on behalf of the patients. The nurses' outstanding therapeutic listening skills truly enhance the quality of care at the outpatient department of this hospital.

Interpreter-mediated health care encounters can be a challenge for therapeutic interchange. The issue of translation and interpretation in health care includes more than the differences in language use. Interpretation should be founded on a word-for-word translation while incorporating nuances and maintaining semantic equivalency of communication. Difficulties in translation and interpretation in health care encounters are illustrated, for example, in a study by Flores et al. (2003) of Spanish–English interpretations in pediatric encounters. The study found that there were, on average, 31 errors in medical interpretation per clinical encounter. Most errors were categorized as "omissions" of important information, and had potential clinical consequences. Those serious errors were more likely to be committed by nonprofessional interpreters—including nurses, social workers, and siblings—as compared with those committed by hospital interpreters. Use of appropriately trained and experienced interpreters is a necessity for clients who have language barriers.

Another study showed that non-English-speaking family members are at increased risk of receiving less information about the patient's condition—as evidenced by less family conference time, and shorter duration and less proportion of clinician speech during a conference (Thornton, Pham, Engelberg, Jackson, & Curtis, 2009). This study also showed that non-English-speaking families receive less reported emotional support from their health care providers, including valuing families' input, easing emotional burdens, and active listening (Thornton et al., 2009). Health care professionals' cultural sensitivity and considerations are vital to promoting quality of care for patients/families with language barriers.

FUTURE RESEARCH

Many research questions have potential for exploration in the area of therapeutic listening. Systematic studies are needed to develop a body of knowledge. The study designs will require new paradigms beyond traditional randomized controlled trials for, among other things, ethical and feasibility reasons. Qualitative studies, case reports, or mixed-method designs may be better options for understanding the nature and effects of therapeutic listening. Some potential questions for future research are:

- Can therapeutic listening via telephone or other interactive technology (synchronous or asynchronous) be effective at a distance?
- What are the effects of the use of listening by health care providers on patient satisfaction and other outcomes of care?
- Are interventions to enhance listening on the part of health care providers cost-effective and legitimate areas on which to focus continuous quality improvement to increase patient safety and quality of care?
- How do multicultural differences manifest themselves in the processes and effectiveness of therapeutic listening?

REFERENCES

Arnold, E. C., & Underman Boggs, K. (2007). *Interpersonal relationships: Professional communication skills for nurses* (5th ed.). London, UK: W. B. Saunders.

Back, A. L., Arnold, R. M., Baile, W. F., Tulsky, J. A., & Fryer-Edwards, K. (2005). Approaching difficult communication tasks in oncology. *CA: A Cancer Journal for Clinicians, 55*(3), 164–177.

Barrere, C. C. (2007). Discourse analysis of nurse-patient communication in a hospital setting: Implications for staff development. *Journal of Nurses in Staff Development, 23*, 114–122.

Battersby, S., & Deery, R. (2001). Midwifery and research: Comparable skills in listening and the use of language. *Practising Midwife, 4*(9), 24–25.

Boudreau, J. D., Cassell, E., & Fuks, A. (2009). Preparing medical students to become attentive listeners. *Medical Teacher, 31*, 22–29.

Bryant, L. (2009). The art of active listening. *Practice Nurse, 37*(6), 49–52.

Burnard, P. (1997). *Effective communication skills for health professionals* (2nd ed.). Cheltenham, UK: Nelson Thornes.

Bush, K. (2001). Do you really listen to patients? *RN, 64*(3), 35–37.

Cherin, D., Enguidanos, S., & Brumley, R. (2001). Reflection in action in caring for the dying: Applying organizational learning theory to improve communications in terminal care. *Home Health Care Services Quarterly, 19*(4), 65–78.

Claveirole, A. (2004). Listening to young voices: Challenges of research with adolescent mental health service users. *Journal of Psychiatric & Mental Health Nursing, 11*(3), 253–260.

Davidhizar, R. (2004). Listening—A nursing strategy to transcend culture. *Journal of Practical Nursing, 54*(2), 22–24.

De Vito, J. A. (2006). *The interpersonal communication book* (11th ed.). Needham Heights, MA: Allyn & Bacon.

Denham, C. R., Dingman, J., Foley, M. E., Ford, D., Martins, B., O'Regan, P., & Salamendra, A. (2008). Are you listening . . . are you really listening? *Journal of Patient Safety, 4*(3), 148–161.

Fassaert, T., van Dulmen, S., Schellevis, F., & Bensing, J. (2007). Active listening in medical consultations: Development of the Active Listening Observation Scale (ALOS-global). *Patient Education and Counseling, 68*(3), 258–264.

Fassaert, T., van Dulmen, S., Schellevis, F., van der Jagt, L., & Bensing, J. (2008). Raising positive expectations helps patients with minor ailments: A cross-sectional study. *BMC Family Practice, 9*, 38. doi:10.1186/1471-2296-9-38

Flores, G., Laws, M. B., Mayo, S. J., Zuckerman, B., Abreu, M., Medina, L., & Hardt, E. J. (2003). Errors in medical interpretation and their potential clinical consequences in pediatric encounters. *Pediatrics, 111*(1), 6–14.

Foy, C. R., & Timmins, F. (2004). Improving communication in day surgery settings. *Nursing Standard, 19*(7), 37–42.

Fredriksson, L. (1999). Modes of relating in a caring conversation: A research synthesis on presence, touch and listening. *Journal of Advanced Nursing, 30*, 1167–1176.

Garcia de Lucio, L., Garcia Lopez, F. J., Marin Lopez, M. T., Mas Hesse, B., & Caamano Vaz, M. D. (2000). Training programme in techniques of self-control and communication skills to improve nurses' relationships with relatives of critically ill patients: A randomized controlled study. *Journal of Advanced Nursing, 32*, 425–431.

Gidron, Y., Gal, R., Freedman, S., Twiser, I., Lauden, A., Snir, Y., & Benjamin, J. (2001). Translating research findings to PTSD prevention: Results of a randomized-controlled pilot study. *Journal of Traumatic Stress, 14*, 773–780.

Harrington, J., Noble, L. M., & Newman, S. P. (2004). Improving patients' communication with doctors: A systematic review of intervention studies. *Patient Education and Counseling, 52*(1), 7–16.

Harris, S. R., & Templeton, E. (2001). Who's listening? Experiences of women with breast cancer in communicating with physicians. *Breast Journal, 7,* 444–449.

Jones, A. C., & Cutcliffe, J. R. (2009). Listening as a method of addressing psychological distress. *Journal of Nursing Management, 17*(3), 352–358.

Kacperek, L. (1997). Non-verbal communication: The importance of listening. *British Journal of Nursing, 6,* 275–279.

Kemper, B. J. (1992). Therapeutic listening: Developing the concept. *Journal of Psychosocial Nursing and Mental Health Services, 30*(7), 21–23.

Kruijver, I. P., Kerkstra, A., Francke, A. L., Bensing, J. M., & van de Wiel, H. B. (2000). Evaluation of communication training programs in nursing care: A review of the literature. *Patient Education and Counseling, 39,* 129–145.

Kubota, S., Mishima, N., & Nagata, S. (2004). A study of the effects of active listening on listening attitudes of middle managers. *Journal of Occupational Health, 46*(1), 66–67.

Lekander, B. J., Lehmann, S., & Lindquist, R. (1993). Therapeutic listening: Key nursing interventions for several nursing diagnoses. *Dimensions of Critical Care Nursing, 12,* 24–30.

Liehr, P., Mehl, M. R., Summers, L. C., & Pennebaker, J. W. (2004). Connecting with others in the midst of stressful upheaval on September 11, 2001. *Applied Nursing Research, 17*(1), 2–9.

Liu, J. E., Mok, E., Wong, T., Xue, L., & Xu, B. (2007). Evaluation of an integrated communication skills training program for nurses in cancer care in Beijing, China. *Nursing Research, 56,* 202–209.

McCambridge, J., Platts, S., Whooley, D., & Strang, J. (2004). Encouraging GP alcohol intervention: Pilot study of change-oriented reflective listening (CORL). *Alcohol & Alcoholism, 39*(2), 146–149.

Molter, N. C. (2003). Creating a healing environment for critical care. *Critical Care Nursing Clinics of North America, 15,* 295–304.

Murphy, D., & Jenkinson, H. (2012). The mutual benefits of listening to young people in care, with a particular focus on grief and loss: An Irish foster carer's perspective. *Child Care in Practice, 18*(3), 243–253.

O'Gara, P. E., & Fairhurst, W. (2004). Therapeutic communication: Part 2. Strategies that can enhance the quality of the emergency care consultation. *Accident and Emergency Nursing, 12,* 201–207.

O'Hagan, B., Webb, L., & Moore, K. (2004). Listening and learning from patients. *Emergency Nurse, 12*(7), 12–14.

Riegel, B., Dickson, V. V., Hoke, L., McMahon, J. P., Reis, B. F., & Sayers, S. (2006). A motivational counseling approach to improving heart failure self-care: Mechanisms of effectiveness. *Journal of Cardiovascular Nursing, 21,* 232–241.

Rogers, C. R. (1957). The necessary and sufficient conditions of therapeutic personality change. *Journal of Consulting Psychology, 21,* 95–103.

Rollnick, S., Allison, J., Ballasiotes, S., Barth, T., Butler, C. C., Rose, G. S., & Rosengren, D. B. (2002). Variations on a theme: Motivational interviewing and its adaptations. In W. R. Miller & S. Rollnick (Eds.). *Motivational interviewing: Preparing people for change* (2nd ed., pp. 270–283). New York, NY: Guilford Press.

Sandelowski, M. (1994). We are the stories we tell: Narrative knowing in nursing practice. *Journal of Holistic Nursing, 12,* 23–33.

Seidel, H. E., Ball, J. W., Dains, J. E., Flynn, J. A., Solomon, B. S., & Stewart, R. W. (Eds.). (2011). Cultural awareness. In *Mosby's guide to physical examination* (7th ed., pp. 32–45). St. Louis, MO: Mosby.

Shannon, S. E., Long-Sutehall, T., & Coombs, M. (2011). Conversations in end-of-life care: Communication tools for critical care practitioners. *Nursing in Critical Care, 16*(3), 124–130.

Shattell, M., & Hogan, B. (2005). Facilitating communication: How to truly understand what patients mean. *Journal of Psychosocial Nursing and Mental Health Service, 43*(10), 29–32.

Strang, J., McCambridge, J., Platts, S., & Groves, P. (2004). Engaging the reluctant GP in care of the opiate users. *Family Practice, 21*(2), 150–154.

Thornton, J. D., Pham, K., Engelberg, R. A., Jackson, J. C., & Curtis, J. R. (2009). Families with limited English proficiency receive less information and support in interpreted intensive care unit family conferences. *Critical Care Medicine, 37*(1), 89–95.

Vitello-Cicciu, J. M. (2002). Exploring emotional intelligence: Implications for nursing leaders. *Journal of Nursing Administration, 32*(4), 203–210.

Wanzer, M. B., Booth-Butterfield, M., & Gruber, K. (2004). Perceptions of health care providers' communication: Relationships between patient-centered communication and satisfaction. *Health Communication, 16*, 363–384.

White, J., Levinson, W., & Roter, D. (1994). "Oh by the way": The closing moments of the medical visit. *Journal of General Internal Medicine, 9*, 24–28.

Williams, K., Kemper, S., & Hummert, M. L. (2004). Enhancing communication with older adults: Overcoming elderspeak. *Journal of Gerontological Nursing, 30*(10), 17–25.

Chapter 5: Creating Optimal Healing Environments

MARY JO KREITZER AND TERRI ZBOROWSKY

Nurses have long been leaders in creating optimal healing environments (OHEs). Florence Nightingale, the founder of modern nursing, described the role of the nurse as helping the patient attain the best possible condition so that nature can act and self-healing can occur (Dossey, 2000). Nightingale recognized the nurse's role in both caring for the patient and managing the physical environment. She wrote about the importance of natural light, fresh air, noise reduction, and infection control as well as spirituality, presence, and caring. Her philosophy embodied the notion that, as nurses, we don't heal our patients: we recognize that healing occurs within a person and our work is to help people tap into their innate capacities.

Increasingly, a base of evidence about the creation of optimal healing environments is emerging from many disciplines, including nursing, interior design, architecture, neuroscience, psychoneuroimmunology, and environmental psychology, among others. Just as evidence-based practice informs clinical decision making, evidence-based design impacts the planning and construction of health care facilities. Nurses need to be taught about the ways in which the physical environment affects health outcomes. First, so that they can contribute to the design of patient care units and clinical facilities that will optimize the health and well-being of patients, their families, and the staff who work in health care environments. Second, nurses are in a unique position to carry on needed research on the impact of specific design interventions on intended outcomes.

DEFINITIONS

The word *healing* comes from the Anglo-Saxon *haelen*, meaning "to make whole." Healing environments are designed to promote harmony or balance of mind, body, and spirit; to reduce anxiety and stress; and to be restorative. The Samueli Institute, a research center focused on the science of healing, defines an optimal healing environment as a place where all aspects of patient care—physical, emotional, spiritual, behavioral, and environmental—are optimized to support and stimulate healing (see Exhibit 5.1).

As illustrated in Exhibit 5.1, within an optimal healing environment, the internal resources—such as the expectations and hopes of all health care providers and of the patients themselves—are recognized as being important. There are opportunities for personal growth and self-care practices that promote wholeness. Healing relationships are cultivated as patients and their families interact with empathetic and compassionate health care providers and staff. A culture is created that supports healing through alignment of the organizational vision, mission, resources, and leadership. Healthy lifestyle behaviors are promoted and patients have options to choose conventional care and/or complementary therapies and healing practices. All of these elements are supported by a physical environment that embodies design characteristics known to promote healing: nature, light, and color, as well as fostering ecological sustainability.

An OHE model developed by Zborowsky and Kreitzer (2009) and depicted in Exhibit 5.2 illustrates that an optimal healing environment is created through a deep and dynamic interplay among people, place, and process. In this model, *people* include the caregivers and support team that surround the patient. The characteristics and competencies of the staff and the knowledge, skills, and attitudes that they embody are some of the most critical elements of an OHE. The *process* element refers to the care processes as well as the leadership processes that support a culture that is aligned with creating an OHE. Care processes include conventional, integrative, and behavioral interventions. The *place* element focuses on the physical space where care is provided and the geography that surrounds the patient, family, and caregiver. Place elements include access to nature, positive distractions, aesthetics, the ambient environment, and ecosystem sustainability.

This model of OHE suggests that optimally, there is good coherence and alignment between the people (nurses and patients) who enact processes (caregiving in the context of patient-centered care) in a place (physical environment) that is designed to maximize positive patient outcomes. The reality is that much of care occurs in old, dysfunctional facilities. Even health care facilities built 20 years ago lack the available space and mechanical systems to function well today due to changes in building codes, guidelines, and best practice in care models. An inadequate space makes it more difficult to attain a truly healing environment, although

Exhibit 5.1. *Optimal Healing Environments Make Healing as Important as Curing*

OPTIMAL HEALING ENVIRONMENTS
MAKING HEALING AS IMPORTANT AS CURING

An Optimal Healing Environment is one that supports and stimulates patient healing by addressing the social, psychological, physical, spiritual and behavioral components of health care and enabling the body's capacity to heal itself.

social, psychological, physical, spiritual, behavioral

INTERNAL	INTERPERSONAL	BEHAVORIAL	EXTERNAL
DEVELOPING HEALING INTENSION	CULTIVATING HEALING RELATIONSHIPS	PRACTICING HEALTHY LIFESTYLES	BUILDING HEALING SPACES
EXPERIENCING PERSONAL WHOLENESS	CREATING HEALING ORGANIZATIONS	APPLYING COLLABORATIVE MEDICINE	FOSTERING ECOLOGICAL SUSTAINABILITY
Expectation	Communication	Diet	Color & Light
Hope	Compassion	Exercise	Art & Architecture
Understanding	Social Support	Relaxation	Aroma & Air
Belief	Empathy	Addiction Management	Music & Sound
Mind	Leadership	Integrative	Eco-friendly
Body	Mission	Person Centered	Green
Spirit	Teamwork	Family Centered	Energy Efficient
Energy	Technology	Culturally Sensitive	Nature

INNER ENVIRONMENTS → TO → OUTER ENVIRONMENTS

SAMUELI INSTITUTE
EXPLORING THE SCIENCE OF HEALING

© 2012 Samueli Institute

Source: Reprinted courtesy of the Samueli Institute.

57

Exhibit 5.2. *People, Place, and Process: The Role of Place in Creating OHEs*

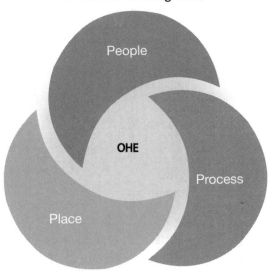

Source: Reprinted from Zborowsky and Kreitzer (2009).

the elements of the caregiver and the care provided are even more critical than the physical place or space. Today, there is a better understanding and rigorous research that describes how to choose elements of place that support and enable an OHE.

The primary emphasis of this volume of *Complementary & Alternative Therapies in Nursing* is on the evidence and clinical applications of complementary and alternative therapies that nurses can use to enhance their practice. This chapter focuses on the dimension of place or space—the physical environment in which care is provided and the ways in which evidence can be used to create environments that contribute to positive health outcomes.

SCIENTIFIC BASIS

There is a growing body of evidence that links the physical environment to health outcomes. According to a review of the research literature on evidence-based health care design (Ulrich et al., 2008), there have been more than 1,000 rigorous empirical studies published that link the design of a hospital's physical environment with health care outcomes. The studies cover a broad scope, with evidence linking:

- *Single-bed rooms* with reduced hospital-acquired infections, reduced medical errors, reduced patient falls, improved patient sleep, and increased patient satisfaction

■ *Decentralized supplies* with increased staff effectiveness
■ *Appropriate lighting* with decreased medical errors and decreased staff stress, and
■ *Ceiling lifts* with decreased staff injuries

Although many of the studies focus on such topics as infection control, patient falls, staff productivity, and staff injuries, a growing number of studies focus on other aspects of the environment that contribute to healing.

As described by Malkin (2008), design strategies that focus on creating healing environments have in common the goal of reducing stress and include:

■ Connections to nature—artwork with a nature theme, views to the outside, interior gardens, plants
■ Options that give patients choices and control—room-service menu, choice of music and art, ability to control lighting and temperature
■ Spaces that provide access to social support—family zones within patient rooms that offer sleeping space, storage, and adequate seating
■ Positive distractions—music, water features, aviaries, videos of nature, aquariums, and sculpture
■ Reductions of environmental stressors such as noise and glare from direct light sources—carpet, indirect lighting, elimination of overhead paging

Theories Related to Healing Environments and Clinical Applications

Biophilia is the inherent human inclination to affiliate with natural systems and processes. The concept, originally proposed by eminent biologist Edward O. Wilson (1984), has grown into a broader framework that increasingly is shaping the design of the man-made environment, including hospitals and other health care facilities. Biophilic design emphasizes the necessity of maintaining, enhancing, and restoring the beneficial experience of nature. It describes attempts to do so through the use of environmental features that embody such characteristics of the natural world as color, water, sunlight, plants, natural materials, and exterior views and vistas (Kellert, 2008). The theory of biophilia has been empirically tested in clinical settings. Outcomes measured most often include stress and pain reduction. For example:

■ A study of elderly residents in an urban long-term-care facility revealed that they attached considerable importance to having access to window views of outdoor spaces with prominent features such as plants, gardens, and birds (Kearney & Winterbottom, 2005).

- Patients in a dental clinic reported less stress on days when a large nature mural was hung in the waiting room, compared to days when there was no nature scene (Heerwagen, 1990).
- In a prospective randomized trial of blood donors, it was found that donors who viewed a wall-mounted television playing a nature videotape had lower blood pressure and pulse rates than subjects who were viewing a television playing either a videotape of urban scenes or game or talk shows (Ulrich, Simons, & Miles, 2003).
- Ulrich, Lunden, and Eltinge (1993) found that patients following heart surgery who viewed photos of trees and water required fewer doses of strong pain medication and reported less anxiety than patients who viewed abstract images or were assigned to a control group with no picture.

There is some evidence that the more engrossing a nature distraction, the greater the potential for pain alleviation. Miller, Hickman, and Lemasters (1992), in a study of burn patients, found that distracting patients during burn dressings by having them view nature scenes, accompanied by music, on a bedside television lessened both pain and anxiety. In a randomized prospective trial of patients undergoing bronchoscopy, those who viewed a ceiling-mounted nature scene and listened to nature sounds reported less pain than subjects in the control group who looked at a blank ceiling. Following a review of the literature on the use of virtual reality as an adjunct analgesic technique, Wismeijer and Vingerhoets (2005) concluded that "nature exposures" might tend to be more diverting—and hence pain-reducing—if they involved sound as well as visual stimulation and maximized realism and immersion. There is emerging research that uses a multimethod approach to understanding the effect nature has on patients. Goto, Park, Tsunetsugu, Herrup, and Miyazaki (2013) found that exposure to organized gardens can affect both the mood and cardiac physiology of elderly individuals. Among other findings, they revealed that a subject's heart rate was significantly lower in the Japanese garden than in the other environments studied. The individual's sympathetic function was significantly lower as well. In this case study of 19 patients in an assisted-living facility, the multimethod approach provided both qualitative and quantitative data.

A number of studies have examined patient preferences for art and the effect of art on stress, recovery, and pain, among other outcomes. Consistently, studies have documented that subjects prefer nature over other subject matter, and that they overwhelmingly prefer realistic art and strongly dislike abstract images (Winston & Cupchik, 1992). Findings such as these, consistent with the theory of biophilia, have led to the use of evidence-based design guidelines in health care facilities to influence the selection of art. According to Ulrich and Gilpin (2003), visual art should be unambiguously positive. Recommended subject matter

includes waterscapes with calm or nonturbulent water, landscap
visual depth or openness, nature settings depicted during warmer
sons when vegetation is verdant and flowers are visible, garden scene
outdoor scenes in sunny conditions, and avoidance of overcast or fore-
boding weather.

Pati and Nanda (2011) utilized a quasiexperimental design to examine pediatric patients' behavior during five distraction conditions ranging
from a slide show to video with music. All distraction conditions were
created on one flat-screen plasma television monitor mounted on a stand
in the waiting areas. Data analysis showed that the introduction of distraction conditions was associated with more calm behavior and less fine and
gross movement, suggesting significant calming effects associated with the
distraction conditions. Data also suggested that positive distraction conditions were significant attention grabbers, and could be an important contributor to improving the waiting experience for children in hospitals by
enhancing environmental attractiveness. Nanda, Zhu, and Jansen (2012)
conducted a systematic review of neuroscience articles on the emotional
states of fear, anxiety, and pain to understand how emotional response is
linked to the visual characteristics of an image at the level of brain behavior. Findings indicated there is a paucity of research in this area; and this is
a compelling field for future research on the direct impact that imagery of
artwork can have on emotional processing centers in the brain.

Chronobiology

Chronobiology is an interdisciplinary field of inquiry that focuses on
biological rhythms. Discoveries in chronotherapeutics have documented
that time patterning of medications in synchrony with body rhythms can
enhance effectiveness and safety. Other studies have targeted the impact
of environmental factors such as light and temperature on body rhythms.
There is a significant body of literature focused on the impact of light
on depression. In a study of psychiatric patients, Beauchemin and Hays
(1996) found that patients in sunnier rooms stayed an average of 2.6 fewer
days than those in sunless rooms. A meta-analysis of 20 randomized controlled trials by Golden et al. (2005) on the impact of light treatment on
nonseasonal and seasonal depression quantified the effect of light treatment as equivalent to that of antidepressant pharmacotherapy trials. Light
has also been found to be related to patients' perception of pain. In a study
(Walch et al., 2005) of postspinal surgery experiences, patients who were
admitted to rooms with greater sunlight intensity reported less pain and
stress and took 22% fewer analgesic medications. Results such as these
support careful site planning to assure adequate access to daylight, and
provide justification for larger windows in patient rooms or the use of
bright (but diffused) artificial light in areas where sufficient daylight is
inaccessible.

/posttest quasiexperimental study in two intensive care ey, Gerbi, Watson, Imgrund, and Sagha-Zadeh (2012) of daylight and window views on patient pain levels, f errors, absenteeism, and vacancy rates. Researchers h levels of natural light and window views may posi- absenteeism and staff vacancy, although factors such patient pain, and length of stay still require additional research. In summary, there is growing evidence that views of nature and light are beneficial for patients as well as staff.

INTERVENTION

Case Study Applications of Optimal Healing Environment

North Hawaii Community Hospital

North Hawaii Community Hospital embodies the culture of the community in the way in which it has operationalized the concept of an optimal healing environment. The footprint of the hospital was aligned so that the front is oriented to the Kohala Mountain, and the back to the Mauna Kea Mountain. Earl Bakken, one of the founders of the hospital, had the vision that the hospital itself would be an "instrument of healing," rather than a "warehouse for sick bodies" (E. Bakken, personal communication, January 2008). All patient rooms are private and have access to views of nature and fresh air through sliding doors that open to the outside. Art in patient rooms is culturally meaningful and can be changed. Hallways are carpeted and there is minimal overhead paging. Soft music plays in public spaces. Familiar cultural patterns, textures, and colors are used in wallpapers, carpeting, and furniture coverings. *Ti* plants at all entrances and corners of the building are believed to filter out bad spiritual energy. An interior bamboo garden also offers spiritual protection and represents strength and resilience. All patient rooms have sleep chairs or extra beds for guests to stay over and there are no limits on the number of visitors or visiting hours. An *ohama* (Hawaiian for family) room includes a kitchen so that families can prepare special meals. Skylights in halls plus windows in the operating rooms were incorporated into the design to enable staff to stay attuned to day/night cycles. In addition to these and many other mechanical, architectural, and engineering adaptations, the hospital embraces a philosophy of blended medicine that encourages the integration of complementary therapies and culturally based healing practices. The vision of North Hawaii Community Hospital is to become the most healing hospital in the world.

Abbott Northwestern Hospital

The design of the Neuroscience/Orthopaedic/Spine Patient Care Center at Abbott Northwestern's new Heart Hospital in Minneapolis, Minnesota, integrates the elements of Abbott Northwestern's healing environment aesthetic standards, including the principles of *feng shui* and patient-centered care, while acknowledging the needs of staff. The 128 inpatient beds are located on two floors of the Heart Hospital, which was designed to incorporate the latest technology to aid in meeting patient and safety requirements as well as implement the organization's holistic approach to healing. To accomplish these goals, patient rooms were zoned so that the needs of each user of the space would be addressed.

■ The *patient zone* provides a view to the outside from every bed, a flower/card shelf, a private safe for valuables, artwork and care-provider information on the footwall, and a small refrigerator for favorite foods.
■ The *family zone* incorporates an upholstered bench seat/sleeper, a reading light with private switch, and a data outlet for Internet access.
■ The *caregiver zone* includes a bedside work area with a sink, computer, and—in each patient room—a ceiling-mounted patient-lift system with a custom track to assist with turning, moving, or toileting a patient.

Other family and patient amenities in the unit include access to a two-story atrium with soothing water walls, a waiting room with a panoramic view of the city, a kitchenette, and a fireplace. In addition to the bedside computer in each patient room, facilities to optimize workflow include decentralized support rooms such as clean utility, soiled utility, nutrition, and medication rooms. A staff-respite area, a private room for staff to use, includes a lounge chair, an ottoman, a phone, and an outside view. Beyond the clinical outcomes, this design provides balance for the psychological, social, and spiritual needs of the staff, the patients, and their families. Ultimately, the new patient care center design aspires to create a unique health care environment at Abbott Northwestern Hospital.

Regions Hospital

A primary objective of a recent building project at Regions Hospital, a large tertiary care facility located in St. Paul, Minnesota, was to replace shared patient rooms with private patient rooms. The new hospital bed tower includes an expansion of the emergency department, replacement of the operating suite, and the addition of 144 private patient rooms. Design principles included an overarching goal to enhance patient safety.

To accomplish this goal in the bed tower, many new features were built into the design:

Patient Safety

- **Standardization of patient rooms.** First, staff realized that standardization of all the patient rooms was imperative. Although each floor has a different service line—even different acuity levels that range from intensive care to orthopedics—all patient rooms are laid out in the same way.
- **Unique staff access and visibility.** Each patient room has a separate doorway for patients and families as well as one for staff. Staff work areas directly adjacent to the patient room include a view window with an integral blind. Staff shares this alcove between two rooms, a design feature particularly important for intensive care unit staff. Patient visibility and ease of access to the patient should enhance patient safety by increasing staff presence.
- **Enhanced family zones.** In addition, family zones in the rooms are spacious, with the intent of encouraging family-centered patient care. Families have the ability to stay overnight in most rooms.
- **Inclusion of acuity-adaptable patient rooms.** Patient rooms on the cardiac unit were designed to be acuity adaptable: allowing patients to stay in the same room as their acuity level varies. This concept is based on data suggesting that decreased transferring of patients lessens medical incidents and errors (Hendrich, Fay, & Sorrels, 2004).
- **Patient access to the toilet.** Finally, because the patient rooms are mirrored, at least one half of the rooms will have direct access to the patient toilet. No studies to date have been able to document that this is a safer layout for patients; however, with a growing number of patient rooms being designed this way, Regions provides the perfect setting to study the impact of this layout on patient safety.

University of Minnesota Amplatz Children's Hospital

The new University of Minnesota Amplatz Children's Hospital opened in Minneapolis in 2011 as Minnesota's first "green" children's hospital. Design of the new hospital included extensive involvement on the part of staff nurses to optimize workflows as well as getting design feedback from children. Highlights of the hospital design include:

- **Natural lighting.** The building was designed with walls of large windows allowing extensive natural lighting. Corridors are positioned to allow the natural light to flow through and across the patient care units. Large windows are not only in patient care rooms but also in conference rooms and staff break rooms to allow staff to take advantage of natural lighting as well.
- **Patient care unit layout.** Design of the pediatric units optimized the concept of minimizing extraneous movement in direct patient care

areas. Patient rooms are clustered in pods of no more than six patient rooms per pod with smaller caregiver workstations and no central unit desk. Access to work rooms, supply rooms, and medication rooms are through a central nonpatient corridor with patient room access on an outer corridor reserved for movement of patients and visitors. This minimizes noise from opening and closing of supply room doors and avoidance of extraneous noise that can occur with the gathering of caregivers at a central desk. Each patient care unit has two supply rooms and two equipment rooms to improve staff workflow efficiencies, thereby allowing staff to be more visible to family and patients. Cabinets were built into the walls to accommodate isolation supplies, minimizing any perceived clutter that can occur from having isolation carts in hallways. There is a greeter stationed at the entrance of each pediatric unit so a friendly, consistent face—rather than a busy central desk with multiple caregivers—greets family and visitors each time they enter the units.

- **Unit aesthetics.** Each pediatric unit has a nature-based theme in the form of drawings and artwork on the walls. Team work areas face toward artwork that features nature scenes such as beautiful flowers. Children gave input into the paint colors chosen for the units.
- **Patient rooms.** All patient rooms are private and large. This allows for distinct parent/family space within the patient room with a couch/ bed for overnight stays, and Internet access. Some patient rooms have a camera in the room giving a direct view of the outside. Each room has a large-screen television, as well as one monitor where patients and families can access a GetWellNetwork—online patient education materials and music and videos to promote relaxation. In addition, some rooms also have the ability for patients and families to Skype with family members who live a distance away, maintaining a patient and family-support system through a difficult time.
- **Nature outdoors.** An outdoor rooftop healing garden allows patients and families an opportunity to spend time outdoors. There is a playground and another garden outside the hospital on the ground level.

A final inclusion in this section is the application of principles for creating a healing environment in the home. These tips for well-being are straightforward and easy to implement (see Exhibit 5.3).

CULTURAL APPLICATIONS AND PRECAUTIONS

The increased diversity of the U.S. population has added a level of complexity to the design of health care environments. As noted by Kopec and Han (2008), entering a health care environment can be frightening and disempowering, particularly when a patient's traditional and

Exhibit 5.3. *Well-Being Tips for the Home*

- *Open a window.* Allowing fresh air to circulate through your home lets you breathe easier. This also rids the air of pollutants, including harmful chemicals that may accumulate from products, equipment such as air conditioners, and furniture.
- *Bring the outside in.* Studies have demonstrated that exposure to nature can reduce stress levels and improve well-being. Viewing nature from a window or looking at nature-related images can give a sense of retreat throughout the day.
- *Create a quiet, comfortable space* that allows you to escape and reflect. Meditation is an important part of overall well-being and has been shown to increase (hard to access) alpha-wave patterns in the brain that have been associated with less stress and anxiety.
- *Use calming colors.* Color can have a wide range of effects on human mood and emotions. Colors with blue undertones have the ability to calm the mind and create a greater sense of relaxation. Light waves corresponding to the color blue are found to have the greatest effect on regulating the circadian rhythms that are directly related to our moods.
- *Avoid clutter in the home*; it can create unnecessary stress! Because our brains are constantly categorizing what we see, it is important to keep the space around us organized and free of clutter.
- *Personalize your space* with items, furnishings, and finishes that bring you joy and that have meaning. Personalizing one's space gives one a sense of control and a deeper connection to a space.
- *Have a sense of control* in your home environment. This can include temperature controls, space allocation and organization, noise levels, security, and safety. Most important, your home should function according to the way you live.

Adapted from Angelita Scott, personal communication, April 1, 2013.

spiritual beliefs differ from those of the dominant culture. Thus, it is becoming increasingly important to carefully weigh all design decisions that impact the physical environment, including the use of color and cultural symbols as well as other visual, auditory, and tactile design elements.

To Asians, for example, the color red symbolizes good luck, whereas the color white is associated with mourning and death. The color green has positive associations within the Islamic tradition because it is associated with vegetation and life and is believed to have been the prophet Mohammed's favorite color. Kopec and Han (2008) have identified a number of ways in which the needs of Muslim patients might be accommodated. A curtain inside the door, for instance, could help patients maintain visual privacy and modesty, while allowing health care providers on rounds to announce their presence, giving patients time to prepare themselves to be seen. Understanding that followers of Islam face the northeast when they pray could be taken into consideration when orienting the bed and furnishings in the room.

Given the diversity of spiritual, religious, and cultural beliefs and practices, however, it would be nearly impossible, from a design perspective (as well as practically and financially), to accommodate all of the specifics and nuances of every tradition. Thus, the goal of design can only be to strive to express core, universal values while seeking to devise design elements that can be flexible. Although the main focus of this chapter has been the physical or built environment, a reminder of the foundational importance of the roles of food, family, and spirituality in the creation of a healing environment is provided in the account of creating a healing environment in Liberia, West Africa (see Sidebar 5.1).

Sidebar 5.1. *Healing Environments in Liberia, West Africa*

Maria Keita, Liberia, West Africa

I am from the Krahn tribe, a small tribe in Liberia, West Africa, which is one of 16 tribes in Liberia. However, I am confident in saying that the healing environment I describe reflects the culture of the Liberian people in general.

When I think of the healing environment in the United States, what comes to mind are the beautiful, well-designed rooms, readily available medications, and high-tech medical devices. The healing environment in my culture consists of four major parts: family presence, food, spirituality, and complementary therapies. When people from Liberia are in the hospital, it is important for staff to understand the importance of presence. Family and friends come in dozens to visit. However, there are always one or two people who stay in the room at all times to support the sick person. The role of the assigned person(s) is to coordinate the care of the patient between hospital caregiver and the family and provide direct support such as encouragement and reassurance to the patient. The presence of friends and family reduces anxiety and builds trust with hospital staff. A healing environment is incomplete without the presence of a family member or a friend with the sick.

It is an expectation in my culture that people stay with one who is ill. The role of the family is to help in the care of the sick with activities of daily living, even when in a formal hospital setting.

(continued)

Sidebar 5.1. *Healing Environments in Liberia, West Africa (continued)*

Food as a Healing Environment

Food is another very important part of the healing environment in my culture. There are special foods that are offered to sick people, such as a pepper soup made with hot spices. If solid food is prepared, it is usually anything that can be easily swallowed. *Depa* and *fufu* are like mashed potatoes made from fresh or dried cassava, yams, or plantains. So-called slippery soups are also easy to swallow. Sick people, it is believed, obtain cleansing and nasal decongestion from various soups.

Complementary Therapy as a Part of a Healing Environment

A warm bath with or without herbs is considered to be very therapeutic in my culture and is therefore offered to sick people. A routine daily bath is an expectation. Herbs are often boiled with the bath water and the hot bath is given to the patient.

Spirituality

Providing regular prayers and the presence of religious symbols is an essential part of the healing environment; however, these may come with different levels of spirituality. Many families may believe that without intervention from above, conventional medicine will not bring about healing.

The combination of conventional medicine and providing a healing environment in the Liberian culture is sometimes a challenge to health care providers in the United States. Family involvement in conventional medicine is limited based on how a healing environment is perceived by Liberians. Hospital staff is usually overwhelmed by the presence of many family members in rooms of patients from Liberia or most African cultures.

More training for nurses and medical staff in the understanding of the healing environment of other cultures will enhance conventional medicine and increase the communication between patient/family and caregivers.

FUTURE RESEARCH

More research is needed to understand the impact of design interventions on the environment of care. Future studies need to rigorously examine the many factors that contribute to healing environments and should include a focus on staff as well as patient outcomes. Health care outcomes for patients may include the reduction of stress, reduced length of stay, decreased incidence of nosocomial infections, less pain, improved sleep, increased patient satisfaction, and fewer patient falls. Outcomes for nursing staff may include fewer staff injuries; decreased staff stress; reduced sick days; and increased staff effectiveness, productivity, and satisfaction.

Hospital construction in the United States is anticipated to increase by 8% by the end of 2013, with costs expected to exceed $44 billion (Giggard, 2013). Nurses must be actively engaged in contributing to the design and evaluation of healing environments that will optimize the health and well-being of patients, family members, and staff.

WEBSITES

Center for Health Design
(www.healthdesign.org)

Center for Spirituality and Healing, University of Minnesota
(takingcharge.csh.umn.edu/therapies/environment/what)

REFERENCES

Beauchemin, K. M., & Hays, P. (1996). Sunny hospital rooms expedite recovery from severe and refractory depressions. *Journal of Affective Disorders, 40*(1/2), 49–51.

Dossey, B. M. (2000). *Florence Nightingale: Mystic, visionary, healer.* Springhouse, PA: Springhouse.

Giggard, J. R., (2013). *FMI's construction outlook. 1st quarter 2013 report.* Raleigh, NC: FMI. Retrieved April 17, 2013, from http://www.fminet.com/media/pdf/forecasts/Outlook_2013Q1_FMI.pdf

Golden, R. N., Gaynes, B. N., Ekstrom, R. D., Hamer, R. M., Jacobsen, F. M., Suppes, T., . . . Nemeroff, C. (2005). The efficacy of light therapy in the treatment of mood disorders: A review and meta-analysis of the evidence. *American Journal of Psychiatry, 162*(4), 656–662.

Goto, S., Park, B-J., Tsunetsugu, Y., Herrup, K., & Miyazaki, Y. (2013). The effect of garden designs on mood and heart output in older adults residing in an assisted living facility. *Health Environments Research & Design Journal 6*(2), 27–42.

Heerwagen, J. H. (1990). The psychological aspects of windows and window design. In K. H. Anthony, J. Choi, & B. Orland (Eds.), *Proceedings of 21st Annual Conference of the Environmental Design Research Association* (pp. 269–280). Oklahoma City, OK: Environmental Design Research Association.

Hendrich, A., Fay, J., & Sorrells, A. (2004). Effects of acuity-adaptable rooms on flow of patients and delivery of care. *American Journal of Critical Care, 113*(1), 35–45.

Kearney, A. R., & Winterbottom, D. (2005). Nearby nature and long-term care facility residents: Benefits and design recommendations. *Journal of Housing for the Elderly, 1*(3/4), 7–28.

Kellert, S. R. (2008). Dimensions, elements and attributes of biophilic design. In S. R. Keller, J. H. Heerwagen, & M. L. Mador (Eds.), *Biophilic design* (pp. 3–20). Hoboken, NJ: John Wiley.

Kopec, D., & Han, L. (2008). Islam and the healthcare environment: Designing patient rooms. *Health Environments Research and Design Journal, 1*(4), 111–121.

Malkin, J. (2008). *A visual reference for evidence-based design.* Concord, CA: The Center for Health Design.

Miller, A. C., Hickman, L. C., & Lemasters, G. K. (1992). A distraction technique for control of burn pain. *Journal of Burn Care and Rehabilitation, 13*(5), 576–580.

Nanda, U., Zhu, X., & Jansen, B. H. (2012). Image and emotion: From outcomes to brain behavior. *Health Environments Research & Design Journal, 5*(4), 40–59.

Pati, D., & Nanda, U. (2011). Influence of positive distraction on children in two clinic waiting areas. *Health Environments Research & Design* (4), 124–140.

Shepley, M. M., Gerbi, R. P., Watson, A. E., Imgrund, S., & Sagha-Zadeh, R. (2012). The impact of daylight and views on ICU patients and staff. *Health Environments Research & Design Journal, 5*(2), 46–60.

Ulrich, R. S., & Gilpin, L. (2003). Healing arts. In S. B. Frampton, L. Gilpin, & P. Charmel (Eds.), *Putting patients first: Designing and practicing patient-centered care* (pp. 117–146). San Francisco, CA: Jossey-Bass.

Ulrich, R. S., Lunden, O. L., & Eltinge, J. L. (1993). Effects of exposure to nature and abstract pictures on patients recovering from heart surgery. *Psychophysiology, 30* (Suppl. 1), 7.

Ulrich, R. S., Simons, R. F., & Miles, M. A. (2003). Effects of environmental simulations and television on blood donor stress. *Journal of Architectural & Planning Research, 20*(1), 38–47.

Ulrich, R. S., Siring, C., Zhu, X., Dubose, J., Seo, H., Choi, Y., ... Anjali, J. (2008). A review of the research literature on evidence-based healthcare design. *Health Environments Research & Design Journal, 1*(3), 61–125.

Walch, J. M., Rabin, B. S., Day, R., Williams, J. N., Choi, K., & Kang, J. D. (2005). The effect of sunlight on post-operative analgesic medication usage: A prospective study of patients undergoing spinal surgery. *Psychosomatic Medicine, 67,* 156–163.

Wilson, E. O. (1984). *Biophilia: The human bond with other species.* Cambridge, MA: Harvard University Press.

Winston, A. S., & Cupchik, G. C. (1992). The evaluation of high art and popular art by naive and experienced viewers. *Visual Arts Research, 18,* 1–14.

Wismeijer, A. J., & Vingerhoets, J. J. (2005). The use of virtual reality and audiovisual eyeglass systems as adjunct analgesic techniques: A review of the literature. *Annals of Behavioral Medicine, 30*(3), 268–278.

Zborowsky, T., & Kreitzer, M. J. (2009). People, place, and process: The role of place in creating optimal healing environments. *Creative Nursing, 15*(4), 186–190.

Part II: Mind–Body–Spirit Therapies

One of the National Center for Complementary and Alternative Medicine (NCCAM) types of complementary/alternative practices is mind and body medicine. According to the NCCAM, "Mind and body practices focus on the interactions among the brain, mind, body, and behavior, with the intent to use the mind to affect physical functioning and promote health" (2012, p. 2). In the 2007 National Health Interview Survey (Barnes, Bloom, & Nahin, 2008), mind and body practices were among the top 10 therapies used, with 12.7% of the subjects using deep-breathing exercises, 9.4% using meditation, and 6.1% practicing yoga. Interestingly, yoga and deep breathing were often used by children.

Because the philosophy of nursing is holistic, "spirit" was added to the title for this part. Not only does the mind affect the body and the body the mind, but the spirit also has an impact on a person's overall functioning. Nursing has moved away from the Cartesian philosophy in which the body and mind (and spirit) were seen as functioning independently of each other. Cartesian philosophy has for centuries dominated Western medicine. Refuting this dichotomy can be seen in the impact that a severe headache has on one's ability to think, to move, and to pray.

A growing body of research supports the use of many of the therapies classified as mind–body–spirit. Since the research of Herbert Benson on transcendental meditation began in the 1960s (Benson, 1975), studies on meditation, music, imagery, and other therapies continue to increase. Of particular help in determining the impact of these therapies on physical, mental, and spiritual well-being has been the development of instruments to not only measure the outcomes of specific therapies, but also to demonstrate the areas of the brain that might be involved. A growing number of researchers are also examining holistic outcomes of these therapies such as improvement of quality of life. However, as could be said for many complementary and alternative therapies, more research needs to be done—especially with populations for whom specific therapies hold promise.

Many of the therapies in this category such as imagery, music, prayer, humor, and meditation have been and continue to be a part of nursing's armamentarium of intervention. Other therapies in this group, such as yoga and journaling, are being used by nurses themselves in self-care.

The integration of mind–body–spirit is an integral part of many healing practices in non-Western and indigenous health care systems. The NCCAM (2012) noted that the mind is important in the healing of illness in traditional Chinese medicine. The spiritual element of a person characterizes many healing practices in Native American cultures. Thus, nurses need to be attentive to therapies that are not discussed in this part of the book but are an integral part of the health care of people from other cultures who may be receiving care in Western health care facilities. The expansion of nursing perspectives can be achieved by reviewing the commentaries, illustrating this point, from other nations in chapter sidebars.

REFERENCES

Barnes, P. M., Bloom, B., & Nahin, R. (2008, December 10). CDC National Health Statistics Report #12. *Complementary and alternative medicine use among adults and children: United States, 2007.* Hyattsville, MD: National Center for Health Statistics.

Benson, H. (1975). *The relaxation response.* New York, NY: Avon.

National Center for Complementary and Alternative Medicine. (2012). *What is complementary and alternative medicine?* Retrieved from http://nccam.nih.gov/health/whatiscam

Chapter 6: Imagery

MAURA FITZGERALD AND MARY LANGEVIN

*I*magery is a mind–body intervention that uses the power of the imagination to bring about change in physical, emotional, or spiritual dimensions. Throughout our daily lives we constantly see images, feel sensations, and register impressions. A picture of lemonade makes our mouths water; a song makes us happy or sad; a smell takes us back to a past moment. Images evoke physical and emotional responses and help us understand the meaning of events.

Imagery is commonly used in health care—most often in the form of guided imagery, clinical hypnosis, or self-hypnosis. In the mid-1950s, the American Medical Association and the American Psychiatric Association recognized hypnosis as a therapeutic tool. Nurses, physicians, psychologists, and others use it with adults and children for treatment of acute and chronic illness, relief of symptoms, and enhancement of wellness. Imagery is a hallmark of stress-management programs and has become a standard therapy to alleviate anxiety, promote relaxation, improve coping and functional status, gain psychological insight, and even to make progress on a chosen spiritual path.

DEFINITION

Imagery is the formation of a mental representation of an object, place, event, or situation that is perceived through the senses. It is a cognitive–behavioral strategy that uses the individual's own imagination and mental processing and can be practiced as an independent activity or guided by a professional. Imagery employs all the senses—visual, aural, tactile, olfactory, proprioceptive, and kinesthetic. Although imagery is often referred to as visualization, it includes imagining through any sense and not just being able to see something in the mind's eye.

Van Kuiken (2004) describes four types of guided imagery: pleasant, physiologically focused, mental rehearsal or reframing, and receptive imagery. While inducing imagery, the individual often imagines seeing, hearing, smelling, tasting, and/or touching something in the image. The image used can be active or passive (playing volley ball versus lying on the beach). Although for many participants physical and mental relaxation tend to facilitate imagery, this is not necessary— particularly for children, who often do not need to be in a relaxed state. Imagery may be receptive, with the individual perceiving messages from the body, or it may be active, with the individual evoking thoughts or ideas. Active imagery can be outcome- or end-state-oriented, in which the individual envisions a goal, such as being healthy and well; or it can be process-oriented, in which the mechanism of the desired effect is imagined, such as envisioning a strong immune system fighting a viral infection or tumor.

Imagery and clinical hypnosis are closely related. Clinical hypnosis is a strategy in which a professional guides the participant into an altered state of deep relaxation, and suggestions for changes in subjective experience and alterations in perception are made. Both hypnosis and guided imagery incorporate the use of relaxation techniques, such as diaphragmatic breathing or progressive muscle relaxation to assist the participant to focus the attention. In hypnosis, this is referred to as an induction. Guided imagery is often used within the context of hypnosis to further deepen the state of relaxation, and in both techniques suggestions for positive growth, change, or improvement are often made. Because of the close association between these two processes, selected studies on hypnosis are discussed in this chapter.

SCIENTIFIC BASIS

Imagery can be understood as an activity that generates physiologic and somatic responses. It is based on the cognitive process known as mental imagery, which is a central element of cognition that operates when mental representations are created in the absence of sensory input. Functional magnetic resonance imaging (fMRI) has demonstrated that the mental construction of an image activates the same neural pathways and central nervous system structures that are engaged when an individual is actually using one or more of the senses (Djordjevic, Zatorre, Petrides,

Boyle, & Jones-Gotaman, 2005; Formisano et al., 2002; Gulyas, 2001; Kosslyn, Ganis, & Thompson, 2001; Kraemer, Macrae, Green, & Kelley, 2005). For example, if an individual is imagining hearing a sound, the brain structures associated with hearing will become activated. Mental rehearsal of movements will activate motor areas and can be incorporated into stroke rehabilitation and sports improvement programs (Braun, Beurskens, Borm, Schack, & Wade, 2006; Lacourse, Turner, Randolph-Orr, Schandler, & Cohen, 2004).

Andrasik and Rime (2007) postulated that cognitive tasks, such as mental imagery, can be conceptualized as neuromodulators. Neuromodulation is generally defined as the interaction between the nervous system and electrical or pharmacological agents that block or disrupt the perception of pain. By distraction, imagery alters processing in the central, peripheral, and autonomic nervous systems. The perception of a symptom such as pain or nausea is reduced or eliminated.

A key mechanism by which imagery modifies disease and reduces symptoms is thought to be by reducing the stress response, which is triggered when a situation or event (perceived or real) threatens physical or emotional well-being or when the demands of the situation exceed available resources. It activates complex interactions between the neuroendocrine system and the immune system. Emotional responses to situations trigger the limbic system and signal physiologic changes in the peripheral and autonomic nervous systems, resulting in the characteristic fight-or-flight stress response. Over time, chronic stress results in adrenal and immune suppression and may be most harmful to cellular immune function, impairing the ability to ward off viruses and tumor cells (Pert, Dreher, & Ruff, 1998).

The complexity of the human response to stress is best understood through psychoneuroimmunology (PNI), an interdisciplinary field of study that explains the mechanisms by which the brain and body communicate through cellular interactions. Early work was based on rat-model research by Robert Ader and Nicholas Cohen, which confirmed that the immune system could be conditioned by expectations and beliefs (Ader & Cohen, 1981; Ader, Felten, & Cohen, 1991; Fleshner & Laudenslager, 2004). Subsequent research focused on the mechanisms of brain and body communication through cellular interactions, and identified receptors for neuropeptides, neurohormones, and cytokines that reside on neural and immune cells and induce biochemical changes when activated by neurotransmitters.

A cascade of signaling events in response to perceived or actual stress results in the release of hormones from the hypothalamus, pituitary gland, adrenal medulla, adrenal cortex, and peripheral sympathetic nerve terminals. Psychosocial and physical stressors have the potential to upregulate this hypothalamic–pituitary–adrenal (HPA) axis. Chronic hyperactivation of the HPA axis and sympathetic nervous system with the associated increased levels of cortisol and catecholamines can deregulate immune function, whereas moderate levels of circulating cortisol may enhance immune function (Langley, Fonseca, & Iphofen, 2006). Cytokines are secreted by cells participating in the immune response and act as messengers between the immune system and the brain (McCance & Huether, 2002). They also function as neurotransmitters crossing the blood–brain barrier or affecting sensory neurons. Through these channels, cytokines induce symptoms of fever, increased sensitivity to pain, anorexia, and fatigue, which are adaptive responses that may facilitate recovery and healing (Langley et al., 2006). These interactions between the brain and the immune system are bidirectional and changes in one system will influence the others. The stress response can therefore become a double-edged sword that can either enhance or suppress optimal immunity (Fleshner & Laudenslager, 2004).

Although immune responses to emotional states are extremely complex, in general, acute stress activates cardiac sympathetic activity and increases plasma catecholamines and natural killer (NK) cell activity, whereas chronic stress (or inescapable or unpredictable stress) is associated with suppression of NK cells and interleukin-1-beta and other pro-inflammatory cytokines (Glaser et al., 2001). These effects appear to be mediated by the influence of stress hormones on T helper components (Th1 and Th2) (Segerstrom, 2010). Imagery, by inducing deep relaxation and reprocessing of stressful triggers, interrupts or alters the stress response and supports the immune system. In a review of guided-imagery studies examining immune system function, Trakhtenberg (2008) concluded that there is evidence to support a relationship between the immune system and stress or relaxation.

The degree of response to stress varies according to many factors, including the nature of the stressor, magnitude and duration, and degree of control over the stressor (Costa-Pinto & Palermo-Neto, 2010). Individuals who have great physiological responses to everyday stressors have high stress reactivity and are at greater risk for disease susceptibility, even when coping, performance, and perceived stress are comparable. One of the goals of imagery is to reduce stress reactivity by reframing stressful situations from negative responses of fear and anxiety to positive images of healing and well-being (Kosslyn et al., 2001). Donaldson (2000) proposed that thoughts produce physiological responses and activate appropriate neurons. Using imagery to increase emotional awareness and restructure the meaning of a remembered situation by changing negative responses to positive images and meaning alters the physiological response and improves outcomes.

INTERVENTION

Techniques and Guidelines

Imagery has been used extensively in children, adolescents, and adults. Children as young as 4 years old, who have language skills adequate to understand the suggestions, can benefit from imagery (Kohen & Olness, 2011). Young children often are better at imagery because of the natural, active use of their imaginations. Imagery may be practiced independently, with a coach or teacher, or with a videotape or audiotape. The most effective imagery intervention is one that is specific to individuals' personalities, their preferences for relaxation and specific settings, their age or developmental stage, and the desired outcomes. The steps of a general imagery session are outlined in Exhibit 6.1.

Imagery sessions for adults and adolescents are usually 10 to 30 minutes in length, whereas most children tolerate 5 to 15 minutes. The session typically begins with a relaxation exercise that enables the participant to focus or "center." A technique that works well both for children and for adults is to engage in slow and expansive breathing, which facilitates relaxation as the breath moves lower into the chest and the diaphragm, while the abdominal muscles begin to be used more than the upper chest muscles. Other techniques include progressive muscle relaxation or focusing on a word or object. Some children may use their bodies to demonstrate or respond to their image. Although most participants close their eyes, some, especially young children, will prefer to have eyes open.

Once the participant is in a relaxed or in an "altered" state, the practitioner suggests an image of a relaxing, peaceful, or comforting place or introduces an image suggested by the client. Scenes commonly used to induce relaxation include watching a sunset or clouds, sitting on a warm beach or by a fire, or floating through water or space. Some participants, particularly young children, may prefer active images that involve motion, such as flying or playing a sport. The scene used is one that the client finds relaxing or engaging. It is often introduced as a favorite place. Huth, VanKuiken, and Broome (2006) interviewed children who were participants in a guided-imagery research study, to determine the content of their imagery. The children reported their favorite images as the park, swimming at a beach, amusement parks, and vacationing. They also visualized a variety of familiar places, such as sports events and places that included pets and other animals.

Although mental relaxation is often accompanied by muscle relaxation, this is not always a goal. Participants of any age, but particularly preschool and school-age children, may imagine in an active state. For example, a group of 9- to 12-year-old boys with sickle cell disease were being taught guided imagery as a pain-control technique. When asked

Exhibit 6.1. *General Guided Imagery Technique*

1. Achieving a relaxed state
   A. Find a comfortable sitting or reclining position (not lying down).
   B. Uncross any extremities.
   C. Close your eyes or focus on one spot or object in the room.
   D. Focus on breathing with abdominal muscles—being aware of the breath as it enters through your nose and leaves through your mouth. With your next breath let the exhalation be longer and notice how the inhalation that follows is deeper. And as you notice that, let your body become even more relaxed. Continue to breathe deeply, gradually letting the exhalation become twice as long as the inhalation.
   E. Bring your mind back to thinking of your breathing and your relaxed body if your thoughts roam.

2. Specific suggestions for imagery
   A. Picture a place you enjoy and where you feel good.
   B. Notice what you see—hear—taste—smell—and feel.
   C. Let yourself enjoy being in this place.
   D. Imagine yourself the way you want to be—(describe the desired goal specifically).
   E. Imagine what steps you will need to take to be the way you want to be.
   F. Practice these steps now—in this place where you feel good.
   G. What is the first thing you are doing to help you be the way you want to be?
   H. What will you do next?
   I. When you reach your goal of the way you want to be—notice how you feel.

3. Summarize process and reinforce practice
   A. Remember that you can return to this place, this feeling, and this way of being anytime you want.
   B. You can feel this way again by focusing on your breathing, relaxing, and imagining yourself in your special place.
   C. Come back to this place and envision yourself the way you want to be every day.

4. Return to present
   A. Be aware again of the favorite place.
   B. Bring your focus back to your breathing.
   C. Become aware of the room you are in (drawing attention to the temperature, sounds, or lights).
   D. You will feel relaxed and refreshed and be ready to resume your activities.
   E. You may open your eyes when you are ready.

what special place they would like to go to, they requested a trip to a local amusement park and a ride on the roller coaster. During the imagery, many of them were physically and vocally active, swaying from side to side and moving their arms up and down. At the end of the visualization they all reported feeling like they had been in the park (absorption) and gave examples of things they felt, saw, heard, or smelled.

For directed imagery, the practitioner guides the imagery, using positive suggestions to alleviate specific symptoms or conditions (outcome or end-state imagery) or to rehearse or walk through an event (process imagery). Images do not need to be anatomically correct or vivid. Symbolic images may be the most powerful healing images because they are drawn from individual beliefs, culture, and meaning. A cancer patient might imagine sweeping cancer cells away or an asthma patient might picture the lungs as an expanding tree.

The ability to use guided imagery is related to the individual's hypnotic ability or the ability to enter an altered state of consciousness and to become involved or absorbed in the imagery (Kwekkeboom, Wanta, & Bumpus, 2008). Studies have demonstrated that responsiveness to hypnosis increases through early childhood, peaking somewhere between ages 7 and 14 and then leveling off into adolescence and adulthood. However, clinicians have argued that in clinical settings, in which techniques are adjusted to the child's development, preschool children and younger can be quite responsive to hypnosis (Kohen & Olness, 2011).

Some individuals have naturally high hypnotic abilities: they recall pictures more accurately, generate more complex images, have higher dream-recall frequency in the waking state, and make fewer eye movements in imagery than poor visualizers. However, most individuals can use imagery if the experience is adjusted to their needs and preferences (Carli, Cavallaro, & Santarcangelo, 2007; Olness, 2008). Recognizing individual, cultural, and developmental preferences for settings, situations, and preference for either relaxation or stimulation can improve the effectiveness of the imagery and reduce time and frustration with learning it. Practicing imagery oneself is extremely helpful in guiding others.

Measurement of Outcomes

Evaluating and measuring outcomes are important in determining the effectiveness and value of imagery in clinical practice. The clinical outcomes of imagery are related to the context in which it is used and include: physical signs of relaxation; lower levels of anxiety and depression; alteration in symptoms; improved functional performance or quality of life; a sense of meaning, purpose, and/or competency; and positive changes in attitude or behavior. Health services benefits may include reduced costs, morbidity, and reduced length of stay.

The outcomes measured should reflect the client's situation and the conceptual framework providing the rationale for the use of imagery. If imagery is used to facilitate rehabilitation or performance, outcomes would include functional measures such as improved gait or ability to perform a specific task. If imagery is used to control symptoms in clients undergoing chemotherapy for cancer, expected outcomes might include reduced nausea, vomiting, and fatigue; enhanced body image; positive mood states; and improved quality of life. When imagery is used to reduce the stress response and promote relaxation, outcomes may include increased oxygen saturation levels, lower blood pressure and heart rate, warmer extremities, reduced muscle tension, greater alpha waves on electroencephalography, and lower anxiety.

Factors that may influence imagery's success include dose, client characteristics, and condition being treated. Great variability exists in how frequently imagery is recommended. In an attempt to quantify this effect, Van Kuiken (2004) conducted a meta-analysis of 16 published studies going back to 1996. Although the final sample of 10 studies was too small for statistical analysis, Van Kuiken concluded that imagery practice up to 18 weeks increases the effectiveness of the intervention. A minimum dose was not determined and further study is needed to explore a dose relationship with outcomes. To help with standardization of imagery interventions and generalizability, other documentation should include a detailed description of the specific interventions used, outcomes affected by the imagery, and factors influencing effectiveness.

Individual differences such as imaging ability, outcome expectancy, preferred coping style, relationship with the imagery practitioner, and disease state may all affect the outcome of an imagery experience. In a crossover-design pilot study comparing progressive muscle relaxation therapy (PMRT) and imagery to a control, the combined intervention groups demonstrated improved pain control (Kweekeboom et al., 2008). However, the individual responder analysis revealed that subjects did not respond equally to each therapy and only one half of the participants had reduced pain from each intervention. Imagery sessions were more likely to have positive results when participants had greater imaging ability, positive outcome expectancy, and fewer symptoms. A study of 323 adult medical patients who received six interactive guided-imagery sessions with a focus on gaining insight and self-awareness demonstrated that participants' ability to engage in the guided-imagery process and the relationship with the practitioner were strong influences on outcome (Scherwitz, McHenry, & Herrero, 2005).

One of the most difficult determinations to make is whether the outcomes are the result solely of imagery or of a combination of factors. Learning and practicing imagery often change other health-related behaviors, such as getting more sleep, eating a healthier diet, smoking cessation, or exercising regularly. The therapist's presence, attention, and compassion also may constitute an intervention independent of the imagery process.

Precautions

Imagery is generally a safe intervention, as noted in a systematic review of guided imagery for cancer, in which there were no reports of adverse events or side effects (Roffe, Schmidt, & Ernst, 2005). However, occasionally a participant will react negatively to relaxation or to the imagery. Subjects may experience anxiety, particularly when using imagery to reduce stress. Huth, Broome, and Good (2004) reported that two children became distressed during guided-imagery practice sessions; hence, the authors encourage prescreening. Some individuals have anecdotally reported increased discomfort, airway constriction, or difficulty breathing when they focus on diaphragmatic breathing. This is most likely to occur if the participant is experiencing a symptom such as abdominal pain or dyspnea. Using another centering method, such as focusing on an object in the room or repeating a mantra, can reduce this distressing response and still induce relaxation. Some participants may report feeling out of control or "spacey" when deeply relaxed. The guide can help participants to become more grounded by focusing on an image such as a tree with strong roots or do more alert relaxation such as having eyes open and focusing on an object. Participants may report dizziness that is often related to mild hyperventilation and can be relieved by encouraging them to breathe slower and less deeply.

The expertise and training of the nurse should guide judgment in using imagery to achieve outcomes in practice. Imagery techniques can be easily applied to managing symptoms (pain, nausea, vomiting) and facilitating relaxation, sleep, or anxiety reduction. Advanced techniques often associated with hypnosis—such as age regression and management of depression, anxiety, or posttraumatic stress disorder—require further training.

USES

Imagery has been used therapeutically in a variety of conditions and populations (Exhibit 6.2). Pain and cancer are two conditions in which imagery has been helpful both in adults and in children.

Pain

Pain is a uniquely subjective experience, and proper management depends on individualizing interventions that recognize determinants affecting the pain response. Age, temperament, gender, ethnicity, and stage of

Exhibit 6.2. *Conditions for Which Imagery Has Been Tested*

Clinical Condition	Selected Sources
In children and adolescents	
Abdominal pain	Anbar (2001a); Ball, Sharpiro, Monheim, and Weydert (2003); Cotton et al. (2010); Galili, Shaoul, and Mogilner (2009); Gottsegen (2011); Vlieger, Blink, Tromp, and Benninga (2008); Weydert et al. (2006); Youssef et al. (2004)
Asthma	Hackman, Stern, and Gershwin (2000)
Cancer	Richardson, Smith, McCall, and Pilkington (2006)
Chronic dyspnea	Anbar (2001b)
Habit cough	Anbar and Hall (2004)
Headache	Fichtel and Larsson (2004)
Hospice care	Russell, Smart, and House (2007)
Pain	Baumann (2002); Culbert, Friedrichsdorf, and Kuttner (2008); Kline et al. (2010); Wood and Bioy (2008)
Periopertive symptom management (pain, nausea, anxiety, behavioral disorders)	Calipel, Lucas-Polomeni, Wodey, and Ecoffey (2005); Huth et al. (2004); Kuttner (2012); Mackenzie and Frawley (2007); Polkki, Pietila, Vehvilainen-Julkunen, Laukkala, and Kiviluoma (2008)
Post-traumatic stress disorder	Gordon, Staples, Blyta, Bytyqi, and Wilson (2008)
Procedural pain	Alexander (2012); Butler, Symons, Henderson, Shortliffe, and Spiegel (2005); Cyna, Tomkins, Maddock, and Barker (2007); Uman, Chambers, McGrath, and Kisely (2008)
Psychiatry	Anbar (2008)
Sickle cell anemia	Gil et al. (2001)
In adults	
Asthma	Epstein et al. (2004)
Autoimmune disorders	Collins and Dunn (2005); Torem (2007)
Cancer treatment—physical and emotional side effects	Leon-Pizarro et al. (2007); Roffe et al. (2005); Sloman (2002); Yoo, Ahn, Kim, Kim, and Han (2005)
Chronic obstructive pulmonary disease	Louie (2004)

(continued)

Exhibit 6.2. *Conditions for Which Imagery Has Been Tested (continued)*

Clinical Condition	Selected Sources
Counseling	Heinschel (2002)
Depression	Chou and Lin (2006)
Fibromyalgia	Creamer, Singh, Hochberg, and Berman (2000); Menzies and Kim (2008); Menzies, Taylor, and Bourguignon (2006)
Health and well-being	Watanabe, Fukuda, Hara, Maeda, and Ohira (2006); Watanabe, Fukuda, and Shirakawa (2005)
Immune response in breast cancer	Lengacher et al. (2008); Nunes et al. (2007)
Medical conditions (general)	Scherwitz et al. (2005); Toth et al. (2007)
Osteoarthritis	Baird and Sands (2004, 2006)
Pain—cancer	Kwekkeboom et al. (2008); Kwekkeboom, Hau, Wanta, and Bumpus (2008); Kwekkeboom, Kneip, and Pearson (2003)
Pain—chronic	Carrico, Peters, and Diokno (2008); Lewandowski, Good, and Draucker (2005); Proctor, Murphy, Pattison, Suckling, and Farquhar (2008); Turk, Swanson, and Tunks (2008)
Pain—phantom limb	Beaumont, Mercier, Michon, Malouin, and Jackson (2011); MacIver, Lloyd, Kelly, Roberts, and Nurmikko (2008); Oakley, Whitman, and Halligan (2002)
Pain—postoperative	Antall and Kresevic (2004); Haase, Schwenk, Hermann, and Muller (2005)
Pain—procedural	Flory, Salazar, and Lang (2007)
Pregnancy	DiPietro, Costigan, Nelson, Gurewitsch, and Laudenslager (2008)
Rehabilitation	Braun et al. (2006); Braun, Wade, and Beurskens (2011); Dunsky, Dickstein, Marcovitz, Levy, and Deutsch (2008); Hovington and Brouwer (2010); Kim, Oh, Kim, and Choi (2011)
Sleep	Krakow and Zadra (2006); Richardson (2003)
Smoking cessation	Wynd (2005)
Sports medicine	Driediger, Hall, and Callow (2006); Newmark and Bogacki (2005)

development are all considerations when developing a pain-management plan (Gerik, 2005; Young, 2005). Whether pain is from illness, side effects of treatment, injury, or physical stress on the body, emotional factors contribute to pain perception, and mind–body interventions such as imagery can help make pain more manageable (Reed, 2007). Stress, anxiety, and fatigue decrease the threshold for pain, making the perceived pain more intense. Imagery can break this cycle of pain–tension–anxiety–pain. Relaxation with imagery decreases pain directly by reducing muscle tension and related spasms and indirectly by lowering anxiety and improving sleep. Imagery also is a distraction strategy; vivid, detailed images using all senses tend to work best for pain control. In addition, cognitive reappraisal/restructuring used with imagery can increase a sense of control over the ability to reframe the meaning of pain.

There is a considerable body of research examining the efficacy of guided imagery as a therapy to treat adult pain. Studies have explored the effectiveness of guided imagery in treating cancer pain (Kwekkeboom et al., 2008), dysmenorrhea (Proctor et al., 2008), orthopedic pain (Antall & Kresevic, 2004), interstitial cystitis (Carrico et al., 2008), and fibromyalgia (Menzies et al., 2006; Menzies & Kim, 2008); among others. Results have been variable but favorable enough to indicate that guided imagery might help to relieve some forms of pain, especially when used as an adjunct to standard care measures. Although Haase et al. (2005) found no change in report of pain or analgesic use in a population of colorectal surgery patients, they noted that patients responded positively to guided imagery—79% perceiving a benefit from listening to tapes of either guided imagery or relaxation.

There are many causes of chronic pain, but, whatever the underlying etiology, it is generally challenging and costly to treat and has an impact on many aspects of an individual's life. Analgesic therapy often falls short of achieving adequate pain relief, and successful management frequently depends on the use of cognitive–behavioral techniques such as imagery (Turk et al., 2008). Two conditions leading to chronic pain in adults are osteoarthritis and fibromyalgia. In a randomized trial of 28 women with osteoarthritis, participants received either standard care or a 12-week program of guided imagery with relaxation (Baird & Sands, 2006). Participants in the intervention group improved in scores of health-related quality of life. Analysis noted that improvement in scores was not completely explained by improved mobility and pain reduction, and that the guided-imagery and relaxation intervention might have had a positive effect on social and emotional functioning.

Fibromyalgia is a condition of chronic widespread pain accompanied by fatigue, disturbed sleep, stiffness, and depression (Menzies & Kim, 2008). In a feasibility study, 20 subjects were enrolled in an 8-week group intervention (Creamer et al., 2000). Each session included education (30 min), relaxation and meditation (1 hr), and Chinese movement therapy—Qigong (1 hr). Significant improvement was seen in a number of indicators, including difficulty in sleeping, fatigue, social functioning, and pain. However, given the small sample, lack of control, and multimodal approach, it is difficult to determine the specific effect of the imagery. Menzies and colleagues investigated the effect of guided imagery on fibromyalgia in a randomized, control trial of 48 subjects (Menzies et al., 2006). Subjects in the intervention group received guided-imagery audiotapes and were instructed to use them daily. The control group received usual care. There was improvement in functional status and self-efficacy in the experimental group, but no change in report of pain. Subsequently a small (10-subject) pilot study of Hispanic adults was conducted to assess a 10-week course of imagery with relaxation (Menzies & Kim, 2008). Improvement was seen in daily pain, functional status, and self-efficacy measures; however, no improvement was seen in psychological distress and other pain measures. This study has limited generalizability due to its small sample size, lack of control, and use of self-report measures.

In spite of the many advances made in the treatment of pediatric pain, the American Academy of Pediatrics and the American Pain Society (2001) reported that children's pain continues to be inadequately assessed and managed. They recommended a multimodal approach to pain management to include both pharmacological and nonpharmacological interventions. There are adverse short-term and long-term effects of inadequate pain management in children, including hypoxemia, immobility, altered pulmonary function, posttraumatic stress, and adverse psychological and behavioral patterns (Grunau, Oberlander, & Whitfield, 2001). Distraction imagery is particularly helpful in getting a child through a medical procedure with a safe and effective level of sedation/analgesia and as little movement as possible (Butler et al., 2005). Suggestions to breathe deeply and to relax or be comfortable are combined with vivid images of a favorite place or pleasant experience that draw the attention away from the pain. It is best to introduce the child to breathing techniques and explore favorite images prior to the procedure. However, in critical or emergency situations imagery has been successfully employed without prework (Kohen, 2000). In a randomized study of 44 children from 4 to 15 years of age undergoing voiding cystourethrography, children who were taught self-hypnotic visual imagery before the procedure were compared with controls that received routine care. Results indicated benefits for the intervention group in the form of parental perception of decreased trauma, decreased observational ratings of distress, increased ease of procedure by physician report, and decreased time to complete the procedure (Butler et al., 2005). In a systemic review of controlled trials of interventions for needle-related procedural pain and distress distraction, combined cognitive–behavioral interventions and hypnosis showed the most promise (Uman et al., 2008).

Chronic abdominal pain in childhood can be challenging to treat and has significant impact on the child's quality of life and engagement in school and social activities. The efficacy of imagery and relaxation on abdominal pain was assessed in two studies. Youssef et al. (2004) reported significant improvement over baseline, with overall improvement of pain, fewer pain episodes, decreased intensity, fewer missed school days per month, and improved quality-of-life scores; however, sample size was small and there was no control group. Weydert et al. (2006), in a randomized trial, compared guided imagery to control group that was taught breathing exercises. The imagery group had significantly fewer days with pain at 1 and 2 months. In addition, children in the imagery group had less than four pain episodes a month and did not miss any activities because of pain. Both of these studies reported no adverse effects.

Huth et al. (2004) examined the use of guided imagery as an adjunct to routine analgesics for postoperative tonsillectomy and/or adenoidectomy pain. Significantly less pain was found in the treatment group 1 to 4 hours after surgery, but not at 22 to 24 hours after surgery. Children in the imagery group had 28% less sensory pain, 10% less anxiety, and 8% less affective pain than the children in the control group. A correlation between state of anxiety and sensory pain was high at both points and there were no differences in analgesic use between groups. The researchers reported two adverse events in which children became distressed during the practice sessions.

Cancer Treatment

Imagery interventions in oncology have focused on physiological and psychological responses to cancer treatment. Areas that have been researched are: efficacy in management of symptoms (pain, nausea), influence on surgical outcomes, improvement in quality of life, and changes in immunity (Roffe et al., 2005). Roffe and colleagues, in a systematic literature search that spanned 3 decades, uncovered 103 articles investigating guided imagery in cancer care. Of these, 27 were case studies, 56 combined imagery with another treatment (e.g., PMRT, music therapy, hypnosis), 12 were uncontrolled trials, and two were nonrandomized. The authors reviewed in detail six randomized control trials. The collective data suggested that guided imagery is most beneficial on psychosocial and quality-of-life indicators. No effects were found on physical symptoms, which may be partially explained by a paucity of distressing symptoms in the subjects. When guided imagery was compared with other relaxation strategies, all study arms did better than the control, indicating that other relaxation strategies are also beneficial or that there is significant overlap among strategies.

In clinical cancer care, relaxation strategies such as PMRT are often paired with imagery. This combination was investigated in a randomized controlled trial of 60 women undergoing chemotherapy treatment for breast cancer (Yoo et al., 2005). Guided imagery was paired with PMRT to determine their effect on nausea, vomiting, and quality of life. Thirty patients received PMRT and guided imagery 1 hour before treatment for six chemotherapy cycles, and were given a tape to use at home. The 30 patients in the control group received standard therapy. Both groups received an antiemetic half an hour before chemotherapy administration. Patients in the intervention group demonstrated improvement in anticipatory nausea, postchemotherapy nausea, and quality of life. Positive treatment effects on quality of life were present at 3 months and 6 months posttherapy. Similarly, Leon-Pizarro et al. (2007) conducted a randomized controlled trial of 66 gynecologic and breast cancer patients who were undergoing brachytherapy (placement of a radioactive source near or within the tumor source). The intervention group had a 10-minute training period in relaxation and guided imagery and an individualized cassette for home use; the control group received standard care. The treatment group had statistically significant reductions in anxiety, depression, and body discomfort.

Guided imagery is a recognized intervention for women receiving treatment for breast cancer. Serra et al. (2012) studied the effect of a guided-imagery intervention during radiation therapy. A convenience sample of 61 women received a guided-imagery session in the radiation oncology setting immediately before their radiation treatment. Physiological and psychological measurements were evaluated. There was a statistically significant improvement in pulse rate, respiratory rate, and blood pressure between sessions one and two. There was also a rise in skin temperature, indicating increased peripheral blood flow and decreased sympathetic response. The guided-imagery intervention was determined to be helpful by 86% of the participants.

In pediatric oncology, the focus of research has largely been on procedural pain and on the use of hypnosis. A review of seven randomized controlled trials and one nonrandomized controlled clinical trial (Richardson et al., 2006) reported reductions in pain and anxiety for hypnosis in pediatric oncology patients undergoing procedures (bone marrow aspiration, lumbar puncture, venipuncture). Both this review and a previous one (Wild & Espie, 2004) cited methodological limitations, including: small, underpowered samples; lack of reporting on the method of randomization; concealment of allocation and/or blinding; lack of information on standard care; and wide variation in procedures used.

The role of imagery in improving cancer outcomes has been studied for more than 2 decades. It continues to be difficult to identify the significance of imagery in long-term survival when so many related factors must be considered in cancer survival. Sahler, Hunter, and Liesveld (2003) showed reduced time to engraftment in 23 patients undergoing bone marrow transplant. A common explanation for how imagery may improve cancer outcomes is postulated through increasing cellular immune function. Some studies have demonstrated increases in natural killer cytotoxicity (Gruzelier, 2002; Lengacher et al., 2008) and NK cell numbers (Bakke, Purtzer, & Newton, 2002), whereas others have found no differences in NK numbers and cytotoxicity (Nunes et al., 2007). Despite inconclusive effects on cancer outcome, imagery interventions have consistently improved coping responses and psychological states in patients with cancer, suggesting that imagery may mediate psychoneuroimmunology outcomes in breast and other cancers (Walker, 2004). Further study is needed to determine the clinical significance of immunological effects.

Guided imagery has been identified on the Internet as one of the 10 most frequently recommended integrative therapies for cancer (Schmidt & Ernst, 2004). The low methodological quality of the studies suggests that rigorous research in imagery for cancer is not as prevalent as actual use in clinical practice.

CULTURAL APPLICATIONS

Modern-day imagery owes it roots to the use of imagery in traditional healing. Achtenberg (1985) described imaging as "the world's oldest and greatest healing resource" (p. 3), and noted that the use of imagery is foundational to the shamanic healing found in many healing traditions. Shamanic healing is a centuries-old practice in which imagery is used within an ecstatic or altered state to access the patient's subconscious mind and belief system (Reed, 2007). This opens communication among mind, body, and spirit in order to cure, alleviate suffering, and facilitate spiritual transformation. Epstein (2004) noted that in spiritual life, experiences are images reflecting us back to ourselves.

The interest in imagery as part of a therapeutic treatment plan is found globally. In addition to the many studies from the United States, research on the use and effectiveness of imagery is prevalent in many other countries: Canada (Beaumont et al., 2011; Kuttner, 2012), Spain (Leon-Pizarro et al., 2007), Brazil (Nunes et al., 2007), Korea (Kim et al., 2011; Yoo et al., 2005), and Japan (Watanabe et al., 2005, 2006). A comparison of the use of imagery versus mindful attention with children in Thailand is described in Sidebar 6.1.

Cultures are broadly categorized as tending toward either individualism or collectivism. La Roche, Batista, and D'Angelo (2010) investigated guided-imagery scripts to determine their level of idiocentrism versus allocentrism. Idiocentrism is the tendency to define oneself in isolation from others and would be found in individualistic societies; allocentrism is the tendency to define oneself in relation to others and would be seen in cultures valuing collectivism. The authors reviewed 123 guided-imagery scripts and found that they tended to be more idiocentric.

The practitioner should be aware that when directing a guided-imagery experience it is always important to consider individual preferences and use images that are understandable and acceptable to the participant. As a rule, the most powerful and meaningful image is one that the participant creates rather than one that is supplied by the guide. Participants will be more likely to choose images that are congruent with their cultural, spiritual, and personal beliefs. The guide or therapist is there to help them use those images.

Sidebar 6.1. *Comparison of the Use of Guided Imagery Versus Mindful Attention With Thai Children With Cancer*

Kesanee Boonyawatanangkool, Khon Kaen University, Thailand

In Thailand, as elsewhere, children with a life-threatening illness such as cancer experience multiple types of distress. These can range from disease symptoms and procedures and treatments to the psychological discomfort of living with a potentially terminal illness. Indeed, there are numerous challenges inherent to the provision of holistic nursing care to these Thai children throughout their illness trajectory. Guided imagery is an independent nursing intervention that uses psychoneuroimmunology principles to help manage distress symptoms such as pain, anxiety, and fear by directing attention away from difficult events. Conversely, mindfulness involves devoting attention to one's experience in an accepting and nonjudgmental way; however, the effect of this instruction on distress symptoms—including pain and other outcomes—is unknown.

The objective we addressed in our clinical work was to examine whether mindful attention could help children focus on pain, anxiety, or fear without increasing their distress symptoms or decreasing their symptom tolerance. In this clinical evaluation, we compared the effects of mindful attention to a well-established intervention for reduction of difficult symptoms (i.e., guided imagery/self-hypnosis)—an intervention that is designed to take attention away from uncomfortable events.

To implement this comparison, anxiety and fear were monitored in children (n = 58), 5 to 18 years of age who were hospitalized and receiving chemotherapy. Each child attended and completed a session of guided imagery. Participants then received either mindful attention or guided-imagery instructions designed to direct attention to focus on or away from their pain, anxiety, and fear, respectively.

Our clinical evaluation revealed that children who received the mindful attention instructions demonstrated more awareness of the physical sensations of pain, anxiety, and fear—including thoughts about those sensations—without decreasing tolerance levels. Some of them said, "I am now feeling better; can you help me do this again please?" (e.g., a 14-year-old boy with palliation of rhabdomyosarcoma pain). There were no interactions observed between baseline characteristics of the children and the specific intervention used to address their symptoms.

From the findings of our clinical observations, we concluded that mindful (trance) attention—compared to guided imagery—was successful in helping the children to focus attention on experiences of pain, anxiety, and fear without increased pain intensity or decreased symptom tolerance.

(continued)

Sidebar 6.1. *Comparison of the Use of Guided Imagery Versus Mindful Attention With Thai Children With Cancer (continued)*

These conclusions were based solely on the clinical experience in my practice setting in Thailand. Factors that we know to be important to the implementation of either intervention with children include: the children's knowledge, their developmental stage, trust and rapport, gender and age, pain and other uncomfortable experiences, coping strategies, disease status, religious and cultural beliefs, and family background. Both interventions appeared to be beneficial in reducing distress in children and included shared strategies such as eye-fixation techniques, taking deep breaths, and progressive muscle relaxation through guided instruction.

FUTURE RESEARCH

Despite documented relationships between the mind and the body, there continues to be a lack of high-quality intervention trials testing the effectiveness of guided imagery and other mind–body interventions. Although the body of evidence is growing, with many reports of clinical efficacy, more scientifically rigorous research testing outcomes are needed. For example, Richardson et al. (2006) concluded that there is sufficient evidence for the efficacy of hypnosis to manage procedural pain in pediatric oncology, but noted a number of methodological limitations. Small sample sizes, lack of standardized control groups, and inadequate reporting of research methods limit the generalizability of the findings of many imagery studies.

Key questions remain to be answered regarding specific physiological responses to imagery, the influence of imagery on clinical outcomes and quality of life, and the effect of individual factors. As a low-cost, noninvasive intervention, imagery has the potential to be effective in reducing symptoms and distress across several conditions. Questions to be pursued include:

- What is the role of imagery in maintaining health and wellness? Should imagery be a component of preventive medicine? Over time, can imagery reduce stress, improve coping, enhance well-being, create healthier lifestyles, and reduce illness in individuals?
- What is the effect of imagery on clinical outcomes relevant to quality-of-life and health/illness states and does it have an impact on cost-effectiveness and quality of care?
- What is the relationship between imagery and other relaxation strategies? Are they more effective when paired or should they be used alone?

- Does the type of imagery (outcome or process) produce different outcomes? What imagery protocols or processes are most appropriate in specific conditions (use of tape recorder or session with a practitioner; duration and number of sessions)?
- Is it possible to predict the usefulness of an imagery intervention in specific individuals? Are there certain characteristics of individuals that determine their ability to respond to imagery and produce desired outcomes? Are there certain individuals or conditions for which imagery should not be recommended?
- What are the long-term effects of imagery?
- What is the role of practitioner characteristics (type of training, practitioner style, number of different practitioners) in outcomes?

ACKNOWLEDGMENT

The authors would like to acknowledge Janice Post-White, PhD, RN, for her past work on this chapter.

WEBSITES

The following websites contain additional information on guided imagery:

Academy for Guided Imagery (2012). Workshops and resources.
(www.acadgi.com)

American Holistic Nurses Association (2012)
(www.ahna.org)

American Society of Clinical Hypnosis (2012). Certification, workshops, and resources.
(www.asch.net)

Association for Music and Imagery (2012). Bonny method of guided imagery and music therapy.
(www.ami-bonnymethod.org)

Imagery International (2012)
(www.imageryinternational.org)

National Center for Complementary and Alternative Medicine (2012). Overview of mind–body medicine and information on relaxation techniques.
(nccam.nih.gov)

National Pediatric Hypnosis Training Institute (2012). Training in pediatric hypnosis. (www.nphti.net)

REFERENCES

Achtenberg, J. (1985). *Imagery in healing: Shamanism and modern medicine.* Boston, MA: Shambhala.

Ader, R., & Cohen, N. (1981). Conditioned immunopharmacologic responses. In R. Ader (Ed.), *Psychoneuroimmunology* (pp. 281–319). New York, NY: Academic Press.

Ader, R., Felten, D. L., & Cohen, N. (1991). *Psychoneuroimmunology* (2nd ed.). San Diego, CA: Academic Press.

Alexander, M. (2012). Managing patient stress in pediatric radiology. *Radiologic Technology, 83*(6), 549–560.

American Academy of Pediatrics Committee on Psychosocial Aspects of Children and Family Health and American Pain Society Task Force on Pain in Infants, Children and Adolescents. (2001). The assessment and management of acute pain in infants, children and adolescents. *Pediatrics, 10*(8), 793–797.

Anbar, R. D. (2001a). Self-hypnosis for the treatment of functional abdominal pain in childhood. *Clinical Pediatrics, 40*(8), 447–451.

Anbar, R. D. (2001b). Self-hypnosis for management of chronic dyspnea in pediatric patients [Electronic version]. *Pediatrics, 107*(2):e21.

Anbar, R. D. (2008). Subconscious guided therapy with hypnosis. *American Journal of Clinical Hypnosis, 50*(4), 323–334.

Anbar, R. D., & Hall, H. R. (2004). Childhood habit cough treated with self-hypnosis. *Journal of Pediatrics, 144,* 213–217.

Andrasik, F., & Rime, C. (2007). Can behavioural therapy influence neuroma dulation? *Neurological Sciences, 28* (Suppl. 2), S124–S129.

Antall, G. F., & Kresevic, D. (2004). The use of guided imagery to manage pain in an elderly orthopaedic population. *Orthopedic Nursing, 23*(5), 335–340.

Baird, C. L., & Sands, L. (2004). A pilot study of the effectiveness of guided imagery with progressive muscle relaxation to reduce chronic pain and mobility difficulties of osteoarthritis. *Pain Management Nursing, 5*(3), 97–104.

Baird, C. L., & Sands, L. (2006). Effect of guided imagery with relaxation on health-related quality of life in older women with osteoarthritis. *Research in Nursing and Health, 29,* 442–451.

Bakke, A. C., Purtzer, M. Z., & Newton, P. (2002). The effect of hypnotic-guided imagery on psychological well-being and immune function in patients with prior breast cancer. *Journal of Psychosomatic Research, 53*(6), 1131–1137.

Ball, T. M., Shapiro, D. E., Monheim, C. J., & Weydert, J. A. (2003). A pilot study of the use of guided imagery for the treatment of recurrent abdominal pain in children. *Clinical Pediatrics, 42*(6), 527–532.

Baumann, R. J. (2002). Behavioral treatment of migraine in children and adolescents. *Pediatric Drugs, 4*(9), 555–561.

Beaumont, G., Mercier, C., Michon P. E., Malouin, F., & Jackson, P. L. (2011). Decreasing phantom limb pain through observation of action and imagery: A case series. *Pain Medicine,* 12, 289-299.

Braun, S. M., Beurskens, A. J., Borm, P. J., Schack, T., & Wade, D. T. (2006). The effects of mental practice in stroke rehabilitation: A systematic review. *Archives of Physical Medicine and Rehabilitation,* 87, 842–852.

Braun, S. M, Wade, D. T., & Beurskens, A. J. (2011). Use of movement imagery in neuro-rehabilitation: Researching effects of a complex intervention. *International Journal of Rehabilitation Research, 34,* 203–208.

Butler, L. D., Symons, B. K., Henderson, S. L., Shortliffe, L. D., & Spiegel, D. (2005). Hypnosis reduces distress and duration of an invasive medical procedure for children. *Pediatrics, 115*(1), e77–e85.

Calipel, S., Lucas-Polomeni, M. M., Wodey, E., & Ecoffey, C. (2005). Premedication in children: Hypnosis versus midazolam. *Pediatric Anesthesia, 15,* 275–281.

Carli, G., Cavallaro, F. I., & Santarcangelo, E. L. (2007). Hypnotizability and imagery modality preference: Do highs and lows live in the same world? *Contemporary Hypnosis, 24*(2), 64–75.

Carrico, D. J., Peters, K. M., & Diokno, A. C. (2008). Guided imagery for women with interstitial cystitis: Results of a prospective, randomized controlled pilot study. *Journal of Alternative and Complementary Medicine, 14*(1), 53–60.

Chou, M. H., & Lin, M. F. (2006). Exploring the listening experiences during guided imagery and music therapy of outpatients with depression. *Journal of Nursing Research, 14*(2), 93–102.

Collins, M. P., & Dunn, L. F. (2005). The effects of meditation and visual imagery on an immune system disorder: Dermatomyositis. *Journal of Alternative and Complementary Medicine, 11*(2), 275–284.

Costa-Pinto, F., & Palermo-Neto, J. (2010). Neuroimmune interactions in stress. *NeuroImmunoModulation, 17,* 196–199.

Cotton, S., Roberts, Y. H., Tsevat, J., Britto, M., Succop, P., McGrady, M. E., & Yi, M. S. (2010). Mind-body complementary alternative medicine use and quality of life in adolescents with inflammatory bowel disease. *Inflammatory Bowel Disease, 16*(3), 501–506.

Creamer, P., Singh, B. B., Hochberg, M. C., & Berman, B. M. (2000). Sustained improvement produced by nonpharmacologic intervention in fibromyalgia: Results of a pilot study. *Arthritis Care and Research, 13*(4), 198–204.

Culbert, T., Friedrichsdorf, S., & Kuttner, L. (2008). Mind-body skills for children in pain. In H. Breivik, W. I. Campbell, & M. K. Nicholas (Eds.), *Clinical pain management: Practice and procedures* (2nd ed., pp. 478–495). London, UK: Hodder Arnold.

Cyna, A. M., Tomkins, D., Maddock, T., & Barker, D. (2007). Brief hypnosis of severe needle phobia using switch-wire imagery in a 5-year-old. *Pediatric Anesthesia, 17,* 800–804.

DiPietro, J. A., Costigan, K. A., Nelson, P., Gurewitsch, E. D., & Laudenslager, M. L. (2008). Fetal responses to induced maternal relaxation during pregnancy. *Biological Psychology, 77,* 11–19.

Djordjevic, J., Zatorre, R. J., Petrides, M., Boyle, J. A., & Jones-Gotaman, M. (2005). Functional neuroimaging of odor imagery. *Neuroimage, 24*(3), 791–801.

Donaldson, V. W. (2000). A clinical study of visualization on depressed white blood cells in medical patients. *Applied Psychophysiology and Biofeedback, 25*(2), 230–235.

Driediger, M., Hall, C., & Callow, N. (2006). Imagery use by injured athletes: A qualitative analysis. *Journal of Sports Sciences, 24*(3), 261–271.

Dunsky, A., Dickstein, R., Marcovitz, E., Levy, S., & Deutsch, J. (2008). Home-based motor imagery training for gait rehabilitation of people with chronic poststroke hemiparesis. *Archives in Physical Medicine and Rehabilitation, 89,* 1580–1588.

Epstein, G. (2004). Mental imagery: The language of spirit. *Advances, 20*(3), 4–10.

Epstein, G. N., Halper, J. P., Barrett, E. A., Birdsal, C., McGee, M., Baron, K. P., . . . Lowenstein, S. (2004). A pilot study of mind–body changes in adults with asthma who practice mental imagery. *Alternative Therapies, 10*(4), 66–71.

Fichtel, A., & Larsson, B. (2004). Relaxation treatment administered by school nurses to adolescents with recurrent headaches. *Headache, 44*, 545–554.

Fleshner, M., & Laudenslager, M. L. (2004). Psychoneuroimmunology: Then and now. *Behavioral and Cognitive Neuroscience Reviews, 3* (2), 114–130.

Flory, N., Salazar, G. M. M., & Lang, E. V. (2007). Hypnosis for acute distress management during medical procedures. *International Journal of Clinical and Experimental Hypnosis, 55*(3), 303–317.

Formisano, E., Linden, D. E. J., DiSalle, F., Trojano, L., Esposito, F., Sack, A. T., . . . Goebel, R. (2002). Tracking the mind's image in the brain: Time-resolved fMRI during visuospatial mental imagery. *Neuron, 35*, 185–194.

Galili, O., Shaoul, R., Mogilner, J. (2009). Treatment of chronic recurrent abdominal pain: Laparoscopy or hypnosis? *Journal of Laparoendoscopic and Advanced Surgical Techniques, 19* (1), 93–96.

Gerik, S. M. (2005). Pain management in children: Developmental considerations and mind–body therapies. *Southern Medical Journal, 98*(3), 295–301.

Gil, K. M., Anthony, K. K., Carson, J. W., Redding-Lallinger, R., Daescher, C. W., & Ware, R. E. (2001). Daily coping practice predicts treatment effects in children with sickle cell disease. *Journal of Pediatric Psychology, 26*(3), 163–173.

Glaser, R., MacCallum, R. C., Laskowski, B. F., Malarkey, W. B., Sheridan, J. F., & Kiecolt-Glaser, J. K. (2001). Evidence for a shift in the Th-1 to Th-2 cytokine response associated with chronic stress and aging. *Journal of Gerontology. A: Biological Science and Medical Science, 56*(8), M477–M482.

Gordon, J. S., Staples, J. K., Blyta, A., Bytyqi, M., & Wilson, A. (2008). Treatment of posttraumatic stress disorder in postwar Kosovar adolescents using mind–body skills groups: A randomized controlled trial. *Journal of Clinical Pyschiatry, 69*(9), 1469–1476.

Gottsegen, D. (2011). Hypnosis for functional abdominal pain. *American Journal of Clinical Hypnosis, 54*, 56–69.

Grunau, R. E., Oberlander, T. F., & Whitfield, M. F. (2001). Demographic and therapeutic determinants of pain reactivity in very low birth weight neonates at 32 weeks postconception age. *Pediatrics, 107*, 105–117.

Gruzelier, J. H. (2002). A review of the impact of hypnosis, relaxation, guided imagery and individual differences on aspects of immunity and health. *Stress, 5*(2), 147–163.

Gulyas, B. (2001). Neural networks for internal reading and visual imagery of reading: A PET study. *Brain Research Bulletin, 54*(3), 319–328.

Haase, O., Schwenk, W., Hermann, C., & Muller, J. M. (2005). Guided imagery and relaxation in conventional colorectal resections: A randomized, controlled, partially blinded trial. *Diseases of the Colon and Rectum, 48*(10), 1955–1963.

Hackman, R. M., Stern, J. S., & Gershwin, M. E. (2000). Hypnosis and asthma: A critical review. *Journal of Asthma, 37*(1), 1–15.

Heinschel, J. A. (2002). A descriptive study of the interactive guided imagery experience. *Journal of Holistic Nursing, 20*, 325–346.

Hovington, C. L., & Brouwer, B. (2010). Guided motor imagery in healthy adults and stroke: Does strategy matter? *Neurorehabilitation and Neural Repair, 24*, 851–856.

Huth, M. M., Broome, M. E., & Good, M. (2004). Imagery reduces children's postoperative pain. *Pain, 110*(1/2), 439–448.

Huth, M. M., VanKuiken, D. M., & Broome, M. E. (2006). Playing in the park: What school age children tell us about imagery. *Journal of Pediatric Nursing, 21*(2), 115–125.

Kim, J. S., Oh, D. W., Kim, S. Y., & Choi, J. D. (2011). Visual and kinesthetic locomotor imagery training integrated with auditory step rhythm for walking performance of patients with chronic stroke. *Clinical Rehabilitation, 25*, 134–145.

Kline, W. H., Turnbull, A., Labruna, V. E., Haufler, L., DeVivio, S., & Ciminera, P. (2010). Enhancing pain management in the PICU by teaching guided mental imagery: A quality-improvement project. *Journal of Pediatric Psychology, 35*(1), 25–31.

Kohen, D. (2000, June). *Integrating hypnosis into practice.* Paper presented at the Introductory Workshop in Clinical Hypnosis. St. Paul, MN: University of Minnesota and the Minnesota Society of Clinical Hypnosis.

Kohen, D., & Olness, K. (2011). *Hypnosis and hypnotherapy with children* (4th ed.). New York, NY: Routledge.

Kosslyn, S. M., Ganis, G., & Thompson, W. (2001). Neural foundations of imagery. *Nature Reviews, 2,* 635–642.

Kraemer, D. J., Macrae, C. N., Green, A. E., & Kelley, W. M. (2005). Musical imagery: Sound of silence activates auditory cortex. *Nature, 434*(7030), 158.

Krakow, B., & Zadra, A. (2006). Clinical management of chronic nightmares: Imagery rehearsal therapy. *Behavioral Sleep Medicine, 4*(1), 45–70.

Kuttner, L. (2012). Pediatric hypnosis: pre-, peri-, and post-anesthesia. *Pediatric Anesthesia, 22,* 573–577.

Kwekkeboom, K., Kneip, J., & Pearson, L. (2003). A pilot study to predict success with guided imagery for cancer pain. *Pain Management Nursing, 4*(3), 112–123.

Kwekkeboom, K. L., Hau, H., Wanta, B., & Bumpus, M. (2008). Patients' perceptions of the effectiveness of guided imagery and progressive muscle relaxation interventions used for cancer pain. *Complementary Therapies in Clinical Practice, 14,* 185–194.

Kwekkeboom, K. L., Wanta, B., & Bumpus, M. (2008). Individual difference variables and the effects of progressive muscle relaxation and analgesic imagery interventions on cancer pain. *Journal of Pain and Symptom Management, 36*(6), 604–615.

Lacourse, M. G., Turner, J. A., Randolph-Orr, E., Schandler, S. L., & Cohen, M. J. (2004). Cerebral and cerebellar sensorimotor plasticity following motor imagery-based mental practice of a sequential movement. *Journal of Rehabilitation Research and Development, 41*(4), 505–524.

Langley, P., Fonseca, J., & Iphofen, R. (2006). Psychoneuroimmunology and health from a nursing perspective. *British Journal of Nursing, 15*(29), 1126–1129.

La Roche, M., Batista, C., & D'Angelo, E. (2010). A content analysis of guided imagery scripts: A strategy for the development of cultural adaptations. *Journal of Clinical Psychology, 67*(1), 45–57.

Lengacher, C. A., Bennett, M. P., Gonzalez, L., Gilvary, D., Cox, C. E., Cantor, A., . . . Djeu, J. (2008). Immune responses to guided imagery during breast cancer treatment. *Biological Research in Nursing, 9*(3), 205–214.

Leon-Pizarro, C., Gich, I., Barthe, E., Rovirosa, A., Farrus, B., Casa, F., . . . Arcusa, A. (2007). A randomized trial of the effect of training in relaxation and guided imagery techniques in improving psychological and quality-of-life indices for gynecologic and breast brachytherapy patients. *Psycho-Oncology, 16,* 971–979.

Lewandowski, W., Good, M., & Draucker, C. B. (2005). Changes in the meaning of pain with the use of guided imagery. *Pain Management Nursing, 6*(2), 58–67.

Louie, S. W. (2004). The effects of guided imagery relaxation in people with COPD. *Occupational Therapy International, 11*(3), 145–159.

MacIver, K., Lloyd, D. M., Kelly, S., Roberts, N., & Nurmikko, T. (2008). Phantom limb pain, cortical reorganization and the therapeutic effect of mental imagery. *Brain, 131,* 2181–2191.

Mackenzie, A., & Frawley, G. P. (2007). Preoperative hypnotherapy in the management of a child with anticipatory nausea and vomiting. *Anesthesia and Intensive Care, 35,* 784–787.

McCance, K. L., & Huether, S. E. (2002). *Pathophysiology: The biologic basis for disease in adults and children* (4th ed.). St. Louis, MO: Mosby.

Menzies, V., & Kim, S. (2008). Relaxation and guided imagery in Hispanic persons diagnosed with fibromyalgia: A pilot study. *Family and Community Health, 31*(3), 204–212.

Menzies, V., Taylor, A. G., & Bourguignon, C. (2006). Effects of guided imagery on outcomes of pain, functional status, and self-efficacy in persons diagnosed with fibromyalgia. *Journal of Alternative and Complementary Medicine, 12*(1), 12–30.

Newmark, T. S., & Bogacki, D. F. (2005). The use of relaxation, hypnosis, and imagery in sport psychiatry. *Clinics in Sports Medicine, 21*, 973–977.

Nunes, D. F. T., Rodriguez, A. L., Hoffman, F. S., Luz, C., Filho, A., Muller, M. C., & Bauer, M. E. (2007). Relaxation and guided imagery program in patients with breast cancer undergoing radiotherapy is not associated with neuroimmunomodulatory effects. *Journal of Psychosomatic Research, 63*, 647–655.

Oakley, D. A., Whitman, L. G., & Halligan, P. W. (2002). Hypnotic imagery as a treatment for phantom limb pain: Two case reports and a review. *Clinical Rehabilitation, 16*, 368–377.

Olness, K. (2008). Helping children and adults with hypnosis and biofeedback. *Cleveland Clinic Journal of Medicine, 75*(Suppl. 2), S39–S43.

Pert, C. B., Dreher, H. E., & Ruff, M. R. (1998). The psychosomatic network: Foundations of mind–body medicine. *Alternative Therapies, 4*(4), 30–41.

Polkki, T., Pietila, A. M., Vehvilainen-Julkunen, K., Laukkala, H., & Kiviluoma, K. (2008). Imagery-induced relaxation in children's postoperative pain relief: A randomized pilot study. *Journal of Pediatric Nursing, 23*(3), 217–224.

Proctor, M. L., Murphy, P. A., Pattison, H. M., Suckling, J., & Farquhar, C. M. (2008). Behavioural interventions for primary and secondary dysmenorrhoea (review). *Cochrane Library, 4*, 1–24.

Reed, T. (2007). Imagery in the clinical setting: A tool for healing. *Nursing Clinics of North America, 42*, 261–277.

Richardson, J., Smith, J. E., McCall, G., & Pilkington, K. (2006). Hypnosis for procedure-related pain and distress in pediatric cancer patients: A systematic review of effectiveness and methodology related to hypnosis interventions. *Journal of Pain and Symptom Management, 31*(1), 70–84.

Richardson, S. (2003). Effects of relaxation and imagery on the sleep of critically ill adults. *Dimensions of Critical Care Nursing, 22*(4), 182–190.

Roffe, L., Schmidt, K., & Ernst, E. (2005). A systematic review of guided imagery as an adjuvant cancer therapy. *Psycho-Oncology, 14*, 607–617.

Russell, C., Smart, S., & House, D. (2007). Guided imagery and distraction therapy in paediatric hospice care. *Paediatric Nursing, 19*(2), 24–25.

Sahler, O. L., Hunter, B. C., & Liesveld, J. L. (2003). The effect of using music therapy with relaxation imagery in the management of patients undergoing bone marrow transplantation: A pilot feasibility study. *Alternative Therapies in Health & Medicine, 9*(6), 70–74.

Scherwitz, L. W., McHenry, P., & Herrero, R. (2005). Interactive guided imagery therapy with medical patients: Predictors of health outcomes. *Journal of Alternative and Complementary Medicine, 11*(1), 69–83.

Schmidt, K., & Ernst, E. (2004). Assessing websites on complementary and alternative medicine for cancer [Electronic version]. *Annals of Oncology, 15*, 733–742.

Segerstrom, S. (2010). Resources, stress, and immunity: An ecological perspective on human psychoneuroimmunology. *Annals of Behavioral Medicine, 40*, 114–125.

Serra, D., Parris, C. R., Carper, E., Homel, P., Fleishman, S. B., Harrison, L. B. & Chadha, M. (2012). Outcomes of guided imagery in patients receiving radiation therapy for breast cancer. *Clinical Journal of Oncology Nursing, 16*(6), 617–623.

Sloman, R. (2002). Relaxation and imagery for anxiety and depression control in community patients with advanced cancer. *Cancer Nursing, 25*(6), 432–435.

Torem, M. S. (2007). Mind-body hypnotic imagery in the treatment of auto-immune disorders. *American Journal of Clinical Hypnosis, 50*(2), 157–170.

Toth, M., Wolsko, P. M, Foreman, J., Davis, R. B., Delbance, T., & Phillips, R. S. (2007). A pilot study for a randomized, controlled trial on the effect of guided imagery in hospitalized medical patients. *Journal of Alternative and Complementary Medicine, 13*(2), 194–197.

Trakhtenberg, E. C. (2008). The effects of guided imagery on the immune system: A critical review. *International Journal of Neuroscience, 118*, 839–855.

Turk, D. C., Swanson, K. S., & Tunks, E. R. (2008). Psychological approaches in the treatment of chronic pain patients—when pills, scalpels and needles are not enough. *Canadian Journal of Psychiatry, 53*(4), 213–223.

Uman, L. S., Chambers, C. T., McGrath, P. J., & Kisely, S. (2008). A systematic review of randomized controlled trials examining psychological interventions for needle-related procedural pain and distress in children and adolescents: An abbreviated Cochrane review. *Journal of Pediatric Psychology, 33*(8), 842–854.

Van Kuiken, D. (2004). A meta-analysis of the effect of guided imagery practice on outcomes. *Journal of Holistic Nursing, 22*(2), 164–179.

Vlieger, A. M., Blink, M., Tromp, E., & Benninga, M. (2008). Use of complementary and alternative medicine by pediatric patients with functional and organic gastrointestinal diseases: Results from a multicenter survey. *Pediatrics, 122*, e446–e451. Retrieved November 2008 from http://www.pediatrics.org/cgi/content/full/122/2/e446

Walker, L. G. (2004). Hypnotherapeutic insights and interventions: A cancer odyssey. *Contemporary Hypnosis, 21*(1), 35–45.

Watanabe, E., Fukuda, S., Hara, H., Maeda, Y., & Ohira, H. (2006). Differences in relaxation by means of guided imagery in a healthy community sample. *Alternative Therapies, 12*(2), 60–66.

Watanabe, E., Fukuda, S., & Shirakawa, T. (2005). Effects among healthy subjects of the duration of regularly practicing a guided imagery program. *BMC Complementary and Alternative Medicine, 5*(21), 1–8.

Weydert, J. A., Shapiro, D. E., Acra, S. A., Monheim, C. J., Chambers, A. S., & Ball, T. M. (2006). Evaluation of guided imagery as treatment for recurrent abdominal pain in children: A randomized controlled trial. *BMC Pediatrics, 6*(29), 1–10.

Wild, M. R., & Espie, C. A. (2004). The efficacy of hypnosis in the reduction of procedural pain and distress in pediatric oncology: A systematic review. *Developmental and Behavioral Pediatrics, 25*(3), 207–213.

Wood, C., & Bioy, A. (2008). Hypnosis and pain in children. *Journal of Pain and Symptom Management, 35*(4), 437–446.

Wynd, C. A. (2005). Guided health imagery for smoking cessation and long-term abstinence. *Journal of Nursing Scholarship, 37*(3), 245–250.

Yoo, H. J, Ahn, S. H, Kim, S. B., Kim, W. K., & Han, O. S. (2005). Efficacy of progressive muscle relaxation training and guided imagery in reducing chemotherapy side effects in patients with breast cancer and in improving their quality of life. *Supportive Care in Cancer, 13*, 826–833.

Young, K. D. (2005). Pediatric procedural pain. *Annals of Emergency Medicine, 45*(2), 160–171.

Youssef, N. N., Rosh, J. R., Loughran, M., Schuckalo, S. G., Cotter, A. N., Verga, B. G., . . . Richard, L. (2004). Treatment of functional abdominal pain in childhood with cognitive behavioral strategies. *Journal of Pediatric and Gastroenterological Nutrition, 39*(2), 192–196.

Chapter 7: Music Intervention

LINDA L. CHLAN AND ANNIE HEIDERSCHEIT

Music has been used throughout history as a treatment modality (Haas & Brandes, 2009). From the time of the ancient Egyptians, the power of music to affect health has been noted (Davis, Gfeller, & Thaut, 2008). Nursing pioneer Florence Nightingale recognized the healing power of music (1860/1969). Today, nurses can use music in a variety of settings to benefit patients and clients.

DEFINITIONS

The *American Heritage Dictionary of the English Language* (2011) defines *music* as "the art of arranging sounds in time so as to provide a continuous, unified and evocative composition, as through melody, harmony, rhythm, and timbre." Crowe (2004) identifies several elements that serve as the building blocks of music.

- **Rhythm** is the timing in music and is a phenomenon that is universal to all music. Rhythm includes: tempo, beat, meter, and the duration of tones. It is what provides the movement in music. Rhythm influences motor skills and activates muscles. Slow rhythms can invoke a sense of peace and calm. Strong and intense rhythms can foster a sense or feelings of energy or power.
- **Melody** is the movement of pitches and tones in time. Melody is the relationship between the pitches. The movement and frequency of these pitches impacts our experience. Frequency and pitch are produced by the number of vibrations of a sound—the highness or lowness of a

musical tone, noted by the letters A, B, C, D, E, F, G. Higher pitches have more rapid vibrations that tend to act as a stimulant, whereas lower pitches have slower vibrations that can bring about relaxation. Melody is often the element in music a listener follows that can serve to engage or distract the mind.

■ **Harmony** is related to melody in that it is the sound produced when pitches are played or sung simultaneously. Harmony communicates a sense of relationship, how the notes connect or relate to one another. Harmony often conveys the emotions in music. When harmony is consonant or pleasing in sound, there is a feeling of calm connection. Harmony that is dissonant creates a sense of tension, conflict, and unpleasantness. It is important to note that cultural norms determine what a listener deems enjoyable and pleasant. Different cultures use different tonal systems.

■ **Timbre** is the characteristic sound of the instrument playing the music or the voice singing. The construction, shape, materials, and the technique of the player impact timbre of an instrument. Timbre of a voice is impacted by the body and technique of the vocalist. The psychological significance of timbre includes the associations with feelings, memories, and events.

■ **Form** is the structure or design of music. It can be considered the container within which music is organized. For example, symphonies follow a form of four movements, whereas in a song there will be lyrics and a chorus. The organization in form provides a sense of comfort and predictability.

■ **Dynamics** in music are the change in sound intensity or volume. Dynamics range from loudness to softness. The intensity in dynamics can impact our experience with music. Softer or quieter music can create a sense of calm, closeness, and intimacy; louder music can create a feeling of energy and power.

Music therapists are well versed in using and implementing the healing elements of music to meet the specific and individualized needs of patients. In the United States and around the world, music therapists are employed in a wide variety of health care settings and facilities. Although music therapists are specifically trained to use music in various therapeutic ways, there are many situations in which nurses can implement music intervention into a patient's plan of care. So as not to confuse the practice of music therapy with the use of music from a nursing perspective, the term *music intervention* will be used in this chapter.

SCIENTIFIC BASIS

Music is a complex auditory stimulus that affects the physiological, psychological, and spiritual dimensions of human beings. Individual responses to music can be influenced by personal preferences, experiences, demographic characteristics, the environment, education, and cultural factors.

Entrainment, a physics principle, is a process whereby two objects vibrating at similar frequencies tend to cause mutual sympathetic resonance, resulting in their vibrating at the same frequency (Dissanayake, 2009). Entrainment also refers to the synchronization of body rhythms to an external rhythm (Crowe, 2004; Hodges & Sebald, 2011). Music and physiological processes (including heartbeat, blood pressure, brain waves, body temperature, digestion, and adrenal hormones) involve rhythms and vibrations that occur in a regular, periodic manner and consist of oscillations (Crowe, 2004). Rhythm and tempo of music can be used to synchronize or entrain body rhythms (e.g., heart rate and respiratory pattern) with resultant changes in physiological states. Certain properties of music (less than 80 beats per minute with fluid, regular rhythm) can be used to promote relaxation by causing body rhythms to slow down or entrain with the slower beat and regular, repetitive rhythm (Robb, Nichols, Rutan, Bishop, & Parker, 1995).

Likewise, music can decrease anxiety by occupying attention channels in the brain with meaningful, distractive auditory stimuli (Bauldoff, Hoffman, Zullo, & Sciurba, 2002). Music intervention provides a patient/client with a familiar, comforting stimulus that can evoke pleasurable sensations while focusing the individual's attention onto the music (distraction) instead of on stressful thoughts, pain, discomfort, or other environmental stimuli.

INTERVENTION

Determining a patient's music preferences through assessment is essential; among the tools developed for this purpose is an assessment instrument by Chlan and Heiderscheit (2009) that elicits information on how frequently music is listened to; the type of music selections, artists, groups, and genres preferred; and the individual's reasons for listening to music. For some people, the purpose of listening to music may be to relax, whereas others may prefer music that distracts, stimulates, and invigorates. After assessment data have been gathered, appropriate techniques with specific music can then be devised and implemented.

Techniques

The use of music for intervention can take many forms, such as (passive) listening to selected compact discs (CDs) or individual music downloads from the Internet, as well as actively singing or drumming. A number of factors should be kept in mind when considering the specific technique: the type of music and personal preferences, active music making versus passive listening, individual versus group involvement, length of time involved with the music, and desired outcomes. Two of the more commonly used music-intervention techniques are discussed here: individual listening and group music making.

Individual Music Listening

Providing the means for patients to listen to music is the intervention technique most frequently implemented by nurses. CDs or MP3 downloads from a reputable Internet source (such as www.MyMusicInc.com or iTunes) make it easy to provide music intervention for patients in a wide range of health care settings. CD/MP3 players are relatively inexpensive; they are small and can be used in even the most crowded confines, such as critical care units. CD/MP3 players have superior sound clarity and track seeking that enables immediate selection of a desired piece of music. Comfortable headphones allow patients private listening that does not disturb others. Equipment selected for music intervention should be easy for patients to use with minimal effort. Small MP3 players, like the Apple iPod® or Apple iPad®, are more expensive than CD/MP3 players and should be reserved for patients with intact dexterity and sufficient visual acuity to operate these units.

Nurses can encourage patients and their family members to bring in their own music from home to use while hospitalized. Patients may already have own their preferred music available via a mobile or digital device. With only a very modest outlay of money, a nursing unit can establish a music library containing a wide variety of selections to suit various musical preferences. The Public Radio Music Source (www.prms.org) offers diverse music for purchase. It is also easy to individualize CDs or MP3 files to accommodate the preferences of each client. Attention to copyright laws is necessary when reproducing CDs or downloading music from Internet sites (for guidance refer to www.copyright.gov).

Although various musical genres are available on the radio or Internet radio (Pandora), commercial messages and talking are deterrents to using these sources for music intervention. Likewise, one cannot control the quality of the radio signal reception or the specific music selections.

Group Music Making

Music can be used for patient groups as a powerful integrating force. Music creates and fosters connection and interrelationships among the members as well as between the listener and the music. One method of group music making is drumming, a form of rhythmic auditory stimulation. Drumming has been found to reduce posttraumatic stress disorder (PTSD) symptoms in a small group of soldiers, both by serving as an outlet for rage and for regaining a sense of control (Bensimon, Amir, & Wolf, 2008). Drumming circles can induce relaxation by entraining theta and alpha brain waves, leading to altered states of consciousness by activation of the limbic brain region with the lower brain (Winkelman, 2003) and by increasing natural killer (NK) cell activity (Bittman et al., 2001; Wachi et al., 2007). Group drumming has been used effectively to reduce burnout and improve mood in nursing students (Bittman et al., 2004), decrease employee burnout and improve mood states of staff working in long-term-care settings (Bittman, Bruhn, Stevens, Westengard, & Umbach, 2003), foster creativity and body movement in long-term-care residents (Bittman et al., 2004), and enhance recovery from a variety of chemical addictions (Winkelman, 2003).

Before implementing this type of group music making, nurses should consult with experts trained in the use of group drumming. The American Music Therapy Association website (www.musictherapy.org) can provide assistance in locating a music therapist for consultation. Interested nurses can visit the HealthRhythms website at Remo.com to locate an endorsed HealthRhythms facilitator in a specific area or to learn more about HealthRhythms training. HealthRhythms is a group-drumming protocol developed by Remo, Inc.; training is offered throughout the United States each year. Further, diversity in the preferences, interests, and abilities of individuals in a group or the difficulties of securing an appropriate site for a group session may necessitate handling music on an individual basis; group sessions also require more planning than individual sessions.

Types of Music for Intervention

Careful attention to the selection of the music contributes to its therapeutic effect. For example, music to induce relaxation has a consistent and steady rhythm (less than 80 beats per minute); melody that is smooth, flowing, and predictable, with a small range of interval dynamics; and harmonic structure that is consonant and pleasing, with instrumentation that the individual enjoys (Grocke & Wigram, 2007). It is important to note that past experiences can influence one's response to music and that music can elicit a powerful emotional response or reaction at times.

Older adults may enjoy patriotic and popular songs from an earlier era (often music from their late teens to early twenties) or hymns with slower tempos played with familiar instruments (Moore, Staum, & Brotons, 1992). Religious music may be preferred and welcomed by those unable to attend spiritual services, and for whom faith is important.

New Age or contemporary music may be preferred by some people. This kind of music differs from traditional music, which is characterized by tension and release. However, some experts think that this type of synthesized music is not appropriate for relaxation because of the novelty of the stimulus and the absence of the usual forms found in more conventional music (Bonny, 1986; Hanser & Thompson, 1994). Music perceived as unfamiliar will cause an orienting response that may undermine goals for intervention (Maranto, 1993).

Guidelines

Music intervention for the purpose of relaxation uses music as a pleasant stimulus to block out sensations of anxiety, fear, and tension and to divert attention from unpleasant thoughts (Thaut, 1990). A minimum of 20 minutes of music is necessary to induce relaxation, along with some form of diversion exercise, such as deep breathing, prior to initiating music intervention (Guzzetta, 1995).

Although the definition of relaxing music may vary by individual, factors affecting response to music include musical preferences, familiarity of selections, and cultural background. Relaxing music should have a tempo at or below a resting heart rate (less than 80 beats per minute); predictable dynamics; fluid melodic movement; pleasing harmonies; regular rhythm without sudden changes; and tonal qualities that include strings, flute, piano, or specially synthesized music (Robb et al., 1995). One of the most widely used classical music selections for relaxation is Pachelbel's Canon in D Major, which is frequently included in commercially available diversion CDs. In the last several years, many music companies have been producing recordings specifically packaged as music for relaxation. There is a wide array of recordings available in various genres and styles that can also include various instrumentation and environmental sounds. Exhibit 7.1 outlines the basic steps for handling music intervention for promoting relaxation.

Measurement of Outcomes

The outcome indices for evaluating the effectiveness of music intervention vary, depending on the purpose for which the music is used. Results may be physiological and/or psychological alterations and include a decrease in anxiety or stress arousal, promotion of relaxation, increase in social interaction, reduction in the need for medications, and increase in overall well-being. The nurse should carefully consider the goals of intervention and select outcome measurements and appropriate instruments accordingly.

Precautions

It is imperative that music preferences be assessed prior to initiating a music-listening intervention. Everyone has "musical memories" and listening to a piece of music can bring up negative emotions that can be detrimental to an individual's well-being and also negatively impact the goals of intervention.

Exhibit 7.1. *Guidelines for Music Intervention for Relaxation*

1. Ascertain that patient has adequate hearing
2. Ascertain patient's like/dislike for music
3. Assess music preferences and previous experience with music for relaxation
4. Provide a choice of relaxing selections; assist with CD/MP3 selections as needed
5. Determine agreed-upon goals for music intervention with patient
6. Complete all nursing care prior to intervention; allow for a minimum of 20 minutes of uninterrupted listening time
7. Gather equipment (CD or MP3 player, CDs, headphones, fresh batteries) and ensure all are in good working order
8. Test volume and comfort of volume level with patient prior to intervention
9. Assist patient to a comfortable position as needed; ensure call-light is within easy reach and assist patient with equipment as needed
10. Enhance environment as needed (e.g., draw blinds, close door, and turn off lights)
11. Post a "Do Not Disturb" sign to minimize unnecessary interruptions
12. Encourage and provide patient with opportunities to practice relaxation with music
13. Document patient responses to music intervention
14. Discuss feelings of patient after using music intervention. Identify whether client encountered any challenges or problems with the equipment
15. Revise intervention plan and goal(s) as needed

Initiating music intervention without first assessing a person's likes and dislikes may produce deleterious effects. Because of music's effect on the limbic system, it can bring about intense emotional responses. Use of portable players with headphones may be inappropriate or prohibited for patients in psychiatric settings, who may use the equipment cords for self-harm.

Likewise, using music for diversion in patients with tenuous or unstable cardiovascular status should be done with extreme caution. Patients should be closely monitored for any untoward cardiovascular responses.

Age-Related Implications or Adjustments Needed for Optimal Implementation

Older adults may require additional precautions prior to using music for therapeutic listening purposes. For instance, volume and bass may need to be adjusted to match hearing acuity. Headphones are ideal for masking background noise that can interfere with hearing acuity. Careful selection of equipment for music-listening interventions requires special attention to dexterity and/or vision impairments. Diminishing dexterity or vision may impact the frequency or use of individual music listening.

USES

Music has been tested as a therapeutic intervention with many different patient populations; a majority of the nursing literature focuses on individualized music listening. Exhibit 7.2 shows those patient populations and the numerous therapeutic purposes that music has served. Two frequent uses are highlighted here.

Exhibit 7.2. *Uses of Music Intervention*

Orientation/Minimizing Disruptive Behaviors

Older adults (Cooke, Moyle, Shum, Harrison, & Murfield, 2010; Hicks-Moore, 2005; Thomas & Smith, 2009)

Decreasing Anxiety

Pediatrics (Barrera et al., 2002; Kemper et al., 2008)

Surgical patients (Johnson, Raymond, & Goss, 2012; Kain, Sevarino, Alexander, Pincus, & Mayes, 2000; Lee, Henderson, & Shum, 2004; Yung et al., 2002)

Cancer patients (Clark et al., 2006; Ferrer, 2007)

Cardiac patients (Hamel, 2001)

Flexible sigmoidoscopy (Chlan, Evans, Greenleaf, & Walker, 2000; Lee et al., 2002)

Ventilator-dependent intensive care unit (ICU) patients (Almerud & Peterson, 2003; Chlan, 1998; Davis & Jones, 2012; Heiderscheit, Chlan, & Donely, 2011; Wong et al., 2001)

Pain Management

Acute pain (Dunn, 2004; Good et al., 2001; Huang, Good, & Zauszniewski, 2010; Koelsch et al., 2011; Laurion & Fetzer, 2003; Shertzer & Keck, 2001)

Chronic pain management (Guetin et al., 2012)

Nursing care procedures/pediatrics (Whitehead-Pleaux, Zebrowski, Baryza, & Sheridan, 2007)

(continued)

Exhibit 7.2. *Uses of Music Intervention (continued)*

Interventional radiological procedures—decrease in pain and sedation (Kulkarni, Johnson, Kettles, & Kasthuri, 2012)

Stress Reduction and Relaxation

Neonatal intensive care (NICU) patients (Kemper et al., 2004); Nursing students (Bittman et al., 2004)

Mechanically ventilated ICU patients (Conrad et al., 2007)

Hospitalized psychiatric patients (Yang et al., 2012)

Stimulation

Cognitive recovery and mood poststroke (Sarkamo et al., 2008)

Sleep disturbances in college students (Harmat, Takacs, & Bodizs, 2008)

Head injury (Formisano et al., 2001)

Distraction

Adjunct to spinal or general anesthesia (Lepage, Drolet, Girard, Grenier, & DeGagne, 2001; Nilsson, Rawal, Unesthahl, Zetterberg, & Unosson, 2001)

Bone marrow biopsy and aspiration (Shabanloie, Golchin, Esfani, Dolatkhah, & Rasoulian 2010)

Burn care (Fratianne et al., 2001; Prensner et al., 2001)

Groin hemostasis with C-clamp application after percutaneous coronary intervention (Chan et al., 2006)

Hemodialysis-associated pain and anxiety (Lin et al., 2012; Pothoulaki et al., 2008)

Cardiac laboratory environmental enhancement (Thorgaard, Henriksen, Pedersbaek, & Thomsen, 2003)

Radiation therapy (Clark et al., 2006)

Decreasing Anxiety and Stress

One of the strongest effects of music is anxiety reduction (Pelletier, 2004). Music can enhance the immediate environment, provide a diversion, and lessen the impact of potentially disturbing sounds for pediatric patients (Barrera, Rykov, & Doyle, 2002), and for patients experiencing a variety of surgical procedures (Ebneshahidi & Mohseni, 2008; Nilsson,

2009). The effect of music intervention on the stress response has been documented in cardiac surgery patients (Yung, Chui-Kam, French, & Chan, 2002), in coronary care unit patients (Hamel, 2001), and in ventilator-dependent ICU patients (Chlan, 1998; Almerud & Peterson, 2003; Conrad et al., 2007; Heiderscheit, Chlan, & Donely, 2011; Wong, Lopez-Nahas, & Molassiotis, 2001). Specially designed music can be effective in enhancing relaxation in an outpatient oncology setting for children (Kemper, Hamilton, McClean, & Lovato, 2008). Music can be an efficient intervention for enriching the NICU environment and reducing stress (Kemper, Martin, Block, Shoaf, & Woods, 2004) with such improvements as enhanced oxygenation during suctioning (Chou, Wang, Chen, & Pay, 2003) and increased feeding rates (Standley, 2003).

Distraction

Music is an effective adjunctive intervention for creating distraction, particularly for procedures that induce untoward symptoms and distress, such as pain and anxiety with hemodialysis (Lin, Lu, Chen, & Chang, 2012; Pothoulaki et al., 2008). It has been found to be an adept diversional adjunct in the care of individuals with burns (Formisano et al., 2001; Prensner, Yowler, Smith, Steele, & Fratianne, 2001), in the management of nausea and pain intensity after bone marrow transplantation (Sahler, Hunter, & Liesveld, 2003), in people undergoing regular hemodialysis (Pothoulaki et al., 2008), and for reduction in the amount of sedation required for adults during colonoscopy (Lee et al., 2002; Smolen, Topp, & Singer, 2002).

How to Locate a Music Therapist for Consult or Collaboration

Given the importance of music preference assessment and knowledge of the physiological and psychological influences of music on the individual listener, it may be appropriate for a nurse to consult or collaborate with a professional music therapist prior to instituting music-listening interventions. One source that nurses can access to locate a music therapist in the United States is:

American Music Therapy Association
8455 Colesville Road, Suite 1000
Silver Spring, MD 20910
www.musictherapy.org
(301) 589-3300

To locate a music therapist internationally, the World Federation of Music Therapy can be accessed at (www.musictherapyworld.net).

CULTURAL ASPECTS

Although music may indeed be considered a universal phenomenon, there is no universal language to music. Various cultures structure music differently from what is usual to the average Western listener. For example, music from Eastern cultures contains very different tone structures and timbre, which can be foreign to the Western listener. Likewise, individuals from a non-Western culture may find the classical music of Mozart or Beethoven as foreign sounding and irritating to the listener. These structural differences in what various cultures consider music are crucial to consider when implementing music-listening interventions.

Across five pain intervention studies, Caucasians preferred orchestral music, African Americans favored jazz, and Taiwanese enjoyed harp music (Good et al., 2000). However, other investigators have found that minority older adults tend to prefer music that is familiar to their own cultural background rather than Western music (Lai, 2004). These disparate findings highlight the need for careful music preference assessment prior to intervention. It is imperative to keep in mind that music intervention should never be used in place of pharmacological therapy for the management of acute pain. Music can, however, serve as an adjunctive intervention for pain management.

There is interest in music for clinical applications around the world, and researchers in the context of their clinical settings are exploring the benefits of music to address patient conditions that they encounter. Sidebar 7.1 provides an example of a program of clinical investigation to determine how music can benefit patients in emergency care.

Sidebar 7.1. *Making a Difference in Emergency Care: Australian Music-Listening Applications*

Alison Short, Sydney, Australia

People search for emergency care when they are sick, in pain, in shock, and distressed. Typically, they find this in a hospital emergency department (ED). Both their health problems and the ED environment may contribute to their experience of stress and anxiety. High noise levels in the ED promote stress, aggravation, and sleep loss, with potential effects on communication and behavior (Ortiga et al., 2013; Short, Ahern, Holdgate, Morris, & Sidhu, 2010; Short, Short, Holdgate, Ahern, & Morris, 2011). Several Australian studies have used music-listening interventions in the ED to reduce anxiety and stress and promote calm (Daly et al., 2012/2013; Short et al., 2010; Weiland et al., 2011). Findings

(continued)

Sidebar 7.1. *Making a Difference in Emergency Care: Australian Music-Listening Applications (continued)*

suggest that music can reduce anxiety and negative affect for moderately anxious patients in triage categories 2 and 3 (Australasian College for Emergency Medicine, 2000), assisting them in feeling better during their stay in the ED (Short et al., 2010; Weiland et al., 2011). For example, patients commented: "Thought it was absolutely fabulous, blocked out conversations"; "Very good idea for passing the time, relaxes you"; "Gives you more time out of here, more peaceful." Combined with other modalities, music may also assist with reducing stress and anxiety levels in emergency nurses (Davis, Cooke, Holzhauser, Jones, & Finucane, 2005).

Planning a music-listening intervention in the ED needs careful consideration regarding the mode of delivery, the type of music to be used, patient choice, and volume levels. It may be difficult or inappropriate to use live music in many ED settings. Open-air broadcast of music may raise noise levels and be unsuitable, given the diverse sociocultural factors of the crowded multiaged and multicultural ED context. Nevertheless, the use of music in the waiting room area is currently being trialed in a major Sydney hospital (Daly et al., 2012/2013). The use of headphones and music-listening equipment require careful consideration of operational and infection-control issues (Short & Ahern, 2009). In addition, decisions about what music to use are complex and need to consider many aspects of patient demographics, including language and ethnicity (Short & Ahern, 2009). Patient choice is generally understood to contribute to improved stress management (Chlan & Heiderscheit, 2014; Short et al., 2010). In using headphones, volume levels need to be tracked to avoid hearing damage; severe distraction by high noise levels may also potentially contribute to falls. As with other innovations, implementation of a music-listening intervention in the ED environment must first begin with a thorough consideration of the local context and its specific needs related to patients, staff, and the organization—as is consistent with the approach at our institution in Sydney, Australia.

References

Australasian College for Emergency Medicine [West Melbourne, Australia]. (2000). *Guidelines on the implementation of the Australasian triage scale in emergency departments.* Retrieved December 14, 2012, from: http://www.acem.org.au/media/policies_and_guidelines/G24_Implementation_ATS.pdf

Chlan, L., & Heiderscheit, A. (2014). Music intervention. In R. Lindquist, M. Snyder, & M. F. Tracy, (Eds.), *Complementary & alternative therapies in nursing* (7th ed., pp. 99–116). New York, NY: Springer Publishing Company.

(continued)

Sidebar 7.1. *Making a Difference in Emergency Care: Australian Music-Listening Applications (continued)*

Daly, B., Hilbers, J., Varndell, W., Chalkey, D., Cudmore, B., & Short, A. (2012/2013). *Auditory environments in healthcare: Reducing chaos and enhancing calm within the emergency department using music and recorded messages* (Study in progress). Sydney, Australia: Australian Institute of Health Innovation, University of New South Wales.

Davis, C., Cooke, M., Holzhauser, K., Jones, M, & Finucane, J. (2005). The effect of aromatherapy massage with music on the stress and anxiety levels of emergency nurses. *Australasian Emergency Nursing Journal, 8,* 43–50.

Ortiga, J., Kanapathipillai, S., Daly, B., Hilbers, J., Varndell, W., & Short, A. (2013). The sound of urgency: Understanding noise in the emergency department. *Music and Medicine, 5*(1), 44–51.

Short, A., & Ahern, N. (2009). Theory into practice: A systematic decision-making process addressing patient needs for relaxing music in the emergency department context. *Australian Journal of Music Therapy, 20,* 3–28.

Short, A., Ahern, N., Holdgate, A., Morris, J., & Sidhu, B. (2010). Using music to reduce noise stress for patients in the emergency department: A pilot study. *Music & Medicine, 2* (4), 201–207.

Short, A., Short, K., Holdgate, A., Ahern, N., & Morris, J. (2011). Noise levels in an Australian emergency department. *Australasian Emergency Nursing Journal, 14* (1), 26–31.

Weiland, T., Jelinek, G., Macarow, K., Samartzis, P., Brown, D., Grierson, E., & Winter, C. (2011). Original sounds compositions reduce anxiety in emergency department patients: A randomised controlled trial. *Medical Journal of Australia, 195* (11/12), 694–698.

FUTURE RESEARCH

Although the evidence base is increasing, the following are areas in which research is needed to further build the science of music intervention:

- Recent meta-analyses have been published on the consistent effects of music intervention on preoperative anxiety (Dileo, Bradt, & Murphy, 2008) and anxiety reduction in critically ill patients receiving mechanical ventilatory support (Bradt, Dileo, & Grocke, 2010). Whereas music consistently induces favorable outcomes, pooled effect sizes can be small. Common limitations are the inconsistent use of instruments to measure phenomena, such as anxiety, and lack of multisite clinical trials. Additional investigation is needed that builds on the findings of these meta-analyses through the consistent use of instruments and the conduct of multisite clinical trials.
- Additional exploration into the management of symptom clusters would enhance the scientific base of music intervention. For example,

persons with cancer typically experience nausea, vomiting, distress, and fatigue with treatments. Can the implementation of carefully selected music and its delivery improve a constellation of symptoms? Can cancer patients be taught symptom management through the self-initiation of tailored or preferred music?

- Cost and cost savings are significant issues in health care today. Little is known about the potential cost savings that could be realized with music intervention. Study is needed to determine whether music is a cost-effective or cost-neutral intervention and, if cost-effective, in which patient-care or symptom-management settings this is so.
- Much of the nursing review focuses on immediate or short-term effects of music intervention. It is not known whether music can be effective for managing symptoms and distress in those with chronic conditions, or improve their quality of life. Appropriate longitudinal research designs are needed to answer these questions.
- There is a paucity of explorations as to the appropriate or optimal timing for delivery of music intervention to enhance effectiveness—and for which specific patient populations or symptoms.
- There is limited research on the impact of music intervention on patient satisfaction or on the patient's overall experience. Client satisfaction with music intervention is an important outcome and quality indicator in a variety of health care settings. Appropriate measures and instruments are needed to capture quality data, which requires further research to develop.

Although intervention study itself is labor intensive, there is a need for additional investigation on music intervention. The knowledge base about music intervention for promotion of patient/client health and well-being can be expanded through high-quality research and by dissemination of those findings in a timely manner. To further build a strong body of knowledge surrounding the implementation and outcomes of music intervention, the authors of this chapter recommend an interdisciplinary approach, including nurses and music therapists conducting collaborative research. From quality evidence, music-intervention implementation guidelines can then be integrated into patient care.

REFERENCES

Almerud, S., & Peterson, K. (2003). Music therapy—A complementary treatment for mechanically ventilated intensive care patients. *International Critical Care Nursing, 19*(1), 21–30.

American Heritage dictionary of the English language (5th ed.). (2011). Boston, MA: Houghton Mifflin.

Barrera, M., Rykov, M., & Doyle, S. (2002). The effects of interactive music therapy on hospitalized children with cancer: A pilot study. *Psycho-Oncology, 11*(5), 379–388.

Bauldoff, G., Hoffman, L., Zullo, T., & Sciurba, I. (2002). Exercise maintenance following pulmonary rehabilitation: Effect of distractive stimuli. *Chest, 122*(3), 948–954.

Bensimon, M., Amir, D., & Wolf, Y. (2008). Drumming through trauma: Music therapy with post-traumatic soldiers. *Arts in Psychotherapy, 35*(1), 34–48.

Bittman, B., Berk, L., Felten, D., Westengard, J., Simonton, O., Pappas, J., & Ninehouser, M. (2001). Composite effects of group drumming music therapy on modulation of neuroendocrine-immune parameters of normal subjects. *Alternative Therapy Health Medicine, 7*, 38–47.

Bittman, B., Bruhn, K., Stevens, C., Westengard, J., & Umbach, P. (2003). Recreational music-making: A cost effective group interdisciplinary strategy of reducing burnout and improving mood states in long-term care workers. *Advances in Mind-Body Medicine, 19*(3/4), 4–15.

Bittman, B. B., Snyder, C., Bruhn, K. T., Liebfreid, F., Stevens, C. K., Westengard, J., & Umbach, P. O. (2004). Recreational music-making: An integrative group intervention for reducing burnout and improving mood states in first-year associate degree nursing students: Insights and economic impact. *International Journal of Nursing Education Scholarship, 1*, Article 12.

Bonny, H. (1986). Music and healing. *Music Therapy, 6*(1), 3–12.

Bradt, J., Dileo, C., & Grocke, D. (2010). Music interventions for mechanically ventilated patients. *Cochrane Database of Systematic Reviews*, Issue 12. Art. No.: CD006902. DOI: 10.1002/14651858.CD006902.pub2.

Chan, M. F., Wong, O. C., Chan, H. L., Fong, M. C., Lai, S. Y., Lo, C. W., … Leung, S. K. (2006). Effects of music on patients undergoing C-clamp procedure after percutaneous coronary interventions. *Journal of Advanced Nursing, 53*(6), 669–679.

Chlan, L. (1998). Effectiveness of a music therapy intervention on relaxation and anxiety for patients receiving ventilatory assistance. *Heart & Lung, 27*(3), 169–176.

Chlan, L., Evans, D., Greenleaf, M., & Walker, J. (2000). Effects of a single music therapy intervention on anxiety, discomfort, satisfaction, and compliance with screening guidelines in outpatients undergoing screening flexible sigmoidoscopy. *Gastroenterology Nursing, 23*(4), 148–156.

Chlan, L., & Heiderscheit, A. (2009). A tool for music preference assessment in critically ill patients receiving mechanical ventilatory support: An interdisciplinary approach. *Music Therapy Perspectives, 27*(1), 42–47.

Chou, L., Wang, R., Chen, S., & Pay, L. (2003). Effects of music therapy on oxygen saturation in premature infants receiving endotracheal suctioning. *Journal of Nursing Research, 11*(3), 209–215.

Clark, M., Isaacks-Donton, G., Wells, N., Redlin-Frazier, S., Eck, C., Hepworth, J. T., & Chakravarthy, B. (2006). Use of preferred music to reduce emotional distress and symptom activity during radiation therapy. *Journal of Music Therapy, 43*(3), 247–265.

Conrad, C., Niess, H., Jauch, K. W., Bruns, C., Hartl, W., & Welker, L. (2007). Overture for growth hormone: Requiem for interleukin-6? *Critical Care Medicine, 35*(12), 2709–2713.

Cooke, M. L., Moyle, W., Shum, D. H., Harrison, S. D., & Murfield, J. E. (2010). A randomized controlled trial exploring the effect of music on agitated behaviours and anxiety in older people with dementia. *Aging & Mental Health, 14*(8), 905–916.

Crowe, B. (2004). *Music and soul making: Toward a new theory of music therapy.* Oxford, UK: The Scarecrow Press.

Davis, W., Gfeller, K., & Thaut, M. (2008). *An introduction to music therapy: Theory and practice.* New York, NY: McGraw-Hill.

Davis, T., & Jones, P. (2012). Music therapy: Decreasing anxiety in the ventilated patient: A review of the literature. *Dimensions of Critical Care Nursing, 31*(3), 159–166.

Dileo, C., Bradt, J., & Murphy, K., (2008) Music for preoperative anxiety (Protocol). *Cochrane Database of Systematic Reviews*, Issue 1. Art. No.: CD006908. DOI: 10.1002/14651858.CD006908.

Dissanayake, W. (2009). Bodies swayed to music: The temporal arts as integral to ceremonial ritual. In S. Malcok & C. Trevarthen (Eds.), *Communicative musicality: Exploring the basis of human companionship* (pp. 17–30). Oxford, UK: Oxford University Press.

Dunn, K. (2004). Music and the reduction of post-operative pain. *Nursing Standard, 18*(36), 33–39.

Ebneshahidi, A., & Mohseni, M. (2008). The effect of patient-selected music on early postoperative pain, anxiety, and hemodynamic profile in Cesarean Section surgery. *Journal of Alternative and Complementary Medicine, 14*(7), 827–831.

Ferrer, A. (2007). The effect of live music on decreasing anxiety in patients undergoing chemotherapy treatment. *Journal of Music Therapy, 44*(3), 242–255.

Formisano, R., Vinicola, V., Penta, F., Matteis, M., Brunelli, S., & Weckel, J. (2001). Active music therapy in the rehabilitation of severe brain injured patients during coma recovery. *Annali Dell InstitutoSuperiore di Sanitá, 37*(4), 627–630.

Fratianne, R., Prensner, J., Huston, M., Super, D., Yowler, C., & Standley, J. (2001). The effect of music-based imagery and musical alternate engagement on the burn debridement process. *Journal of Burn Care & Rehabilitation, 22*(1), 47–53.

Good, M., Picot, B., Salem, S., Chin, C., Picot, S., & Lane, D. (2000). Cultural differences in music chosen for pain relief. *Journal of Holistic Nursing, 18*(3), 245–260.

Good, M., Stanton-Hicks, M., Grass, J., Anderson, G. C., Lai, H., Roykulcahroen, V., . . . Adler, P. A. (2001). Relaxation and music to reduce postsurgical pain. *Journal of Advanced Nursing, 33*(2), 208–215.

Grocke, D., & Wigram, T. (2007). *Receptive methods in music therapy. Techniques and clinical applications for music therapy clinicians, educators and students.* London, UK: Jessica Kingsley.

Guetin, S., Ginies, P., Siou, D. K., Picot, M. C., Pommie, C., Guldner, E., . . . Touchon, J. (2012). The effects of music intervention in the management of chronic pain: A single-blind, randomized, controlled trial. *Clinical Journal of Pain, 28*(4), 329–337.

Guzzetta, C. (1995). Music therapy: Hearing the melody of the soul. In B. Dossey, L. Keegan, C. Guzzetta, & L. Kolkmeier (Eds.), *Holistic nursing* (pp. 670–698). Gaithersburg, MD: Aspen.

Haas, R., & Brandes, V. (Eds.). (2009). *Music that works: Contributions of biology, neurophysiology, psychology, sociology, medicine and musicology.* New York, NY: SpringerWien.

Hamel, W. (2001). The effects of music intervention on anxiety in the patient waiting for cardiac catheterization. *Intensive and Critical Care Nursing, 17*(2), 279–285.

Hanser, S., & Thompson, L. (1994). Effects of a music therapy strategy on depressed older adults. *Journal of Gerontology, 49*(6), 265–269.

Harmat, L., Takacs, J., & Bodizs, R. (2008). Music improves sleep quality in students. *Journal of Advanced Nursing, 62*(3), 327–335.

Heiderscheit, A., Chlan, L., & Donely, K. (2011). Instituting a music listening intervention for critically ill patients receiving mechanical ventilation: Exemplars from two patient cases. *Music and Medicine, 3*(4), 239–245.

Hicks-Moore, S. (2005). Relaxing music at mealtime in nursing homes. *Journal of Gerontological Nursing, 31*(12), 26–32.

Hodges, D., & Sebald, D. (2011). *Music in the human experience: An introduction to music psychology.* New York, NY: Routledge.

Huang, S., Good, M., & Zauszniewski, J. (2010). The effectiveness of music in relieving pain in cancer patients: A randomized controlled trial. *International Journal of Nursing Studies, 47*(11), 1354–1362.

Johnson, B., Raymond, S., & Goss, J. (2012). Perioperative music or headsets to decrease anxiety. *Journal of Perianesthesia Nursing, 27*(3), 146–154.

Kain, Z., Sevarino, F., Alexander, G., Pincus, S., & Mayes, L. (2000). Preoperative anxiety and post-operative pain in women undergoing hysterectomy. A repeated-measures design. *Journal of Psychosomatic Research, 49*, 417–422.

Kemper, K., Hamilton, C., McClean, T., & Lovato, J. (2008). Impact of music on pediatric oncology patients. *Pediatric Research, 64*(1), 105–109.

Kemper, K., Martin, K., Block, S., Shoaf, R., & Woods, C. (2004). Attitudes and expectations about music therapy for premature infants among staff in the neonatal intensive care unit. *Alternative Therapies in Health & Medicine, 10*(2), 50–54.

Koelsch, S., Fuermetz, J., Sack, U., Bauer, K., Hohenadel, M., Wiegel, M., & Heinke, W. (2011). Effects of music listening on cortisol levels and propofol consumption during spinal anesthesia. *Frontiers in Psychology, 2*, Article 58.

Kulkarni, S., Johnson, P. C., Kettles, S., & Kasthuri, R. S. (2012). Music during interventional radiological procedures, effect on sedation, pain and anxiety: A randomized controlled trial. *British Journal of Radiology, 85*(10), 1059–1063.

Lai, H. L. (2004). Music preference and relaxation in Taiwanese elderly people. *Geriatric Nursing, 25*(5), 286–291.

Laurion, S., & Fetzer, S. J. (2003). The effect of two nursing interventions on the post-operative outcomes of gynecologic laparoscopic patients. *Journal of Perianesthesia Nursing, 18*(4), 254–261.

Lee, D. W. H., Chan, K., Poon, C., Ko, C., Cha, K., Sin, K., . . . Chan, A. C. W. (2002). Relaxation music decreases the dose of patient-controlled sedation during colonoscopy: A prospective randomized controlled trial. *Gastrointestinal Endoscopy, 55*(1), 33–36.

Lee, D., Henderson, A., & Shum, D. (2004). The effect of music on preprocedure anxiety in Hong Kong Chinese day patients. *Journal of Clinical Nursing, 13*, 297–303.

Lepage, C., Drolet, P., Girard, M., Grenier, Y., & DeGagne, R. (2001). Music decreases sedative requirements during spinal anesthesia. *Anesthesia and Analgesia, 93*, 912–916.

Lin, Y. J., Lu, K. C., Chen, C., & Chang, C. C. (2012). The effects of music as therapy on the overall well-being of elderly patients on maintenance hemodialysis. *Biological Research for Nursing, 14*(3), 277–285.

Maranto, C. (1993). Applications of music in medicine. In M. Heal & T. Wigram (Eds.), *Music therapy in health and education* (pp. 153–174). London, UK: Jessica Kingsley.

Moore, R., Staum, M., & Brotons, M. (1992). Music preferences of the elderly: Repertoire, vocal ranges, tempos, and accompaniments for singing. *Journal of Music Therapy, 29*(4), 236–252.

Nightingale, F. (1969). *Notes on nursing.* New York, NY: Dover. (Original work published 1860)

Nilsson, U. (2009). Soothing music can increase oxytocin levels during bed rest after open-heart surgery: A randomized control trial. *Journal of Clinical Nursing, 8*, 2153–2161.

Nilsson, U., Rawal, N., Unesthahl, L., Zetterberg, C., & Unosson, M. (2001). Improved recovery after music and therapeutic suggestions during general anesthesia: A double-blind randomized controlled trial. *Acta Anesthesiologica Scandinavica, 45*, 812–817.

Pelletier, C. (2004). The effect of music on decreasing arousal due to stress: A meta-analysis. *Journal of Music Therapy, 41*, 192–214.

Pothoulaki, R., MacDonald, P., Flowers, E., Stamataki, V., Filiopoulos, D., Stamatiadis, D., & Stathakis, C. (2008). An investigation of the effects of music on anxiety and pain perception in patients undergoing haemodialysis treatment. *Journal of Health Psychology, 13*(7), 912–920.

Prensner, J. D., Yowler, C. J., Smith, L. F., Steele, A. L., & Fratianne, R. B. (2001). Music therapy for assistance with pain and anxiety management in burn treatment. *Journal of Burn Care & Rehabilitation, 22*(1), 83–88.

Public Radio Music Source. Retrieved from www.prms.org

Robb, S., Nichols, R., Rutan, R., Bishop, B., & Parker, J. (1995). The effects of music-assisted relaxation on preoperative anxiety. *Journal of Music Therapy, 32*(1), 3–12.

Sahler, O., Hunter, B., & Liesveld, J. (2003). The effect of using music therapy with relaxation imagery in the management of patients undergoing bone marrow transplantation: A pilot feasibility study. *Alternative Therapies in Health & Medicine, 9*(6), 70–74.

Sarkamo, T., Tervaniemi, M., Laitinen, S., Forsblom, A., Soinila, S., Mikkonene, M., . . . Hietanen, M. (2008). Music listening enhances cognitive recovery and mood after middle cerebral artery stroke. *Brain, 131*, 866–876.

Shabanloei, R., Golchin, M., Esfani, A., Dolatkhah, R., & Rasoulian, M. (2010). Effects of music therapy on pain and anxiety in patients undergoing bone marrow biopsy and aspiration. *AORN Journal, 91*(6), 746–751.

Shertzer, K., & Keck, J. (2001). Music and the PACU environment. *Journal of Peri Anesthesia Nursing, 16*(2), 90–102.

Smolen, D., Topp, R., & Singer, L. (2002). The effect of self-selected music during colonoscopy on anxiety, heart rate and blood pressure. *Applied Nursing Research, 16*(2), 126–130.

Standley, J. M. (2003). The effect of music-reinforced nonnutrative sucking on feeding rate of premature infants. *Journal of Pediatric Nursing, 18*(3), 169–173.

Thaut, M. H. (1990). Physiological and motor responses to music stimuli. In R. F. Unkefer (Ed.), *Music therapy in the treatment of adults with mental disorders: Theoretical bases and clinical interventions* (pp. 33–49). New York, NY: Schirmer Books.

Thomas, D., & Smith, M. (2009). The effect of music on caloric consumption among nursing home residents with dementia of the Alzheimer's type. *Activities, Adaptation & Aging, 33*, 1–16.

Thorgaard, B., Henriksen, B., Pedersbaek, G., & Thomsen, I. (2003). Specially selected music in the cardiac laboratory—An important tool for improvement of the well-being of patients. *European Journal of Cardiovascular Nursing, 3*(1), 21–26.

Wachi, M., Koyama, M., Utsuyama, M., Bittman, B., Kitagawa, M., & Hirokawa, K. (2007). Recreational music-making modulates natural killer cell activity, cytokines, and mood states in corporate employees. *Medical Science Monitor, 13*(2), 57–70.

Whitehead-Pleaux, A., Zebrowski, N., Baryza, M., & Sheridan, R. (2007). Exploring the effects of music therapy on pediatric pain: Phase 1. *Journal of Music Therapy, 34*(3), 217–241.

Winkelman, M. (2003). Complementary therapy for addiction: "Drumming out drugs." *American Journal of Public Health, 93*(4), 647–651.

Wong, H., Lopez-Nahas, V., & Molassiotis, A. (2001). Effects of music therapy on anxiety in ventilator-dependent patients. *Heart & Lung, 30*(5), 376–387.

Yang, C. Y., Chen, C. H., Chu, H., Chen, W. C., Lee, T. Y., Chen, S. G., & Chou, K. R. (2012). The effect of music therapy on hospitalized psychiatric patients' anxiety, finger temperature, and electroencephalography: A randomized clinical trial. *Biological Research for Nursing, 14*(2), 197–206.

Yung, P., Chui-Kam, S., French, P., & Chan, T. (2002). A controlled trial of music and pre-operative anxiety in Chinese men undergoing transurethral resection of the prostate. *Journal of Advanced Nursing, 39*(4), 352–359.

Chapter 8: Humor

Shirley K. Trout

There seems to be nearly universal consensus that humor and laughter are good for humans and that good humor promotes good health. The phrase "laughter is the best medicine" has been tossed about as proven as the sun rising in the east each morning. But is it? And if laughter *should be* the best medicine, does that mean therapeutic humor would be, as well? Does the medicine help just the body, or could laughter—and perhaps humor—help the whole person in other ways? The fact is, there is very little conclusive evidence that definitively demonstrates that either laughter or humor can improve physical health.

Despite the existence of only limited research that supports the use of humor as a healing modality, many professions have an interest in its role in maintaining and promoting health and healing. Interestingly, it was Norman Cousins's personal story, an anecdote in research terms, that launched today's interest in humor and laughter as a viable therapy for healing (Cousins, 1979). His intriguing experience with using laughter to overcome illness helped initiate today's emerging interdisciplinary fields of psychoneuroimmunology and, somewhat less directly, positive psychology. There is a growing body of evidence that validates humor as an appropriate complementary therapy.

DEFINITION

Too often, the two related yet far different terms *laughter* and *humor* are used interchangeably as though they are one and the same. Even authors of peer-reviewed publications are sometimes guilty of this error.

117

To use the two terms interchangeably reflects a common lack of serious consideration of either, and completely ignores specifics within each. For example, when referring to laughter, do authors mean mirthful laughter or nonemotional laughter? Referring to humor, is it comedy, wit, or mirth? Regarding therapeutic humor, is the study about coping humor, sense of humor, or types of humor? In general, are researchers asking the right questions and using rigor in their study design and analyses?

Humor

Although the term *humor* has never been definitively defined by experts, it is clearly distinct from the personality-based consideration of sense of humor (Svebak, Kristofersen, & Aasarod, 2006). Any definition of humor must be developed from a particular theory, such as superiority/disparagement, arousal, incongruity–resolution, or reversal, each of which has its respective body of theory-development literature. The definition of humor selected for this chapter is based on the incongruity theory. Humor is defined as "simply one element of the comic—as are wit, fun, nonsense, sarcasm, ridicule, satire, or irony—and basically denotes a smiling attitude toward life and its imperfections: an understanding of the incongruities of existence" (Ruch, 1998, p. 6).

Therapeutic Humor

When defining therapeutic humor, it helps to make clear what it is *not*. Therapeutic humor is not laughter, which is a physiological phenomenon (although laughter almost always becomes a part of the consideration of humor). It is not comedy, which has a singular purpose of making people laugh. Humor may be used to poke fun *at* the illness or some other element of the health condition or environment, and *not* used to poke fun at an individual. Humor helps people laugh *with* each other.

Psychotherapist Steve Sultanoff clarifies the key difference between, for example, comedy-club humor and therapeutic humor, "the purposeful intention of using therapeutic humor as a complementary therapy must clearly be *for the benefit of the client or patient* [emphasis added] and not for the therapist's [i.e., nurse's] personal gratification or merely for pleasure" (Steve Sultanoff, personal communication, December 4, 2012). Therapeutic humor has been defined as "any intervention that promotes health and wellness by stimulating a playful discovery, expression, or appreciation of the absurdity or incongruity of life's situations. This intervention may enhance health or be used as a complementary treatment of illness to facilitate healing or coping, whether physical, emotional, cognitive, social, or spiritual" (AATH [Association for Applied and Therapeutic Humor], 2000).

SCIENTIFIC BASIS

To put the evidence into perspective, it is important to understand some of the history of today's interest in therapeutic humor and laughter. In 1963, psychiatric researcher Dr. William Fry published a small book, *Sweet Madness: A Study of Humor*, in which he organized his personal thoughts about humor's relationship to mental health. This theoretical publication and its author were mostly confined to the academic community. Sixteen years later, in 1979, *Saturday Review* editor Norman Cousins (1915–1990) introduced to popular culture his award-winning book *Anatomy of an Illness as Perceived by the Patient*. In this work, Cousins recounts his personal journey forcing a debilitating and painful illness, ankylosing spondylitis, into remission by using a self-prescribed (with his physician's approval) regimen of mirthful laughter and megadoses of vitamin C. His thought for trying this was: if negative thinking can make you ill (validated by research by that time), then could positive thinking make you well? Interestingly, Mr. Cousins's book is credited with launching today's growing interest in humor and laughter as complementary therapies in health care.

The International Society for Humor Studies (ISHS; www.hnu.edu/ishs) is a scholarly organization specifically dedicated to furthering the study and understanding of humor in a wide range of disciplines, including therapeutic humor-related areas. This community of scholars has helped aggregate and strengthen research efforts within this emerging field. As with all professional development, nurses are encouraged to examine original research works as they gain knowledge. This organization allows firsthand connection with the international community of scholars informing the conversations around therapeutic humor.

In general, it is agreed that humor is fundamentally a social phenomenon. However, because it involves cognitive processing, it is available to individuals in isolation as well. Some of the most compelling qualitative examples of humor's value as a coping mechanism for individuals, as well as groups, are revealed by those who have experienced captivity. Lipman's (1991) compilation of interviews with Holocaust survivors serves as a powerful testimony to how valuable humor is to human survival. Lipman noted that "during the Holocaust, religion and humor served a like—though not identical—purpose" (p. 11). He concluded that "the former [religion] oriented one's thoughts to a better existence in the next world, the latter [humor] pointed to emotional salvation in this one" (p. 11).

Within the realm of social interaction, researchers have worked to understand how humor is used to incorporate, embrace, and even celebrate the contradictions, incongruities, and ambiguities inherent in interpersonal relationships (Mulkay, 1988). Within this sphere, Martin (2007) cautions that more study is required before the full extent of the interpersonal, cognitive, mental health, coping, and other psychological impacts of humor can be fully understood.

One finding that appears to be building empirical support of late is that the mere *anticipation* of a humorous or laughter event triggers at least as much positive impact on a variety of health indicators as does mirthful laughter. Additionally, there appears to be a secret weapon available to nurses that may, one day, undergird the connection between therapeutic humor and the effectiveness of nursing care: *get the patient to smile!* And the more pleasant (mirthful) the emotion accompanying the smile, the greater the positive responses. Researchers do not yet fully understand everything about why and how this works, but even simply moving one's facial muscles into a smiling position appears to improve stress- and mood-related indicators, similar to what happens in anticipation of a joyful event. In one revealing study, subjects who simply held a pencil in their mouths to stimulate the facial muscles used in smiling rated cartoons as funnier and reported greater increases in positive mood (compared to subjects who held the pen in a way that inhibited such muscle contractions) (Strack, Martin, & Stepper, 1988).

Martin (2007) concludes that "of all the health benefits claimed for humor and laughter, the most consistent research support has been found for the hypothesized analgesic effects" (p. 331). Further, he goes on to say "Although humor may not produce all the health benefits that have been claimed, at least it is not likely to be harmful and it can enhance people's enjoyment if not the duration of their lives" (p. 331).

As is understandably the case with studying a phenomenon as complex as humor, one can certainly find arguments against virtually every finding published. Exhibit 8.1 provides some of the significant findings related to therapeutic humor, along with at least one citation related to that finding that is representative of the body of research examining and exploring the respective conclusions. The citations included were selected to include one or more of the key scholars involved in this area of study.

INTERVENTION

Therapeutic humor is as much of an art as it is a science. Therefore, with practice, study, and self-reflection, individuals can find their own personal rhythm and style for how, when, and with whom to engage in this complementary therapy. Genuinely therapeutic humor requires a caring heart, keen attention to detail, considerate timing, and creativity. What works for one person may not work for another: a one-size-fits-all formula may never exist. Furthermore, humor will not always work, regardless of how well-intentioned the nurse who employs it. In time, however, one will get better by being willing to learn from past experiences, being open to feedback, and striving to improve practice.

Humor typically works because of an incongruence that surprises the receiver. Few people enter a health care setting focused on anything but

Exhibit 8.1. *Humor and Laughter Research Relevant to Therapeutic Humor*

Empirical Facts	Selected Citations	Comments
Smiling (Duchenne smile) is virtually universally interpreted as a positive communication indicating cheerfulness or playful emotions. This smile has been the only *positive* emotion facial expression to be interpreted with such universal consistency, although several *negative* emotions have been recognized across cultures.	Ekman and Friesen (1978)	Marked the creation of the Facial Action Coding System (FACS), which has been used extensively in a wide range of research and continues to demonstrate significant reliability.
Humor appreciation and comprehension evolve from physical to cognitive over one's developmental years.	McGhee (1979)	A foundational humor piece to explore humor's impact on the mind and body. More recently, McGhee is designing research-based applications of humor (see www. laughterremedy.com)
The Duchenne (enjoyment) smile has been shown to be even more responsible for increasing pain tolerance than actual laughing.	Zweyer, Velker, and Ruch (2004)	Enjoyment that was expressed facially was found to be the mediator between perceiving a humorous film and the change in pain perception.
Sense of humor tends to moderate one's reaction to stress or self-reported level of stress, and humor types appear to be related, although results are inconclusive at this time.	Martin and Dobbin (1988)	Many interesting, albeit not absolutely conclusive, findings are emerging related to humor type and a range of psychological outcomes, such as coping and pain tolerance.
Mirthful laughter has been shown to increase HDL cholesterol and decrease LDL immediately and, in one study, improved conditions remained at 4 months follow-up. The *anticipation* of a laughter event has demonstrated similar results in a growing number of studies.	Berk, Tan, and Berk (2008); Berk, Tan, and Tan (2008); Mahony, Burroughs, and Hieatt (2001)	Patients in the laughter groups had lower EP and NEP levels by 2 months; increased HDL cholesterol; decreased TNF-α, IFN-γ, IL-6, and CRP levels by 4 months; and a lower incidence of MI (1/10) than the control group (3/10). Authors concluded: Addition of mirthful laughter may be an effective CV (cardiovascular) preventive adjunct in diabetes mellitus and metabolic syndrome care. Effects may contribute to lower MI occurrence. Note: The *anticipation* of a pleasant (laughter) event resulted in changes at least as strong as and consistent with the laughter event itself, suggesting the benefits of therapeutic humor may extend beyond humor or laughter, per se.

(continued)

Exhibit 8.1. *Humor and Laughter Research Relevant to Therapeutic Humor (continued)*

Empirical Facts	Selected Citations	Comments
A complex relationship exists between behavior associated with emotion and the human CV system.	Miller and Fry (2009)	Dr. Fry continues to contribute to the science of humor.
The positive emotion elicited by humor appears to be closely related to the pleasurable feelings associated with other agreeable, emotionally rewarding activities, including ingestion of mood-altering drugs (heroin or alcohol), eating, sexual activity, enjoyable music, or video games.	Schultz (2002)	Much remains to be understood about how the brain processes complexities of humor. This research has introduced intriguing findings.
Humor and creativity are closely related in that they both involve a switch of perspective or a new way of seeing things, most convincingly through the positive emotion of mirth.	Isen (2003)	Positive emotional states, including mirth, affect various cognitive processes such as memory, judgment, risk-taking and decision making.

Note: CRP, C-reactive protein; EP, epinephrine; HDL, high-density lipoprotein; IFN-γ, interferon-gamma; IL-6, interleukin-6; LDL, low-density lipoprotein; MI, myocardial infarction; NEP, norepinephrine; TNF-α, tumor necrosis factor alpha.

the health concern that brought them there. This provides ample opportunities to shift the wit of patients and their families. The comedic gap that is associated with incongruities may be used in many situations.

Incongruity

Although many forms of humor exist, incongruity of some sort is considered an essential element of humor (Martin, 2007). The term *incongruity* is familiar in discussions of both humor and comedy, especially regarding the word's definition of being incompatible. That is, when two realities lack harmony or are incompatible with each other, it creates a juxtaposition that can lead to humor, a chuckle, or even a hardy belly laugh. In comedy, incongruity is the key to creating jokes that resonate with an audience and result in laughter. Comedy writers consider the gap between the *reality* (real or perceived) and the *ideal* state (real or perceived). In this gap or space, jokes reside.

Using humor involves a cognitive shift in perspective that allows one to distance oneself from the immediate threat of a problem situation (Berk, 2001). Indeed, humor and wit may make tolerable the intolerable;

in humor, one can speak the unspeakable that one suffers. In health care, incongruity and the space that is ripe for humor lie between the present reality for the person or family, and the illness condition or even the health care institution itself. By laughing at the gap that exists, several socioemotional and cognitive things happen. The *elephant in the room* is acknowledged by making some element of the ideal become the butt of the joke. This reduces the emotion (e.g., fear, anger) created by the perceived size of the gap, which leads to creative thoughts about alternative ways to see, think, or feel. This shift reduces the amount of power given to the *perception* of the ideal, which switches, at least, the cognitive or emotional power to the individual so there can be movement toward solutions that can actually reduce the size of the gap, even if only emotionally.

Technique

It may be as subtle as a smile and a quick glance that assures the other you caught what he just did or said, or as overt as donning a red nose or Spock ears. Several intervention starter ideas are provided in Exhibit 8.2. The ideas presented are merely starting suggestions. Personal preferences and skill levels will determine what eventually gets added to each nurse's humor toolbox.

Exhibit 8.2. *Simple Therapeutic Humor—Starter Ideas*

Brief Descriptions	Comments
Set your heart to focus on others.	An "other" focus is always the place to begin.
View humorous videos.	Much humor and laughter research compares data between subjects who have and have not viewed funny videos. Funny videos positively affect people in many physiological and emotional ways.
Read and listen to funny material.	Internet sites have boosted volume and access to a wide array of fun resources. Old standards written or recorded by funny authors, including Erma Bombeck, Bill Cosby, Dave Barry, and Steve Allen, can also be used.
Take time to do something fun.	It is beneficial if the nurse considers: when was the last time I did something fun just because it would be fun to do?
Share something funny with another person.	Humor is a seed that, when sown, might grow to be even funnier next time it appears.

(continued)

Exhibit 8.2. *Simple Therapeutic Humor—Starter Ideas (continued)*

Brief Descriptions	Comments
Lead or join a Laughter Club.	Visit www.worldlaughtertour.com for details.
Create your own personal humor collection.	Find small items that can fit into your pocket. Red noses can be a staple because they are small and inexpensive; clean ones may be used and new ones given away. Puppets can be great and come in a wide range of types, sizes, and characters.
Dress up your uniform and/ or accessories.	Paint a smiley face on your stethoscope; embroider or draw a silly name onto your uniform pocket; have a certain pair of scrubs that you have patients sign at a certain milestone.
Hold silly parades.	These are fun, especially if census is low and you are aware of every patient's ability to enjoy it.
Create a list of caring clowns.	Call on them for special as well as ordinary days. A number of websites can help you get connected. Search the Internet: "caring clowns."
Keep an eye out for the perfect time.	Remember the element of surprise. If a humor intervention becomes too predictable, it will lose some of its effectiveness. Just be aware of situations. When you see an opportunity, *take it*; use humor while the timing is right.
Think in terms of . . .	. . . fill in the blanks. Explore all six senses (sight, hearing, touch, smell, taste, and *humor*) as you consider these starter ideas: rhyming words, nonsensical explanations, facial expressions, made-up (or not) songs, physical incongruities such as entering a room walking backward rather than forward, repetition and overexaggeration (until they get it that you're joking), balloons or other soft-tossing items. The list is endless once your imagination is engaged.
Be open to their leads.	Does your patient tell jokes? Then laugh at the punch line and come up with your own in response (that day or the next). The principle is that when they give you the lead, *respond*.

There are numerous resources available to use to develop one's humor intervention potential. Search the Internet for resources that can help you with your particular area of interest, such as cancer or aging. Selected sources that are readily available and provide direct access to reliable researchers and practitioners, including pioneers in the field, are listed in Exhibit 8.3.

Exhibit 8.3. *Selected Humor Resources*

For comprehensive academic study, consider taking the online course created by one of the first contemporary humor researchers, Paul McGhee: Humor and Nursing I: Impact of Humor and Laughter on Physical Health: (www.corexcel.com/courses4/humor.nursing.part1.title.htm)

Association for Applied and Therapeutic Humor (AATH) conferences explore therapeutic humor in a range of disciplines (e.g., health, education, business, and leadership). These conferences are relevant to professionals in applied fields and include many how-to sessions: (www.aath.org/humor-academy)

International Society for Humor Studies (ISHS) is an organization to join to interact with and be informed by the leading researchers in the field. The international and multidisciplinary nature of this organization helps deepen one's scholarly understanding of humor theories, how humor and comedy work, and how deeply humor exists in and impacts the human condition. (www.hnu.edu/ishs)

Journal of Nursing Jocularity (JNJ) is a site developed by Karyn Buxman to blog humor-in-nursing stories, to read other nurses' stories, and review occasional educational articles. (www.journalofnursingjocularity.karynbuxman.com)

World Laughter Tour, Inc. This organization provides certification for Certified Laughter Leaders, and academic credit from Columbus State Community College, Columbus, OH. (www.worldlaughtertour.com)

Guidelines

Regardless of the technique, the primary considerations when applying therapeutic humor should be:

- *Have your heart right.* Focus on the needs of the patient and family members. Keep *their* best interests at the center of your decisions.
- *Tune your senses.* Be keen to patients' present situation or condition so the humor initiated is appropriate, at least to the extent you are able to assess the environment.
- *Be quick to accept their invitation.* While attending to the patient's and/ or the family's needs, pay close attention so, when patients and/or their family members initiate or plant a humorous seed, you can respond and give the moment real life. One of the truly genius benefits of therapeutic humor is the planting of the seed for an eventual twist, or in the way some simple element from a collective past emerges in a different context, this time as humor, as illustrated in the "Circle of Laugh" (see Sidebar 8.1). Accepting their invitation

Sidebar 8.1. *The "Circle of Laugh" in the Far East*

Interview with Deb Gauldin, Raleigh, NC, United States

Deb Gauldin is a nurse–humorist who has entertained and inspired hardworking nurses across the Far East. Concerned about language barriers, cultural differences, and whether Asian nurses would even relate to her stories, Deb was prepared for a reserved response at best during her first visit.

In large conference-type settings, where nurses typically expect serious, didactic content, Deb found simply approaching the platform carrying her guitar was enough to elicit cheering. Even with translation delays, the nurses wiped tears from their eyes and laughed with abandon.

Among small groups of non-English-speaking nurses in Vietnam, Cambodia, China, and Bali, the nurses would follow along and pantomime their understanding with equal enthusiasm. Even in the most primitive or remote surroundings, there was never a time when this therapeutic humor specialist felt culture was a barrier to sharing laughter and appreciation. There was, however, a time when politics interfered.

Deb was to meet with nurses who were traveling into Katmandu, Nepal, via bus. A frantic call came from one of the nurses coordinating the evening. The main road into the city had been barricaded with burning tires as part of a demonstration against Communist authority. It was logistically impossible and moreover unsafe for the Nepali nurses to proceed.

According to Deb, those who did attend seemed unshaken. Katmandu was a city where electric power was only available 4 hours per day. Abandoned children lay in doorways huddled with stray dogs for warmth. "These nurses define resiliency," Deb recalls. Everywhere she went, they greeted her with warmth and openness and laughed heartily.

At one point Deb asked about general working conditions and whether they viewed their workplaces as positive environments. After a pause, an older woman described an incident. A nurse working at the nearby Public Hospital was pushed through a patient's room window by a disgruntled family member.

Deb said if she had any doubt about how humor serves as a universal bond among nurses, it was put to rest later in the evening. Just before her closing song—in which she sang of wistfully imagining a school of nursing where orphaned children could study at no charge—she interrupted herself to inquire about whether there was, in fact, a shortage of nurses in Nepal.

(continued)

Sidebar 8.1. *The "Circle of Laugh" in the Far East (continued)*

From a far corner came the voice of a young nurse who had been quiet throughout the evening. "I hear there is an opening for a nurse at the Public Hospital," she said, grinning.

This quip illustrates how humor emerges when something (initially humorous or not) circles back into the conversation. In essence, it becomes the "Circle of Laugh."

With the reassurance that smiling and laughter are universal languages indicating positive emotions, nurses can feel quite confident that humor is, in fact, an appropriate complementary therapy. As a rule, however, nurses should begin initial humor interactions with new patients from other cultures with respectful caution.

---

to lighten up serves at least two purposes. First, it helps you pass their test to see whether you are there for the patient or for the illness (or the hospital's rules, the head nurse, the end of your shift, and so on). It is a subtle difference, but humor can help assure the patient and family that your presence is for *their* well-being. Second, it communicates to them that you not only have a sense of humor, but that it is available to be shared. In other words, you're not just a competent nurse, you're fun as well (and competent, fun nurses make it easier to trust).

Beyond the three core guidelines, retain eye contact. This is important so you can gauge your effectiveness. Keep eye contact long enough for the recipient to *get it*—that the humor gesture you just shared was from a caring place in your heart. This is where the therapy demonstrates itself as an art form. Study the style of famous comedians such as Jack Benny, Johnny Carson, or David Letterman, for example. When they expect a laugh that hasn't come yet, the comic just stares at the audience or into the camera until the audience gets it and laughs. In much the same way, the eye contact, even if subtle, sends a powerful message and confirms that one's application of humor was received as intended.

Measurement of Effectiveness

Measurements can be made that are appropriate to the patient's condition and consistent with the intent or goal for which the intervention was delivered—measurements appropriate to judge the outcome for which therapeutic humor was used. For example, if the intent of the use of therapeutic humor was to reduce stress, a measure of perceived stress could be used such as the Perceived Stress Scale (Cohen, 2012). If therapeutic humor is used to promote comfort (or pain reduction) or positive emotions (or relief of negative emotions), self-report scales of comfort, pain relief, or emotions/mood may be used such as a visual analog scale for pain, or the Profile of Mood States™ (Heuchert & McNair, 2012) for moods. A number of biophysiological measures could also be used (e.g., blood pressure or heart rate). In conducting research, a number of serum measures that have been used by investigators are described in Exhibit 8.1. The timing of measurement may be immediately on completion of the intervention or at a later time, keeping in mind that the benefits of therapeutic humor may extend beyond humor or laughter.

If the humor attempt does not appear to be working, be prepared to shift quickly and gauge what adjustments need to be made. Some logical first steps include:

- Soften your approach
- Imply that you recognize your attempt at humor wasn't the right call at that moment
- Offer an apology and return to the patient's medical needs

If a patient or family does not respond to an initial humor attempt, this does not necessarily mean humor will never be appropriate with these individuals. Such a determination only can be made once the nurse has spent more time with the client, and after the nurse has had the opportunity to develop a trusting relationship.

PRECAUTIONS

As with any procedural intervention, nurses using therapeutic humor must remain sensitive to the reaction and receptivity of the patient and family members. The nurse must know the health condition of the client and what is appropriate. Other than with an asthmatic patient or another compromised pulmonary condition such as chronic obstructive pulmonary disease (COPD)—or with a few other conditions such as those affecting the CV system, or a person with fresh stitches or fractured ribs—therapeutic humor carries little risk for serious adverse health impacts. It is possible that the nurse's well-intended use of therapeutic humor may not always be well received. Although this may undermine relationship-building efforts, no lasting physical harm is done; the relationship can be built and nourished in other ways over time. Six caveats are identified.

- Although humor itself is not physically dangerous, nurses should use care if extended, mirthful laughter is initiated with patients with pulmonary (Lebowitz, Suh, Diaz, & Emery, 2011) or heart conditions.

Because laughter is a physiological process that involves the entire pulmonary and cardiovascular systems, care must be taken so humor interventions do not stimulate considerable, sustained laughter unless authorized and under careful monitoring. Brutsche and colleagues (2008) found similar results to Lebowitz et al. (2011), but also found that smiling induced by a humor intervention was able to reduce hyperinflation in patients with severe COPD. Their work suggests that smiling-derived breathing techniques may complement pursed-lips breathing. When providing nursing care to these patients, be confident that the smile, chuckle, and emotional boosts from a humor intervention can provide considerable benefit; however, be cautious when a patient begins to laugh exuberantly.

■ Some unknown considerations when interacting with new patients involve their personal history with humor, sense of humor, or humor style. One woman shared that when her brother broke his arm, the entire family was doubled over with laughter—even as they reached the hospital. Emergency department staff had trouble identifying whom to treat amid the hysteria of the family interaction. The woman clarified that it was the family's typical [unusual] response to when a family member gets hurt. Indeed, some families laugh hysterically at and with each other, even during stressful times; others become serious and believe being ill or injured is no laughing matter. Paying close attention to the cues they provide (verbal and nonverbal, including items they carry with them or post nearby) and spending time with patients and their families will help you pick up the clues you need to make the correct decisions most of the time.

■ As with all humor attempts early in a nurse–patient relationship, if the patient fails to chuckle as a result, it's not a full picture of the patient's receptivity to or capacity for humor; however, it can provide a starting point for further assessments as your engagement with this client continues. *Start slowly.* As your relationship with the patient matures, humor can be developed in the context of the therapeutic relationship.

■ Beware of the potential for a clash of the humor styles. High-humor nurses should be careful to read their patients or other audience carefully so low-humor patients are not disenfranchised by someone who is overly chipper or attempting humor too soon.

■ Watch the noise. Because most health care environments need to remain quiet out of respect for other patients (Maser, 2012), use caution to engage techniques that, most predictably, will result in volume appropriate for the setting.

■ In general, the results of a therapeutic humor intervention are easiest to predict when shared among people with a somewhat similar culture and ethnicity. In these situations, people tend to share values, beliefs, and norms that help them understand and contribute to shared humor. In essence, the language is familiar enough so everyone understands how to interpret the words or actions. When interacting with people of other cultures, it is also important to remember another law of comedy that, again, can be explained by using the gap described earlier. Individuals in a lesser position, whether real or perceived (e.g., social, economic, political, hierarchical), may laugh at or make fun of people or situations of The Ideal/The Powerful, but they may not make fun *downward*. For example, a high-income (real or perceived), 45-year-old Caucasian male is fair game for most of the world, but such men may *not*, publicly, make fun of persons of lower condition—determined by the receiver's perception (e.g., lower income, different race, poorer health, noticeably older or younger). Such a politically incorrect attempt at humor hurts and is sure to erase the opportunity to build a trusting relationship, possibly for a long time. People of higher status within any given interaction are free to make fun of themselves or their situation, but they may not make fun of a person or the condition of one of a less-fortunate status. Similarly, professionals should avoid the three most sensitive subjects—politics, religion, and race—when choosing where to find their humor. These are sure to serve a contrary purpose every time.

USES

Given these caveats, when used correctly, humor can be offered as a signal to a patient that "you and I are on the same plane." Elaine Tagliareni, RN, chief program officer with the National League for Nursing, has studied the concept of *other*, and how individuality and personhood are intimately tied to relationships. "Relationships with others involve an ethic of caring and responsibility, vulnerability, and being touched in a unique way, all elements that are at the very core of the nursing experience" (Tagliareni, 2008). Regarding the use of humor: if you considered the other person as different, then you would not attempt the humor because you would assume the recipient would not understand it enough to respond appropriately. Humor communicates, "We may be different in some ways, but not so many that we can't share a smile together." In any new relationship, it is wise to employ the complementary therapy with some extra care; however, therapeutic humor still holds considerable power to bridge gaps and build relationships, even among people of differing ethnic backgrounds, cultures, and ages.

Therapeutic Humor With Children

Regardless of age, humor provides important social and emotional functions in children. Joking and laughing about taboo topics and things that make them anxious help children manage negative emotions—especially in unfamiliar and threatening environments, as is often the case involving health care.

Just as children have cognitive and physical stages of development, they also have developmental stages in understanding and applying humor—from physical to cognitive. In general, infants understand touch signals (snuggles that make them giggle, playful tickling); toddlers respond with glee to physical humor ranging from peek-a-boo to pratfalls. Preschoolers and early-elementary-age children love more cognitive types of humor, such as rhyming, knock-knock jokes, and nonsense. Middle-elementary-age children are progressively more capable of creating, recognizing, and appreciating incongruity. This age range is also very rigid regarding rules, especially when they see others breaking them. Nurses are wise to make up rules, some general and others personal, for patients in this age range. Young boys age 9 and older will generally respond to "disgusting" body humor, but nurses will want to take some cues from the parents before encouraging this type humor. It may be an effective way to build a relationship with patients of this age.

Children will typically give cues early in their interaction with you as to whether or not they have coping humor strategies that can help them moderate the stress of a hospital visit or medical procedure. Children get somewhat the same benefits from coping humor as adults, such as stress reduction, pain tolerance, and relationship building, but their coping techniques tend to be fairly specific. Those with available coping skills will ask questions and seek information; use problem-focused methods (e.g., behavioral distraction); or engage in positive self-talk. They tend to not dwell on negative emotions or use catastrophic thinking (Goodenough & Ford, 2005).

Some typical humor interventions with children include hospital clowns, humor carts, clown noses and other props, puppets, funny age-appropriate videos, finger play, making funny sounds, making up funny names for some medical device or for the doctor, and creating alternative reality stories. The list is limited only to one's imagination. Whereas an initial humor intervention with lower-humor children may not be as successful as those with a higher sense of humor, it can work.

When engaging a child in therapeutic humor, be sure to watch both the reaction of the child and that of the parents. If parents are indicating any concern, provide a wink or other signal so they understand you are doing this deliberately and you need them to follow your lead to the end of the ruse, or whatever method you are using. If the parent doesn't respond, shift quickly, respecting the cue that your approach is not fitting at this time. Humor with children can result in loud reactive outbursts that may need to be toned down to appropriate noise levels for the environment.

Therapeutic Humor With the Older Individual

Older adults also deserve some special considerations when applying humor to strengthen the healing environment. Obviously, as laughter is a physiological activity, respect should be given to the patient's skeletal, cardiovascular, and pulmonary limitations. However, because humor works so well as a social bonding agent, it can be an especially effective intervention when matched with the physical, cognitive, and emotional needs of the patient—such as depression or lack of appetite.

People older than age 65 make up about 13% of the population of the United States and in 2010 were the fastest growing segment of the U.S. population (U.S. Census Bureau, 2010). Humor appreciation has been shown to diminish beyond age 65, especially; however, causes may be due to conditions as diverse as hearing loss, deteriorating mental capacity, dementia, or even because the icons from their earlier days are unknown by the younger generations, thus creating the absence of cultural cohesion—the infamous generation gap.

As one engages with patients from this population, they or their families will help others to understand their physical reasons for needing services, but they may not think to provide clues about their cognitive, social, or emotional condition that can help to determine how best to help them with their original health concern.

Nursing education typically provides considerable attention to the physical care needs of the aging person, including how to manage those with declining cognition and deteriorating skeletal–muscular conditions. Little, if any, attention is given to an important self-perception that therapeutic humor can overcome in an instant—their feelings of invisibility (Bunkers, 2001). Spontaneous humor calls for keen attention to detail. By picking up on or initiating humor with older patients, you are saying to them, "I notice you, you are 'normal' to me, and I care about your well-being—physical and emotional." In short, humor provides the opportunity to connect as real people.

Well-placed humor can be used as an effective initial assessment that can impact your ability to engage older patients fully in care that optimizes their health. The easiest assessment will be if the patient or family initiates the humor. In this case, respond and appreciate the ease with which the family is setting you up for a positive interaction. As a professional assessment, their humor initiation also provides an indication of this patient's cognitive capacity and social well-being, at least as an initial indicator.

If the humor is not patient initiated, then continue with your nursing procedures, staying ever-aware of the first opportunity to test the waters for an appropriate, well-timed humor *test*. A simple test for cognition could be a silly incongruity joke such as: *Q: Where do you take a sick boat? A: To a dock.* As with all humor attempts early in a nurse–patient relationship, if the patient fails to chuckle as a result, it's not a full picture of the client's cognitive capabilities or overall sense of humor, but it can provide a starting point for understanding and knowing this person. Beyond the covert assessment value, the older patient may especially appreciate the humor intervention simply because it can stimulate further conversation, allow the other to be heard, and it communicates an extra measure of caring.

At the very least, older patients will look forward to seeing you again. In this way, you not only will be assuring these patients of their visibility, importance, and that they are deserving of the best care possible, you will be sharing that little secret weapon for the benefit of their health—you got them to smile. In this smile, you improved the well-being of their minds and bodies.

Self-Care

Therapeutic humor is not only for the benefit of patients. Given the intense, highly unpredictable and ever-changing environment of today's health care settings, nurses can use humor for personal benefits as well. Nurses are encouraged to make and find humor resources that suit their personal tastes. As has been repeated throughout this chapter, even the anticipation of humorous activities can help relieve stress. By using humor to help balance one's own well-being, one becomes more understanding of how therapeutic humor can benefit others.

Therapeutic humor helps reassure the ill and ailing that they are people, first. It enhances a nurse's ability to connect with patients quickly and in ways not yet fully understood. However, therapeutic humor is gaining ground as one of the therapies nurses can call on as a caring professional. Even as empirical evidence continues to reveal the strengths and limitations of this intriguing human phenomenon, nurses are encouraged to build their knowledge and skills so therapeutic humor can be accountably and artfully applied as a responsible complementary therapy.

CULTURAL CONSIDERATIONS

Therapeutic Humor With East Asian Populations

Although humor within populations is a universal social phenomenon, it is also culturally specific, based on that group's own set of values, beliefs, and norms. Verbal humor requires knowledge of word meaning—an obvious barrier across cultural lines. For humor to work therapeutically requires an understanding of the culture's interpretation of nonverbal cues, as well as the culture's relationship with humor, health care, and illness. Complicating the impact further is the patient's biophysical, psychological, and spiritual states of being at that moment (Pasquali, 1990). Therapeutic humor in care situations that involve non-English-speaking patients and clients from foreign countries requires extra consideration. Athough humor may work well as a healing modality in one cultural context, one cannot be assured that it will work the same way in another.

Josepha Campinha-Bacote (2007), an expert in cultural competence in health care, defines cultural competence in terms of four constructs: cultural awareness, cultural knowledge, cultural skill, and cultural encounter. In advocating for cultural competence, she acknowledges it is a lifelong undertaking, characterized by, among other things, humility, curiosity, and building cross-cultural skills. Interestingly, in one preliminary study of cultural differences in therapeutic humor in nursing education (Chiang-Hanisko, Adamle, & Chiang, 2009) investigators explored the linkage between nursing theory and practice among three nursing education programs, two in the United States and one in Taiwan. This study found that the Taiwanese faculty members teach more classroom theory and concepts about therapeutic humor than the U.S.-based faculty, but that they observe and practice less therapeutic humor in clinical settings.

Zen Buddhism authority D. T. Suzuki (1971) suggests that humor is prominent in the Zen tradition. Clasquin (2001) adds that Buddhism embraces incongruity-based humor because humor helps transcend the "absurdity of the human condition" and life's incongruities by bringing Buddhists "down to earth" (p. 113). Regardless of whether Buddhism supports the principles of therapeutic humor or whether or not nursing education in East Asian countries teach it, for a variety of reasons, nurses may find it difficult to employ therapeutic humor techniques in many health care settings.

For example, despite including therapeutic humor in the didactic instruction, the Taiwanese participants in the above study indicated they practice therapeutic humor less, out of respect for the "reverence of illness" that pervades their culture. This reverence is founded in Confucianism, which, as early as the second century BCE, purported that illness may be seen as a failure to meet the obligations of filial piety. Chinese philosopher Chu His (960–1279 CE) wrote that "when a parent is ill, the son should look upset; he should neither amuse himself. . . . Only after his parent had recovered may he resume his normal way of life" (Ebrey, 1991, p. 28). Chiang-Hanisko et al. (2009) conclude that, when serving Taiwanese patients and their families, "Nurses and caregivers are expected to view hospital and clinical settings as places to uphold the cultural value of reverence of illness. This outlook must be considered before attempting to use therapeutic humor" (p. 57).

Universality of Smiling and Laughter

Sauter, Eisner, Ekman, and Scott (2010) examined the interpretation of vocalizations of emotional cues between Americans and Namibian villagers. They found that a number of negative emotions have vocalizations recognized by both cultures, but only one type of positive vocalization—laughter—was recognized by both groups. Laughter has been interpreted as a playful communication signaling joy in this and most other similar types of studies. This finding is especially meaningful when placed alongside the decades of work on facial display recognition across cultures in which the Duchenne smile is repeatedly recognized as a visual signal of amusement or joy (Elfenbein & Ambady, 2002). These findings are consistent with the experiences of nurse–humorist Deb Gauldin, who shares her story in Exhibit 8.1.

FUTURE RESEARCH

Little definitive research exists to support the use of humor as a complementary therapy. However, many professions have an interest in humor and its effects, and multidisciplinary traditions may shape the questions asked. The truth of any social science can be revealed more deeply when informed from both empirical, quantitative research—founded in experimentation (Western principles)—*and* inquiry-based, qualitative research—founded in exploring the lived experience and personal stories (Eastern principles) (Creswell, 2010). Therapeutic humor, especially in nursing, is a field ripe for mixed methods because it affects, and is affected by, physiological, socioemotional, psychological, intellectual, and even spiritual considerations specific to health and healing.

Indeed, much remains to be discovered about the impact of therapeutic humor on human health, and how to use it effectively with people with specific mental and physical health conditions. Future research should use validated scales (e.g., Ruch & Deckers, 1993; Svebak, 1974; Thorson & Powell, 1991), so the evidence base for intervention can be strengthened. Building on or using well-constructed theoretical foundations can also help to increase empirical knowledge about the effects of humor on human health. For example, the promising work within the frameworks of two other emerging interdisciplinary fields—positive psychology and caring nursing practices—may go far toward advancing knowledge in the area. Jean Watson's (1988) caring theory places the client/patient, rather than the technology, as the focus of practice and offers considerable possibilities for understanding how therapeutic humor can contribute to caring nursing practices. There is a need to connect these to fields of study: "like caring, therapeutic humor is part of the 'dance' of making a personal connection with a patient. When you can get them to smile, you have some hope of making more of that personal touch" (Dr. Jan Boller, personal communication, December 3, 2012). This sentiment is especially poignant in light of the power of the smile, an expression of positive affect. Selected areas in which nursing research is needed include the following:

■ How may humor be used to build bridges of communication and understanding in the therapeutic relationships in health care when patients and providers speak different languages, or when they are from different cultures?

■ What are the best ways to operationalize humor to promote health and healing in the context of different patient situations and circumstances such as coping with chronic health conditions (e.g., emphysema) or undergoing difficult therapies (e.g., chemotherapy)?

■ What biopsychosocial outcomes should be selected as standard measures in humor research so that more robust comparisons across studies can be made?

REFERENCES

Association for Applied and Therapeutic Humor. (2013). *What is therapeutic humor?* Retrieved from www.aath.org/general-information

Berk, L. S., Tan, S. A., & Berk, D. (2008). Cortisol and catecholamine stress hormone decrease is associated with the behavior of perceptual anticipation of mirthful laughter. *FASEB Journal, 22* (Meeting Abstract Supplement), 946.11.

Berk, L. S., Tan, L., & Tan, S. (2008). Mirthful laughter, as adjunct therapy in diabetic care, attenuates catecholamines, inflammatory cytokines, C-RP, and myocardial infarction occurrence. *FASEB Journal, 22* (Meeting Abstract Supplement), 1226.2.

Berk, R. A. (2001). The active ingredients in humor: Psychophysiological benefits and risks for older adults. *Educational Gerontology, 27,* 323–339.

Brutsche, M. H., Grossman, P., Muller, R. E., Wiegand, J., Pello, B., Baty, F., & Ruch, W. (2008). Impact of laughter on air trapping in severe chronic obstructive lung disease. *International Journal of Chronic Obstructive Pulmonary Disorders, 3*(1), 185–192.

Bunkers, S. S. (2001). Becoming invisible: Elder as teacher. *Nursing Science Quarterly, 14*(2), 115–119.

Campinha-Bacote, J. (2007). *The process of cultural competence in the delivery of health-care services: The journey continues* (5th ed.). Cincinati, OH: Transcultural C.A.R.E. Associates.

Chiang-Hanisko, L., Adamle, K., & Chiang, L. (2009). Cultural difference in therapeutic humor in nursing education. *Journal of Nursing Research, 17*(1), 52–61.

Clasquin, M. (2001). Real Buddhas don't laugh: Attitudes towards humor and laughter in ancient India and China. *Social Identities, 7*(1), 97–116.

Cohen, S. (2012). *Dr. Cohen's scales: Perceived stress scale (PSS).* Retrieved November 15, 2012, from http://www.psy.cmu.edu/~scohen/scales.html

Cousins, N. (1979). *Anatomy of an illness as perceived by the patient.* New York, NY: Norton.

Creswell, J. W. (2010). *Research design: Qualitative, quantitative and mixed methods approaches.* Thousand Oaks, CA: Sage.

Ebrey, P. B. (1991). *Chu Hsi's family rituals.* Princeton, NJ: Princeton University Press.

Ekman, P., & Friesen, W. V. (1978). *Facial action coding system (FACS).* Palo Alto, CA: Consulting Psychologists Press.

Elfenbein, H. A., & Ambady, N. (2002). On the universality and cultural specificity of emotion recognition: A meta-analysis. *Psychological Bulletin, 128,* 203–235.

Fry, W. (1963). *Sweet madness: A study of humor.* Palo Alto, CA: Pacific Books.

Gilbert, D. T., Fiske, S. T., & Lindzey, G. (1998). *The handbook of social psychology* (4th ed.). Boston, MA: McGraw-Hill.

Goodenough, B., & Ford, J. (2005). Self-reported use of humor by hospitalized pre-adolescent children to cope with pain-related distress from a medical intervention. *Humor, 18*(3), 279–298.

Heuchert, J. P., & McNair, D. M. (2013). *Profile of mood states*^{TM} (2nd ed.). North Tonawanda, NY: Multi-Health Systems, Inc. Retrieved from http://www.mhs .com/product.aspx?gr=cli&prod=poms2&id=resources

Isen, A.M. (2003). Positive affect as a source of human strength. In L. G. Aspinwall & U. M. Staudinger (Eds.), *A psychology of human strengths: Fundamental questions and future directions for a positive psychology* (pp. 179–195). Washington, D.C.: American Psychological Association.

Lebowitz, K. R., Suh, S., Diaz, P. T., & Emery, C. F. (2011). Effects of humor and laughter on psychological functioning, quality of life, health status, and pulmonary functioning among patients with chronic obstructive pulmonary disease: A preliminary investigation. *Heart & Lung, 40*(4), 310–319.

Lipman, S. (1991). *Laughter in hell: The use of humor during the Holocaust.* North Vale, NJ: Jason Aronson.

Mahony, D. L., Burroughs, W. J., & Hieatt, A. C. (2001). The effects of laughter on discomfort thresholds: Does expectation become reality? *Journal of General Psychology, 128*(2), 217–222.

Martin, R. A. (2007). *The psychology of humor: An integrative approach.* Burlington, MA: Elsevier.

Martin, R. A., & Dobbin, J. P. (1988). Sense of humor, hassles, and immunioglobulin-A: Evidence for a stress-moderating effect of humor. *International Journal of Psychiatry in Medicine, 18*, 93–105.

Maser, S. E. (2012). *Nursing, noise, and norms: Why Nightingale is still right.* Healing HealthCare Systems. Retrieved December 29, 2012, from www.healinghealth.com

McGhee, P. (1979). *Humor: Its origin and development.* San Francisco, CA: Freeman.

Miller, M., & Fry, W. F. (2009). The effect of mirthful laughter on the human cardiovascular system. *Medical Hypotheses, 73*(5), 636–639.

Mulkay, M. (1988). *On humor: Its nature and its place in modern society.* New York, NY: Basil Blackwell.

Pasquali, E. A. (1990). Learning to laugh: Humor as therapy. *Journal of Psychosocial Nursing and Mental Health Services, 28*(3), 31–35.

Ruch, W. (Ed.). (1998). *The sense of humor: Explorations of a personality characteristic.* New York, NY: Mouton de Gruyter.

Ruch, W., & Deckers, L. (1993). Do extraverts "like to laugh"? An analysis of the Situational Humor Response Questionnaire (SHRQ). *European Journal of Personality, 7*(4), 211–220.

Sauter, D. D., Eisner, F., Ekman, P., & Scott, S. K. (2010). Cross-cultural recognition of basic emotions through non-verbal emotional vocalizations. *Proceedings of the National Academy of Sciences, 107*(6), 2408–2412. Retrieved December 28, 2012, from www.pnas.org/cgi/doi/10.1073/pnas.0908239106

Schultz, W. (2002). Getting formal with dopamine and reward. *Neuron, 36*(2), 241–263.

Strack, F., Martin, L. L., & Stepper, S. (1988). Inhibiting and facilitating conditions of the human smile: A nonobtrusive test of the facial feedback hypothesis. *Journal of Abnormal & Social Psychology, 54*(5), 278–281.

Suzuki, D. T. (1971). *Sengai: The Zen master.* Greenwich, CT: New York Graphic Society.

Svebak, S. (1974). Revised questionnaire on the sense of humor. *Scandinavian Journal of Psychology, 15*, 328–331.

Svebak, S., Kristoffersen, B., & Aasarod, K. (2006). Sense of humor and survival among a county cohort of patients with end-stage renal failure: A two-year prospective study. *International Journal of Psychiatry in Medicine, 36*(3), 269–281.

Tagliareni, M. E. (2008). More like me than different: Reflections on the notion of other. *Nursing Education Perspectives, 29*(6), 322.

Thorson, J. A., & Powell, F. C. (1991). Measurement of sense of humor. *Psychological Reports, 69*, 691–702.

U.S. Census Bureau. (2010). *The older population: 2010.* Retrieved December 25, 2012, from http://www.census.gov/prod/cen2010/briefs/c2010br-09.pdf

Watson, J. (1988). *Nursing: Human science and human care. A theory of nursing.* Burlington, MA: Jones & Bartlett Learning.

Zweyer, K., Velker, B., & Ruch, W. (2004). Do cheerfulness, exhilaration, and humor production moderate pain tolerance? *Humor, 17*(1/2), 85–119.

Chapter 9: Yoga

mind body universe

Anyone can benefit from yoga, regardless of health, beliefs, age, or culture (White, 2012). The systematic practice of yoga heals body and mind. Yoga's do-it-yourself prescription for stress management and well-being has no side effects and does not require medications or expensive treatments and equipment (Noggle, Steiner, Minami, & Khalsa, 2012). Nurses practice yoga themselves and also use it as a complementary and primary therapy. Around the world, millions of people do yoga primarily for physical fitness and relaxation (Sibbritt, Adams, & van der Riet, 2011); however, yoga has a much deeper dimension (Cameron & Parker, 2004).

Yoga is a way of life to transform consciousness, as yogis for centuries have advocated and Western researchers now are discovering (Bachman, 2011). As practitioners let go of ego, which yoga teaches underlies suffering and most dis-ease, they realize that they are linked to every being, the environment, and larger forces in the universe. Grateful for this vast interconnectedness, they reach out to relieve suffering in other living beings. They sort out the unreal from the real and allow their true natures to shine. Their inner wisdom flows spontaneously through all cells of the body, promoting optimal health, inner freedom, creativity, peace, and joy (Cameron, 2002).

DEFINITION

Yoga, an ancient art and science that originated in India, means integration of mind, body, and universe. Two millennia ago, Indian sage Patanjali systematized yoga into the *Yoga Sutra*, a treatise of 196

Theory & practice

compact observations called sutras (Ravindra, 2009). This unique blend of theoretical knowledge and practical application is the primary textbook for all schools of yoga. In the *Yoga Sutra*, Patanjali analyzed how we know what we know and why we suffer. He explained that the primary purpose of consciousness is to see things as they really are and to achieve freedom from suffering. Through yoga, we can rein in our tendency to seek happiness through external phenomena. Only by turning inward and becoming aware of one's true nature, Patanjali wrote, can we understand how to develop wisdom and happiness. By becoming still, we can abide in this deep, absorptive knowing (White, 2012).

In the *Yoga Sutra*, Patanjali described yoga as consisting of eight inter-connected limbs, or aspects of the whole. Practicing these limbs simul-taneously leads to progressively higher stages of ethics, spirituality, and healing. The first five limbs still the mind and body in preparation for the last three limbs. The eight limbs, their Sanskrit names, and definitions (Ravindra, 2009) are:

1. Ethical behavior (*yama*)—nonharming, truthfulness, nonstealing, responsible sexuality, and nonacquisitiveness
2. Personal behavior (*niyama*)—purity, commitment, contentment, self-study, and surrender to the whole; *niyama* includes *sattvic* (pure) mind, food, beverages, air, and environment
3. Posture (*asana*)—physical poses that stretch, condition, and massage the body
4. Breath regulation (*pranayama*)—regulation and refinement of the breath to expand *prana* (life force) and get rid of toxins
5. Sensory inhibition (*pratyahara*)—temporary withdrawal of the senses from the external environment to the inner self, for example, by closing the eyes and looking inward
6. Concentration (*dharana*)—locking attention on an object or field, such as the breath, mantra, or image
7. Meditation (*dhyana*)—increasingly sustained attention, leading to a profound state of peace and awareness
8. Integration (*samadhi*)—a transcendent state of oneness, wisdom, and ecstasy.

The ancient Indian sacred text, *Bagavad Gita* (Mitchell, 2007), describes schools of yoga and their focus: *Kundalini Yoga*: energy; *Jnana Yoga*: knowledge; *Mantra Yoga*: recitation of sacred syllables; *Tantra Yoga*: technique; *Bhakti Yoga*: devotion; *Karma Yoga*: action, good deeds; *Raja Yoga*: control of mind and body through the eight limbs; and *Hatha Yoga*: willpower.

Hatha Yoga, which is popular in the West, consists primarily of physical postures, breathing techniques, and relaxation, despite yoga's historic quest for inner development. Hatha Yoga has many styles, including a Himalayan tradition, Tibetan Yoga, Iyengar, Ashtanga, Viniyoga, Sivananda, Kripalu, Kundalini, and hot yoga. Even when Hatha Yoga classes focus on physical fitness, they can open the door to yoga's deeper dimension (Cameron, McCall, & Prasek, 2012).

SCIENTIFIC BASIS

Yoga is based on ancient observations, principles, and theories of the mind–body connection. For thousands of years, yogis have passed down this precise knowledge from one generation to the next. Western researchers are now validating many of these health claims. Studies have found that yoga generally is a safe, therapeutic intervention that treats symptoms and/or prevents their onset and recurrence. Yoga practices are hypothesized to reduce allostatic load in stress-response systems and restore optimal homeostasis (Streeter, Gerbarg, Saper, Ciraulo, & Brown, 2012). After reviewing a variety of studies, two different research teams concluded that yoga produced considerable health benefits (Boehm, Ostermann, Milazzo, & Bussing, 2012); yoga improved cognition, respiration, immunity, and joint disorders, as well as reducing cardiovascular risk, body mass index, blood pressure, and diabetes (Balaji, Varne, & Ali, 2012).

Poor body alignment and improper breathing are major factors in health problems. Yoga decreases fatigue and improves physical fitness, balance, strength, flexibility, body alignment, and use of extremities (Galantino et al., 2012). Vital organs and endocrine glands became more efficient and the autonomic nervous system stabilizes (Büssing, Khalsa, Michalsen, Sherman, & Telles, 2012). Yoga improves quality of life and reduces anxiety (Chung, Brooks, Rai, Balk, & Rai, 2012). The systematic practice of yoga promotes a healthy lifestyle; increases exercise; and reduces smoking, alcohol consumption, and stress (Penman, Cohen, Stevens, & Jackson, 2012).

Because of these and other therapeutic effects, yoga therapy (www .iayt.org) has emerged as a discipline. Yoga practitioners use it for healing and health promotion. In several studies, yoga therapy was an effective sole or additional intervention for individuals with depression, anxiety, and schizophrenia (Bangalore & Varambally, 2012). Okonta (2012) reviewed 10 randomized controlled trials, quasiexperimental studies, and pilot studies; yoga therapy modulated the physiological system of the body, including the heart rate, and also reduced blood pressure, blood glucose levels, cholesterol levels, and body weight.

INTERVENTION

Technique

Each of Patanjali's eight limbs is a potential nursing intervention for children, adults, older subjects, pregnant women, people with a disability and/or illness, and individuals who are dying (Bryant, 2009; Ravindra, 2009). Some people need encouragement to behave with nonviolence and compassion toward self and others (limb 1). Other individuals benefit from teachings about cleanliness, nutrition, and self-discipline (limb 2). Nurses can suggest yogic poses (limb 3) and breathing techniques (limb 4) to relax and replenish body and mind (see Exhibits 9.1 and 9.2). Withdrawal of the senses can help individuals to let go of external stimuli and sleep (limb 5). Learning to concentrate and meditate can create meaning in suffering and motivation to develop optimal health (limbs 6 and 7). Through a moment of integration, individuals can experience oneness and joy, even when seriously ill or dying (limb 8) (see Exhibit 9.3).

Guidelines

The best way to learn yoga is to do it. Yoga publications, videos, online postings, and modules (www.csh.umn.edu/Integrativehealingpractices) describe guidelines for beginning through advanced levels. Some individuals use these resources to learn yoga on their own. Other people benefit from yoga classes and individual instruction. Qualified teachers can assist nurses to do yoga themselves and to use yoga as a nursing intervention (Cameron, McCall, & Prasek, 2012).

Exhibit 9.1. *Corpse Pose or Deep Relaxation* (Savasana)

1. Lie on your back with arms relaxed near your sides, palms up, and head, trunk, and legs straight. If you are uncomfortable, put a pillow or blanket under your head and/or knees.
2. Close your eyes, relax, and let your body sink.
3. Breathe in a circular manner: slowly, evenly, deeply through nostrils, from the abdomen, with the in-breath the same length as the out-breath, and no break in between.
4. When ready, open your eyes, bend your knees, turn to your right, and get up.

Corpse pose promotes deep relaxation and decreases hypertension, anxiety, insomnia, stress, and fatigue (Cameron, 2008; McCall, 2007).

Exhibit 9.2. *Alternate Nostril Breathing* (Nadi Shodhana)

1. Sit comfortably with straight back; breathe in a circular manner, as in Exhibit 9.1.
2. Place right thumb on right nostril, ring finger on left nostril, and inhale through both nostrils.
3. Use thumb to close right nostril; exhale slowly through left nostril, and then inhale slowly through left nostril.
4. Use ring finger to close left nostril; exhale slowly through right nostril, and then inhale slowly through right nostril.
5. This sequence constitutes one round; repeat for five more rounds.

This *pranayama* technique promotes balance, gives each side of the body equal time, and strengthens the breath in the weaker nostril (Cameron, 2008; McCall, 2007).

Exhibit 9.3. *Withdrawal of Senses, Concentration, Meditation*

1. Lie in corpse pose or sit comfortably with a straight back in a chair or on a meditation cushion; close eyes, relax, look inward, and breathe in a circular manner, as described in Exhibit 9.1.
2. Focus on your breath. As you inhale through your nose, silently count "one." Exhale. On the next in-breath, count, "two," and so on. When your mind wanders away, bring it back to your breath and start with one again. At 10, go back to one again.
3. When you are deeply relaxed and focused, open up to your inner experience; simply observe and let go of whatever arises, without attachment, judgment, or direction.

Concentration and meditation promote deep relaxation, healing, balance, replenishment, and development of insight and joy (Cameron, 2008; McCall, 2007).

Measurement of Outcomes

Nurses can determine the effectiveness of yoga by asking individuals how they feel after doing it. Most health problems develop over time, and yoga may not alleviate them immediately. Minor health issues may improve quickly, but serious problems require sustained, patient practice. Yoga advocates gradual change. Optimal benefits occur from systematic practice. Short-term outcomes, however—including a more relaxed attitude, decreased anxiety, improved balance, and increased musculoskeletal flexibility—are notable. Faithful practice can produce long-term outcomes of better physical, spiritual, and mental health (McCall, 2007).

Precautions

Injuries may result from doing yoga poses and breathing techniques in a harmful manner: straining to do them, competing with someone, doing them right after eating, breathing stale air while doing them, and doing them fast in a heated environment (Broad, 2012). Yoga discourages anything unnatural, competitive, or hurtful. To avoid injury, nurses can encourage gentleness, mindfulness, self-compassion, and moderation. Although teachers and other aids can be helpful, individuals must listen to their own inner wisdom (Cameron, 2008).

Currently, Hatha Yoga teachers and yoga therapists are not licensed in the United States. Some states, such as Minnesota, have passed statutes (www.revisor.mn.gov/statutes/?id=146A) to regulate unlicensed providers of complementary and alternative therapies. Ordinarily, registered nurses who use yoga as a nursing therapy are not covered by these state statutes; instead, they must adhere to the higher requirements of their state board of nursing.

Standards of Hatha Yoga schools and qualifications of yoga teachers and therapists vary widely. Yoga Alliance (www.yogaalliance.org) has developed standards for registering Hatha Yoga teachers at the 200- and 500-hour levels. Some Hatha Yoga schools use their own standards. The International Association of Yoga Therapists (www.iayt.org) has created standards for yoga therapy schools and yoga therapists. Yoga education (www.csh.umn.edu/thi/Courses/index.htm) is moving from community yoga centers into academia. Now university faculty and PhD students conduct yoga research. Teaching yoga and conducting yoga research in academic settings promote standardization and evolution of yoga into a profession.

USES

Yoga is an excellent fit with nursing because both disciplines treat the whole individual and not just the disease (Okonta, 2012). Nurses can use yoga as a separate therapy or as part of an integrated health plan. Yoga can help nurses to become healthier themselves and be a healing presence. By doing yoga and using it as an intervention, nurses promote nonreactivity of the mind and inner calmness that embraces (rather than denies) difficult circumstances in a healing manner (Cameron, 2002). Exhibit 9.4 lists recent studies about the use and effectiveness of yoga.

All over the world, people adapt yoga to their culture and values (Dalai Lama, 2011). Yoga is integral to many traditional healing systems such as Tibetan medicine and Ayurveda from India. Tibetan medicine and Ayurveda teach the importance of creating a healthy

Exhibit 9.4. *Recent Studies About Effectiveness of Yoga for Individuals With Health Issues*

Anxiety: Katzman et al. (2012); Nidhi, Padmalatha, Nagarathna, and Amritanshu (2012); Rani, Tiwari, Singh, Singh, and Srivastava (2012); Telles, Bhardwaj, Kumar, Kumar, and Balkrishna (2012); Yadav, Magan, Mehta, Mehta, and Mahapatra (2012)

Asthma: Bidwell, Yazel, Davin, Fairchild, and Kanaley (2012)

Attention and awareness: Ross, Friedmann, Bevans, and Thomas (2012); Telles, Joshi, and Somvanshi (2012)

Cancer: Bower et al. (2012); Dhruva et al. (2012)

Cardiac function: Muralikrishnan, Balakrishnan, Balasubramanian, and Visnegarawla (2012)

Chronic obstructive pulmonary disease: Fulambarker et al. (2012); Soni, Munish, Singh, and Singh (2012)

Cognition and quality of life: Froeliger, Garland, Modlin, and McClernon (2012); Rocha et al. (2012)

Depression: Chan, Immink, and Hillier (2012)

Diabetes: Jyotsna et al. (2012); Madanmohan, Bhavanani, Dayanidy, Sanjay, and Basavaraddi, (2012)

Elders' mobility and fear of falling: Galantino et al. (2012)

Inguinal hernia: Alagesan, Venkatachalam, Ramadass, and Mani (2012)

Insomnia: Kudesia and Bianchi (2012)

Intellectual disabilities: Hawkins, Stegall, Weber, and Ryan (2012)

Low back pain: Tekur, Nagarathna, Chametcha, Hankey, and Nagendra (2012)

Motor skills and visual discrimination: Telles, Singh, and Balkrishna (2012a)

Obesity: Seo et al. (2012)

Organ transplantation: Dolgoff-Kaspar, Baldwin, Johnson, Edling, and Sethi (2012)

Osteoarthritis: Ebnezar, Nagarathna, Yogitha, and Nagendra (2012)

Neurological, mental, psychiatric disorders: Meyer et al. (2012); Telles, Singh, and Balkrishna (2012b)

Pain: Sakuma et al. (2012)

(continued)

Exhibit 9.4. *Recent Studies About Effectiveness of Yoga for Individuals With Health Issues (continued)*

Palliative care: Selman, Williams, and Simms (2012)

Physical inactivity: Bryan, Pinto Zipp, and Parasher (2012)

Relaxation: Melville, Chang, Colagiuri, Marshall, and Cheema (2012)

Restless leg syndrome: Innes and Selfe (2012)

Smoking cessation: Bock et al. (2012)

Spirituality: Bussing, Hedtstuck, Khalsa, Ostermann, and Heusser (2012)

Stress and inflammation: Michalsen et al. (2012); Shankarapillai, Nair, and George (2012); Yadav, Magan, Mehta, Sharma, and Mahapatra (2012)

Well-being: Bowden, Gaudry, An, and Gruzelier (2012)

body and mind in order to live a yogic life (Cameron et al., 2012; Ninivaggi, 2008). In Sidebar 9.1, Tashi Lhamo, a Tibetan registered nurse and doctor of Tibetan medicine, explains how she uses yoga in her life and work.

Sidebar 9.1. *Use of Yoga Foundations From Tibet and India*

Tashi Lhamo, Tibet and India

My parents grew up in Tibet. Because I wanted to help others, I decided to become a doctor of Tibetan medicine. I graduated from the Tibetan Medical Institute of His Holiness the Dalai Lama in Dharamsala, India. After practicing Tibetan medicine in a clinic in India, I immigrated to the United States, worked as a nursing assistant, and studied nursing. Now I work as a registered nurse on a busy medical–surgical unit of a large metropolitan hospital. I do Tibetan medicine consultations on the side. Yoga is essential to my practice of nursing and Tibetan medicine.

Yoga means to unite or join physical, mental, and spiritual faculties mindfully. Integration and harmony promote optimal health. Down

(continued)

Sidebar 9.1. *Use of Yoga Foundations From
Tibet and India (continued)*

through the ages, the great Indian and Buddhist yogis have devoted
their lives to training the body and mind in order to develop physical,
mental, and spiritual balance. These sages have engaged in yoga practices to keep themselves healthy while pursuing their spiritual quest.
The scientific community has started to take this ancient wisdom seriously. Recently, scores of scientific studies have been published that document the effectiveness of yoga on body and mind. Increasingly, nurses
and other health care providers, athletes, business people, leaders in
various disciplines, and everyday individuals are embracing yoga as a
means to optimize their productivity and well-being.

Yoga and Tibetan medicine share the same principles about balancing vital energies and creating equilibrium. In my 13 years of practicing Tibetan medicine and 4 years of working as a nurse, yoga not only
has helped me to provide quality care for my patients but also to keep
myself healthy physically, mentally, and spiritually. Yoga teaches me to be
mindful of my surroundings while caring for patients, and to treat each
one with genuine compassion, love, and equanimity. Medical–surgical
nursing can be very stressful. Yoga can help stressed-out nurses to care
for their patients and themselves, and to increase their productivity and
happiness.

FUTURE RESEARCH

Research studies about yoga generally report positive effects. The benefits of yoga in each study may depend on participants' characteristics
(age, gender, health status, and diagnosis), study entry criteria, type and
duration of the yoga intervention, compliance, attrition, and related factors. Because yoga is a relatively new field of research, most studies are
pilot studies with small sample sizes, short study periods, methodological
flaws, inadequate control groups, and other limitations. The lack of standardized practices and the variety of yoga styles complicate applicability
of the results (Büssing et al., 2012).

Yoga's holistic, integrated approach poses challenges for conducting
scientific research. Yoga practices affect body and mind in a manner that
may not be reproducible and quantifiable. Teasing out specific aspects of
yoga is difficult and may not produce statistically significant results. Even
so, the National Center for Complementary and Alternative Medicine
(NCCAM, 2013) at the National Institutes of Health is funding many yoga
studies with promising results (see reference for NCCAM website listing).

Nursing would benefit from well-designed studies that address these research questions:

- Which yoga practices are therapeutic for which health issues?
- How can individuals be encouraged to do yoga regularly?
- Why do some people experience injuries from yoga, and what can be done to decrease the incidence of yoga injuries?
- What are effective strategies for teaching nurses to do yoga?
- What qualifications and standards are needed for nurses to teach and do yoga effectively, ethically, and safely?
- How can yoga therapy be integrated into nursing?

Qualitative methodologies are needed to study yoga as a holistic healing system. Studying the deeper dimension of yoga, rather than focusing on postures and breathing, will enrich the findings. Additional research will promote understanding and use of this fascinating therapy in nursing.

REFERENCES

Alagesan, J., Venkatachalam, S., Ramadass, A., & Mani, S. B. (2012). Effect of yoga therapy in reversible inguinal hernia: A quasi experimental study. *International Journal of Yoga, 5*(1), 16–20.

Bachman, N. (2011). *The path of the yoga sutras: A practical guide to the core of yoga.* Boulder, CO: Sounds True.

Balaji, P. A., Varne, S. R., & Ali, S. S. (2012). Physiological effects of yogic practices and transcendental meditation in health and disease. *North American Journal of Medical Sciences, 4*(10), 442–448.

Bangalore, N. G., & Varambally, S. (2012). Yoga therapy for schizophrenia. *International Journal of Yoga, 5*(2), 85–91.

Bidwell, A. J., Yazel, B., Davin, D., Fairchild, T. J., & Kanaley, J. A. (2012). Yoga training improves quality of life in women with asthma. *Journal of Alternative & Complementary Medicine, 18*(8), 749–755.

Bock, B. C., Fava, J. L., Gaskins, R., Morrow, K. M., Williams, D. M., Jennings, E., . . . Marcus, B. H. (2012). Yoga as a complementary treatment for smoking cessation in women. *Journal of Women's Health, 21*(2), 240–248.

Boehm, K., Ostermann, T., Milazzo, S., & Bussing, A. (2012). Effects of yoga interventions on fatigue: A meta-analysis. *Evidence-Based Complementary & Alternative Medicine: ECAM, 2012*: 124703.

Bowden, D., Gaudry, C., An, S. C., & Gruzelier, J. (2012). A comparative randomised controlled trial of the effects of brain wave vibration training, Iyengar Yoga, and mindfulness on mood, well-being, and salivary cortisol. *Evidence-Based Complementary & Alternative Medicine: ECAM, 234713.*

Bower, J. E., Garet, D., Sternlieb, B., Ganz, P. A., Irwin, M. R., Olmstead, R., . . . Greendale, G. (2012). Yoga for persistent fatigue in breast cancer survivors: A randomized controlled trial. *Cancer, 118*(15), 3766–3775.

Broad, W. (2012). *The science of yoga: Risks and rewards.* New York, NY: Simon & Schuster.

Bryan, S., Pinto Zipp, G., & Parasher, R. (2012). The effects of yoga on psychosocial variables and exercise adherence: A randomized, controlled pilot study. *Alternative Therapies in Health & Medicine, 18*(5), 50–59.

Bryant, E. F. (2009). *The yoga sutras of Patanjali: A new edition, translation, and commentary.* New York, NY: North Point Press.

Büssing, A., Hedtstuck, A., Khalsa, S. B., Ostermann, T., & Heusser, P. (2012). Development of specific aspects of spirituality during a 6-month intensive yoga practice. *Evidence-Based Complementary & Alternative Medicine: ECAM,* 981523.

Büssing, A., Khalsa, S. B. S., Michalsen, A., Sherman, K. J., & Telles, S. (2012). Yoga as a therapeutic intervention. *Evidence-Based Complementary & Alternative Medicine: ECAM,* 174291.

Cameron, M. (2008). The essence of yoga: Ethics, spirituality, and healing. *Wellnessworks, 3*(1), 18–20.

Cameron, M. E. (2002). *Karma & happiness: A Tibetan odyssey in ethics, spirituality, and healing* (Foreword by His Holiness the Dalai Lama). New York, NY: Rowman & Littlefield.

Cameron, M. E., McCall, T., & Prasek, A. (2012). *Yoga.* University of Minnesota, Center for Spirituality & Healing online module: http://www.csh.umn.edu/Integrativehealingpractices/

Cameron, M. E., & Parker, S. A. (2004). The ethical foundation of yoga. *Journal of Professional Nursing, 5,* 275–276.

Cameron, M. E., Torkelson, C., Haddow, S., Namdul, T., Prasek, A., & Gross, C. R. (2012). Tibetan medicine and integrative health: Validity testing and refinement of the constitutional self-assessment tool and lifestyle guidelines tool. *EXPLORE: The Journal of Science and Healing, 8*(3), 158–171.

Chan, W., Immink, M. A., & Hillier, S. (2012). Yoga and exercise for symptoms of depression and anxiety in people with poststroke disability: A randomized, controlled pilot trial. *Alternative Therapies in Health & Medicine, 18*(3), 34–43.

Chung, S. C., Brooks, M. M., Rai, M., Balk, J. L., & Rai, S. (2012). Effect of sahaja yoga meditation on quality of life, anxiety, and blood pressure control. *Journal of Alternative & Complementary Medicine, 18*(6), 589–596.

Dalai Lama. (2011). *Beyond religion: Ethics for a whole world.* New York, NY: Houghton Mifflin Harcourt.

Dhruva, A., Miaskowski, C., Abrams, D., Acree, M., Cooper, B., Goodman, S., & Hecht, F. M. (2012). Yoga breathing for cancer chemotherapy-associated symptoms and quality of life: Results of a pilot randomized controlled trial. *Journal of Alternative & Complementary Medicine, 18*(5), 473–479.

Dolgoff-Kaspar, R., Baldwin, A., Johnson, M. S., Edling, N., & Sethi, G. K. (2012). Effect of laughter yoga on mood and heart rate variability in patients awaiting organ transplantation: A pilot study. *Alternative Therapies in Health & Medicine, 18*(5), 61–66.

Ebnezar, J., Nagarathna, R., Yogitha, B., & Nagendra, H. R. (2012). Effects of an integrated approach of hatha yoga therapy on functional disability, pain, and flexibility in osteoarthritis of the knee joint: A randomized controlled study. *Journal of Alternative & Complementary Medicine, 18*(5), 463–472.

Froeliger, B. E., Garland, E. L., Modlin, L. A., & McClernon, F. J. (2012). Neurocognitive correlates of the effects of yoga meditation practice on emotion and cognition: A pilot study. *Frontiers in Integrative Neuroscience, 6,* 48.

Fulambarker, A., Farooki, B., Kheir, F., Copur, A. S., Srinivasan, L., & Schultz, S. (2012). Effect of yoga in chronic obstructive pulmonary disease. *American Journal of Therapeutics, 19*(2), 96–100.

Galantino, M. L., Green, L., Decesari, J. A., Mackain, N. A., Rinaldi, S. M., Stevens, M. E., . . . Mao, J. J. (2012). Safety and feasibility of modified chair-yoga on functional outcome among elderly at risk for falls. *International Journal of Yoga, 5*(2), 146–150.

Hawkins, B. L., Stegall, J. B., Weber, M. F., & Ryan, J. B. (2012). The influence of a yoga exercise program for young adults with intellectual disabilities. *International Journal of Yoga, 5*(2), 151–156.

Innes, K. E., & Selfe, T. K. (2012). The effects of a gentle yoga program on sleep, mood, and blood pressure in older women with restless legs syndrome (RLS): A preliminary randomized controlled trial. *Evidence-Based Complementary & Alternative Medicine: ECAM, 294058.*

Jyotsna, V. P., Joshi, A., Ambekar, S., Kumar, N., Dhawan, A., & Sreenivas, V. (2012). Comprehensive yogic breathing program improves quality of life in patients with diabetes. *Indian Journal of Endocrinology and Metabolism, 16*(3), 423–428.

Katzman, M. A., Vermani, M., Gerbarg, P. L., Brown, R. P., Iorio, C., Davis, M., . . . Tsirgielis, D. (2012). A multicomponent yoga-based, breath intervention program as an adjunctive treatment in patients suffering from generalized anxiety disorder with or without comorbidities. *International Journal of Yoga, 5*(1), 57–65.

Kudesia, R. S., & Bianchi, M. T. (2012). Decreased nocturnal awakenings in young adults performing Bikram Yoga: A low-constraint home sleep monitoring study. *ISRN Neurology Print, 2012,* 153745.

Madanmohan, Bhavanani, A. B., Dayanidy, G., Sanjay, Z., & Basavaraddi, I. V. (2012). Effect of yoga therapy on reaction time, biochemical parameters and wellness score of peri and post-menopausal diabetic patients. *International Journal of Yoga, 5*(1), 10–15.

McCall, T. (2007). *Yoga as medicine.* New York, NY: Bantam Books.

Melville, G. W., Chang, D., Colagiuri, B., Marshall, P. W., & Cheema, B. S. (2012). Fifteen minutes of chair-based yoga postures or guided meditation performed in the office can elicit a relaxation response. *Evidence-Based Complementary & Alternative Medicine: ECAM, 501986.*

Meyer, H. B., Katsman, A., Sones, A. C., Auerbach, D. E., Ames, D., & Rubin, R. T. (2012). Yoga as an ancillary treatment for neurological and psychiatric disorders: A review. *Journal of Neuropsychiatry & Clinical Neurosciences, 24*(2), 152–164.

Michalsen, A., Jeitler, M., Brunnhuber, S., Ludtke, R., Bussing, A., Musial, F., . . . Kessler, C. (2012). Iyengar yoga for distressed women: A 3-armed randomized controlled trial. *Evidence-Based Complementary & Alternative Medicine: ECAM, 408727.*

Mitchell, S. (2007). *Bhagavad Gita: A new translation.* New York, NY: Three Rivers Press.

Muralikrishnan, K., Balakrishnan, B., Balasubramanian, K., & Visnegarawla, F. (2012). Measurement of the effect of Isha Yoga on cardiac autonomic nervous system using short-term heart rate variability. *Journal of Ayurveda and Integrative Medicine, 3*(2), 91–96.

National Center for Complementary and Alternative Therapies (NCCAM). (2013). *Yoga.* Retrieved from search2.google.cit.nih.gov/search?q=yoga&site=NCCAM&client=NCCAM_frontend&proxystylesheet=NCCAM_frontend&output=xml_no_dtd&filter=0&getfields=*&proxyreload=1&x=7&y=8

Nidhi, R., Padmalatha, V., Nagarathna, R., & Amritanshu, R. (2012). Effect of holistic yoga program on anxiety symptoms in adolescent girls with polycystic ovarian syndrome: A randomized control trial. *International Journal of Yoga, 5*(2), 112–117.

Ninivaggi, F. J. (2008). *Ayurveda: A comprehensive guide to traditional Indian medicine for the West.* Westport, CT: Praeger.

Noggle, J. J., Steiner, N. J., Minami, T., & Khalsa, S. B. (2012). Benefits of yoga for psychosocial well-being in a US high school curriculum: A preliminary randomized controlled trial. *Journal of Developmental & Behavioral Pediatrics, 33*(3), 193–201.

Okonta, N. R. (2012). Does yoga therapy reduce blood pressure in patients with hypertension? *Holistic Nursing Practice, 26*(3), 137–141.

Penman, S., Cohen, M., Stevens, P., & Jackson, S. (2012). Yoga in Australia: Results of a national survey. *International Journal of Yoga, 5*(2), 92–101.

Rani, K., Tiwari, S., Singh, U., Singh, I., & Srivastava, N. (2012). Yoga Nidra as a complementary treatment of anxiety and depressive symptoms in patients with menstrual disorder. *International Journal of Yoga, 5*(1), 52–56.

Ravindra, R. (2009). *The wisdom of Patanjali's Yoga Sutras: A new translation and guide.* Sandpoint, ID: Morning Light Press.

Rocha, K. K., Ribeiro, A. M., Rocha, K. C., Sousa, M. B., Albuquerque, F. S., Ribeiro, S., . . . Silva, R. H. (2012). Improvement in physiological and psychological parameters after 6 months of yoga practice. *Consciousness & Cognition, 21*(2), 843–850.

Ross, A., Friedmann, E., Bevans, M., & Thomas, S. (2012). Frequency of yoga practice predicts health: Results of a national survey of yoga practitioners. *Evidence-Based Complementary & Alternative Medicine: ECAM, 12*, 2012: 983258.

Sakuma, Y., Sasaki-Otomaru, A., Ishida, S., Kanoya, Y., Arakawa, C., Mochizuki, Y., . . . Sato, C. (2012). Effect of a home-based simple yoga program in child-care workers: A randomized controlled trial. *Journal of Alternative & Complementary Medicine, 18*(8), 769–776.

Selman, L. E., Williams, J., & Simms, V. (2012). A mixed-methods evaluation of complementary therapy services in palliative care: Yoga and dance therapy. *European Journal of Cancer Care, 21*(1), 87–97.

Seo, D. Y., Lee, S., Figueroa, A., Kim, H. K., Baek, Y. H., Kwak, Y. S., . . . Han, J. (2012). Yoga training improves metabolic parameters in obese boys. *Korean Journal of Physiology & Pharmacology, 16*(3), 175–180.

Shankarapillai, R., Nair, M. A., & George, R. (2012). The effect of yoga in stress reduction for dental students performing their first periodontal surgery: A randomized controlled study. *International Journal of Yoga, 5*(1), 48–51.

Sibbritt, D., Adams, J., & van der Riet, P. (2011). The prevalence and characteristics of young and mid-age women who use yoga and meditation: Results of a nationally representative survey of 19,209 Australian women. *Complementary Therapies in Medicine, 19*(2), 71–77.

Soni, R., Munish, K., Singh, K., & Singh, S. (2012). Study of the effect of yoga training on diffusion capacity in chronic obstructive pulmonary disease patients: A controlled trial. *International Journal of Yoga, 5*(2), 123–127.

Streeter, C. C., Gerbarg, P. L., Saper, R. B., Ciraulo, D. A., & Brown, R. P. (2012). Effects of yoga on the autonomic nervous system, gamma-aminobutyric-acid, and allostasis in epilepsy, depression, and post-traumatic stress disorder. *Medical Hypotheses, 78*(5), 571–579.

Tekur, P., Nagarathna, R., Chametcha, S., Hankey, A., & Nagendra, H. R. (2012). A comprehensive yoga program improves pain, anxiety and depression in chronic low back pain patients more than exercise. *Complementary Therapies in Medicine, 20*(3), 107–118.

Telles, S., Bhardwaj, A. K., Kumar, S., Kumar, N., & Balkrishna, A. (2012). Performance in a substitution task and state anxiety following yoga in army recruits. *Psychological Reports, 110*(3), 963–976.

Telles, S., Joshi, M., & Somvanshi, P. (2012). Yoga breathing through a particular nostril is associated with contralateral event-related potential changes. *International Journal of Yoga, 5*(2), 102–107.

Telles, S., Singh, N., & Balkrishna, A. (2012a). Finger dexterity and visual discrimination following two yoga breathing practices. *International Journal of Yoga, 5*(1), 37–41.

Telles, S., Singh, N., & Balkrishna, A. (2012b). Managing mental health disorders resulting from trauma through yoga. *Depression Research and Treatment, 2012*: 401513.

White, D. G. (Ed.). (2012). *Yoga in practice.* Princeton, NJ: Princeton University Press.

Yadav, R. K., Magan, D., Mehta, M., Mehta, N., & Mahapatra, S. C. (2012). A short-term, comprehensive, yoga-based lifestyle intervention is efficacious in reducing anxiety, improving subjective well-being and personality. *International Journal of Yoga, 5*(2), 134–139.

Yadav, R. K., Magan, D., Mehta, N., Sharma, R., & Mahapatra, S. C. (2012). Efficacy of a short-term yoga-based lifestyle intervention in reducing stress and inflammation: Preliminary results. *Journal of Alternative & Complementary Medicine, 18*(7), 662–667.

Chapter 10: Biofeedback

MARION GOOD AND JACLENE A. ZAUSZNIEWSKI

This chapter provides an overview of biofeedback, its scientific basis, health conditions in which it is useful, and a technique that can be used by nurses trained in its practice.

DEFINITION

Biofeedback is based on holistic self-care perspectives in which the mind and body are not separated, and people can learn ways to improve their health and performance. Biofeedback therapists use instruments and teach self-regulation strategies to help individuals to increase voluntary control over their internal physiological and mental processes. Biofeedback instruments measure physiological activity such as muscle tension, skin temperature, cardiac activity, and brainwaves, and then provide immediate and real-time feedback to the people in the form of visual and/or auditory signals that increase their awareness of internal processes. The biofeedback therapist then teaches individuals to change these signals and to take a more active role in maintaining the health of their minds and bodies. The holistic and self-care philosophies underlying biofeedback and its focus on helping subjects gain more control over personal functioning make the intervention an appropriate one for nurses to use. Over time, a person can learn to maintain these changes without continued use of an instrument (Biofeedback Certification International Alliance, 2012).

SCIENTIFIC BASIS

The following data provide the basis for the use of biofeedback:

- Biofeedback originated from research in the fields of psychophysiology, learning theory, and behavioral theory. It has been used by nurses for decades and is consistent with self-care nursing theories.
- For centuries it was believed that responses such as heart rate were beyond the individual's control. In the 1960s scientists found that the autonomic nervous system (ANS) had an afferent as well as a motor system, and control of ANS functioning was possible with instrumentation and conditioning.
- Heart rate variability (HRV) biofeedback was first studied by Soviet scientists in the 1980s. HRV is the amount of fluctuation from the mean heart rate. It represents the interaction between sympathetic and parasympathetic systems and specifically targets autonomic reactivity. HRV biofeedback is based on the premise that slowed breathing will increase the HRV amplitude, strengthen baroreflexes, and improve ANS functioning (McKee, 2008). HRV biofeedback is easy to learn and can be used with inexpensive, user-friendly devices, some of which can be used independently in the home.
- Neurofeedback uses electroencephalogram (EEG) feedback that shows people their real-time patterns in cortical functioning (Yucha & Montgomery, 2008).
- The model for biofeedback is a skills-acquisition model in which individuals determine the relationship between ANS functioning and their voluntary muscle or cognitive/affective activities. They learn skills to control these activities, which are then reinforced by a visual and/or auditory display on the biofeedback instrument. The display informs the person whether control has been achieved, reinforcing learning.
- Behavioral strategies, such as relaxation or muscle strengthening, are often part of biofeedback treatment to modify physiological activity.
- Biofeedback with relaxation strategies can be used to control autonomic responses that affect brain waves, peripheral vascular activity, heart rate, blood glucose, and skin conductance.
- Biofeedback combined with exercise can strengthen muscles weakened by conditions such as chronic pulmonary disease, knee surgery, or age.

INTERVENTION

Nurses are ideal professionals to provide biofeedback because of their knowledge of physiology, psychology, and health and illness states. However, to use biofeedback they need to acquire special information, skills, and equipment. It is recommended that information be gained from classes and workshops available in many locations in the United States, a few other countries, and online. Nurses using biofeedback should become certified by the Biofeedback Certification International Alliance (BCIA, www.bcia.org), which offers certifications in general biofeedback, neurofeedback, and pelvic muscle dysfunction biofeedback. People in the following countries have received BICA certificates: Australia, Austria, Brazil, Canada, China, Egypt, El Salvador, Germany, Greece, Ireland, Israel, Jamaica, Japan, Mexico, the Netherlands, Poland, Republic of Korea, Republic of Singapore, Slovakia, South Africa, Taiwan, Turkey, the United Kingdom, the United States , and Venezuela. The Association for Applied Psychophysiology and Biofeedback (AAPB) (303-422-8436, www.aapb. org) is also an excellent resource for information and can be contacted at 10200 W. 44th Avenue, Wheat Ridge, CO 80033.

For professionals in Europe, North and South America, Asia, and Africa, the Biofeedback Foundation of Europe (BFE) sponsors education, training, and research activities in biofeedback. On their website (www.bfe.org) BFE lists these opportunities in the form of conferences, workshops, Internet courses, courseware, and other materials. Both AAPB and BFE recommend a book that can be used for teaching and self-directed learning (Peper, Tylova, Gibney, Harvey, & Combatalade, 2009). Biofeedback Resources International (BRI), (www.bio feedbackinternational.com/smart/smart0.html), another company, offers self-directed online courses that meet the didactic requirements for BCIA certification and also offers software, books, and compact disks (CDs) of biofeedback treatment programs for anxiety, addiction, anger, and pain. Face-to-face training programs with hands-on training and mentoring, however, are strongly recommended, and biofeedback equipment for sale can be found on the AAPB and the BRI websites.

The International Society for Neurofeedback and Research (ISNR) is a nonprofit member organization for health professionals, researchers, educators and other individuals who are interested in the promotion of self-regulation of brain activity for healthier functioning. The major goal of the Society is "to promote excellence in clinical practice, educational applications, and research in applied neuroscience in order to better understand and enhance brain function." Although it is based in McLean, Virginia, Society members gather from around the globe for their annual scientific meetings.

Technique

A biofeedback unit consists of a sensor that monitors the patient's physiological activity and a transducer that converts what is measured into an electronic visual or auditory display. Frequently measured physiological parameters include muscle depolarization, which is monitored by electromyelogram (EMG) and peripheral temperature.

Biofeedback provides information about changes in a physiological parameter when behavioral treatments such as relaxation or strengthening exercises are used for a health problem. For example, a relaxation tape helps patients relax muscles, whereas the EMG biofeedback instrument informs the learner of progress (i.e., reduced tension in the muscle). Temperature feedback is also used with relaxation treatments. As muscles relax, circulation improves and the fingers and toes become warmer. When exercises are used to strengthen perineal muscles in preventing urinary incontinence, success in contracting the correct muscles may be monitored by a pressure sensor inserted into the vagina. In health conditions exacerbated by stress, biofeedback is often combined with stress-management counseling.

Biofeedback is most frequently used in an office or clinic setting in eight to twelve 30-minute training sessions (McKee, 2008). Prior to beginning training at the initial session, the therapist and patient should decide on the number of sessions. If the patient has not achieved mastery or control of a function by the end of the agreed-upon number of sessions, the reasons and the need for further sessions should be discussed. Both the behavioral and feedback aspects of the therapy should be identified to patients.

The first session is devoted to assessing the patient, choosing the appropriate mode of feedback, discussing the roles of the nurse and the patient, and obtaining baseline measurements. Measuring several parameters helps in getting valid baseline data. Because success will be determined by changes from baseline, it is essential that these are accurate and reflect the true status of the parameter being used. The first session will be longer than subsequent ones, perhaps lasting 1 to 2 hours. Behavioral exercises are provided.

The therapist plays a key role in the success of biofeedback. It is helpful for the nurse to have advanced training in relaxation, imagery, and stress-management counseling. Because practice of the behavioral techniques is vital, the nurse who succeeds in motivating patients to practice at home is most likely to have patients who achieve their goals.

The final sessions focus on integration of the learning into the person's life. The patient is connected to the machine, but does not receive feedback while practicing the technique; the nurse monitors the degree of control achieved. Descriptions of stressful situations are provided, and the person is asked to practice the procedure as if in those situations. Final measurements are taken. Follow-up sessions at 1 month and 6 months are advocated.

Guidelines for Biofeedback-Assisted Relaxation

A protocol for using biofeedback with cognitive–behavioral interventions for relaxation and stress management is found in Exhibit 10.1. This technique could be used for hypertension, anxiety, asthma, headache, or pain because muscle relaxation improves these conditions. The protocol should be tailored to the patient, condition, and type of feedback.

Exhibit 10.1. *Biofeedback Protocol*

1. **Before first session**
   - Determine health problem for which biofeedback treatment is sought.
   - Ask for physician's name so care can be coordinated. Give information on location, time commitment, and cost.
   - Request a 2-week patient log with medications and the frequency and severity of the health problem (e.g., number, intensity, and time of headaches).
   - Answer questions.

2. **First session**
   - Interview patient for a health history; include the specific health condition.
   - Assess abilities for carrying out current medical regimen and behavioral intervention. Assess cultural preferences for behavioral treatments.
   - Discuss rationale for biofeedback, type of feedback, and behavioral intervention.
   - Explain that the role of the nurse is to provide ten 50-minute sessions once a week, using the biofeedback instrument to supply physiological information.
   - Explain that the patient is the major factor in the successful use of biofeedback and that it is important to continue to keep a log of the health problem, including home practice sessions. The patient should consult the physician if other health problems occur.
   - Explain the procedure. If using frontal muscle tension feedback, apply three sensors to the forehead after cleaning the skin with soap and water and applying gel. Set the biofeedback machine and operate according to instructions.
   - Obtain baseline EMG readings of frontal muscle tension for 5 minutes while the patient sits quietly with closed eyes.
   - Instruct the patient to practice taped relaxation instructions for 20 minutes while the EMG sensors are on the forehead. Ask the patient to watch the biofeedback display for information on the decreasing level of muscle tension.
   - Review the 2-week record of the health problem and set mutual goals.
   - Give a tape or compact disc and instructions for practicing relaxation at home. Provide a log to record practice and responses. Discuss timing, frequency, length, and setting for practice.
   - Discuss self-care for any possible side effects to the behavioral intervention.

(continued)

Exhibit 10.1. *Biofeedback Protocol (continued)*

3. **Subsequent sessions**
- Open the session with a 20-minute review of the health-problem log, stressors, and ways used for coping in the past week; provide counseling for adaptive coping.
- Apply sensors and earphones and let the patient practice relaxation for 20 minutes while watching the display. Quietly leave the room after the patient masters the technique.
- Vary relaxation techniques to maintain interest and increase skill.
- Give instructions for incremental integration of relaxation into daily life. For example, add 30-second mini-relaxation exercises for busy times of the day (e.g., touch thumbs to middle fingers, close eyes, and feel relaxation spreading through the body).

4. **Final session**
- Conduct the session as above; obtain final EMG readings.
- Discuss a plan for ongoing practice and stress management after treatment ends.

Various types of relaxation exercises, such as autogenic phases or systematic relaxation, may be used. To increase patient awareness of the relaxed state versus the state of tension, progressive muscle relaxation with alternate contraction and relaxation may be helpful. Imagery may relax patients by distracting the mind and reducing negative or stressful thoughts. Hypnosis and self-hypnosis also produce an alternative state of mind. Soft music relaxes and distracts and may be used with relaxation or imagery.

It is important to keep the requirements for home practice simple, interesting, and meaningful. Boredom with the same relaxation tape, failure to find a convenient time to practice, and lack of noticeable improvements may decrease adherence to home practice. Changing to a new relaxation technique can revive interest. To integrate new skills into daily life, patients can progress to mini-relaxation and use of cues (thoughts, positions, or activities) to signal relaxation. Other interventions and biofeedback modalities appropriate for children can be found in the literature (Olness, 2008).

Although some patients have multiple symptoms that all require treatment, training should only address one symptom at a time. Other symptoms can be treated sequentially after mastery of the first one is attained. The patient can decide which symptom will be treated first.

Exhibit 10.2. *Parameters Used for Feedback to Patients*

Airway resistance
Blood pressure
Blood volume
Bowel sounds
EEG neurofeedback
EMG muscle feedback
Forced expiratory volume
Galvanic skin response
Gastric pH
Heart rate
Heart rate variability
Peripheral skin temperature
Pneumography
Tidal volume
Tracheal noise
Vagal nerve stimulation

Measurement of Outcomes

Feedback parameters that reflect mastery of the behavioral intervention are found in Exhibit 10.2. Frequently used mastery parameters include heart rate, muscle tension, peripheral temperature, blood pressure, heart rate variability, and EEG neurofeedback. For learning purposes, it is important that the nurse be clear about mastery parameters that consist of ongoing feedback to the patient and outcome parameters that reflect the desired health improvement. For example, temperature feedback is used in peripheral vascular problems, but health care outcomes may result in fewer episodes of painful vasoconstriction. Both EMG feedback and temperature feedback are learning modalities used in those with diabetes mellitus, tension headache, and chronic pain. Outcomes may include decreased glycosylated hemoglobin, fewer and/or less severe headaches, cessation of urinary incontinence, or relief of pain.

Precautions

Biofeedback should be used cautiously, if at all, in persons with depression psychosis, seizures, and hyperactive conditions. Those with rigid personalities may be unwilling to change their mode of functioning. The nurse should consider that negative reactions may also be related to relaxation rather than to biofeedback. Relaxation-related reactions may be avoided by means of patient education and the type of relaxation used (Schwartz & Andrisik, 2003).

Biofeedback-assisted relaxation is expected to lower blood pressure and heart and respiratory rates. Excessive decreases should be avoided in patients with cardiac conditions, hemodynamic instability, or multiple illnesses.

Use of relaxation therapies may also reduce the amount of medication needed to control diabetes mellitus, hypertension, and asthma. This should be discussed with patients and physicians, and responses to therapy should be carefully monitored. For example, in individuals with diabetes there is the potential for hypoglycemic reactions to occur if patient education is not provided or if adjustments in insulin or diet are not made. Patients should be taught to manage hypoglycemia and blood glucose. The nurse should keep simple carbohydrates, glucagon, and a blood glucose monitor in the office and have the expertise to administer them. Home practice can be timed to avoid low blood glucose (McGrady & Bailey, 2005).

Nurses should therefore consider the person, his or her health problem, any known adverse reactions to the behavioral intervention used, and negative reactions to the biofeedback itself. For example, perineal muscle strengthening exercises for stress incontinence carry the risk of "accidents," during the muscle strengthening process, which can be compensated for with padding; however, pharyngeal muscle exercises for dysphasia following stroke carry the more serious risk of aspiration as strength is slowly regained. Finally, although there are generally few side effects to using biofeedback, along with relaxation or exercises to improve function, ineffectiveness is always possible with some people. Nurses should be cautioned to consider the risks of using a mild intervention with variable effectiveness and also assess for age and culture-related acceptability and effectiveness as the patient tries biofeedback with the nonpharmacological treatment. On the other hand, the nurse and patient should consider the learning benefits of using nondrug methods and receiving biological feedback on the patient's efforts to improve body functioning.

Electric shock is a potential hazard when any electrical equipment is used. Dangerous levels of current flow may arise from equipment malfunction or operator error. The AAPB publishes a list of companies whose products have met their safety code.

Although biofeedback is noninvasive, cost-effective, and very promising in the treatment of many conditions, it is not a miracle intervention. It requires that the therapist be knowledgeable about the health problem, intervention, and medication effects, with a sincere interest in patient outcome. It requires the patient to contribute time, attention, and motivation for success of the biofeedback practice. To control the condition, ongoing use of the behavioral technique may be needed after biofeedback sessions end. This should be made very clear before training is initiated.

USES

Biofeedback has been used in the treatment of many medical and psychological problems. For example, neurofeedback is used for attention and learning disabilities, seizures, depression, brain injury, substance abuse, and anxiety. HRV biofeedback, another relatively new approach, is possibly efficacious for depressive disorders, asthma, coronary heart disease, and myocardial infarction (Yucha & Montgomery, 2008). The AAPB website lists 37 conditions in which biofeedback has been empirically studied, and has resulted in an efficacy rating of 3 (probably efficacious) to 5 (efficacious and specific). Biofeedback has been shown to be efficacious in multiple observational, clinical, and wait-list controlled studies, including replications. A visitor to the AAPB website can click on the health condition of interest and obtain information on the level of evidence, the reason biofeedback would help this condition, and the supporting evidence.

Researchers reviewed the efficacy ratings for many disorders that have been treated with biofeedback (Yucha & Montgomery, 2008). The health condition for which the best evidence is available is urinary incontinence in women (level 5—efficacious and specific). Biofeedback treatment of hypertension in adults, anxiety, and chronic pain are at level 4 (efficacious), whereas diabetes mellitus, fecal incontinence, and insomnia are at level 3 (probably efficacious).

Inspection of the PubMed database reveals that nurses have authored biofeedback studies on health problems that are of interest to nurses and are commonly seen in nursing care. These problems include: labor stress, pelvic floor muscle strength after delivery, poststroke footdrop, chemotherapy, stress in mastectomy, climacteric symptoms, incontinence, blood glucose in diabetes, stress in nurses, pediatric migraine, hemodialysis, overactive bladder, hypertension, movement in hemiplegia, anxiety, and chronic lumbar pain.

Tension Headache

Controlled clinical and follow-up studies have shown that biofeedback reduces tension headaches in adults and children. Tension headaches are caused by prolonged tension in the face, jaws, neck, and shoulders. Muscle tension feedback is used to teach patients to recognize their level of tension and relax the muscles using relaxation therapy. Yucha and Montgomery (2008) found that several meta-analyses reported that biofeedback has a stable medium-effect size for migraine and is as good as current medications for both migraine and tension headaches. (Andrasik, 2007; Nestoriuc & Martin, 2007). The effects last for most people as long as they continue to practice the behavioral techniques they have learned.

Fecal Incontinence

A *Cochrane Review* of 21 eligible randomized or quasirandomized trials evaluated biofeedback and/or anal sphincter exercises in 1,525 adults with fecal incontinence. They reported that the limited number of trials and their methodological weaknesses do not allow a definitive assessment of the possible role of anal sphincter exercises and biofeedback therapy in this population (Norton & Cody 2012). These findings were supported by other reviews (Yucha & Montgomery, 2008).

Motor Function After Stroke

An early *Cochrane Review* found that 13 small trials of EMG biofeedback plus standard physiotherapy (269 people) provided weak evidence of effectiveness. Nevertheless, a small number of individual studies continued to suggest that EMG biofeedback plus standard physiotherapy improved motor power, functional recovery, and gait quality when compared with physiotherapy alone (Woodford & Price, 2007; Yucha & Montgomery, 2008). A recent systematic review with meta-analysis of randomized trials found that biofeedback was superior to usual therapy/placebo in improving lower limb activities following stroke. Furthermore, these benefits were largely maintained in the longer term (Stanton, Ada, Dean, & Preston, 2011). Recent studies continue to be conducted for various post-stroke issues such as dysphasia (Bogaardt, Grolman, & Fokkens, 2009), hand motion (Hsu, et al. 2012), and locomotion by using cycling (Ferrante et al., 2011) or a treadmill (Druzbicki, Kwolek, Depa, & Przysada, 2010).

Children and Adolescents

Age-appropriate biofeedback can be used to treat many conditions in children and adolescents, such as migraine, hypertension, and fecal incontinence. Biofeedback, combined with self-hypnotherapy, helps them change their thoughts and bring about changes in their bodies. Olness (2008) describes special biofeedback equipment, explanations, and inductions for children. And she reports her use of many imaginative techniques that appeal to children.

International Use

Biofeedback therapy has been used and studied around the world. In Thailand, for example, it has been used for a variety of conditions, as shown in Sidebar 10.1.

Sidebar 10.1 *Use of Biofeedback in Thailand*

Nutchanart Bunthumporn, Klong Luang, Pathum Thani, Thailand

Currently, many kinds of biofeedback—including galvanic skin response, electromyography, electroencephalography, and heart rate variability—are used in Thailand. However, electromyography feedback is used most widely. In Thailand, biofeedback is most often used with relaxation techniques to decrease stress and anxiety in students, staff nurses, and patients with chronic diseases. Along with autogenic training, it has also helped to decrease aggressive behaviors in drug abusers, and improve behaviors in children with attention-deficit/hyperactivity disorder. A heart rate variability biofeedback training program with support for paced breathing, in a randomized study, decreased older patients' depressive symptoms, negative affect, and depressive cognitions, while it enhanced their resourceful behaviors ($N = 100$; Bunthumporn, 2012).

The benefits of biofeedback are limited by practitioner issues such as complexity of use, availability of training, and the overall cost of the device. To improve the training issues, biofeedback concepts have been integrated into courses for nursing and psychology graduate students. Interestingly, challenges of biofeedback technology did not deter Thai older adults, as there was no attrition during the study (Bunthumporn, 2012).

There are national biofeedback associations in 15 countries in North and South America, Europe, Asia, the Middle East, and Russia (Biofeedback International Resources, 2008). Although the number of articles published outside the United States cannot be easily estimated, the PubMed database identifies scientific articles about biofeedback that have been written in Japanese, German, Dutch, French, Spanish, Chinese, Norwegian, Finnish, Czech, Hebrew, Korean, Russian, and other languages. In the Russian and Japanese languages, for example, there are studies on many different health problems, including epilepsy, asthma, itch, sleep, and mandibular dysfunction. Many of these studies are written in English.

Using their native languages, nurses have authored or coauthored research reports on biofeedback for a variety of health problems of interest to nurses. In the Korean language, nurses have reported biofeedback studies of abdominal breathing training for quality of life after mastectomy (Kim et al., 2005), extremity movement in hemiplegic patients

(continued)

Sidebar 10.1. *Use of Biofeedback in Thailand (continued)*

(Kim, Kim, & Kang, 2003), and progressive muscle relaxation for stress and climacteric symptoms (Jeong, 2004). In Japanese, nurses reported that combined autogenic relaxation training and biofeedback relieved chronic lumbar pain (Yamazaki, Hoshino, Ito, Matsuo, & Katsura, 1985). In the German language, nurses reported a home biofeedback training program for fecal incontinence in older patients (Musial, Hinninghofen, Frieling, & Enck, 2000). In the French language, nurses wrote that biofeedback and relaxation were used for patients with hypertension (Brassard & Couture, 1993). The knowledge and use of biofeedback and behavioral therapies by nurses has spanned many countries of the world.

FUTURE RESEARCH

There continues to be great need for randomized controlled clinical trials to determine the effectiveness, acceptability, and durability of biofeedback in treating physiological and psychological conditions in adults, children, and minorities worldwide. Biofeedback studies of prevalent local health problems are needed in developing countries; however, large multicenter studies with similar inclusion criteria, biofeedback protocol, and research methods are needed to show overall efficacy (Yucha, 2002). Nurses can address the following questions:

- What is the availability of biofeedback training in various countries?
- What culturally acceptable behavioral treatments can be provided along with biofeedback?
- What are the predictors of improvement in using biofeedback for managing health?

REFERENCES

Andrasik, F. (2007). What does the evidence show? Efficacy of behavioural treatments for recurrent headaches in adults. *Neurological Sciences, 28*(Suppl. 2), S70–S77.

Association for Applied Psychophysiology and Biofeedback (AAPB). Retrieved December 8, 2012, from http://www.aapb.org

Biofeedback Certification International Alliance (BCIA). Retrieved December 8, 2012, from www.bcia.org

Biofeedback Foundation of Europe (BFE). Retrieved December 8, 2012, from www.bfe .org

Biofeedback Resources International (BRI). *Frequently asked questions.* Retrieved December 8, 2012, from http://biofeedbackinternational.com/faqs.htm

Bogaardt, H. C., Grolman, W., & Fokkens, W. J. (2009). The use of biofeedback in the treatment of chronic dysphagia in stroke patients. *Folia Phoniatrica et Logopaedica, 61*(4), 200–205.

Brassard, C., & Couture, R. T. (1993). Biofeedback and relaxation for patients with hypertension. *Canadian Nurse, 89*(1), 49–52.

Bunthumporn, N. (2012). *Effects of biofeedback training on negative affect, depressive cognitions, resourceful behaviors, and depressive symptoms in Thai elders.* Retrieved December 20, 2012, from OhioLINK ETD Center (case1333479530).

Druzbicki, M., Kwolek, A., Depa, A., & Przysada, G. (2010). The use of a treadmill with biofeedback function in assessment of relearning walking skills in post-stroke hemiplegic patients—A preliminary report. *Neurologia i neurochirurgia polska, 44*(6), 567–573.

Ferrante, S., Ambrosini, E., Ravelli, P., Guanziroli, E., Molteni, F., Ferrigno, G., & Pedrocchi, A. (2011). A biofeedback cycling training to improve locomotion: A case series study based on gait pattern classification of 153 chronic stroke patients. *Journal of Neuroengineering and Rehabilitation, 8,* 47.

Hsu, H. Y., Lin, C. F., Su, F. C., Kuo, H. T., Chiu, H. Y., & Kuo, L. C. (2012). Clinical application of computerized evaluation and re-education biofeedback prototype for sensorimotor control of the hand in stroke patients. *Journal of Neuroengineering and Rehabilitation, 9*(1), 26.

Jeong, I. S. (2004). Effect of progressive muscle relaxation using biofeedback on perceived stress, stress response, immune response and climacteric symptoms of middle-aged women. *Taehan Kanho Hakhoe Chi, 34*(2), 213–224.

Kim, K. S., Kim, K. S., & Kang, J. Y. (2003). Effects of upper extremity exercise training using biofeedback and constraint-induced movement on the upper extremity function of hemiplegic patients. *Taehan Kanho Hakhoe Chi, 33*(5), 591–600.

Kim, K. S., Lee, S. W., Choe, M. A., Yi, M. S., Choi, S., & Kwon, S. H. (2005). Effects of abdominal breathing training using biofeedback on stress, immune response and quality of life in patients with a mastectomy for breast cancer. *Taehan Kanho Hakhoe Chi, 35*(7), 1295–1303.

McGrady, A., & Bailey, B. (2005). Diabetes mellitus. In M. S. Schwartz & F. Andrisik (Eds.), *Biofeedback: A practitioner's guide* (3rd ed., pp. 727–750). New York, NY: Guilford Press.

McKee, M. G. (2008). Biofeedback: An overview in the context of heart-brain medicine. *Cleveland Clinic Journal of Medicine, 75*(Suppl. 2), S31–S34.

Musial, F., Hinninghofen, H., Frieling, T., & Enck, P. (2000). Therapy of fecal incontinence in elderly patients: Study of a home biofeedback training program. *Zeitschrift fur Gerontologie und Geriatrie, 33*(6), 447–453.

Nestoriuc, Y., & Martin, A. (2007). Efficacy of biofeedback for migraine: A meta-analysis. *Pain, 128*(1/2), 111–127.

Norton, C., & Cody, J. D. (2012). Biofeedback and/or sphincter exercises for the treatment of faecal incontinence in adults. *Cochrane Database Systematic Review, 7,* CD002111.

Olness, K. (2008, March). Helping children and adults with hypnosis and biofeedback. *Cleveland Clinic Journal of Medicine, 75*(Suppl. 2), S39–S43.

Peper, E., Tylova, H., Gibney, K. H., Harvey, R., & Combatalade, D. (2009). *Biofeedback mastery—An experiential teaching and self-training manual.* Wheat Ridge, CO: Association for Applied Psychophysiology and Biofeedback.

Schwartz, M. S., & Andrisik, F. (Eds.). (2003). *Biofeedback: A practitioner's guide* (3rd ed.). New York, NY: Guilford Press.

Stanton, R., Ada, L., Dean, C. M., & Preston, E. (2011). Biofeedback improves activities of the lower limb after stroke: A systematic review. *Journal of Physiotherapy, 57*(3), 145–155.

Woodford, H., & Price, C. (2007, April 18). EMG biofeedback for the recovery of motor function after stroke. *Cochrane Database of Systematic Reviews, 2*, CD004585.

Yamazaki, C., Hoshino, N., Ito, C., Matsuo, T., & Katsura, T. (1985). Nursing of a patient with chronic lumbar pain—Success with autogenic training combined with biofeedback. *Kango Gijutsu. Japanese Journal of Nursing Art, 31*(5), 628–634.

Yucha, C., & Montgomery, D. (2008). *Evidence-based practice in biofeedback and neurofeedback.* Wheat Ridge, CO: Association for Applied Psychophysiology and Biofeedback.

Yucha, C. B. (2002). Problems inherent in assessing biofeedback efficacy studies. *Applied Psychophysiology and Biofeedback, 27*(1), 99–106.

Chapter 11: Meditation

CYNTHIA R. GROSS, MICHAEL S. CHRISTOPHER,
AND MARYANNE REILLY-SPONG

Meditation has numerous attributes that make it particularly appealing for nurses. Meditation training can be provided to patients across the life span with a wide spectrum of conditions, without any equipment or expensive technology, and presented one on one or in a group setting. Moreover, meditation is a pathway for attaining emotional regulation and insight, and a building block for forming self-sustaining skills to cope with life and health challenges. Many nurses and nursing students use meditation skills for stress reduction, enhancing relationships, and building resilience. Nursing is a stressful profession in which symptoms of burnout are not uncommon. In this chapter meditation practices for health are described, the state of the art of meditation research is summarized, and new directions are outlined. Readers are also encouraged to read *Leaves Falling Gently: Living Fully with Serious and Life-Limiting Illness through Mindfulness, Compassion, and Connectedness* (Bauer-Wu, 2011). This slim, exquisitely written text by Susan Bauer-Wu, a nurse and researcher from Emory University, has detailed examples of how to integrate mindfulness into one's life and health care practice, and it is based on her experiences teaching meditation practices to hundreds of patients, including bone-marrow transplant recipients.

Meditation is the quintessential mind–body practice and the foundation for a number of widely used training programs, each with a rapidly growing evidence base to support health benefits. In the past decade, the number of U.S. adults turning to meditation for health reasons has significantly increased—from 7.2% in 2002, to 9.4% in 2007—with the primary reasons for use being control of symptoms such as pain and anxiety, and self-management of chronic conditions (Barnes, Bloom, & Nahin, 2008). Among the most widely used and well-researched meditation programs are mindfulness-based stress reduction (MBSR) and transcendental meditation (TM®). In this section, the focus is on these and closely related programs. This chapter also discusses new experimental findings of structural, physiological, cognitive, and emotional effects from meditation training with a standardized brief meditation instruction protocol, integrative body–mind training (IBMT). Although inclusive definitions of mindfulness consider practices such as yoga, Tai Chi, and Qigong as meditative practices, in this book these movement-focused practices are described separately and in-depth, and therefore they are not included in this segment on meditation. Many religious traditions incorporate meditation within the context of religious observance and prayer (e.g., chanting, use of prayer [Rosary] beads, walking the labyrinth); however, these practices are also not included in this chapter.

Research published since 2005 is emphasized in this section. In 2007, a major evidence report concluded that no firm conclusions could be drawn regarding the therapeutic impacts of any meditative practice or program based on available evidence (Ospina et al., 2007). However, the 2007 review evaluated only work published through 2005, and in the ensuing years there has been a veritable explosion of research on meditation—particularly mindfulness meditation (Bohlmeijer, Prenger, Taal, & Cuijpers, 2010; Chiesa & Serretti, 2009; Fjorback, Arendt, Ornbol, Fink, & Walach, 2011; Hofmann, Sawyer, Witt, & Oh, 2010; Shennan, Payne, & Fenlon, 2011).

DEFINITION

Meditation practices have played an important role in many civilizations for thousands of years for religious purposes and as a means of cultivating well-being. In this chapter meditation is defined as a set of attentional practices leading to an altered state or trait of consciousness characterized by expanded awareness, greater presence, and a more integrated sense of self (Davis, Lau, & Cairns, 2009). These procedures are used to self-regulate the mind and body, thereby affecting mental events by engaging a specific attentional set. There are many distinct meditative techniques, but given that self-regulation of attention is a major component that is common among all of them, it is possible to classify meditative style on a continuum, depending on how attentional processes are directed (Cahn & Polich, 2006). Lutz, Slagter, Dunne, and Davidson (2008) proposed a theoretical framework in which meditation practices are categorized in two main groups: mindfulness and concentration. Mindfulness meditation strategies involve bringing one's attention in a nonjudgmental or accepting way to whatever experience arises in the present moment.

Mindfulness

In mindfulness, practitioners are instructed to allow any thought, feeling, or sensation to arise in consciousness while maintaining a nonreactive awareness to what is being experienced. Mindfulness practice was primarily developed in Buddhism, where it has been an integral component of a 2,500-year-old system of training that leads to insight and the overcoming of suffering (Bodhi, 2011). In the West, mindfulness has been integrated into medicine, nursing, psychology, and related fields, with the goal of teaching patients a more mindful approach to reducing distress, preventing relapse, and enhancing quality of life (e.g., MBSR; Kabat-Zinn, 1990). Concentrative meditation processes involve focusing attention on a selected mental or sensory object. The object of focus may be breath or body sensations, a subvocal repeated sound or word (mantra), or an imagined mental image. In concentration meditation, awareness is narrowed so that the mind only attends to the object of focus. The mind is gently returned to the object of meditation when the meditator notices that it has wandered. Similar to mindfulness, concentration meditation was primarily developed in Buddhism, but it is also a core element in Sufism, Hinduism, and many other religious traditions. It has also become a widely practiced meditation in the West, beginning in the 1960s with the development of TM (Yogi, 1963). In comparing the two types of meditation, Germer (2005) noted that mindfulness meditation is akin to a searchlight that illuminates a wider range of objects as they arise in awareness, one at a time, whereas concentration meditation is like a laser light beam that highlights whatever object on which it is directed. It has been hypothesized that meditators pass through stages, from effortful to effortless maintenance of a meditative state (Tang & Posner, 2013). Consistent with this conceptualization, the concentrative and guided-meditation techniques, which are taught to novices, have been termed "scaffolding" by Jon Kabat-Zinn, and others have commented on mantras with the phrase "you use it to lose it."

SCIENTIFIC BASIS

Understanding how meditation works is the basis for groundbreaking research by leading neuroscientists, including collaborators Yi-Yuan Tang and Michael Posner. In a recent review, Tang summarized the findings from a series of clinical trials they conducted to examine the effects of IBMT, a brief meditation training program that he developed (Tang, 2011). In the first trial, 80 undergraduate students in China were randomly assigned to 5 days of 20 minutes training per day with IBMT, or to relaxation training. Findings showed that meditation, compared to relaxation, improves mood and abilities to self-regulate emotions and efficiently deploy cognitive resources. The IBMT group had significantly better attentional control (important for executive functioning); more energy/vigor; plus less anxiety, depression, anger, and fatigue on the profile of mood states (POMS). Less stress reactivity to a mental arithmetic stressor based on cortisol levels; and greater immunoreactivity. Additional clinical trials have been conducted using the same treatment and a range of outcomes, including brain imaging (measures of regional cerebral blood flow), electroencephalography (EEG), heart rate, and respiratory rate. Findings supported hypotheses that meditation improved regulation of the autonomic nervous system via systems in the ventral midfrontal brain system. In more recent studies, these investigators have begun to explore neuroplasticity: changes in brain morphology following meditation training.

Hölzel and colleagues recently summarized and integrated self-report, brain imaging and experimental evidence from Tang's group and others (Hölzel et al., 2011). Based on the evidence found, these authors proposed four distinct but interrelated mechanisms of action for mindfulness meditation: attention regulation, body awareness, emotional regulation, and change in perspective on the self. These authors note that mindfulness techniques may differ in the extent they activate each mechanism, which suggests an opportunity to tailor practices to specific health needs. Both Tang (2011) and Hölzel et al. (2011) state that research to establish the mechanisms responsible for the health benefits of meditation is in its early stages.

Although the mechanisms of action have not been established, considerable empirical research has been conducted to identify the health impacts of meditation. A comprehensive review of the literature on the health effects of meditation practices funded by the Agency for Healthcare Research and Quality examined studies of MBSR, TM, yoga, and other meditation-related procedures with caregivers, students, and people in the general community published between 1956 and 2005 (Ospina et al., 2007). Whereas multiple conditions and outcomes were studied, meta-analytic results were available only for hypertension and cardiovascular diseases. Meta-analyses of studies of TM compared to progressive muscle relaxation for hypertensive patients showed potentially clinically significant benefits to blood pressure (systolic blood pressure [SBP] and diastolic blood pressure [DBP]) with TM, and for Zen Buddhist meditation versus blood pressure checks (DBP only); other meta-analyses of studies with healthy people showed significant benefits to blood pressure and cholesterol (low-density lipoprotein [LDL-C]) for TM, but findings were qualified due to heterogeneity across studies. Considering all the collective evidence through 2005, these authors concluded that, "the therapeutic effects of meditation practices cannot be established based on the current literature."

A more recent comprehensive meta-analysis examined the effects of meditation on psychological outcomes in healthy adults (Sedlmeier et al., 2012). This review included 163 studies of concentrative, mindfulness, or guided-meditation interventions conducted between 1970 and 2011.

Outcomes evaluated included measures of emotion, personality, cognition, affect, behavior, and well-being. To provide an overall summary of impact, effects were pooled across all outcomes where meditation could be regarded as having either a positive or negative impact. This global analysis revealed medium-sized beneficial effects for meditation compared to active controls (such as relaxation) and no-treatment comparison groups. Examination of individual outcomes showed the largest effect sizes were for emotional (e.g., anxiety reduction) and relationship outcomes. Findings varied by type of meditation. Authors of both of these meta-analyses identified flawed methodology in the conduct of the clinical trials and a significant lack of quality (Ospina et al., 2007; Sedlemeier et al., 2012), including issues such as wait-list control groups, lack of double-blind procedures, and small sample sizes.

Recent reviews and meta-analyses of the impacts of mindfulness meditation training with MBSR, MBCT (mindfulness-based cognitive therapy), and related programs have generally found small to medium treatment effects, but also noted gaps and methodological flaws in the meditation literature. Shennan and colleagues (2011) reviewed the evidence for use of mindfulness-based interventions in cancer. They identified 13 studies, published from 2007 to 2009, in patients with varying types of cancer. They included quantitative, qualitative, and mixed-methods reports, concluding that mindfulness interventions have promising results for subjectively (e.g., anxiety, sexual dysfunction) and objectively (e.g., physiologic arousal, immune function) measured outcomes. Their findings suggest that mindfulness interventions may be useful across the cancer trajectory.

Bohlmeijer et al. (2010) conducted a meta-analysis to estimate the impact of mindfulness training on anxiety, depression, and psychological distress in adults with chronic medical diseases. They identified eight randomized, controlled clinical trials of MBSR or related adaptations published between 2000 and 2008. Study populations included patients with chronic back pain, heart disease, chronic fatigue syndrome, fibromyalgia, rheumatoid arthritis, and cancer. Outcomes were assessed with widely used, psychometrically strong self-report measures such as the State-Trait Anxiety Inventory Scale (STAI-S), Hospital Anxiety and Depression Scale (HADS), POMS, and SF-36 Mental Component Score (MCS). Criteria proposed by the Cochrane Collaborative were used to evaluate study quality. Initial meta-analytic effect sizes were small to medium-sized ($d = 0.26$ for depression, $d = 0.47$ for anxiety, and $d = 0.32$ for overall psychological distress), but varied with study quality. When only studies of high or medium quality were included, all effect sizes were significant but smaller. These authors suggested that integrating mindfulness with other behavioral therapies specific for each condition may enhance efficacy.

A meta-analysis of MBSR programs for stress reduction in healthy people by Chiesa and Serretti (2009) identified 10 comparative trials published between 1997 and 2008, most with wait-list controls. They concluded that evidence supported nonspecific beneficial effects for MBSR on measures of stress and increased spirituality compared to inactive controls, but there was limited evidence for specific effects when compared to an active control, relaxation training.

Hoffman and colleagues (2012) led a randomized, wait-list controlled trial of the impact of MBSR on mood and quality of life, assessed by well-validated instruments, including the POMS (primary outcome), Functional Assessment of Cancer Therapy–Breast (FACT-B), Functional Assessment of Cancer Therapy–Endocrine Symptoms (FACT-ES) scales, and the World Health Organization Well-Being Questionnaire (WHO-5). The sample comprised 229 women with breast cancer (stages 0 to III, 2 months to 2 years after cancer treatment, ages between 18 and 80). Women were randomized to the MBSR group or to the wait-list control group. The intervention followed the standard MBSR curriculum. Twelve MBSR groups (10 to 20 participants) were conducted by Hoffman. Findings showed MBSR provided significant benefits compared to wait-list for essentially all POMS, FACT, and WHO outcomes at posttreatment, 12-week follow-up, or both. MBSR treatment effects reached the accepted level for clinical importance for the FACT-B. Practice and participation time during the 8-week intervention period was associated with greater benefit. Novel and notable results were MBSR-related improvements in endocrine-related symptoms. It was noted that those with stage III cancer and those who had received more extensive chemotherapy and hormone therapies were less willing to join this study. Hoffman and colleagues conclude that MBSR can benefit mood and quality of life for women with breast cancer, including those who receive hormone therapy.

Two randomized trials of meditation training in patients with diabetes were published in the past year. These were the Heidelberger Diabetes and Stress Study (HEDIS; Hartmann et al., 2012) clinical trial in Heidelberg, Germany, and the DiaMind (van Son et al., 2012) trial of MBCT in the Netherlands. HEDIS is a 5-year trial of MBSR to reduce emotional distress and progression of nephropathy in patients with type 2 diabetes and albuminuria. Patients were randomized to the MBSR group or the treatment-as-usual control group. All participants received standard diabetes care. The primary outcome was change in albuminuria, a measure of nephropathy and a risk factor for cardiovascular disease. Secondary outcomes included the Patient Health Questionnaire (PHQ)-9 depression scale and the SF-12 (German version). Groups of six to eight participants attended 8 weekly MBSR sessions plus a booster session at 6 months, led by a psychologist and a resident in internal medicine. The MBSR curriculum was integrated with discussion about diabetes-specific thoughts and feelings. Findings at year 1 showed no differences in progression of albuminuria, based on intent-to-treat analyses adjusted for baseline values, age, and gender. However, the MBSR group reported less depression, better mental health, and lower diastolic blood pressures. Because HEDIS is a 5-year study, the authors remain optimistic The year-1 treatment impact on albuminuria was in the correct direction and encouraging in magnitude (effect size of 0.40). Unlike some interventions, which wane with time, it has been posited that MBSR's benefits increase with time.

DiaMind (van Son et al., 2012) was designed to test the short-term effectiveness of MBCT on stress, mood, and health-related quality of life in patients with diabetes. The study sample comprised 139 outpatients with type 1 or type 2 diabetes, who reported low levels of emotional well-being. Participants were randomized to either MBCT or treatment as usual; all received standard diabetes care throughout the study. MBCT consisted of 8 weekly, 2-hour group sessions with four to eight participants led by certified mindfulness instructors who were also psychologists with a personal mindfulness practice. Program adaptations specific to diabetes were detailed in the design paper (van Son, Nyklíček, Pop, & Pouwer, 2011). Results indicated better outcomes for the MBCT group compared to controls for measures of stress, depression, anxiety, fatigue, and health-related quality of life with medium to large effects from baseline to postintervention based on mixed models and an intent-to-treat sample. Most outcomes showed some improvement by 4 weeks (mid intervention), and greater improvement by 8 weeks, the end of the intervention period. HbA1c results were not significant. Inability to detect improvements in HbA1c levels may be partly explained by relatively good glycemic control at baseline (mean HbA1c = 7.6%). There is also some question about the acceptability of the intervention because about 80% of those eligible declined to participate. These authors conclude the MBCT adapted for diabetes may be effective in reducing emotional distress and enhancing health-related quality of life for patients with diabetes.

Findings of medium to large effects for psychosocial outcomes from the Hoffman, HEDIS, and DiaMind trials are encouraging; however, enthusiasm must be tempered by the fact the each used an inactive control. Treatment effects tend to be biased upward when there are no controls for nonspecific effects such as the time and attention from an instructor, group support, or expectations of benefit (placebo effect; Chiesa & Serretti, 2009; Ospina et al., 2007). Establishing active control groups for meditation interventions is feasible, as evidenced by the work of Tang et al. (2012; Tang & Posner, 2013) and by another trial, which tested the impact of MBSR on symptoms of anxiety, depression, and insomnia in solid organ transplant recipients (Gross et al., 2010). In the latter trial, 150 recipients were randomized into one of three groups: MBSR; Health Education—a peer-led chronic disease self-management program conducted to match MBSR for time, attention, and group support; and a wait-list. Primary outcomes were the STAI, Center for Epidemiologic Studies Depression Scale (CESD), and the Pittsburgh Sleep Quality Inventory (PSQI). Results demonstrated that those receiving active interventions had better outcomes than those on the wait-list at 8 weeks (the end of the active intervention period). Over 1 year, MBSR ($n = 63$) was superior to Health Education

($n = 59$) in reducing anxiety and sleep dysfunction based on mixed-model regression analyses. A notable finding in this trial was that outcomes continued to improve in the MBSR group over the entire follow-up period, whereas the active control group had an initial benefit but then returned to baseline levels.

The final study is a randomized, controlled prevention clinical trial to evaluate the impact of TM on cardiovascular mortality in African Americans with cardiovascular disease (Schneider et al., 2012). Participants were 201 African Americans with angiographic evidence of 50% or more stenosis of at least a coronary artery. Secondary outcomes included nonfatal cardiovascular events and lifestyle variables (smoking, alcohol use, diet, body mass index, and psychological distress). Participants were randomized to either TM or cardiovascular health education. The TM technique was taught by a certified instructor in a series of six 90-minute to 2-hour individual or group meetings, with home practice expectations of 20 minutes per day throughout follow-up. The health education program comprised information about diet, exercise, and stress, and was taught by professional health educators in a format designed to be similar in time and attention to the TM intervention. With an average of 5.4 years of follow-up, the TM group had a significant 42% risk reduction for cardiovascular mortality in a survival analysis stratified by age, gender, and lipid-lowering medications. Significant impacts for TM were also found for systolic blood pressure and the Anger Expression Scale. Both groups showed improvement in exercise and decreased alcohol consumption. No serious adverse events related to the interventions were reported. Study limitations include variations in follow-up procedures and substantial rates of nonparticipation (19% for the TM group and 10% for health education). The authors conclude that TM may be clinically useful in the secondary prevention of cardiovascular disease among African Americans.

INTERVENTION

Techniques and Guidelines

Although there are numerous meditation programs, four of the most widely used and researched meditation programs in Western health care were selected for description below: MBSR (and several related programs), IBMT, TM, and loving-kindness.

Mindfulness-Based Stress Reduction and Related Programs

MBSR was developed by Jon Kabat-Zinn at the Stress Reduction Clinic at the University of Massachusetts Medical Center (www.umassmed .edu/cfm/home/index.aspx) more than 30 years ago. It is a particular

way of learning mindfulness meditation that emerged in a hospital system and was fashioned as a complement to traditional medical care for
patients with chronic pain conditions (Kabat-Zinn, 1990). The program
is theoretically grounded in secularized Buddhist meditation practices,
mind–body medicine, and the transactional model of stress that suggests
people can be taught to manage their stress by adjusting their cognitive
perspective and increasing their coping skills to build self-confidence in
handling external, stressful situations. MBSR is an 8-week generic skills-
based program led by an instructor in a classroom format. The course
comprises eight weekly 2.5-hour classes, one 7.5-hour meditation retreat,
and 30 minutes to 45 minutes of daily homework practicing the techniques learned in the course. Sessions include information about stress,
cognition, and health, but primarily concentrate on learning to focus
attention through a variety of meditative techniques, such as focusing
on the breath, body-scan, sitting and walking meditations, and gentle
yoga. Participants are trained to perceive their immediate emotional and
physical state, including pain or discomfort, and to let thoughts come and
go into awareness with no attempt to change, suppress, or ruminate on
these thoughts.

Through mindfulness training, participants come to view their
thoughts as temporary mental events. In this way, they become exposed
to the positive and negative content of their thoughts, but do not get
absorbed in thought—caught up in planning for the future, or worry-
ing about the past. By incorporating mindfulness techniques into their
daily lives, practitioners learn to find breathing space to respond skillfully to stressors with appropriate action, as opposed to reacting on automatic pilot with conditioned responses that can be emotionally arousing
or unhelpful. The goal of MBSR is lifelong self-management. Although
MBSR was originally developed for people with chronic pain, it was later
applied to patients with a variety of conditions, such as cancer (Hoffman
et al., 2012), diabetes (Hartmann et al., 2012), fibromyalgia (Schmidt et al.,
2011), irritable bowel syndrome (Gaylord et al., 2011), and social anxiety
(Goldin & Gross, 2010). Moreover, MBSR has expanded beyond medical
settings, and courses are now widely available in community settings, at
universities, and in the workplace. Referral by a health provider and medical oversight are not required. Becoming a certified MBSR instructor (for
details see www.umassmed.edu/cfm/certification/index.aspx) requires
intensive experiential and didactic training, including a practicum and
supervised work.

Over the past decade, a number of similar programs have been
developed that integrate core elements of MBSR with existing evidence-
based therapies. Unlike MBSR, which is a generic stress-reduction program, most of these programs target a specific physical or mental illness.
The first of these to emerge was mindfulness-based cognitive therapy
(MBCT) (Segal, Teasdale, & Williams, 2012). MBCT is an 8-week group

intervention that integrates elements of cognitive therapy (CT) with the MBSR program to prevent depressive relapse in patients with a history of major depressive disorder. Unlike CT, there is no attempt to challenge or change the content of thoughts; rather, the emphasis is on changing the awareness of and relationship to thoughts, feelings, and bodily sensations. Aspects of CT included in MBCT are primarily those designed to facilitate a detached or decentered view such as "thoughts are not facts" and "I am not my thoughts." Increased mindfulness allows early detection of relapse-related patterns of negative thinking, feelings, and bodily sensations, thus allowing them to be nipped in the bud at a stage when this may be much easier than if such warning signs were not noticed or ignored (Segal, Teasdale, & Williams, 2004, p. 56). The MBCT program has added several techniques to MBSR that have been widely disseminated, including the 3-minute breathing space (see Exhibit 11.1). Additionally, the MBCT protocol is clear and concise, and includes all necessary materials to begin an MBCT group.

Exhibit 11.1. *Intervention Techniques*

Breath awareness is a practice in which passive breathing is carefully observed. Breath awareness may be used as needed or can be practiced as a technique to promote awareness and health. Continued practice of breath awareness is an anchor for mindfulness, which helps the practitioner to remain in the moment, bringing calm and creativity to situations requiring perspective (Kabat-Zinn, 1990). The practice of breath awareness requires a beginner's mind, open to observation without attempting to change the breath. Kabat-Zinn (1990) describes a simple process that can be used to teach breath awareness to patients:

1. Sit or lie in a comfortable position. If sitting, keep a straight spine and let the shoulders drop.
2. Close your eyes if that is comfortable, or gaze ahead without focusing.
3. Bring attention to your full in-breath and out-breath. Notice the sensation of the breath, especially in the rising and falling abdomen.
4. Don't try to change the breath, just notice the waves of your own breathing.
5. When your mind wanders away from the breath (e.g., you notice that you are thinking of something else) just return your focus to the breath.

Body scan is a technique that promotes the mind's ability to focus and adapt, and is a powerful tool for reconnecting with the body. This

(continued)

Exhibit 11.1. *Intervention Techniques (continued)*

practice involves lying down or sitting comfortably in a chair and focusing attention through the parts of the body, noticing the sensations there and directing the breath, as if breathing in and out of each body part. In this practice, unwelcome sensations like discomfort, tension, or fatigue are noticed and let go, or are imagined to flow out of the body with the breath. The typical sequence for the scan is: toes of left foot, left foot, left ankle, leg, pelvis, then toes of the right foot progressing up to the right hip, pelvis, low back and belly, high back and chest, fingers of both hands (simultaneously), and then both arms, shoulders, neck, face, back of the head, and top of the head (Kabat-Zinn, 1990). At the end of the body scan, one visualizes that the breath goes through the whole body, through the toes, and in and out of an imaginary blow hole at the top of the head. As in other mindfulness practices, unrelated thoughts or interruptions are noted and let go, and the practitioner brings attention back to the scan. The body scan is deeply relaxing for some, and so taking some time to move slowly afterward is helpful. Meditation novices may find that they fall asleep while practicing body scan, or have concerns they are not doing it right. These are normal responses, and practitioners may be encouraged to continue practicing, and to bring themselves back to the scan with awareness and acceptance when they notice that their minds have wandered.

Breathing space can be used routinely to cultivate awareness and self-compassion, or can be used as needed when experiencing unwanted thoughts or feelings. A three-step, 3-minute Breathing Space practice designed by Segal and colleagues is part of MBCT (Segal, Teasdale, & Williams, 2002).

1. Awareness: Bring awareness to the breath and thoughts, feelings and sensations of this moment, observing carefully and describing the experience silently, in words (e.g., "Noticing tension in the body and feeling anxious.").
2. Redirecting attention: Bring your attention to the breath and experience it fully.
3. Expanding attention: Let awareness grow to include the whole body, breathing into areas of discomfort (thoughts, feelings, sensations), breathing out discomfort, and making accepting statements (e.g., "Whatever it is, it's okay.").

Similar to MBCT, mindfulness-based relapse prevention (MBRP) (Witkiewitz, Marlatt, & Walker, 2005) was developed to integrate mindfulness into the cognitive–behavioral treatment (CBT) of substance use, and the prevention of relapse in particular. In MBRP mindfulness practices provide a unique opportunity to decrease habitual responding and avoidance by cultivating an attitude of curiosity and attention to ongoing cognitive, affective, and physical stimuli (Bowen, Chawla, & Marlatt, 2011). The goal of MBRP is to develop awareness of thoughts, feelings, and sensations (including urges or cravings) by developing mindfulness skills that can be applied in high-risk situations for relapse.

Last, mindfulness-based eating awareness training (MB-EAT; Kristeller & Hallet, 1999) was developed by integrating elements from MBSR and CBT with guided-eating meditations. The program draws on traditional mindfulness meditation techniques, as well as guided meditation to address specific issues pertaining to shape, weight, and eating-related self-regulatory processes such as appetite, and both gastric and taste-specific satiety (Kristeller, Baer, & Quillian-Wolever, 2006). The meditative process is integrated into daily activity related to food craving and eating. Similar to MBCT and MBRP, mindfulness meditation is conceptualized as a way of training attention to help individuals first to increase awareness of automatic patterns and then to disengage from undesirable reactivity. Adaptations have also been developed or are in the developmental process for specific populations such as adolescents, pregnant women, and couples, and for health conditions such as cancer, diabetes, insomnia, and posttraumatic stress disorder (PTSD).

Integrative Body–Mind Training

Integrative body–mind training (IBMT; Tang, 2011) originates from traditional Chinese medicine, and also uses the idea of humans in harmony with nature from Taoism and Confucianism. IBMT was developed in the mid-1990s and the goal of the practice is to enhance self-regulation for body–mind health, balance, and well-being (Tang et al., 2012). IBMT involves body relaxation, mental imagery, breath adjustment, and mindfulness training, which are accompanied by background music. It achieves the desired state by "initial mind setting" with a brief period of instructions, to induce a cognitive or emotional set that will influence the training. The method does not stress the control of thoughts, but instead provides a state of restful alertness that allows a high degree of awareness of the body, breathing, and external instructions. IBMT stresses a balanced state of relaxation while focusing on attention. This is achieved gradually through posture and relaxation, body–mind harmony, and balance with the help of the coach rather than by making the trainee attempt an internal struggle to control thoughts. For adults, IBMT has three levels of training: body–mind health, body–mind balance, and body–mind purification. For children, there are two levels: health and wisdom. Across age groups, in each level there are several core techniques packaged in compact discs or audiotapes that are instructed and guided by a qualified coach. A person who achieves the three levels of full training after theoretical and practical tests can apply for instructor (for details see www.yi-yuan.net/english/tyy.asp) status.

Transcendental Meditation

The TM technique is the principal mind–body modality of the Maharishi Vedic Approach to Health, a comprehensive traditional system of natural health care derived from the ancient Vedic tradition. A much-publicized program, TM was developed and introduced into the United States in the early 1960s by Maharishi Mahesh Yogi. It is estimated that there are now more than 5 million practitioners worldwide and the TM organization has grown to include educational programs, health products, and related services (Rosenthal, 2011). According to the TM movement, it is a method for relaxation, stress reduction, and self-development. Certified instructors teach TM in a seven-step course that is outlined on the TM (www.tm.org) website. A TM teacher presents general information about the technique and its effects during a 90-minute introductory lecture. This is followed by a second 60-minute lecture in which more specific information is given. People interested in learning the technique then attend a 10- to 15-minute interview and a 1- to 2-hour session. Following a brief ceremony, the prospective practitioner receives a mantra, which he or she is told to keep confidential. Over the next 3 days, the learner attends three more 1- to 2-hour sessions. In these sessions, the teacher explains the practice in greater detail, offers corrective advice if needed, and provides information about the benefits of regular practice. Over the next several months, the teacher regularly meets with practitioners to ensure correct technique.

TM practice involves two components: a suitable sound (mantra) specifically chosen for its facilitation of the process of settling the mind, and a precise technique for using it (Haaga et al., 2011). Thinking the sound leads the meditator to experience quieter and quieter aspects of his or her awareness, eventually experiencing complete silence (Nidich et al., 2009). In this way, the mantra serves as scaffolding for the developing practice, but eventually fades away as the practitioner's skills are enhanced. TM practice is intended to take the mind from active levels of thinking to the state of least mental activity. This is practiced for 20 minutes, twice per day (in the morning, and in the evening). The TM technique can only be taught by a certified instructor through the seven-step course of instruction outlined above.

Loving-Kindness Meditation

Loving-kindness meditation (LKM) is a core Buddhist meditation practice and it refers to a mental state of unselfish and unconditional kindness to all beings. It is used to develop an affective state of increased feelings of

warmth and caring for self and others (Salzberg, 1995). Like other meditation practices, LKM involves quiet contemplation in a seated posture, often
with eyes closed and an initial focus on the breath. Whereas mindfulness
and similar types of meditation encourage nonjudgmental awareness of
experiences in the present moment by focusing on bodily or other sensorial
experience, affective states, thoughts, or images, LKM focuses on loving and
kind concern for well-being. During LKM, the person typically proceeds
through a number of stages that differ in focus and generally become more
challenging. These include: (a) focus on self, (b) focus on a good friend (i.e.,
a person who is still alive and who does not invoke sexual desires), (c) focus
on a neutral person (i.e., a person who typically does not elicit either particularly positive or negative feelings but who is commonly encountered
during a normal day), (d) focus on a difficult person (i.e., a person who is
typically associated with negative feelings), and eventually (e) focus on the
entire universe (Hofmann, Grossman, & Hinton, 2011). As can be seen from
this sequence, typically warm feelings are initially directed toward oneself
and then extended to an ever-widening circle of others, ultimately radiating
them in all directions (north, south, east, west, and so on), although the order
can be changed to accommodate individual preferences. In LKM, people
cultivate the intention to experience positive emotions during the meditation itself, as well as in their life more generally. Within traditional Buddhist
practice, LKM is considered particularly helpful for people who have a
strong tendency toward hostility or anger (Anālayo, 2003). Although there
are no training requirements or guidelines for LKM, there are a number of
Buddhist and secular resources available to help develop one's practice.

Measurement of Outcomes

Meditation training with programs such as MBSR or TM is a low-risk activity that complements regular medical treatments, diet, exercise and other
lifestyle changes prescribed for known health conditions. Because these
meditation practices have no known serious adverse effects, recommendations for monitoring patients who report engaging in meditation are
consistent with general practice guidelines. Regular assessments to screen
for depression, pain control, and changes in disease-specific symptoms
are warranted. In research studies, meditation has been found to have
impacts on mood, perceived stress, physiological markers of stress, including blood pressure, respiration, heart rate, and cortisol levels, and global
indicators of health-related quality of life. Due to meditation's physiological effects, meditators with hypertension should be regularly monitored
for possible dose adjustments (reductions). And nurses should be alert
to changes in other conditions because anecdotal evidence suggests that
meditation practice enhances adherence, enabling practitioners to better
tolerate intrusive treatments such as nocturnal oxygen (continuous positive airway pressure [cPAP]) for obstructive sleep apnea or "put pain in

its place" without exacerbating suffering with worries. One would specu-late that present-moment attention and awareness lead to better symptom awareness and attention to cues to treat symptoms that wax and wane, and to recognize health changes in conditions such as asthma or diabe-tes. In the earlier Scientific Basis section, several specific instruments and methods to measure these effects in a research setting were mentioned. Some instruments, like the Patient Health Questionnaire (PHQ-9; avail-able from the MacArthur Initiative on Depression and Primary Care at www.depression-primarycare.org/clinicians/toolkits/materials/forms/ phq9), are appropriate for clinical practice as well as for research. Other brief, valid, and reliable self-report instruments appropriate for measur-ing patient outcomes in clinical practice or research are available (www .nihpromis.org/about/overview) at no cost through the National Institutes of Health PROMIS® project.

Precautions

Meditation practices are considered generally safe as a complementary therapy. They are appealing in medical settings because they are inherently portable, do not require a prescription, and can be personalized to meet the needs of the individual. Clinical research supports the use of awareness meditation combined with other behavioral approaches for the treatment of serious disorders like Borderline Personality Disorder (Dialectical Behavior Therapy; Linehan et al., 1999) and addictions or psychosis (Acceptance and Commitment Therapy; Hayes, Wilson, & Strosahl, 1999). There are few condi-tions for which we do not recommend meditation at bedside: delirium, psycho-sis, drug or alcohol intoxication, and mania. People experiencing symptoms of posttraumatic stress or grief may find it difficult to practice awareness exercises, because meditation might intensify their negative experience, and research in this area is ongoing; consultation with a mental health provider is encouraged. People who practice meditation may experience decreased blood pressure, reduced need for insulin or cardiovascular medications. Patients with low blood pressure or who are dizzy or light-headed should not meditate, and medication dose and levels should be considered if their effects could be potentiated by the relaxation response. In our studies of organ transplant recipients, kidney transplant candidates, and people with chronic insomnia, no adverse events related to meditation were encountered (Gross et al. 2010; Gross et al., 2011).

USES

Meditation's health benefits are largely attributed to two over-arching, interacting mechanisms—reduced physiologic arousal and increased men-tal clarity. These factors are thought to combine to change how individuals respond to the stress in their lives, and thereby reduce the harmful effects of stress on their health and well-being. In *Full Catastrophe Living*, Jon Kabat-Zinn (1990) provides an overview of how stressors can trigger automatic "fight or flight" reactions causing rise in blood pressure, pulse rate, and stress hormones, and igniting feelings of fear, anxiety, and anger. He goes on to describe how hyperarousal can become "a way of life," eventually leading to maladaptive, self-destructive behaviors and poor health outcomes. Kabat-Zinn proposes that practice of mindful meditation can prevent this harmful cycle of stress reactivity. He posits that with present-centered attention and awareness, choices can be made and actions taken to skillfully respond to potential stressors. These choices allow the meditator to maintain balance and equanimity, and thereby avoid or diminish the negative impacts of stress that over time erode health and well-being.

The physiological processes leading to stress-induced disease and how meditation may change these processes are detailed in Vernon Barnes and David Orme-Johnson's (2012) bio-behavioral model of how TM works to treat and prevent hypertension and cardiovascular disease. They explain that environmental and psychosocial stress contribute to the development of hypertension and cardiovascular disease through pathways of excessive cardiovascular reactivity, chronic sympathetic nervous system activation, hypothalamic-pituitary-adrenal dysfunction, and increased circulation of neurohormones. These processes cause vasoconstriction, increase blood pressure and, if sustained or repeated, lead to the structural changes of hypertension and cardiovascular disease. Barnes and Orme-Johnson posit that TM practice provides periods of "deep metabolic rest" that result in numerous psychological and physiological changes working in an integrated fashion to enable the body's homeostatic mechanisms to resume normal functioning. Herbert Benson, a pioneer in mind–body research, termed this the "relaxation response," a state of physiologic quietude in which blood pressure, metabolic rate, and respiratory rate are matched to physiological needs—essentially the opposite of the stress response (Benson & Klipper, 2000). Benson has shown that any number of meditative practices, as well as yoga, qigong, or recitation of a prayer (e.g., Hail Mary full of grace; Our Father who art in heaven), can induce the relaxation response; however, Benson's initial work was conducted with TM (Wallace & Benson, 1972).

Proposed physiological mechanisms responsible for meditation's effects on health are reductions in stress reactivity and sympathetic tone. Meditation practice reduces acute and chronic stress reactivity and sympathetic nervous system activity, thereby lowering the load on the heart and lowering blood pressure levels. As a result, risks for hypertension and cardiovascular disease are reduced. In their review, Barnes and Orme-Johnson (2012) cite evidence of the immediate and long-term physiological effects of TM that is consistent with their model. This evidence includes studies of adolescents at risk for hypertension who were trained in TM and demonstrated reduced ambulatory and resting blood pressures, no enlargement of left ventricular mass or increase in cardiovascular reactivity, and studies of hypertensive adults that demonstrated reductions in blood pressure and use of blood-pressure control medications.

The psychological processes that enable meditators to change how they respond to stress have not been established. A series of cognitive and behavioral mechanisms include:

■ attention control
■ attention switching
■ meta-cognition (how one views one's thoughts)
■ meta-cognitive awareness (insight about one's attitudes and beliefs)
■ cognitive restructuring (changing one's perspective on events/thoughts)
■ emotional regulation
■ decreased rumination
■ exposure and desensitization (to enable recognition and exposure to painful states or discomfort without heightened arousal from "catastrophizing," as opposed to avoidance behaviors; Kabat-Zinn, 1990)
■ nonattachment (not relying on objects or events to attain happiness)
■ acceptance
■ present-moment orientation

All these have been proposed to account for the impact of mindfulness meditation on health outcomes (Baer, 2003; Bishop, 2002; Segal et al., 2012; Teasdale, Segal, & Williams, 1995). There are varying levels of evidence to support each of these mechanisms, mostly derived from longitudinal intervention trials using self-report scales to measure mechanisms such as rumination or avoidance. Causal modeling of self-report data using structural equation models is another source of support for some of these mechanisms. Thus far there have been few qualitative studies to contribute to our understanding of the effects of meditation.

Web Resources

Tools for meditation instruction and practice are increasingly available as portable applications. Although many argue that the use of technology has resulted in a culture that is constantly wired or plugged-in, these electronic resources can be useful to introducing patients to meditation practices at bedside. It is recommended that practitioners always familiarize themselves with and use these tools before providing them to patients (see Exhibit 11.2). Professionals should also carefully consider the source when evaluating the potential benefits of these aids. Helpful guidelines for selecting resources on the web are available at nccam.nih.gov/health/webresources, the website of the National Center for Complementary and Alternative Medicine (NCCAM). Selected resources are provided. Additional resources are

Exhibit 11.2. *Web Resources for Meditation*

Resource	Tool, Technology, Source	Description
Diaphramatic breathing exercise	Breathe2Relax (iPhone app); National Center for Telehealth & Technology (t2health.org/apps/ breathe2relax)	Includes instructions with diagrams, practice with an adjustable breath timer, audio prompts with music choices and nature scenery choices. Free.
Mindfulness meditation tracks	Mindfulness Awareness Research Center (MARC) Mindfulness Meditation (podcasts and iTunes downloads); UCLA Mindful Awareness Center (marc.ucla.edu)	Instructions, 5-minute breathing meditation, loving-kindness meditation (LKM), body scan for sleep. Free.
MBSR information, training, and classes	Center for Mindfulness (CFM) at the University of Massachusetts Medical School (www.umassmed.edu/cfm)	Search engine will identify MBSR programs worldwide, by state, or country. CFM offers MBSR teacher training, annual scientific conference, and MBSR courses.
TM information, training, and classes	The Transcendental Meditation Program (www.tm.org)	Search engine will identify TM teachers and programs.

described by Dr. Ruth Buczynski (www.nicabm.com/nicabmblog/) on her blog at the National Institute for the Clinical Application of Behavioral Medicine.

CULTURAL APPLICATIONS

Several meditation practices have been examined across a variety of different populations. For example, several small-sample quantitative and qualitative studies have generated some promising preliminary findings regarding the effectiveness of the standard MBSR protocol with ethnic minorities. Roth and colleagues (Roth & Creaser, 1997; Roth & Robbins, 2004) found that a Spanish version of MBSR for inner-city patients resulted in significant decreases in reported anxiety and medical symptoms, and a significant increase in self-esteem. Similarly, in a randomized controlled trial (RCT), Palta et al. (2012) found statistically significant improvements in systolic and diastolic blood pressure among African American female MBSR group members compared to a social support control group. Sbinga et al. (2011) found reductions in hostility, general discomfort, and emotional discomfort among HIV-infected or at-risk African American youth after participating in an MBSR group. Several qualitative studies among racial and ethnic minority participants have also identified important benefits to MBSR, including receiving social support from other group members (Abercrombie, Zamora, & Korn, 2007; Szanton, Seplaki, Thorpe, Allen, & Fried, 2010) and positive impact on family relationships (Sbinga et al., 2011). In addition to these quantitative and qualitative findings, several authors have suggested possible modifications to the standard MBSR protocol to enhance its appeal and effectiveness among racial and ethnic minority participants. These modifications include delivering the program in the native language of participants (if relevant to a particular group), locating the group at a community agency or center that is trusted by patients, and facilitating increased interaction among group members (Abercrombie et al., 2007; Roth & Robbins, 2004).

Meditation is practiced in countries around the globe. The experience and use of meditation in Thailand, including Thai studies and a case report, are described in Sidebar 11.1.

Sidebar 11.1. *Meditation as a Nursing Intervention in Thailand*

Sukjai Charoensuk, Chon Buri, Thailand

Meditation has long been considered to be a religious practice in Thailand. The application of meditation as a nursing intervention was first documented in 1992 when, for her master's thesis (Jitsuwan, 1992), Pattaya Jitsuwan examined the effects of *Anapanasati* (mindfulness of breathing) training on anxiety and depression in 35 chronic renal failure patients. The effect of Anapanasati was found to decrease anxiety and depression, as well as to improve mental health. Since then, there has been a strong trajectory of studies by faculty and students at a number of Thai universities that have added to the evidence base for the use of meditation for a variety of conditions among a variety of populations in Thailand. These universities include, Ramkhamheng University, Mahidol University, Mahasarakham University, Khon Kaen University, Ratchabhut Nakhon Ratchasima University, Phuket Rajabhat University, and Chiangmai University.

The practice of Anapanasati has been used to improve the mental state of students, and meditation combined with cognitive behavior therapy has been used for depressive disorders. Meditation has been studied with Thai youth and adolescents to enhance happiness, improve emotional well-being, and promote self-esteem and self-control. Studies have also used meditative practices to target indicators of poor health, including hypertension, hemoglobin A1c, hypercholesterolemia, tachycardia, anxiety, and pain. Meditation has also been used in Thailand for specific patient groups with disease conditions such as diabetes, rheumatoid arthritis, end-stage cancer, and depression.

(continued)

Sidebar 11.1. *Meditation as a Nursing Intervention in Thailand (continued)*

Types of Practice in Thailand

The most common type of meditation examined in Thai research has been Anapanasati. In the studies described above, meditation practice times ranged from 30 minutes to 90 minutes daily. In Thailand, meditation includes sitting practices, like Anapanasati, and movement meditation, like Qigong. Recently, meditation interventions have been incorporated into palliative care as a spiritual dimension; meditation has been applied with other medical treatments and complementary therapies in the care of patients with end-stage cancer to improve clinical status and quality of life.

A Case Study of Arokaya Sala

Arokaya Sala is a natural recovery center located at Kam Pramong temple in Sakol Nakorn province, Thailand. It was established to provide help and integrated treatments for cancer patients—including those who are in the final stages of illness—to aid in relief from stress and pain, and to improve patients' quality of life. Religious ceremonies, including chanting, sitting meditation, and walking meditation, are organized to cultivate faith and encourage patients to treat the illness. Arokaya Sala has served more than 3,300 cancer patients from across Thailand and from other countries since it was established.

Reference

Jitsuwan, P. (1992). *Effect of anapanasati practice on anxiety and depression of chronic renal failure patients with dialysis* (Unpublished master's thesis). Mahidol University, Thailand.

FUTURE RESEARCH

To survey the lines of research being actively pursued at this time, we searched the database of U.S. federal funded grants using keywords of meditation or mindfulness, and identified 137 active grants (projectreporter .nih.gov/reporter.cfm, searched January 2013). These included intervention development studies to create or adapt meditation programs to particular populations. There were also clinical trials of MBSR, MBCT, and other meditation programs in diverse populations (including children, older adults, veterans, the underserved, urban minorities) and conditions. Many had the hallmarks of methodological rigor: randomization, adequate statistical power, active comparison groups, an array of self-reported and physiological outcomes, and longer follow-up to establish durability of impact. There were also experiments and imaging studies to elucidate mechanisms. However, few of the grants represented studies described as using qualitative or mixed-methods approaches, and none appeared to be of the scope and magnitude of multicentered pharmaceutical intervention trials.

To maximize the potential for meditation to improve health, more research is needed about *how* it works and to identify *who* is most likely to benefit. Meditation is unlikely to be one size fits all. It is not known whether the quality of the meditation state achieved differs by technique (concentration, mindfulness, or other), and to what extent all meditation approaches engage common pathways versus distinct cognitive and physiological systems. This information could form the foundation for matching specific meditative techniques to particular health problems. Specific personality or genetic factors may predict ability to learn and use each type of meditation. The roles of personal characteristics such as age, gender, personality traits, and genetics could be evaluated to determine the best age to begin meditation training or to tailor programs. With this information, it may be possible to match people to the type of meditation training most likely to work best for them.

REFERENCES

Abercrombie, P. D., Zamora, A., & Korn, A. P. (2007). Lessons learned: Providing a mindfulness-based stress reduction program for low-income multiethnic women with abnormal pap smears. *Holististic Nursing Practice, 21*(1), 26–34.

Anãlayo. (2003). *Satipatthãna: The direct path to realization.* Cambridge, UK: Windhorse Publications.

Baer, R. A. (2003). Mindfulness training as a clinical intervention: A conceptual and empirical review. *Clinical Psychology Science and Practice, 10*(2), 125–143.

Barnes, P. M., Bloom, B., & Nahin, R. (2008). *Complementary and alternative medicine use among adults and children: United States, 2007.* (Center for Disease Control National Health Statistics Report #12). Retrieved from http://nccam.nih.gov/news/camstats/2007/72_dpi_CHARTS/chart6.htm

Barnes, V. A., & Orme-Johnson, D. W. (2012). Prevention and treatment of cardiovascular disease in adolescents and adults through the Transcendental Meditation® Program: A research review update. *Current Hypertension Reviews, 8*(3), 227–242.

Bauer-Wu, S. (2011). *Leaves falling gently: Living fully with serious and life-limiting illness through mindfulness, compassion, and connectedness.* Oakland, CA: New Harbinger.

Benson, H., & Klipper, M. Z. (2000). *The relaxation response- updated and expanded.* New York, NY: HarperCollins.

Bishop, S. (2002). What do we really know about mindfulness-based stress reduction? *Psychosomatic Medicine, 64,* 71–84.

Bodhi, B. (2011). What does mindfulness really mean? A canonical perspective. *Contemporary Buddhism, 12*(1), 19–39.

Bohlmeijer, E., Prenger, R., Taal, E., & Cuijpers, P. (2010). The effects of mindfulness-based stress reduction therapy on mental health of adults with a chronic medical disease: A meta-analysis. *Journal of Psychosomatic Research, 68*(6), 539–544.

Bowen, S., Chawla, N., & Marlatt, G. A. (2011). *Mindfulness-based relapse prevention for addictive behaviors: A clinician's guide.* New York, NY: Guilford Press.

Cahn, B. R., & Polich, J. (2006). Meditation states and traits: EEG, ERP, and neuroimaging studies. *Psychological Bulletin, 132*(2), 180–211.

Chiesa, A., & Serretti, A. (2009). Mindfulness-based stress reduction for stress management in healthy people: A review and meta-analysis. *Journal of Alternative and Complementary Medicine, 15*(5), 593–600.

Davis, K. M., Lau, M. A., & Cairns, D. R. (2009). Development and preliminary validation of a trait version of the Toronto Mindfulness Scale. *Journal of Cognitive Psychotherapy, 23*(3), 185–197.

Fjorback, L. O., Arendt, M., Ornbol, E., Fink, P., & Walach, H. (2011). Mindfulness-based stress reduction and mindfulness-based cognitive therapy: A systematic review of randomized controlled trials. *Acta Psychiatrica Scandinavica, 124*(2), 102–119.

Gaylord, S. A., Palsson, O. S., Garland, E. L., Faurot, K. R., Coble, R. S., Mann, J. D., . . . Whitehead, W. E. (2011). Mindfulness training reduces the severity of irritable bowel syndrome in women: Results of a randomized controlled trial. *American Journal of Gastroenterology, 106*(9), 1678–1688.

Germer, C. K. (2005). Mindfulness: What is it? What does it matter? In C. K. Germer, R. D. Siegel, & P. R. Fulton (Eds.), *Mindfulness and psychotherapy* (pp. 3–27). New York, NY: Guilford Press.

Goldin, P. R., & Gross, J. J. (2010). Effects of mindfulness-based stress reduction (MBSR) on emotion regulation in social anxiety disorder. *Emotion, 10*(1), 83–91.

Gross, C. R., Kreitzer, M. J., Reilly-Spong, M., Wall, M., Winbush, N. Y., Patterson, R., . . . Cramer-Bornemann, M. (2011). Mindfulness-based stress reduction versus pharmacotherapy for chronic primary insomnia: A randomized controlled clinical trial. *Explore (NY), 7*(2), 76–87.

Gross, C. R., Kreitzer, M. J., Thomas, W., Reilly-Spong, M., Cramer-Bornemann, M., Nyman, J. A., . . . Ibrahim, H. N. (2010). Mindfulness-based stress reduction for solid organ transplant recipients: A randomized controlled trial. *Alternative Therapies in Health and Medicine, 16*(5), 30–38.

Haaga, D. A. F., Grosswald, S., Gaylord-King, C., Rainforth, M., Tanner, M., Travis, F., . . . Schneider, R. H., (2011). Effects of the Transcendental Meditation Program on substance use among university students. *Cardiology Research and Practice, 2011,* 5371–5301.

Hartmann, M., Kopf, S., Kircher, C., Faude-Lang, V., Djuric, Z., Augstein, F., . . . Nawroth, P. P. (2012). Sustained effects of a mindfulness-based stress-reduction intervention in type 2 diabetic patients: Design and first results of a randomized controlled trial (the Heidelberger Diabetes and Stress-study). *Diabetes Care, 35*(5), 945–947.

Hayes, S. C., Wilson, K. G., & Strosahl, K. (1999). *Acceptance and commitment therapy: An experiential approach to behavior change.* New York, NY: Guilford Press.

Hoffman, C. J., Ersser, S. J., Hopkinson, J. B., Nicholls, P. G., Harrington, J. E., & Thomas, P. W. (2012). Effectiveness of mindfulness-based stress reduction in mood, breast- and endocrine-related quality of life, and well-being in stage 0 to III breast cancer: A randomized, controlled trial. *Journal of Clinical Oncology, 30*(12), 1335–1342.

Hofmann, S. G., Grossman, P., & Hinton, D. E. (2011). Loving-kindness and compassion meditation: Potential for psychological interventions. *Clinical Psychology Review, 31*(7), 1126–1132.

Hofmann, S. G., Sawyer, A. T., Witt, A. A., & Oh, D. (2010). The effect of mindfulness-based therapy on anxiety and depression: A meta-analytic review. *Journal of Consulting and Clinical Psychology, 78*(2), 169–183.

Hölzel, B. K., Lazar, S. W., Gard, T., Schuman-Olivier, Z., Vago, D. R., & Ott, U. (2011). How does mindfulness meditation work? Proposing mechanisms of action from a conceptual and neural perspective. *Perspectives on Psychological Science, 6*(6), 537–559.

Kabat-Zinn, J. (1990). *Full catastrophe living: Using the wisdom of your body and mind to face stress, pain, and illness.* New York, NY: Bantam Dell.

Kristeller, J. L., Baer, R. A., & Quillian-Wolever, R. (2006). Mindfulness-based approaches to eating disorders. In R. A. Baer (Ed.), *Mindfulness-based treatment approaches: A clinician's guide to evidence base and applications* (pp. 75–91). San Diego, CA: Academic Press.

Kristeller, J. L., & Hallet, B. (1999). Effects of a meditation-based intervention in the treatment of binge eating. *Journal of Health Psychology, 4*(3), 357–363.

Linehan, M. M., Schmidt, H., Dimeff, L. A., Craft, J. C., Kanter, J., & Comtois, K. A. (1999). Dialectical behavior therapy for patients with borderline personality disorder and drug-dependence. *American Journal of Addictions, 8*(4), 274–292.

Lutz, A., Slagter, H. A., Dunne, J. D., & Davidson, R. J. (2008). Attention regulation and monitoring in meditation. *Trends in Cognitive Science, 12*(4), 163–169.

Nidich, S. I., Rainforth, M. V., Haaga, D. A. F., Hagelin, J., Salerno, J. W., Travis, F., . . . Schneider, R. H. (2009). A randomized controlled trial on effects of the Transcendental Meditation Program on blood pressure, psychological distress, and coping in young adults. *American Journal of Hypertension, 22*(12), 1326–1331.

Ospina, M., Bond, K., Karkhaneh, M., Tjosvold, L., Vandermeer, B., Liang, Y., . . . Klassen, T. (2007). *Meditation practices for health: State of the research.* (Evidence Report/Technology Assessment). June (155), 1–263.

Palta, P., Page, G., Piferi, R. L., Gill, J. M., Hayat, M. J., Connolly, A. B., & Szanton, S. L. (2012). Evaluation of a mindfulness-based intervention program to decrease blood pressure in low-income African-American older adults. *Journal of Urban Health, 89*(2), 308–316.

Rosenthal, N. E. (2011). *Transcendence: Healing and transformation through transcendental meditation.* New York, NY: Tarcher.

Roth, B., & Creaser, T. (1997). Mindfulness meditation-based stress reduction: Experience with a bilingual inner-city program. *Nurse Practitioner, 22*(3), 150–152, 154, 157 passim.

Roth, B., & Robbins, D. (2004). Mindfulness-based stress reduction and health-related quality of life: Findings from a bilingual inner-city patient population. *Psychosomatic Medicine, 66*(1), 113–123.

Salzberg, S. (1995). *Loving-kindness: The revolutionary art of happiness.* Boston, MA: Shambhala.

Sbinga, E. M. S., Kerrigan, D., Stewart, M., Johnson, K., Magyari, T., & Ellen, J. M. (2011). Mindfulness-based stress reduction for urban youth. *Journal of Alternative and Complementary Medicine, 13*, 213–218.

Schmidt, S., Grossman, P., Schwarzer, B., Jena, S., Naumann, J., & Walach, H. (2011). Treating fibromyalgia with mindfulness-based stress reduction: Results from a 3-armed randomized controlled trial. *Pain, 152*(2), 361–369.

Schneider, R. H., Grim, C. E., Rainforth, M. V., Kotchen, T., Nidich, S. I., Gaylord-King, C., . . . Alexander, C. N. (2012). Stress reduction in the secondary prevention of cardiovascular disease: Randomized, controlled trial of transcendental meditation and health education in Blacks. *Circulation: Cardiovascular and Quality Outcomes, 5*(6), 750–758.

Sedlmeier, P., Eberth, J., Schwarz, M., Zimmermann, D., Haarig, F., Jaeger, S., & Kunze, S. (2012). The psychological effects of meditation: A meta-analysis. *Psychological Bulletin, 138*(6), 1139–1171.

Segal, Z. V., Teasdale, J. D., & Williams, J. M. G. (2002). *Mindfulness-based cognitive theory therapy for depression: A new approach to preventing relapse.* New York, NY: Guilford.

Segal, Z. V., Teasdale, J. D., & Williams, J. M. G. (2004). Mindfulness-based cognitive therapy: Theoretical rationale and empirical status. In S. C. Hayes, V. M. Follette, & M. Linehan (Eds.), *Mindfulness and acceptance: Expanding the cognitive–behavioral tradition* (pp. 45–65). New York, NY: Guilford Press.

Segal, Z. V., Teasdale, J. D., & Williams, J. M. G. (2012). *Mindfulness-based cognitive theory therapy for depression: A new approach to preventing relapse* (2nd ed.). New York, NY: Guilford Press.

Shennan, C., Payne, S., & Fenlon, D. (2011). What is the evidence for the use of mindfulness-based interventions in cancer care? A review. *Psycho-Oncology, 20*(7), 681–697.

Szanton, S. L., Seplaki, C. L., Thorpe, R. J., Allen, J. K., & Fried, L. P. (2010). Socioeconomic status is associated with frailty: The women's health and aging studies. *Journal of Epidemiology and Community Health, 64*(1), 63–67.

Tang, Y. Y. (2011). Mechanism of integrative body-mind training. *Neuroscience Bulletin, 27*(6), 383–388.

Tang, Y. Y., Lu, Q., Fan, M., Yang, Y., & Posner, M. I. (2012). Mechanisms of white matter changes induced by meditation. *Proceedings of the National Academy of Sciences, USA, 109*(26), 10570–10574.

Tang, Y. Y., & Posner, M. I. (2013). Tools of the trade: Theory and method in mindfulness neuroscience. *Social Cognitive and Affective Neuroscience, 8*(1), 118–120.

Teasdale, J. D., Segal, Z., & Williams, J. M. (1995). How does cognitive therapy prevent depressive relapse and why should attentional control (mindfulness) training help? *Behaviour Research and Therapy, 33*(1), 25–39.

van Son, J., Nyklíček, I., Pop, V. J., Blonk, M. C., Erdtsieck, R. J., Spooren, P. F., . . . Pouwer, F. (2012). The effects of a mindfulness-based intervention on emotional distress, quality-of-life, and HbA1c in outpatients with diabetes (DiaMind): A randomized controlled trial. *Diabetes Care, 36*(4), 823–830.

van Son, J., Nyklíček, I., Pop, V. J., & Pouwer, F. (2011). Testing the effectiveness of a mindfulness-based intervention to reduce emotional distress in outpatients with diabetes (DiaMind): Design of a randomized controlled trial. *BMC Public Health, 11*, 131.

Wallace, R. K., & Benson, H. (1972). The physiology of meditation. *Scientific American, 226*, 84–90.

Witkiewitz, K., Marlatt, G. A., & Walker, D. (2005). Mindfulness-based relapse prevention for alcohol and substance use disorders. *Journal of Cognitive Psychotherapy, 19*(3), 211–228.

Yogi, M. M. (1963). *The science of being and art of living.* New York, NY: Meridien Press.

Chapter 12: Prayer

MARIAH SNYDER AND LAURA LATHROP

Although prayer is not included in the most recent list of complementary therapies of the National Center for Complementary and Alternative Medicine (NCCAM; 2012), it has been included on many surveys that have been done on use of complementary procedures. However, controversy exists when surveys include prayer within the scope of complementary therapies as the rate of use of therapies increases dramatically and at times even doubles (Tippens, Marsman, & Zwickey, 2009). Because spiritual care, of which prayer may be a component, is inseparable from nursing, prayer is included in this text as a complementary treatment.

Tippens et al. (2009) contend that inclusion of prayer as a complementary therapy on surveys requires consideration of four points:

- Need for a clearer standard for classifying therapies that are and are *not* part of the NCCAM classification
- Distinction between prayer and other diverse forms of spiritual healing used by practitioners
- Recognition that the inclusion of prayer as a complementary therapy increases the percentage of people using complementary therapies
- Understanding that prayer is often used more by individuals of certain groups and hence this is reflected in elevated use of complementary therapies by these groups (e.g., African Americans)

Some contend that prayer, given its philosophical basis, cannot be studied using randomized clinical trials because the person praying may be seeking to conform to God's will, and the outcome being prayed for is not in accordance with God's will at this point in time (Dusek, Astin, Hibberd, & Krucoff, 2003). Control groups present another concern because it is almost impossible to ferret out whether others outside of the study are praying for the individuals in the control group. After an extensive review of studies on prayer, Roberts, Ahmed, and Hall (2009) noted that the evidence found is "interesting enough" to prompt further studies on prayer. However, they further stated that the effects of prayer cannot be proven or disproven as the perceived results are dependent on God.

People often equate prayer with religion; yet prayer, like spirituality, transcends religion. Prayer and spirituality acknowledge the existence of a Greater or Supreme Being and humans have a connectedness with this Being. Cultural and religious groups have different names for this Higher Being such as God, Supreme Being, Mother Earth, Master of the Universe, Creator, Absolute, El, or Great Spirit. Islam has 99 names for the Supreme Being. Although recognizing that there are many names for this Higher Being, *God* will be used throughout this chapter.

Early studies on prayer largely focused on use of Christian prayer and were conducted using Western populations. A growing number of studies have now been administered in the use of prayers in diverse religions and cultures: Muslim prayer (Badsha & Tak, 2008; Doufesh, Faisal, Lim, & Ibrahim, 2012), Jewish prayer (Milevsky & Eisenberg, 2012), Hispanic migrants (Bergland, Heuer, & Lausch, 2007), and Native Americans (Walton, 2007). Thus, the universality of prayer as a complementary therapy is being established.

With the growing number of persons without a specific religious affiliation and those who do not attend a church on a regular basis, attention needs to be given to secular spirituality that postulates that the universe is a coherent whole with interconnectedness without ties to traditional religious groups. The Pew Forum survey (2013) found that 16% of Americans identify themselves as unaffiliated with a specific religion. This finding suggests that there are those who make sense of their lives without relying on a specific religious belief system. Ai and colleagues (1998) assessed reverence as a broad experience involving a sense of self-transcendence not exclusively related to religious involvement. They explored *secular reverence* and frequency of prayer on postoperative complications. Patients using secular reverence had a shorter hospital length of stay following coronary artery bypass graft surgery than did those using prayer. However, the study had a small sample size and there was homogeneity of beliefs among the participants. Thus, prayer as a complementary therapy needs to be examined in a broader context than solely within established religions.

DEFINITION

The word *prayer* comes from the Latin *precarius*, which means to obtain by begging, and from *precari*, which means to entreat. Many definitions for prayer can be found. Stabile (2013) defines prayer as:

> [S]imply communication between humans and God (or whatever label a person gives to the Ultimate Reality that transcends human existence), a mutual communication that includes speaking to God and listening to God, and that sometimes uses words and sometimes is wordless. (pp. 55–56)

Prayer and meditation (Chapter 11) share many commonalities. Whereas the object of meditation for the person frequently gives attention to a word or object so as to become more attentive and aware, the focus of prayer is on communication with a Higher Being. There are many forms of meditation and some of these, such as centering, are used in prayer.

Many different types of prayer have been described in the literature. Exhibit 12.1 provides a description of types of prayer that are commonly used. Banzinger, Van Uden, and Janssen (2008) note that persons may view prayer as being in collaboration with God in which they are in contact and communion with God. Prayer may be done on an individual basis, within a group, or as part of a faith or religious community. Prayer

Exhibit 12.1. *Types of Prayer*

Adoration or praise: Acknowledging the greatness of God

Collaborative: Person works with God

Colloquial: Communicating informally with God

Directed: Requesting a specific outcome

Intercessory: Communicating with God for a specific outcome for others or self

Lamentation: Communicating to God during loss or difficult times

Nondirected: Requesting the best thing to occur in a given situation

Petition: Asking God for a personal request; person asking for God's intervention

Ritual: Using set words and/or practices often within a specific religious faith

Thanksgiving: Offering gratitude to God for a request or gift received

is unique to an individual in that each person establishes his or her relationship with God. Many of the studies that have been conducted on prayer have used intercessory prayer in which prayers are offered for persons.

SCIENTIFIC BASIS

Despite the concern of some that it is oxymoronic to explore the effects of prayers from a scientific perspective, as prayer appears to have a different philosophical basis from physiological phenomena, numerous studies on prayer have been implemented. Moher et al. (2010) recommend that studies of prayer should adopt the Consolidated Standards of Reporting Trials guidelines. Since the seminal research by Joyce and Welldon (1965), research on prayer has continued but great diversity exists in the quality of studies that have been conducted. Comparisons across studies are difficult to make because of differing methodologies and outcome measures (Olver & Dutney, 2012). For example, Harris et al. (1999) sought to replicate the work of Byrd (1998). However, comparisons were difficult to make because of differences in methodologies and measurement.

A conceptual model regarding the nature of prayer and its relationship to health has been developed by Breslin and Lewis (2008). They identify four variables that may have an impact on positive health outcomes from prayer: physiological, psychological, placebo, and social support. Physiologically, prayer may promote a relaxation response that lowers heart rate, decreases muscle tension, and slows breathing. The feelings of peace and relaxation produced may stimulate endorphins that have an impact on the autonomic nervous system's reaction to stress. On the psychological level, prayer may create positive emotions and increase a sense of meaning, hope, empathy, and forgiveness. For some, prayer may be viewed as a placebo or a positive form of a self-fulfilling prophecy. The social support that may accompany some prayers may serve as a protective factor against illness. Knowing that others are praying for you provides a form of social support and may have a positive effect on health and well-being. Social support may also encourage the use of health behaviors. These aspects of the model may be considered the *causal* mechanisms of the model because effects can be more easily measured.

In contrast, the *spiritual* pathways identified by Breslin and Lewis (2008) in their model are variables that may influence health outcomes; however, it is difficult to prove or reject their influence because Divine intervention is not readily measureable. Some believe that prayer works subliminally or below the perception of the person. What the *pray-er* believes will be the result of prayer is difficult to research because of the difficulty in understanding what the *pray-er* believes. Likewise the belief that prayer activates energies such as *chi* and thus impacts health outcomes has not been experimentally verified. Another possible spiritual mechanism is that prayer moves across time and space and the universe to have positive effects on health. This may produce a connection between the *pray-er* and *pray-ee* leading to a unity of consciousness and promoting healing. However, this is difficult to measure because one does not always know who or how many persons are praying for an individual.

Olver and Dutney (2012) attempted to incorporate the Consolidated Standards of Reporting Trials guidelines in examining the impact of intercessory prayer on improvement in spiritual well-being. A triple-blinded methodology was used with a Christian prayer group praying for the subjects in the experimental groups. Only the principal investigator communicated with those praying for the experimental group; first names, ages, marital status, occupations, and types of cancer were provided so as to enable the prayer group to personalize their prayers for the well-being of the subjects. Outcome measures included the Functional Assessment of Chronic Illness Therapy-Spiritual Well-Being (FACIT-Sp) scale (Peterman, Fitchett, Brady, Hernandez, & Cella, 2002), which is a part of a general quality of life (QOL) scale that incorporated questions on physical, functional, social/family, and emotional well-being and included 12 additional items on spiritual well-being measurement. These factors covered items on peace, meaning, and faith; the instrument has shown good internal reliability and convergent validity. Subjects in the intercessory prayer group had a small but statistically significant improvement in spiritual well-being as well as improvement in emotional well-being. The control group manifested a decrease in functional well-being during the 6-month period, whereas the experimental group showed an improvement.

New techniques in brain imaging hold promise for detailing areas of the brain involved in prayer. When Tibetan monks and Franciscan nuns were invited to pray or meditate inside a single proton emission computed tomography machine (SPECT), Newberg, D'Aquili, and Rause (2001) found that activity shifted in specific regions in the brain. These shifts included: a decrease in the activity of the left hemisphere language centers indicating a silencing of brain "chatter," and a decrease in the activity in the posterior parietal gyrus of the left hemisphere. This latter area is a place that helps individuals identify physical boundaries, so that they lose an awareness of where their boundaries begin and end relative to the surrounding space.

A number of studies have documented the effectiveness of prayer as a coping strategy. From a review of studies on prayer, Hollywell and Walker (2009) concluded that prayer was a coping strategy that helps to mediate between religion and well-being.

Positive results from prayer have not been found in all of the studies reviewed. In a meta-analysis of studies in which prayer was used as the intervention, Masters and Spielmans (2007) found no evidence that distant intercessory prayer had any impact on health outcomes. Blumenthal et al. (2007) reported that prayer, meditation, and church attendance contributed minimally to decreased cardiac morbidity in patients who had an acute myocardial infarction, and who had depression or low levels of social support.

The mechanism of how prayer works, whether intercessory on behalf of others or for oneself, is not known. The person praying for another person does not have to be in proximity to the person for whom they are praying for prayer to be effective. A question about whether the person being prayed for must believe in the efficacy of prayer or be receptive to it for prayer to be effective has not been explored. In most research studies, patients have given consent to be the recipient of prayers. However, in daily life, many prayers are offered for others without their knowledge. Therefore, it is difficult to design studies on prayer that would control for intercessory prayers outside of the research being done.

INTERVENTION

When prayer is discussed in terms of health, intercessory prayer—prayer for others or for self in relation to a particular problem—is often the type of prayer being used. Less attention has been given to exploring the impact of overall prayerfulness on the lives of individuals.

Assessment

Spiritual assessment should be part of a patient's health history obtained by nurses or other health professionals. Many spiritual assessments include information about the beliefs people hold, how they address God, and things that are important to them in order to pray. The Joint Commission Standards for Patient Care (2012) includes elements on spiritual and emotional care of patients. The standards note that the spiritual assessment should obtain information about the faith community or denomination, if any, of the patient and the beliefs and spiritual practices that may be important to the person. Examples of other questions that may provide information that would be helpful to the health team in planning holistic care include:

- Does the patient use prayer in life?
- How does the individual express spirituality?
- What provides the patient with strength and hope?
- What meaning does the person find concerning the disease process?
- How does the subject cope with illness or difficulties?
- Is the person at peace?

Findings from the spiritual assessment will guide the nurse in deciding if, when, and how to use prayer as an intervention. Prayers are often appreciated when a diagnosis has been made, during times of high anxiety, prior to and after diagnostic tests and surgery, when giving birth, and when death is imminent. Prayers of thanksgiving should not be forgotten in times of recovery or when the findings from a diagnostic test show no serious condition.

Increased attention is being paid to health professionals praying for their patients (Schroder, 2011). Praying is closely linked to caring for a person. Praying for patients can be as simple as asking God to bless the patients and families you meet during each day, or it may be a short prayer as one enters a room. Little information about the dose of prayer needed for effectiveness exists. Are long prayers better than short ones? Remen (2000), a physician, commented that caring for the souls of patients is as important as caring for their bodies.

Technique

If nurses feel comfortable doing so, they can ask whether patients would like the nurse to join them in praying. Reading scripture or reading from a holy book is one way to pray with a person. The nurse can create an environment conducive to prayer: playing meditative music, preventing interruptions, and obtaining books or supplies needed for the person to pray such as a yarmulke for a Jewish man or a rosary for a person of the Catholic faith. Many hospitals, nursing homes, and clinics have a chapel or room for prayer and meditation. The health status of many patients in acute care settings often does not allow them to go to a chapel; however, family members may find peace and comfort in this space.

Patients with a religious affiliation may wish to use the formal prayers of their faith tradition. For example, Christians may find the Lord's Prayer comforting. Patients of the Jewish faith may want to read the Psalms or have them read to them, and Muslims may choose to recite prayers from the Qur'an (Koran). Giving praise to the four directions may be a prayer form that people of Native American ancestry desire to use. Nurses need to respect whatever form or ritual the prayer takes. Exhibit 12.2 provides short prayers from different faith traditions. Websites provide prayers of many religions that can be shared with patients. A website (www. sacredspace.ie) contains Christian prayers and meditations for each day. Also, chaplains are an excellent resource for nurses.

Measurement of Outcomes

Although many studies have examined the impact of prayer on indices related to improvement in health, others have explored the effect prayer has on psychological and spiritual variables. The purpose for which prayer

Exhibit 12.2. *Prayers of Other Cultures*

Lakota Indian Prayer

Wakan Tanka, Great Mystery, teach me how to trust my heart, my mind, my intuition, my inner knowing, the senses of my body, the blessings of my spirit. Teach me to trust these things so that I may enter my sacred space and love beyond my fear, and thus walk in balance with the passing of each glorious sun (www.goodreads.com/quotes/160438-wakan-tanka) (2012).

Prayer From Qur'an (Muslim)

In the name of God, Most Gracious, Most Merciful. Praise be to GOD, Lord of the universe. Most Gracious, Most Merciful. Master of the day of Judgment. You alone we worship. You alone we ask for help. Guide us in the right path; the path of those whom You blessed; not of those who have deserved wrath, nor of the strayers (1:1–7) (www.submission.info/God/prayers_from_Quaran.html) (2012).

---

is being used will dictate the specific outcomes to be measured. Because of the mind–body–spirit interactions, nurses may want to include holistic measures rather than simply a measurement of physiological, psychological, or spiritual status. Olver and Dutney (2012) examined the impact of prayer on quality of life. Spiritual variables that have been measured include contentment, being more at peace, and acceptance of status.

Precautions

Because of the highly personal nature of faith, spirituality, religious beliefs, and practices, it is important for nurses to assess both the prayer preferences of patients and their own personal beliefs and comfort with using prayer. Knowledge about the beliefs and practices of other faith traditions and about secular spirituality is imperative in our pluralistic society. Using prayer improperly may offend others, awaken old antipathies, and make patients uncomfortable. Assessment and then offering possibilities are paramount. Ethical issues related to health professionals praying for patients are being discussed with no definitive directions at this time (Bremmer, Koole, & Bushman, 2011).

Because prayer is to God and the "result" depends on what God determines is best for the person, the outcome is outside the person praying. When the outcome is not the one desired by the patient or family, the nurse must be careful not to use platitudes, such as "God knows what is best," but rather provide comfort and support.

USES

Prayer has been used with persons having many illnesses, of all age groups, and from all cultures. Exhibit 12.3 lists selected conditions for which studies on the use of prayer have been conducted. The literature also contains many anecdotal accounts about the efficacy of prayer in indivduals who are ill. In a number of surveys, prayer has been the most frequently used complementary therapy (Brown, Barner, Richards, & Bohman, 2007; King & Pettigrew, 2004).

Research has been conducted on the use of prayer with patients having chronic conditions. In a study of adults who were HIV-1-positive and who engaged in spiritual activities such as prayer, subjects had a reduced risk of death (Fitzpatrick et al., 2007). Konkle-Parker, Erlen, and Dubbert (2008) reported that prayer and spirituality were facilitators of persons with HIV adhering to their medication regimen. Likewise, people with depression and anxiety who had participated in six weekly 1-hour prayer sessions showed improvement in depression and anxiety compared to subjects in the control group (Boelens, Reeves, Replogle, & Koenig, 2009). In a 1-year follow-up study, the investigators reported similar findings (Boelens et al., 2012).

The efficacy of prayer is beginning to be explored in areas such as decreasing aggression and promoting forgiveness (Bremmer et al., 2011; Marschall, Toussaint, Stuart, & Gates, 2012). Armstrong (2011) provides 12 steps to help individuals lead a more compassionate life, including

Exhibit 12.3. *Selected Studies Documenting the Use of Prayer*

Alcoholism (Lambert, Fincham, Marks, & Stillman, 2010)

Cancer (Rezaei, Adib-Hajbaghery, Seyedfatemi, & Hoseini, 2008)

Cardiac conditions (Blumenthal et al., 2007)

Caregivers (Wilks & Vonk, 2008)

Community-dwelling older adults (Cheung, Wyman, & Halcon, 2007)

Diabetes (Yeh, Eisenberg, Davis, & Phillips, 2002)

Forgiveness (Marschall et al., 2012)

Hemodialysis (Walton, 2007)

HIV-1 adults (Fitzpatrick et al., 2007)

Medication adherence (Konkle-Parker et al., 2008)

Poststroke (Robinson-Smith, 2002)

Reduction of anxiety and depression (Boelens et al., 2012)

a compassion prayer in which one prays for people—both those loved and those hated or disliked. In our world, where aggression and violence are so prevalent and often result in increased stress and sometimes serious injury or death, ways to promote a sense of universal peace would have a profound impact on overall health.

As noted earlier, prayer is universal across the globe. Sidebar 12.1 describes how prayer is part of health care in Japan.

Sidebar 12.1. *Buddhist Prayer in Health Care in Japan*

Konomi Nakashima, Kyoto, Japan

Overall, nurses in Japan are skeptical about the use of prayer. However, nurses and paramedical staff are beginning to give more attention to prayer. Japanese nurses do not treat prayer as care, but see it in terms of an amulet or talisman. They are also giving more attention to the religious feelings of their patients.

It would not be an exaggeration to say that most Japanese people took shelter in Buddhism in earlier times. Prayer helps a person to obtain enlightenment by abandoning worldly desires. In Buddhism, the Buddhas take vows to save all living beings. People believe that the Buddhas are there to save them ultimately, and they believe in their power. This unconditional faith of individuals establishes the power of prayer. There are three types of Buddhist prayer:

- Prayer to fulfill worldly desires
- Prayer to obtain enlightenment
- Prayer to help others as vowed by Bodhisattvas

Hospice care is one area in which prayer is becoming visible. In Nagaokanishi Hospital in Niigata prefecture, a Buddhist altar room is in the center of the hospice unit. Patients and family members from other units also come to the prayer room. During the morning and evening prayers, patients, family members, and hospital staff listen to the Buddhist priest's prayer. When a patient dies, the farewell ceremony is held in the altar room and other patients attend. The ceremony is televised so all patients can participate in the prayer service.

Although Japanese nurses have not, to any great degree, included prayer in the care of patients, prayer rituals are a part of many aspects of life. For example, parents visit a Shinto shrine after the birth of a baby, and for the safety and peace in a family. Prayers are also offered for a long life, to die without pain, and to avoid dementia.

FUTURE RESEARCH

Prayer continues to be a frequently used complementary therapy. In implementing research on prayer, especially using randomized clinical trials, many challenges are encountered. The following are several areas in which study is needed:

- Most of the reported research on prayer has been from a Christian perspective. As noted, more studies are beginning to be published about the use of prayer in other religions and cultures. Continued explorations will help health care professionals provide holistic care to patients from many backgrounds. Investigation of prayer by those who have no specific religious affiliation is also needed.
- Initial studies on use of prayer in promoting forgiveness and decreasing aggression point to the need for further exploration in this area because hatred and violence are so much a part of societies.
- In many regions, particularly in the West, major religions are playing less of a role in the lives of individuals, particularly the young. What are the spiritual practice needs of this group as they face illness and loss?

REFERENCES

Ai, A., Dunkle, R., Peterson, C., & Bolling, S. (1998). The role of private prayer in psychological recovery among midlife and aged patients following heart surgery. *The Gerontologist, 38*, 591–601.

Armstrong, K. (2011). *Twelve steps to a compassionate life.* New York, NY: Alfred A. Knopf.

Badsha, H., & Tak, P. (2008). Can Islamic prayer benefit spondyloarthritis? Case report of a patient with anklyosing spondylitis and increased spinal mobility after an intensive regimen of Islamic prayer. *Rheumatology International, 28*, 1057–1059.

Banzinger, S., Van Uden, M., & Janssen, J. (2008). Praying and coping: The relation between varieties of praying and religious coping styles. *Mental Health, Religion & Culture, 11*, 101–118.

Bergland, J., Heuer, L., & Lausch, C. (2007). The use of prayer by Hispanic migrant farmworkers with type 2 diabetes. *Journal of Cultural Diversity, 14*, 164–168.

Boelens, P., Reeves, R., Replogle, W., & Koeig, H. (2009). A randomized trial of the effect of prayer on depression and anxiety. *International Journal of Psychiatry in Medicine, 39*, 377–392.

Boelens, P., Reeves, R., Replogle, W., & Koeig, H. (2012). The effect of prayer on depression and anxiety: Maintenance of positive influence one year after prayer intervention. *International Journal of Psychiatry in Medicine, 43*, 85–98.

Blumenthal, J. A., Babyak, M. A., Ironson, G., Thoresen, C., Powell, L., Czajkowski, S., . . . Catellier, D. (2007). Spirituality, religion, and clinical outcomes in patients recovering from an acute myocardial infarction. *Psychosomatic Medicine, 69*, 501–508.

Bremmer, R., Koole, S., & Bushman, B. (2011). "Pray for those who mistreat you": Effect of prayer on anger and aggression. *Personality & Social Psychology Journal, 37*, 830–837.

Breslin, M. J., & Lewis, C. A. (2008). Theoretical models of the nature of prayer and health: A review. *Mental Health, Religion & Culture, 11*, 9–21.

Brown, C. M., Barner, J. C., Richards, K. M., & Bohman, T. M. (2007). Patterns of complementary and alternative therapy medicine use in African Americans. *Journal of Complementary & Alternative Medicine, 12*, 751–758.

Byrd, R. (1998). Positive therapeutic effects of intercessory prayer in a coronary care unit population. *Southern Medical Journal, 81*, 826–829.

Cheung, D. K., Wyman, J. F., & Halcon, L. L. (2007). Use of complementary and alternative therapies in community-dwelling older adults. *Journal of Alternative & Complementary Medicine, 13*, 997–1006.

Doufesh, H., Faisal, T., Lim, K., & Ibrahim, F. (2012). EEG spectral analysis on Muslim prayer. *Applied Psychophysiology & Biofeedback, 37*, 11–8.

Dusek, J. A., Astin, J. A., Hibberd, P. L., & Krucoff, M. W. (2003). Healing prayer outcome studies. *Alternative Therapies in Health and Medicine, 9* (Suppl. A.), A44–A53.

Fitzpatrick, A. L., Standish, L. J., Berger, J., Kim, J. G., Calabrese, C., & Polissar, N. (2007). Survival in HIV-1-positive adults practicing psychological or spiritual activities for one year. *Alternative Therapies in Health & Medicine, 13*(5), 18–20, 22–24.

Harris, W. S., Gowda, M., Kolb, J. W., Strychacz, C. P., Vacek, J. L., & Jones, P.G. (1999). A randomized, controlled trial of the effects of remote, intercessory prayer on outcomes in patients admitted to the coronary care unit. *Archives of Internal Medicine, 159*, 2273–2278.

Hollywell, C., & Walker, J. (2009). Private prayer as a suitable intervention for hospitalized patients: A critical review of the literature. *Journal of Clinical Nursing, 18*, 637–651.

Joint Commission Standards for Patient Care. (2012). *Spiritual assessment*. Retrieved October 31, 2012, from http://www.jointcommission.org/AcreditationPrograms

Joyce, C. R., & Welldon, R. M. (1965). The objective efficacy of prayer. *Journal of Chronic Disease, 18*, 367–376.

King, M. O., & Pettigrew, A. C. (2004). Complementary and alternative therapy use by older adults in three ethnically diverse populations: A pilot study. *Geriatric Nursing, 25*(1), 30–37.

Konkle-Parker, D. J., Erlen, J. A., & Dubbert, P. M. (2008). Barriers and facilitators to medication adherence in a southern minority population with HIV disease. *Journal of the Association of Nurses in AIDS Care, 19*, 98–114.

Lambert, N., Fincham, F., Marks, L., & Stillman, T. (2010). Invocations and intoxication: Does prayer decrease alcohol consumption? *Psychology of Addictive Behaviors, 24*, 209–219.

Marschall, J., Toussaint, L., Stuart, K., & Gates, L. (2012). Say your prayers, but make 'em quick: Replicating the effects of three minutes of prayer on forgiveness. *Explore, 8*, 249–251.

Masters, K. S., & Spielmans, G. I. (2007). Prayer and health: Review, meta-analysis, and research agenda. *Journal of Behavioral Medicine, 30*, 329–338.

Milevsky, A., & Eisenberg, M. (2012). Spiritually oriented treatment with Jewish clients: Meditative prayer and religious texts. *Professional Psychology: Research and Practice, 43*, 336–340.

Moher, D., Hopewell, S., Schulz, K. F., Monton, V., Gotzsche, P., Devereaux, P. J., . . . Altman, D. (2010). *Consort 2010 explanation and elaboration: Updated guidelines for reporting parallel group randomized trials*. Retrieved December 17, 2012, from http://www.bmj.com/content/340/bmj.c869

National Center for Complementary and Alternative Medicine. (2012). *What is CAM?* Retrieved August 21, 2008, from http://nccam.nih.gov/health/whatiscam

Newberg, A., D'Aquili, E., & Rause, V. (2001). *Why God won't go away*. New York, NY: Ballantine Books.

Olver, J., & Dutney, A. (2012). A randomized, blinded study of the impact of intercessory prayer on spiritual well-being in patients with cancer. *Alternative Therapies, 18*, 18–27.

Peterman, A. H., Fitchett, G., Brady, M. J., Hernandez, L., & Cella, D. (2002). Measuring spiritual well-being in people with cancer: The Functional Assessment of Chronic Illness Therapy-Spiritual Well-Being Scale (FACIT-Sp). *Annals of Behavioral Medicine, 24*, 49–58.

Pew Forum. (2013). *Church statistics and religious affiliations-U.S. religious landscape*. Retrieved March 1, 2013, from http://religions.pew.forum.org/affiliations

Remen, R. N. (2000). *My grandfather's blessings*. New York, NY: Riverhead Books.

Rezaei, M., Adib-Hajbaghery, M., Seyedfatemi, N., & Hoseini, F. (2008). Prayer in Iranian cancer patients undergoing chemotherapy. *Complementary Therapies in Clinical Practice, 14*, 90–97.

Roberts, L., Ahmed, I., & Hall, S. (2009). *Intercessory prayer for the alleviation of ill health*. (Cochrane Database of Systematic Reviews 2009(2), CD000368:10:1002/14651858. CD 000368. Pub. 3.) Retrieved October 23, 2012, from www. Cochrane.org/reviews

Robinson-Smith, G. (2002). Prayer after stroke: Its relationship to quality of life. *Journal of Holistic Nursing, 20*, 352–366.

Schroder, D. (2011). Presidential address: Can prayer help surgery? *American Journal of Surgery, 201*, 275–278.

Stabile, S. (2013). *Growing in love & wisdom*. New York, NY: Oxford University Press.

Tippens, K., Marsman, M.A., & Zwickey, H. (2009). Paradigms: Is prayer CAM? *Journal of Alternative and Complementary Medicine, 15*, 435–438.

Walton, J. (2007). Prayer warriors: A grounded theory study of American Indians receiving dialysis. *Nephrology Nursing Journal: Journal of the American Nephrology Nurses' Association, 34*, 377–386.

Wilks, S. E, & Vonk, M. E. (2008). Private prayer among Alzheimer's caregivers: Mediating burden and resiliency. *Journal of Gerontological Social Work, 50*, 113–131.

Yeh, G. Y., Eisenberg, D. M., Davis, R. B., & Phillips, R. S. (2002). Use of complementary and alternative medicine among persons with diabetes mellitus: Results of a national survey. *American Journal of Public Health, 92*, 1648–1652.

not a diary. more introspective

Chapter 13: Journaling

MARIAH SNYDER

Journal writing is one of a group of therapies that provides an opportunity for persons to reflect on and analyze their lives and the events and people surrounding them, and to get in touch with their feelings. Memoirs, life review, and storytelling are other interventions that use a similar scientific basis. All of these therapies require individuals to be engaged in reflecting on and gaining insights about their lives and experiences.

From the beginning of history, people have recorded the events of their lives, first in pictures and then in words. Reeve Lindbergh (2008) states:

> To write as honestly as I can in my journals about my everyday life and the thoughts and feelings I have as I go along is an old tenacious yearning, maybe due [to] an early discomfort with the oddly intangible [enormities] of my family history. Or perhaps this effort is just something else my mother left to me; her belief that writing is the way to make life as perceptible as life can be perceived. (p. 80)

Although much anecdotal evidence exists about the beneficial effects of journaling, research on the use of journals is sparse. However, results of studies revealing the positive outcomes of journaling have been published (Petrie, Fontanilla, Thomas, Booth, & Pennebaker, 2004; Proctor, Hoffmann, & Allison, 2012; Smith, Anderson-Hanley, Langrock, & Compas, 2005). Most journaling research has explored the efficacy of reflective writing in education.

Diary—events encounters
Journal—processes of life

DEFINITION

The terms *journaling, diary, reflective writing,* and *expressive writing* are often used interchangeably. Diaries more often focus on the recording of events and encounters, whereas journaling serves as a tool for recording the process of one's life (Cortright, 2008). Events and experiences are noted in journals, with emphasis on the person's reflections about these events and the personal meaning assigned to them. In journal writing, interplay between the conscious and unconscious often occurs. Forms of expressive writing such as poetry, stories, and scrapbooking are methods an individual may use to explore inner feelings and thoughts. Journaling is used in this chapter to encompass writing for therapeutic purposes.

SCIENTIFIC BASIS

Journaling is a holistic therapy because it involves all aspects of a person—physical (muscular movements), mental (thought processes), emotional (getting in touch with or expressing feelings), and spiritual (finding meaning). Through journal recordings, people are able to connect with the continuity of their lives and thus enhance wholeness. Writing may also aid individuals in identifying unconscious ideas and emotions that may be influencing their behaviors and lives. Awareness of these is furthered as subjects reflect on specific events, thoughts, or feelings while recording them; link them with past feelings and meanings; and consider present and future implications.

Progoff (1975), a Jungian psychologist, developed a systematized method for journaling called "the intensive journal." He noted that this transpsychological approach provided active strategies that enable participants to draw on their inherent resources to become whole. Through journaling, Progoff maintained, people become more self-reliant as they develop their inner strengths and draw on these when faced with problems and challenges such as stress or illness.

Journaling provides an opportunity for catharsis related to traumatic events in one's life (Sealy, 2012). Unlike merely venting one's feelings, journaling furnishes the avenue for a person to explore causes and solutions and gain insights. Sealy noted that "reflective journaling and meditation can provide an opportunity to 'socially reconstruct' past psychological injury" (p. 38).

Inhibiting expression of emotions may result in increased autonomic activity that may have long-lasting harmful effects on the body, such as precipitating hypertension. Therapies that assist one in venting feelings in a healthy manner may help to improve a person's health. Ulrich and Lutgendorf (2002) reported that students who journaled about cognitive and emotional aspects of a stressful event developed a greater awareness of the positive aspects of the event, as compared with students who wrote only about the associated emotions or about overall events. Further support for the efficacy of writing about traumatic events was documented in a second study in which persons with HIV infections wrote about emotional topics versus neutral topics; journaling about emotional topics resulted in a heightened immune function (Petrie et al., 2004).

Some hypotheses for why journaling may be helpful in bringing about positive physical and emotional outcomes include:

1. The physical act of writing (or typing) occupies the left brain and leaves the right brain free to examine emotions and seek insights.
2. Journaling assists in discovering patterns in one's life, particularly those that have a negative impact.
3. Journaling assists in the discernment process by helping to clarify thoughts and the emotions that are generated through encounters with specific events or persons. It also assists in generating possible solutions and identifying which solution(s) might be the best option.

INTERVENTION

Various techniques for journaling exist—free-flowing writing, topical or focused journaling, and creative writing. The length of time journaling is carried out (weeks, months, or years) will depend on the specific purpose of the journaling. Sometimes people initially write during a stressful situation or transition in their lives, but become hooked and continue writing after the initial event has ended.

Some general guidelines for journaling or writing are found in Exhibit 13.1. What is most important for journaling is that the person be honest with self when writing. Knowing that the content is private and to be shared only if the writer so desires, allows the individual to write about difficult topics or feelings. If, on the other hand, participants know that what they are writing has to be shared, an internal censor may be activated that impedes them from writing their true feelings.

Entries should be made in a special notebook. This may be a book designed exclusively for journaling or an inexpensive spiral notebook. Plain notebooks can be personalized by putting pictures on the cover, or using pictures and colored markers throughout the notebook. Because pencil recordings fade over time, a pen should be used because the person may want to reread past entries.

Developments in media have created many new avenues for journal writing. Some may prefer using the computer to make entries. With the advent of iPads and iPhones, there is an ease in making entries during

Exhibit 13.1. *Guidelines for Journaling*

Date entries.

Choose a time of day to write, such as morning or evening.

Select a specific place to write, if possible, where there will be few interruptions.

Use a pen, not a pencil.

Leave what you write; do not cross out or erase words.

Use a notebook specific to journaling; if desired, personalize the notebook.

Remember, journaling is for you and does not need to be shared unless you choose to do so.

short breaks. Some may wish to use blogs to share their reflections with others. Shepherd and Aagard (2011) described the use of web 2.0 tools with older adults to promote health.

When to write and for how long are questions each person needs to answer. Journaling for 15 minutes to 30 minutes each day is recommended by a number of sources (Pennebaker, 2012). Journaling needs to be the servant and not the master. Establishing a specific time of day to make entries is helpful. Some find early morning a good time to write, when information in the unconscious seems to be closest to the surface. Others prefer to do journaling in the evening, to resolve pent-up anger or troublesome events of the day before retiring.

Techniques

Free-Flow Journaling

Free-flow journaling is the most common type of journaling. Cortright (2008) suggested writing quickly and allowing words to just fall onto the page, without attention to grammar, punctuation, or spelling. The main goal is to put one's thoughts and feelings on paper. Journaling provides a vehicle to uncover the wisdom one already possesses and the feelings that have been dormant. Sometimes a person will write pages and pages on one topic or event. At other times, one's mind flits from topic to topic. The latter may happen when one is highly distressed, and concentrating on one topic is difficult. There is no right or wrong way to journal. The main goal is to put words into written form and then reflect on them. One suggestion is, upon finishing the day's entry, to reread it and then jot down an "insight line" about what your entry is telling you (Cortright, 2008).

Topical Journaling

This type of journaling focuses on a specific event or situation. The focus can be the person's illness or that of a family member. Individuals are asked to write about their feelings, how they perceive the illness will be affecting their lives or how it has affected their lives, and fears they have about the treatments or outcomes. Instructions may include specific questions to which the person is to respond. For example, in using journaling with people who desire to lose weight, the following are a sample of questions that could be posed:

- What are your eating habits? For example, do you eat large meals or snack throughout the day?
- What is the meaning of food in your life?
- What are your favorite foods and why?

Often topical journaling is used in conjunction with support groups.

Creative Writing

Some people may be more comfortable writing in story form or in poetry rather than focusing on specific events or emotions in their lives. This type of writing can assist persons in uncovering deeper thoughts or emotions in a safe manner because a story may have characters saying things that individuals would feel uncomfortable attributing to themselves. Stories allow for feelings to be seen initially in the people in the story and then as they relate to oneself. Pictures may be used as an initiator of a story.

Some prefer to do free-flowing journaling in a poetic form. This type of writing allows one to be creative and still explore feelings. Using short lines and spreading the content over a page make it easier to examine thoughts and emotions.

Combining journaling and art is another form of creative writing. Several authors described using scrapbooking and journaling for therapeutic purposes (Davidson & Robison, 2008; Subhani & Ifrah, 2012). Pictures or items used in creating the scrapbook served as the trigger for the journaling for the participants. Digital online pictures could be used for the journaling stimulus. Infinite possibilities exist and can be adapted to the preferences of the patient.

A number of websites provide helpful information about journaling. Some of these are noted in Exhibit 13.2.

Measurement of Outcomes

Many outcomes from journal writing may not be immediately discernible. Some of the possible areas to measure are improvement in self-esteem or quality of life, reduction in anxiety and/or negative feelings, and adapting

Exhibit 13.2. *Online Resources About Journaling*

Conversations within: Journal writing and inner dialog (www.journal-writing.com)

Journal for you (www.journalforyou.com)

Top 10 miraculous benefits of keeping a personal journal (www.mymotivator.com/journal_top 10.htm)

Writing and health: Some practice advice (homepage.psy.utexas.edu/Faculty/Pennebaker/Homepage)

Writing the journey (www.writingthejourney.com)

to a chronic condition. Physiological measures such as the immune system, weight loss, and blood pressure have also been used to determine the efficacy of journaling. Unless patients share their journals, nurses are not aware of the content or focus of the journaling. In some studies in which journaling was used, content analysis was carried out on journal entries to determine themes (DiNapoli, 2004).

Precautions

Fear that others will find and read journal entries is a common concern and may deter persons from being open in expressing themselves in a journal. A concern expressed at a corrections facility was that the journals would be confiscated and used in court. Care needs to be taken if individuals appear to be extremely introspective or scrupulous, as journaling may deepen this inward focus. Passwords on computers will help ensure privacy of entries when this form is used for journaling.

USES

Journaling has been used with various conditions and populations, both in illness and to promote health. Exhibit 13.3 lists some of the populations for whom journaling has been used. In those newly diagnosed with a chronic illness, journaling about their perspectives on how the illness may affect their lives may help them uncover fears that could then be discussed with a health professional. Journaling also provides an avenue for people to identify hidden resources or strengths they may possess that will assist them in living with a chronic illness. Writing positive affirmations and then reading the statements may help them gain confidence in their abilities to manage the chronic condition. Tanabe et al. (2010) reported that journaling was one of the therapies that adults with sickle

Exhibit 13.3. *Uses of Journaling*

Assist with transitions (Rancour & Brauer, 2003)
Decrease anxiety (Ulrich & Lutgendorf, 2002)
Decrease depression (Smith et al., 2005)
Decrease jail recidivism (Proctor et al., 2012)
Decrease use of tobacco (DiNapoli, 2004)
Improve community problem solving (Aronson, Wallis, O'Campo, Whitehead, & Schafer, 2006)
Improve well-being and personal growth (Ulrich & Lutgendorf, 2002; Wagoner & Wijekumar, 2004)
Increase creativity (Dowrick, 2009)
Palliative care (Penz & Duggleby, 2012)
Posttraumatic stress disorder (Davidson & Robison, 2008)
Spiritual growth (Chittister, 2004)

cell disease used to successfully manage their condition. Other researchers (Rancour & Brauer, 2003) used journaling to assist patients with cancer adjust to changes in their body image.

Research and anecdotal evidence support the use of journaling to improve well-being. DiNapoli (2004) found that journaling assisted adolescent girls with a smoking history to lessen their use of tobacco. Ulrich and Lutgendorf (2002) reported that journaling about stressful events resulted in positive growth and health outcomes. Journaling helped older patients adapt to changes occurring with aging (Caplan, Haslett, & Burelson, 2005). Other investigators found that interactive journaling was helpful in reducing recidivism in jail inmates (Proctor et al., 2012).

Although not specifically journaling, diaries have been used in intensive care units (Storlie, Lind, & Viotti, 2003). Nurses and families kept a record of the patients' stays. These were then used in a follow-up program to help subjects gain an understanding of their time in the intensive care unit, including dreams and times when patients were confused or unconscious. The program proved valuable for participants and staff.

Journal writing has also been used to help people develop spiritually. Chittister (2004) related how journaling on quotations or sayings of others helped her gain new perspectives. Journaling may also be helpful in praying. The act of writing helps keep a person centered on conversation with God. As suggested by Chittister, a passage from a holy book may be the stimulus for using journaling to pray.

CULTURAL ASPECTS

Although journaling is a therapy that many find helpful, others, particularly those from oral-based cultures, may find it daunting to reflect on their thoughts and experiences in writing. Painting and other forms of art may be alternative mechanisms that can be used to express feelings. The Hmong culture, an Asian ethnic group, has been a nonoral culture. The embroidery pieces of art created by Hmong women depict the history of the Hmong. This representational embroidery, or "story cloths," is used by members, especially women, to convey experiences of the Hmong and their history to future generations (Arkenberg, 2007).

Sidebar 13.1 describes the consideration of the use of journaling in Perú. It is clear that the intervention would need to be adapted in an oral culture such as in Perú, and potentially in other nations and peoples.

Sidebar 13.1. *The Potential Use of Journaling in Perú*

Sasha Orange, Lima, Perú

As a Peruvian, and as a student in a nursing school in the United States, I have carefully considered the potential applicability of journaling as a nursing intervention in Perú. The journaling intervention as described in this chapter is not in widespread use, nor could it easily be transferred to Perú and widely applied. The Peruvian culture is primarily an oral culture. Many people are not accustomed to writing as a means of natural communication, even though many know how to read and write; the preference is to communicate orally. For example, our bus system lists the destinations on the side of the bus. In addition, there is a person whose job it is to shout the destinations for the people who cannot or do not read them. In my experience, I have heard of journaling being used among psychiatrists with their patients. This therapy is useful among a scholarly population; however, it is perhaps not the best therapy to implement broadly among the population in Perú. For people—children and adults—who cannot read or write, drawing therapies are used instead. Specifically, in the Andes, many of the indigenous people living there do not possess the necessary skill set, and they speak different languages. In order to overcome this language barrier it is easier to implement drawing therapy as opposed to journaling.

If journaling is used, it is most likely to be used with women as opposed to men. In our culture, men are taught at a young age that they are not allowed to express their feelings and that they need to prove their

(continued)

Sidebar 13.1. *The Potential Use of Journaling in Perú (continued)*

manhood. Aside from this, there is less need for a journal because there are close family connections in which people can share their feelings. In Perú, there is a large emphasis on extended family, so most likely there will always be someone to talk to. Our culture is very open, and sharing feelings and problems with family and friends is common. I recall as a child being included in adult conversations in which my family discussed life issues. Perhaps such conversations are therapeutic and serve as a replacement for the use of journaling.

FUTURE RESEARCH

Exploration in the efficacy of journaling in health care is in its infancy. Journaling has often been used in conjunction with other therapies and hence its specific impact has been difficult to extract. Some of the areas in which research is needed include:

- Technology offers numerous possibilities for new avenues for journaling. Few studies have explored the use of technology as a means for journaling. Investigations in this arena are particularly needed with younger populations.
- Ethical and legal implications for journaling require study and need to be resolved, especially for those who are incarcerated. Fears about their journals being "used against them" may inhibit persons from being honest in their journaling.
- Reviewing the research base on the use of journaling in education may reveal strategies for its use in health care.

REFERENCES

Arkenberg, R. (2007). Hmong story cloths. *SchoolArts: The Art Magazine for Teachers, 107*(2), 32–33.

Aronson, R. E., Wallis, A. B., O'Campo, P. J., Whitehead, T. L., & Schafer, P. (2006). Ethnographically informed community evaluation: A framework and approach for evaluating community-based initiatives. *Maternal and Child Health Journal, 11,* 97–109.

Caplan, S. E., Haslett, B. J., & Burelson, B. R. (2005). Telling it like it is: The adaptive function of narratives in coping with loss in later life. *Health Communication, 17,* 233–251.

Chittister, J. (2004). *Called to question.* Lanham, MD: Sheed & Ward.

Cortright, S. M. (2008). *Journaling: A tool for your spirit.* Retrieved September 3, 2008, from http://www.journalforyou.com/full_article.php?article_id=7

Davidson, J., & Robison, B. (2008). Scrapbooking and journaling interventions for chronic illness: A triangulated investigation of approaches in the treatment of PTSD. *Kansas Nurse, 83*(3), 6–11.

DiNapoli, P. P. (2004). The lived experience of adolescent girls' relationship with tobacco. *Issues in Comprehensive Pediatric Nursing, 27,* 19–26.

Dowrick, S. (2009). *Creative journal writing: The art and heart of reflection.* New York, NY: Penguin.

Lindbergh, R. (2008). *Forward from here.* New York, NY: Simon & Schuster.

Pennebaker, J. (2012) *Writing and health: Some practical advice.* Retrieved October 20, 2012, from http:www. Homepage.psy.utexas.edu/homepage/Faculty/Pennebaker/ Homepage

Penz, K., & Duggleby, W. (2012) "It's different in the home. . . ." The contextual challenges and rewards of providing palliative care in community settings. *Journal of Hospice and Pailliative Care, 14,* 365–373.

Petrie, K. J., Fontanilla, I., Thomas, M. G., Booth, R. J., & Pennebaker, J. W. (2004). Effect of written emotional expression on immune function in patients with human immunodeficiency virus infection: A randomized trial. *Psychosomatic Medicine, 66,* 272–275.

Proctor, S., Hoffmann, N., & Allison, S. (2012). The effectiveness of interactive journaling in reducing recidivism among substance-dependent jail inmates. *International Journal of Offender Therapy and Comparative Criminology, 56,* 317–332.

Progoff, I. (1975). *At a journal workshop.* New York, NY: Dialogue House Library.

Rancour, P., & Brauer, K. (2003). Use of letter writing as a means of integrating body image: A case study. *Oncology Nursing Forum, 30,* 841–846.

Sealy, P. (2012). Autoethnography: Reflective journaling and meditation to cope with life-threatening breast cancer. *Clinical Journal of Oncology Nursing, 16,* 38–41.

Shepherd, C., & Aagard, S. (2011). Journal writing with Web 2.0 tools: A vision for older adults. *Educational Gerontology, 37,* 606–620.

Smith, S., Anderson-Hanley, C., Langrock, A., & Compas, B. (2005). The effects of journaling for women with newly diagnosed breast cancer. *Psycho-Oncology, 14,* 1075–1082.

Storlie, S. L., Lind, R., & Viotti, I. (2003). Using diaries in intensive care: A method for following up patients. *Connect: The World of Critical Care Nursing, 2*(4), 103–108.

Subhani, M., & Ifrah, I. (2012). Digital scrapbooking as a standard of care in neonatal intensive care units: Initial experience. *Journal of Neonatal Nursing, 31,* 162–168.

Tanabe, P., Porter, J., Creary, M., Miller, S., Ahmed-Williams, E., & Hassell, K. (2010). A qualitative analysis of best self-management practices: Sickle-cell disease. *Journal of National Medical Association, 102*(11), 1033–1041.

Ulrich, P. M., & Lutgendorf, S. K. (2002). Journaling about stressful events: Effects of cognitive processing and emotional expression. *Annals of Behavior Medicine, 24,* 244–250.

Wagoner, D., & Wijekumar, K. (2004). Improving self-awareness of nutrition and life style practices through on-line journaling. *Journal of Nutrition Education & Behavior, 36,* 211–212.

Chapter 14: Storytelling

MARGARET P. MOSS

*T*he art and science of storytelling is presented in this chapter as a mechanism that can be used in alternative or complementary therapy. Its historical roots in orality (also known as oralism) are defined and explicated through examples from primary oral cultures. These are cultures that do not have a written language system (Sampson, 1980). In direct contrast, taking the art form into the future, digital storytelling is explored. Storytelling is then connected to its use as an alternative method in which to affect the path of one's health in terms of education, prevention, and intervention. Finally, concrete recommendations for health professionals close out the chapter.

DEFINITIONS

Orality

"The narratives we live and share everyday are our identity as a storied people and make visible what matters most in our lives" (Heliker, 2007, p. 21). Although there are around 3,000 languages in existence today, only 106 have ever been written and less than one half of those are said to have literature (Edmondson, 1971). Orality is defined as a mostly verbal communication system employed by whole cultures and devoid of the conventions or use of the written word (Olson & Torrance, 1991). The connection of orality or oralism to storytelling is intuitive. Storytelling is as universal in human communication as "the basic orality of language is permanent" (Ong, 2002, p. 7).

Literate societies evolved from oral societies. Each literate individual evolved from an oral beginning (Olson & Torrance, 1991). That is not to say that the formal and informal rules of orality are not as intricate as those in written communication. However, the vast majority of languages have never been translated into a written language (Edmondson, 1971).

The speaker, the process, and the aesthetics of orality are keys to imparting information (Lord, 1960). The rules concerning who speaks and when are defined by the culture. For instance, in some American Indian tribes, certain stories can only be told in the winter, others in the summer. Some words are not to be spoken at certain times of the day or to certain listeners. The process may be as in a prayer, a dance, or a story, and can be in front of a large audience or one on one. Aesthetics may involve the use of masks, rattles, costumes, or specific surroundings. Finally, orality uses postural and gestural tools, as well as silence, as paralinguistic features in the transmission of the communication (Tedlock, 1983). "Formulaicness is valued when wisdom is seen as knowledge passed down through generations. Novelty is valued when wisdom is viewed as new information" (Tannen, 1982, p. 6). Therefore, anyone wishing to impart information through purposive oral means, such as through storytelling, needs to understand the key components, rules, and assigned power of oralism.

Storytelling

Storytelling is defined as the art or act of telling stories (Dictionary.com, 2013). A story is "a narrative, either true or fictitious, in prose or verse, designed to interest, amuse, or instruct the hearer or reader; [a] tale." Sociolinguist William Labov (as cited in Sandelowski, 1994) states that a complete story typically is composed of the:

- Abstract—what the story is about
- Orientation—the "who, when, where, and what" of the story
- Complicating action—the "then-what-happened" part of the story
- Evaluation—the "so-what" of the story
- Resolution—the "what-finally-happened" portion of the story
- Coda—the signal a story is over
- Return to the present (Sandelowski, 1994, p. 25)

It is the instructive nature of storytelling that is of interest for health care as an alternative means to an outcome: improved health. But it must also be understood that lives, including our health, are "shaped by the stories we live" (Heliker, 2007, p. 21). Stories have shaped patients' current selves; and it is through stories that nurses can "interest, amuse, or instruct" them as listeners. Storytelling has paralleled human endeavors and will continue to evolve through future mechanisms.

Digital Storytelling

Digital storytelling is "the modern expression of the ancient art of story-telling. Digital stories derive their power by weaving images, music, narrative, and voice together, thereby giving deep dimension and vivid color to characters, situations, experiences, and insights" (Rule, 2009).

Although technology in digital storytelling provides the processes and aesthetics, it can also present some difficulties. For those cultures with restrictions on word use, the 24-hour, 365-day availability of words via computer technology brings uncertainty. Matching the listener and the teller and their implicit contract is of utmost importance when choosing the type of conveyance.

Storytelling, whether traditional or digital, whether oral or written, serves multiple purposes across the life span and can be used by nurses. Nurses listen to stories whenever patients tell them what is going on in their lives; and they tell and retell stories every time they pass on information about patients (Fairbairn & Carson, 2002). Whether it is the person being cared for or the nurse, each individual telling the story "is" the story being told (Sandelowski, 1994). It is in the unfolding, intertwining, and connecting that a story becomes my story, your story, or our story. Stories are woven into the threads of life's fabric in our daily lives (Barton, 2004). We are all connected on a deeper or—if you prefer—higher level and storytelling can take us to these levels.

SCIENTIFIC BASIS

Storytelling "is one of the world's most powerful tools for achieving astonishing results" in almost any industry (Guber, 2007, p. 55). Through an implicit contract between the storyteller and the listener (Guber, 2007), time is always a necessary ingredient. The storyteller must take the time to fully tell a story through all of its parts, using the necessary gestures, processes, and aesthetics. A story, as a sequence of events with discernible relations between those events and culminating in some conclusion, is a cognitive package (Bergner, 2007) that can be given to the listener. The listener must make time available to be present within the story to *hear* the message and absorb it. Successful transmission will allow the listener to repeat the story to others in some form. Repetition, of course, leads to stronger transmission on both sides.

Effective storytellers understand their listener(s) and what they already know, what they care about, and what they want to hear (Guber, 2007). The great storyteller will guide the story through essential elements based on the listener's understanding that the story is larger than the teller (Guber, 2007).

Language and Healing Beyond Health Literacy

"One of the few universals is that humans in all known cultures use language and tell stories" (Ramirez-Esparza & Pennebaker, 2006, p. 216). Storytelling without language is not possible. "Language embodies cultural reality" (Kramsch, 1998, p. 3). Language *itself* and healing may have a connection not yet fully explored or understood, beyond health literacy bounds. Most of the literature involving language and health surround the idea of health literacy, which has been defined as, "the degree to which individuals have the capacity to obtain, process, and understand basic health information and services needed to make appropriate health decisions" (Nielsen-Bohlman, Panzer, & Kindig, 2004, p. 4). Although evidence points to greater understanding of health services and all that entails when spoken in the receiver's primary language (Koh et al., 2012), language as a healing tool and force are offered for consideration in this section.

In many indigenous cultures, for example, medicine and religion lines blur (Moss, 2000). Healing prayers are taken as a means toward optimum health whether in the physical, mental, spiritual, or emotional domain (Moss, 2000). These prayers are likely conducted in the traditional language. A recent study from South Africa offers that, "language creates an image of the unknown to which people attach meaning" (Lourens, 2013, abstract). There is comfort in hearing one's own language. It takes away a struggle and the required energy needed to accept either information or prayer, presumably then, allowing more energy to be used for healing.

Whereas indigenous examples of language use in prayer and healing may be specifically seen as other examples, the dominant cultures also use language in healing and prayer beyond their use as delivery of information only. We see this in the change in tone, speed, earnestness, and length of delivery that exceeds any aesthetic needed to merely deliver information. This can be from a mother to a sick child, a prayer group to a member, or other cultural convention or relationship.

American Indian Exemplar

The Zuni Indians of New Mexico use storytelling through all parts of their lives. It is used casually and formally. It is used in secular and sacred telling. The teller can be a priest, a *kiva* group, a grandmother, or another person. A *kiva* is a "medicine (i.e., priestly) society" to which men are initiated as youths and remain to carry out the work of the *kiva* (Moss, 2000). The purpose of the dances they perform can be solely to heal listeners from sickness. Through word of mouth, the news may spread that a Rain Dance is called. Unlike what Hollywood portrays, this dance calls listeners to one of the small plazas (flat dirt squares) in the village where they can receive needed healing prayers.

Time is part of the contract. The listener arrives at a loosely determined time and waits. The dancers and lead teller arrive some time later.
The teller knows why the listeners are there: the contract is intact. There
is respectful listening and targeted telling. The telling is in the form of
prayer, song, and dance. The team is in full regalia, with masks and dress
from centuries of performances. A formula is employed in the telling.
It can take hours. The teller(s), the process, and the aesthetics all come
together in dance, silence, and singing to heal the listener.

INTERVENTION

Bergner (2007) writes about the "staying power of stories," which has
obvious benefits when delivering therapeutic messages. He tells of stories
that patients have recounted as far back as 8 years earlier.

Technique

Stories in therapy draw from the general culture of the patient, integrate
common knowledge sequences, and therefore do not require the acquisi-
tion of new knowledge to participate (Bergner, 2007). Code words can then
be used to recall the entire story for the patient at later dates. Stories can be
targeted to specific diagnoses in increasing meaning for the patient. This
allows taking away aspects that do not apply and bringing in aspects that
may be unique to the patient.

Guidelines

The following guideline sequence has been presented in the literature for
storytelling in therapy: present the story, elaborate as needed to increase
understanding, and then discuss application to this particular patient situation (Bergner, 2007). In some cultures, there are situations in which reality can be "spoken into being." Again, often these are strongest in oral
cultures. However, even in the dominant culture in the United States, people will shush a person if he or she speaks about death, cancer, or some
bad thing happening.
    In primarily oral cultures, such as traditional indigenous societies,
it would be difficult to explain advance directives or informed consent
in the manner in which they are presented in Western medical facilities.
This applies whether in caring for a patient or in conducting research. As
an example, it might be the task of a health care provider to tell a traditional American Indian older adult from the Southwest that this individual could die, or lose a leg, or get an infection if the suggested traditional
treatments were completed. The patient would perceive harm in even
hearing this message. The subject certainly would not want to review or
sign a consent form that contained these facts. In this case, one would

be wise to use a hypothetical story instead. The harm would be taken away from the patient and, instead, the teller would describe to the listener facts about "another" person in a similar situation, drawing from cultural norms and common knowledge and asking the listener whether the hypothetical person would be willing to go through the procedure.

Using the above guidelines, there would be elaboration as needed in a context familiar to the patient. For instance, one might describe the following:

> Mr. Vigil was an older Pueblo man who had diabetes. He had it for 20 years and lived fairly comfortably with his family on the pueblo and saw his doctor regularly. There came a time when Mr. Vigil's leg began to bother him more and more. He tried several things with his doctor to increase blood flow and promote nerve health. Even though he did what he could for his health, it became apparent that he might have to lose the leg to continue living and being with his family. The doctor told him that he would still be able to participate in ceremonies and get around after the surgery with the use of a prosthetic leg and physical therapy. Mr. Vigil was worried. What do you think he was worried about? What do you think he might have decided? What questions would you ask if you were Mr. Vigil?

The use of vignettes such as the preceding one has been introduced in research as well as in practice.

When using stories as an intervention, one should use the ideas of orality, where repetition, setting, aesthetics, and process are important in the transmission of information. Implementing these will assist the listener in retaining the information.

Suggestions for Implementing Storytelling

Suggestions for health care practitioners, educators, or researchers contemplating using storytelling include:

■ Learn the difference between orality and literacy:
  - It is much more than: one group reads and the other writes.
  - A whole system of rules for use of each exists.
  - Each uses differing paths to arrive at the desired outcomes.
  - Orality and literacy may be used separately or together.
  - Understand the parts and mechanisms for telling the story:
  - The right person tells the right patient the right set of facts at the right time, in the right way, and the right place.
■ Understand differences in response to storytelling by age and culture:
  - Younger *and* older patients may be more attuned to traditional, oral, face-to-face storytelling.
  - The teenage through middle-adult patient may be more open and attuned to digital storytelling techniques.

- – Using vignettes and anecdotes in the third person takes the pressure off the listener.
- Use technology as appropriate:
  - – Certain cultures may not access the computer for fear of encountering a word deemed inappropriate at certain times or to certain people.
  - – Interactive media can be used with almost all persons *if geared specifically to* their age, culture, and level of technological proficiency.

Measurement of Outcomes

A variety of tools can be used to measure outcomes of storytelling. Depending on the purpose for which storytelling is being used, instruments that measure anxiety, depression, social isolation, spirituality, caring, and sense of well-being may be appropriate. Qualitative research methods may also be used to measure the effectiveness or changes brought about through storytelling, including increased understanding of the information.

Precautions

Those using storytelling need to be prepared to deal with the strong emotions stories may evoke. Health professionals should be ready to assist and support the participants, as diverse reactions can occur. A list of available resources for making referrals for follow-up will be helpful. Only persons trained in psychotherapy should use storytelling with people who have psychological problems. The health sciences represent disciplines that attempt to understand humans from their various perspectives and philosophies, but these disciplines have grown so specialized in their jargon that the message to the patient may easily be lost (Evans, 2007). The use of storytelling in common vernacular can be an antidote to this loss of message.

USES

The use of storytelling in health care settings, health care research, and teaching is unlimited. This section will share some examples of the use of storytelling. Nurses can use storytelling in multiple situations across the life span for a variety of purposes. Stories can be used in family therapy and can assist members in tapping into the flow of meaning of the past, present, and future, and help patients open up possibilities for "making meaning" and healing (Roberts, 1994).

Another aspect of using storytelling is when the *teller* of the story is the one to benefit from it. In Ramirez-Esparza and Pennebaker's (2006) article

"Do Good Stories Produce Good Health?," evidence for a link between expressive writing (storytelling) and markers for both mental and physical health are described. The stories do not even have to be coherent but just the ability of the person to express his or her story is beneficial (Ramirez-Esparza & Pennebaker, 2006). Analysis of the story down to which type of pronoun is used (i.e., first person or not) can point to health indicators around depression, for example (Ramirez-Esparza & Pennebaker, 2006).

This use and resulting phenomena have been seen in digital storytelling as well. The *teller* of the story receives a feeling of greater well-being or other health-related benefit. Sharing experiences, lightening a burden, and helping others allowed participants to report feeling better (www.patientvoices.org.uk) (Haigh & Hardy, 2011).

Older Persons: Practice

To increase the reciprocity of care between nursing home staff and residents, *story sharing* has been used as an intervention strategy. To lessen the almost totally task-oriented nature of caring, the use of story sharing has been shown to increase the quality of life of residents in six different nursing homes (Heliker, 2007). Through story sharing, the staff was encouraged to come to know the patients, their backgrounds, interests, and likes. Active listening and expressions of concern are key elements. This is a mutual process in which each learns about the other and trust and shared experiences become evident. The intervention suggested by Heliker used three 1-hour sessions between six nurse aides and a facilitator. In session 1, staff learn about confidentiality, respectful and attentive listening, and role playing. In session 2, staff bring an object that holds personal meaning for themselves, to better understand the residents and what few possessions residents may have with them, and the monumental meaning of these possessions. In session 3, staff learn about "sharing informs care" practices. Both residents and aides reported being in a better relationship with each other, which can be seen as a "best practice" in the care of older, frail adults (Heliker, 2007).

Older Persons: Education

"Many older adults were raised in an era when learning occurred primarily through reading, discussion, and retelling stories" (Cangelosi & Sorrell, 2008, p. 19). Often it is through storytelling, whether formal or informal, that otherwise missed information will be shared. Many older patients detail numerous topics and events until they hit on pertinent information in describing their current problem. Unless this wandering is not only allowed but encouraged, especially with older subjects, crucial data needed for their care will be missed. When questions requiring only *yes* and *no* answers are asked and are hurried in encounters with older clients, they will not be able to share information with the health care professional that is vital to their health story. Probing questions require time, patience, and empathy. In addition, older persons will need time to *hear* and process what the health care provider is telling them. One strategy is to share health information in a group setting allowing for support from others in the group (Cangelosi & Sorrell, 2008). But by using storytelling as an intervention for teaching older individuals, unique learning needs will be met (Cangelosi & Sorrell, 2008).

Digital Storytelling

Digital storytelling may be an effective way to educate younger people, whether in the classroom or in patient education, in this world of ever-changing technology. Visual and audio media may stimulate deeper learning in this population, which is largely familiar and comfortable with the use of technology (Sandars, Murray, & Pellow, 2008). Sandars and colleagues have used digital storytelling with medical students. As a guideline, they suggest the following 12-step sequence of events for digital storytelling:

1. Decide on the topic of the story.
2. Write the story.
3. Collect a variety of multimedia to create a story.
4. Select which to use to create the story.
5. Create the story.
6. Present the digital story.
7. Encourage reflection at each stage of the project.
8. Avoid being too ambitious.
9. Provide adequate technical support.
10. Develop a relevant assessment framework.
11. Embed it within existing teaching and learning approaches.
12. Persuade others of its value.

Here, building the story encourages active learning and constant reflection for the teller. This process could be used with other populations such as patient groups. Although the storyteller is in many ways the learner in this situation, the same orality notions are in play. The storyteller, the process, and the aesthetics are of great import. Here, rather than regalia, video and audio supply the aesthetics.

When looking ahead to digital delivery and/or storytelling in the future, it is probable that, "growth in technology is actually likely to increase health disparities for those with limited health, computer, and reading literacy, unless effort is devoted to the development of IT [information technology] specifically designed for these disadvantaged groups, and issues of technology access are addressed" (Bickmore & Paasche-Orlow, 2012, p. 23).

CULTURAL APPLICATIONS

In many indigenous societies, especially when they are described as primarily oral cultures, Western health practices will be seen as the alternative and complementary modalities (Moss, 2000). This is important because the practitioner—or here, the storyteller—must understand that to patients coming from a basically oral culture, storytelling is already seen as primary to their well-being. There have been a number of health-related studies that use storytelling in various cultures (Crawford O'Brien, 2008; Finucane & McMullen, 2008; Inglebret, Jones, & Pavel, 2008; Larkey & Gonzalez, 2007; Leeman, Skelly, Burns, Carlson, & Soward, 2008).

In a narrative analysis of 115 stories of women of African descent, Banks-Wallace (2002) found storytelling useful for learning more about the historical and contextual factors affecting the well-being of these women. The major functions storytelling served were: contextual grounding, bonding with others, validating and affirming experiences, venting and catharsis, resisting oppression, and educating others. See Sidebar 14.1 for a vivid personal account of the use of storytelling in Kenya illustrating these major functions.

Rogers (2004) found storytelling at the heart of 11 Pacific Northwest African American widows, 55 years of age and older, who described their experiences of bereavement after their husbands' deaths. During the interviews, the widows took on various mannerisms and speech patterns of people who were part of the story. These included changed tones; mimicking the voices of those involved; and use of hands, body language, and

---

Sidebar 14.1. *Healing Through the Oral Tradition in Kenya and Beyond*

Eunice M. Areba, Kenya

Presenting health messages in a manner that patients can easily understand and incorporate into their lives is usually challenging. Communicating effectively means *transforming* health messages into pieces of information that are not only easily understood but can also be put into *action* by the recipient to attain mutually agreed-upon health outcomes (Silver, 2001). A cornerstone to effective communication is use of mechanisms already familiar to the members of the target community, which also ensures sustainability of the message. A notable example is the use of oral narratives (folklore) or simply storytelling: an art that has been used for eons in communities across the world. Nurses and other health care providers in Kenya and beyond have been great proponents and facilitators of storytelling, especially in chronic disease management. These stories are usually real-life accounts of the patients.

(continued)

Sidebar 14.1. *Healing Through the Oral Tradition in Kenya and Beyond (continued)*

I grew up surrounded by stories depicting characters that I could easily relate to and children were encouraged to participate in the storytelling process through song, dance, and rehearsed phrases such as these roughly translated ones:

Paukwa? Pakawa! (Who wants to be served? Me!)

Sahani? Ya mchele! (A plate? Of rice!)

Needless to say, I vividly remember not just the stories but also the lessons that were imparted. The storyteller is most often an elder who aims to instill a virtue, rectify a vice, and educate the young on the history or origin of a community. Some examples in the Kisii, Luhya, and coastal tribes in Kenya, respectively, include *the prophetess Moraa and Otenyo* (a historical event), *Simbi and Nashikufu* (beauty and humility), and *Abunuwasi* (social justice). Over time, oral narratives—especially from tribes whose mother tongue might soon become extinct—are being recorded both on paper and digital platforms. Storytelling in any form is a powerful and versatile health-teaching tool that can easily be implemented by health care providers across many settings, as illustrated in these examples.

HIV is not killing anybody unless you close your mouth (Leon, 2012, p. 28). HIV-positive women are healing with the help of their peers whose stories have helped them conquer social stigma, fear, and denial. Participants in the programs organized by the nongovernmental organization (NGO) Women Fighting Aids in Kenya (WOFAK) and its affiliates draw strength from one another's stories and, in so doing, develop a shared identity that comforts and assures them that they are not alone (Leon, 2012). Storytelling in this setting takes on a communal nature and encourages them to adhere to treatment programs. Health care providers also organize storytelling workshops targeting high-risk groups such as transport workers in specific geographical locations.

Peace building and mental health. No matter where or how it happens, those exposed to violence experience traumatic events that can significantly hamper their psychosocial, emotional, and physical well-being. In war, social institutions are destroyed and the tapestry of shared values in the community is torn. Stories utilized by both perpetrators and victims have been used to try and achieve peace by rebuilding relationships and reestablishing trust. Storytelling occurs in the form of people giving their accounts of atrocities committed in a communal setting (e.g., in Rwanda's gacaca courts post the 1994 genocide). Storytelling is seen as *familiar ground*, a tradition that many are exposed to during their upbringing, and is in turn perceived as *safe ground*. Some participants

(continued)

Sidebar 14.1. *Healing Through the Oral Tradition in Kenya and Beyond (continued)*

in these traditional set-ups have expressed feelings of relief, empowerment, and personal and communal healing. In cases of community reintegration, storytelling has been critical in accepting people back into the community. Conversely, there is the danger of re-traumatization and, therefore, adequate provisions for mental health care have to be instituted.

Creating a space for storytelling empowers patients, creates rapport, is easy to replicate, and places decisions in the hands of the patients—thus building the capacity for a community to identify, acknowledge, and come up with solutions for the problems they face.

References

Leon, K. (2012). *Storytelling and healing: The influence of narrative on identity construction among HIV positive individuals in Kisumu, Kenya*. Unpublished manuscript. Retrieved from http://digitalcollections.sit.edu/isp_collection/1385

Silver, D. (2001). Songs and storytelling: Bringing health messages to life in Uganda. *Education for Health, 14*, 51–60.

facial expressions. Nurses should be aware of storytelling as a means to gain in-depth understanding and cultural insight into African American experience.

Culturally appropriate communication methods, such as storytelling, have been found to be effective in health-promotion activities. The *talking circle* is one format in which the art of storytelling occurs. Indigenous Ojibwa and Cree women healers use talking circles as instruments of healing and storytelling in their everyday traditional practice (Struthers, 1999). Storytelling was preferred as a natural pattern of communication for Yakima Indians to learn about health promotion related to cervical cancer prevention (Strickland, Squeoch, & Chrisman, 1999).

FUTURE RESEARCH

Technology will certainly play a larger role in storytelling in the future. However, the orality of storytelling with which we are familiar will always be retained. Therefore, integrating future trends will keep the modality in line with evolving human endeavors. Wyatt and Hauenstein (2008) explore "how technology and storytelling can be joined to promote positive health outcomes" (p. 142). They recognize that although storytelling is widely used to teach children in the classroom, it has been minimally used in the health arena as a teaching–learning tool. With advances in technology—and its ubiquitous presence—interactive, digital storytelling may provide one mechanism to help enhance health promotion.

Explorations are needed to determine the efficacy of vignettes in both research and practice, particularly with individuals from other cultures and with older adults. Triangulation of qualitative and quantitative measures will provide a more complete examination of a patient's reflection, understanding, and outcomes. Specific questions that require investigation include:

- What are strategies to use to help nurses become more comfortable using storytelling as an intervention?
- What are some ways in which vignettes can be used with people from diverse cultures and age groups?

REFERENCES

Banks-Wallace, J. (2002). Talk that talk: Storytelling and analysis rooted in African American oral tradition. *Qualitative Health Research, 12*(3), 410–426.

Barton, S. S. (2004). Narrative inquiry: Locating aboriginal epistemology in a relational methodology. *Journal of Advanced Nursing, 45*(5), 519–526.

Bergner, R. M. (2007). Therapeutic storytelling revisited. *American Journal of Psychotherapy, 61*(2), 149–162.

Bickmore, T. W., & Paasche-Orlow, M. K. (2012). The role of information technology in health literacy research. *Journal of Health Communication: International Perspectives, 17*(Suppl. 3), S23–S29.

Cangelosi, P. R., & Sorrell, J. M. (2008). Storytelling as an educational strategy for older adults with chronic illness. *Journal of Psychosocial Nursing and Mental Health Services, 46*(7), 19–22.

Crawford O'Brien, S. (Ed.). (2008). *Religion and healing in Native America: Pathways for renewal.* Westport, CT: Praeger.

Dictionary.com. (2013). *Story.* Retrieved February 28, 2013, from: http://dictionary .reference.com/search?q=story&db=luna

Edmondson, M. E. (1971). *Lore: An introduction to the science of folklore and literature.* New York, NY: Holt, Rinehart, & Winston.

Evans, J. (2007). The science of storytelling. *Astrobiology, 7*(4), 710–711.

Fairbairn, G. J., & Carson, A. M. (2002). Writing about nursing research: A storytelling approach. *Nurse Researcher, 10*(1), 7–14.

Finucane, M. L., & McMullen, C. K. (2008). Making diabetes self-management education culturally relevant for Filipino Americans in Hawaii. *Diabetes Educator, 34*(5), 841–853.

Guber, P. (2007). The four truths of the storyteller. *Harvard Business Review, 85*(12), 52–59, 142.

Haigh, C., & Hardy, P. (2011). Tell me a story—A conceptual exploration of storytelling in healthcare education. *Nurse Education Today, 31*(4), 408–411.

Heliker, D. (2007). Story sharing: Restoring the reciprocity of caring in long-term care. *Journal of Psychosocial Nursing and Mental Health Services, 45*(7), 20–23.

Inglebret, E., Jones, C., & Pavel, D. M. (2008). Integrating American Indian/Alaska native culture into shared storybook intervention. *Language, Speech, and Hearing Services in Schools, 39*(4), 521–527.

Koh, H. K., Berwick, D. M., Clancy, C. M., Baur, C., Brach, C., Harris, L. M., & Zerhusen, E. G. (2012). New federal policy initiatives to boost health literacy can help the nation move beyond the cycle of costly 'crisis care'. *Health Affairs, 31*(2), 434–443.

Kramsch, C. (1998). *Language and culture.* Oxford, UK: Oxford University Press.

Larkey, L. K., & Gonzalez, J. (2007). Storytelling for promoting colorectal cancer prevention and early detection among Latinos. *Patient Education and Counseling, 67*(3), 272–278. doi:10.1016/j.pec.2007.04.003

Leeman, J., Skelly, A. H., Burns, D., Carlson, J., & Soward, A. (2008). Tailoring a diabetes self-care intervention for use with older, rural African American women. *Diabetes Educator, 34*(2), 310–317.

Lord, A. (1960). *The singer of tales* (2nd ed.). Cambridge, MA: Harvard University Press.

Lourens, M. M. (in press). An exploration of Xhosa speaking patients' understanding of cancer treatment and its influence on their treatment experience. *Journal of Psychosocial Oncology.*

Moss, M. P. (2000). *Zuni elders: Ethnography of American Indian aging* (Unpublished doctoral dissertation). University of Texas Health Science Center at Houston, Houston, TX. Retrieved from http://digitalcommons.library.tmc.edu/dissertations/AAI9974591

Nielsen-Bohlman, L., Panzer, A., & Kindig, D. (Eds.). (2004). *Health literacy: A prescription to end confusion* (National Research Council). Washington, DC: National Academies Press.

Olson, D. R., & Torrance, N. (Eds.). (1991). *Literacy and orality.* Cambridge, UK: Cambridge University Press.

Ong, W. J. (2002). *Orality and literacy.* New York, NY: Routledge.

Pilgrim Projects Limited. (2013). *Patient Voices.* Retrieved March 2013, from http://patientvoices.org.uk

Ramirez-Esparza, N., & Pennebaker, J. W. (2006). Do good stories produce good health?: Exploring words, language, and culture. *Narrative Inquiry, 16*(1), 211–219.

Roberts, J. (1994). Tales and transformations: Stories in families and family therapy. New York, NY: Norton.

Rogers, L. S. (2004). Meaning of bereavement among older African American widows. *Geriatric Nursing, 25*(1), 10–16.

Rule, L. (2009). *Digital storytelling.* Retrieved January 9, 2009, from http://electronic portfolios.com/digistory

Sampson, G. (1980). *Schools of linguistics.* Stanford, CA: Stanford University Press.

Sandars, J., Murray, C., & Pellow, A. (2008). Twelve tips for using digital storytelling to promote reflective learning by medical students. *Medical Teacher, 30*(8), 774–777.

Sandelowski, M. (1994). We are the stories we tell: Narrative knowing in nursing practice. *Journal of Holistic Nursing, 12*(1), 23–33.

Strickland, C. J., Squeoch, M. D., & Chrisman, N. J. (1999). Health promotion in cervical cancer prevention among the Yakima Indian women of the Wa'Shat Long-house. *Journal of Transcultural Nursing, 10*(3), 190–196.

Struthers, R. (1999). *The lived experience of Ojibwa and Cree women healers* (Unpublished doctoral dissertation). University of Minnesota, Minneapolis.

Tannen, D. (Ed.). (1982). *Spoken and written language: Exploring orality and literacy.* New York, NY: Ablex.

Tedlock, D. (1983). *The spoken word and the work of interpretation.* Philadelphia, PA: University of Pennsylvania Press.

Wyatt, T. H., & Hauenstein, E. (2008). Enhancing children's health through digital story. *Computers, Informatics, Nursing: CIN, 26*(3), 142–148; quiz, 149–150.Dictionary. com. (2013). *Story.* Retrieved February 28, 2013, from: http://dictionary .reference.com/search?q=story&db=luna

Chapter 15: Animal-Assisted Therapy

Susan O'Conner-Von

The domestication of animals began more than 12,000 years ago and continues today as animals play a significant role in human life (Lindsay, 2000). Much of what was known about the animal–human bond was anecdotal in nature until recently (Pavlides, 2008). Research examining the use of animals as a complementary or alternative therapy is based on studies about pet ownership. It is evident—with approximately 70 million pet dogs and 74 million pet cats in the United States—that pets play an important role in people's lives (American Veterinary Medical Association, 2012a). Pets can help provide companionship, promote dialogue and social interaction, facilitate exercise, increase feelings of security, mitigate the effects of stress, be a source of consistency, and be a comfort to touch (Arkow, 2011). The healing power of pets is "their capacity to make the atmosphere safe for emotions, the spiritual side of healing; whatever you are feeling, you can express it around your pet and not be judged" (Becker, 2002, p. 80).

In a comparative study examining the impact of pet ownership in childhood on young adults' social characteristics and professional choices, those who owned a pet in childhood retrospectively rated their pet higher than television, relatives, and neighbors in terms of social support received during childhood (Vizek, Arambasic, Kerestes, Kuterovac & Vlahovic-Stetic, 2001). The sample comprised 356 college students at a mean age of 21 years (68% women, 32% men). A total of 74% of the sample had pets (mostly dogs) during childhood and were found to be more empathetic and expressed more altruistic attitudes than those students who did not own a pet in childhood. Moreover, those students who had a pet in childhood were more likely to choose a career in the helping professions.

The role that animals play in healing environments was first documented in records from 9th-century Belgium where animals were used with persons with physical disabilities, followed by 18th-century England where animals were used with people with mental illness (Pavlides, 2008). Florence Nightingale wrote of the connection between animals and health in 1860 by suggesting that pets were perfect companions for the sick, especially those individuals with chronic health conditions (Nightingale, 1859/1992).

The 1970s launched the beginning of widespread interest in the interaction between animals and humans in the health care setting. In 1976, Elaine Smith, an American registered nurse, observed the benefits of pets in the health care setting while working in England. She noticed how patients reacted positively to the visits of a chaplain and his golden retriever. Upon returning to the United States, Smith introduced the concept of pet therapy into health care settings and founded Therapy Dogs International (2012). The goal of creating Therapy Dogs International was to formally test dogs so they could be certified, insured, and registered as volunteer therapy dogs. In 1977, the Delta Foundation was established to study the human–animal bond and the potential use of animal-assisted therapy (AAT). Scientific research in this area began in the 1980s, with an important step forward by the National Institutes of Health convening a conference in 1987 on the health benefits of pets (Fine & Beck, 2010). During the 1990s the focus was the establishment of professional standards and guidelines with the development of the *Standards of Practice for Animal-Assisted Activities and Animal-Assisted Therapy* (Delta Society, 1996). In 2008, the National Institute of Child and Human Development convened a conference to discuss the need for clarity and well-designed research examining the animal/human bond (Fine & Beck, 2010). Carefully designed studies provide the evidence needed to increase acceptance of AAT as a credible complementary therapy.

DEFINITIONS

Animal-Assisted Therapy

Animal-assisted therapy is defined as a goal-directed intervention that uses the human–animal bond as an integral part of the treatment process (American Veterinary Medical Association, 2012b). Although a variety of animal species and breeds, such as cats, birds, rabbits, horses, and dolphins, are involved in AAT, dogs account for the highest percentage of animals used for AAT (Hart, 2000).

Some key features of AAT are: (a) specific goals and objectives are set for each patient, (b) progress is measured, and (c) interactions are documented. The goals are designed by a nurse, occupational therapist, physical therapist, counselor, physician, or other health care professional who uses AAT in the treatment process (American Veterinary Medical Association, 2012b). A physical goal would include, for example, improved mobility by walking with a dog. Examples of cognitive goals include improved verbal expression (via normal interaction with the animal) and improved short- and long-term memory (via recalling the animal's name and activity at last visit). Social goals could include improved social skills and building rapport with others through the animal. Animals may also help to increase socialization by facilitating discussion of pets one may have had in the past. Finally, one illustration of an emotional goal would be improved motivation shown by getting dressed or walking to see the animal.

Animal-Assisted Activity

Animal-assisted activity (AAA) is defined as the use of the animal–human bond to promote activities to improve a patient's quality of life; however, the activity is not necessarily directed by a health professional and is not evaluated (American Veterinary Medical Association, 2012b).

Some key features of AAA are: (a) specific goals and objectives are not planned for each patient, (b) visit activities are spontaneous and last as long as needed, and (c) interactions are not necessarily documented. AAAs are less structured and provide human and animal contact for recreation, education, or pleasure. Examples include an informal visit by a friendly pet to a residential care center, hospital, school, or prison with the intent to bring joy and companionship to the residents (Rivera, 2010).

SERVICE ANIMAL

A service animal was originally defined in the Americans with Disabilities Act of 1990 as any animal trained to do work for the benefit of a person with a physical or emotional disability (U.S. Department of Justice, 2010). As of March 15, 2011, only dogs are recognized as service animals under Title II (state and local government services) or Title III (public accommodations and commercial facilities) of the Americans with Disabilities Act. Service dogs or guide dogs are trained specifically for the service they are providing: sight, sound, movement, or support. Once service animals are certified, they have federally approved access to accompany their owners anywhere. Service dogs are considered working animals, not pets. Although there is increased awareness and acceptance of therapy dogs in health care and public settings, such dogs do not receive federal protection or the same rights as service dogs who assist people with physical or emotional disabilities (U.S. Department of Justice, 2010).

SCIENTIFIC BASIS

Many studies indicate that there are physical and/or psychological benefits derived from human–animal bonds. Most of the research that has examined the physical benefits of AAT has focused on an animal's ability to attenuate a person's response to stress. When an individual becomes stressed, the sympathetic nervous system releases a cascade of hormones such as cortisol, aldosterone, and adrenaline. Stress-reduction strategies, such as petting an animal, can assist in reducing the build-up of these stress hormones (Wolff & Frishman, 2005). Likewise, the hormone oxytocin can lower blood pressure, lower cortisol levels, increase the pain threshold and have an antianxiety effect. One of the best ways to increase oxytocin levels is through positive physical touch, such as petting an animal (Chandler, 2012). Research that has examined the psychological benefits of AAT has explored the stress-reducing benefits the animal provides through social support (Arkow, 2011).

PHYSICAL CONDITIONS

The research investigating the impact of AAT on physical conditions has concentrated on cardiovascular disease, seizure disorders, dementia, and pain management.

Cardiovascular Disease

The study of the relationship between pets and their positive health effects on a human's cardiovascular system dates back to 1929 (Wolff & Frishman, 2005). Several studies demonstrated the effect of pet ownership on survival after myocardial infarction. Friedmann, Katcher, Lynch, and Thomas (1980) conducted the seminal longitudinal research examining the effect of pet ownership on survival for 92 adult patients after myocardial infarction. Only 5% of the subjects who owned pets died within 1 year after hospitalization, whereas 28% of those who were not pet owners died during the same interval.

Another study by Friedmann and Thomas (1995), examining pet ownership and 1-year survival after myocardial infarction, included the severity of cardiac disease. For the 368 patients in this investigation, disease severity and pet ownership were found to positively affect survival, whereas marital status and living situations did not.

In the Cardiac Arrhythmia Suppressions Trial (CAST) by Friedmann and Thomas (2003), the investigators examined the effect of owning a pet on heart rate variability (HRV) for patients after recovery from a myocardial infarction. As a noninvasive method of showing risk assessment after myocardial infarction, a depressed HRV predicts cardiac complications and increased mortality. Pet owners in this study had a higher HRV, thus supporting the hypothesis that survival differences between pet owners and non–pet owners were due to differences in the autonomic modulation of the heart, therefore providing long-term cardiac benefits and increased survival rates.

In work specifically examining the effects of AAT on hemodynamic measures and state anxiety, 76 adult patients (44 men and 32 women) with advanced heart failure were randomized to: (a) a 12-minute AAT session with a therapy dog; (b) a 12-minute visit with a volunteer; or (c) the control group, which included usual care (Cole, Gawlinski, Steers, & Kotlerman, 2007). Using a repeated-measures experimental design, data were collected at baseline, 8 minutes, and 16 minutes. The results revealed that, compared with the control group, the AAT group had significantly greater decreases in systolic pulmonary artery pressure during and after the AAT intervention and significantly greater decreases in pulmonary capillary wedge pressures during and after the AAT intervention. Moreover, after the intervention, patients in the AAT group had the greatest decrease in state anxiety, compared with the other two groups.

Seizure Disorders

The use of animals as an important component of the treatment plan for subjects with epilepsy was first documented in 1867 in Germany (Fontaine, 2011). Over the last several decades, a number of investigations have examined the value of dogs in the care of patients with seizure disorders. A survey of 122 families who had a child with epilepsy reported that, of those living with a dog, 15% of the dogs could predict seizure onset at least 80% of the time (Kirton, Wirrell, Zhang, & Hamiwka, 2004). In addition, 50% of the dogs exhibited behaviors that were protective of the child, such as lying on top of the child during a seizure or pushing the child away from stairs.

Dementia

For more than 2 decades, studies have supported the use of AAT with patients with degenerative cognitive disorders. For patients with dementia, interacting with an animal can improve short-term memory and communication (Tyberg & Frishman, 2008) and trigger long-term memory (Laun, 2003). The presence of a therapy dog can decrease agitation and aggression, while increasing social behaviors among patients with dementia (Filan & Llewellyn-Jones, 2006). Indeed, the presence of fish aquariums in a long-term-care facility was associated with increased weights and improved nutritional status among 62 patients with Alzheimer's disease. These residents were more attentive in the presence of the aquarium, stayed at the dining room table longer, and required less nutritional supplements (Edwards & Beck, 2002). Research specifically examining problem behaviors in patients with dementia found significantly fewer problem behaviors after placement of a dog in the health care facility (McCabe, Baun, Speich, & Agrawal, 2002).

Pain Management

Adult Pain Management

Nurses are acutely aware of the importance of including complementary therapies in providing pain management for patients. Most studies examining animal-assisted therapy in health care have been conducted in acute care settings. Marcus et al. (2012a) evaluated the effects of brief therapy dog visits in an outpatient adult chronic pain clinic compared to time spent in a waiting room without a therapy dog. The sample consisted of 235 patients, 34 family/friends, and 26 staff for a total of 295 therapy dog visits. Participants were able to spend clinic waiting time with a certified therapy dog or in the clinic waiting room. Significant improvements were reported on pain, mood, and other measures of distress among those patients who spent time with the therapy dog, compared to those who chose to remain in the clinic waiting room. Significant improvements were also reported by family/friends and staff after therapy dog visits. Study results revealed that therapy dog visits can significantly improve the feelings of well-being in this patient population.

Pediatric Pain Management

Sobo, Eng, and Kassity-Krich (2006) examined the effectiveness of canine visitation therapy (CVT) on children's postoperative pain in a pediatric hospital. The convenience sample consisted of 25 English-speaking children, ages 5 years to 18 years. Each patient received a one-time visit after surgery by a West Highland terrier named Lizzy and could choose the level of interaction with the dog. In high interaction, the child actively played and walked with the dog; in low interaction, the dog would do an occasional trick for the child; and in passive interaction, the dog would sit quietly with the child. Despite the small sample size, there was a significant decrease in pain perception after the dog visitation. Moreover, post-CVT interviews with each child revealed eight themes, the dog (1) brought pleasure or happiness, (2) provided distraction from the pain, (3) was fun, (4) provided company, (5) was calming, (6) reminded them of home, (7) was nice to cuddle with, and (8) eased the pain.

PSYCHOLOGICAL CONDITIONS

The use of animals for treatment of people with mental conditions dates back to 1792 at the York Retreat in England. It was observed that the farm animals helped to enhance the humanity of those with emotional disorders (Altschiller, 2011). The goal was to lessen the use of medications and physical restraints by helping residents learn self-control through the care of animals (Fontaine, 2011). More recently, in 1964, American child psychotherapist Boris Levinson (who is considered to be the father of animal-assisted therapy) coined the term "pet therapy." Levinson first described the therapeutic effects of companionship with his dog, Jingles, for withdrawn children living in a residential mental health program. The dog served as an ice-breaker and opened communication to establish a positive relationship for effective therapy (Altschiller, 2011). Since the 1960s, a number of studies have been conducted to examine the effects of AAT for patients hospitalized on psychiatric units. It has been found that AAT can promote feelings of safety and comfort along with a nonevaluative external focus for patients who are not fearful of animals or have a negative attitude toward them (Odendaal, 2000). Specifically, older patients with schizophrenia who were exposed to AAT showed growth in communication, interpersonal contact with others, and activities of daily living (Barak, Savorai, Mavashev, & Beni, 2001).

Military Personnel

Veterans can experience negative physical, emotional, and psychological effects from their experiences in war. As early as the 1940s, the beneficial effect of working with animals was evident in returning World War II veterans who recovered at the Army Air Corps Convalescent Hospital in New York (Fontaine, 2011). Today, there are several million veterans in our country, many of whom suffer from posttraumatic stress disorder (PTSD) (Matuszek, 2010). Over the past decade, animal-assisted therapy has become more commonplace in veterans' hospitals, with the Department of Defense allocating funding to examine the effectiveness of its use. In addition, in March 2011, the Americans with Disabilities Act approved PTSD as a qualification of need for a service dog (Arkow, 2011). Veterans suffering with PTSD can apply for a service dog through organizations such as Veterans Moving Forward (2012) (www.vetsfwd.org). Although research to support the use of a service or therapy dog for individuals with PTSD is at an early stage, veterans report that these dogs help to manage their PTSD symptoms such as anxiety, panic attacks, and fear (Arkow, 2011).

A recent pretest, posttest nonrandomized control group study evaluated the effects of animal-assisted therapy on Wounded Warriors in transition (N = 24) attending an Occupational Therapy Life Skills Program (Beck et al., 2012). Although significant differences were not found between the groups on most measures (mood, stress, resilience, fatigue, and function), anecdotal information indicated the participants expressed pleasure being with the dogs and did not want the experience to end.

INTERVENTION

AAT has been shown to be a successful intervention for patients of all ages with a variety of physical and psychological conditions. This intervention can be provided in many settings, including private homes, acute care and rehabilitation facilities, long-term and group care homes, schools, and correctional facilities.

Guidelines

Selecting an animal for AAT requires careful screening and extensive training (American Veterinary Medical Association, 2012b; Granger & Kogan, 2006). Although there is no ideal animal for AAT, the animal must be calm, tolerant, and reliable (Arkow, 2011). Further, all animals must complete yearly veterinary screening to ensure they are healthy, current on vaccinations, and parasite free.

AAT requires that the animal and handler work together as a team. To provide safe and effective AAT, the AAT team should abide by established standards of practice for AAA and AAT. Examples from the Standards of Practice (Delta Society, 1996) for the handler include: (a) demonstrating appropriate treatment of people and animals, (b) using appropriate social skills, (c) acting as the animal's advocate, (d) having the ability to read the animal's cues, and (e) maintaining confidentiality.

AAT Training

Most national therapy dog organizations require the Canine Good Citizen test (American Kennel Club [AKC], 2011) as a basic skills requirement for acceptance into a therapy dog training program. The Canine Good Citizen test, developed by the AKC in 1989, is a certification program that tests dogs in everyday situations and requires a dog to have mastered a basic set of skills (Exhibit 15.1).

Exhibit 15.1. *Canine Good Citizen Test*

Ten Required Exercises

1. Accepting a friendly stranger

2. Sitting politely for petting

3. Appearance and grooming

4. Walking with a loose leash

5. Walking through a crowd

6. Sit and stay on command, staying in place

7. Coming when called

8. Reacting politely to another dog

9. Reacting to distraction without panic or aggression

10. Supervised separation without fear or agitation

From the American Kennel Club (2011).

Additional requirements may include didactic content for the human partner to understand the theory and research supporting AAT, standards of practice, and ethical considerations. The animal partner receives training in simulated health care settings that include such activities as (a) learning how to leave an object alone, such as food or medication; (b) being bumped while walking in a crowded space; (c) being comfortable around hospital equipment such as wheelchairs, walkers, or crutches; (d) receiving petting from several people at once; and (e) sitting quietly as paws, ears, and tail are examined.

Measurement of Outcomes

The effects of AAT have been measured through qualitative and quantitative means. A variety of outcomes have been examined such as cardiovascular benefits, decreased pain, lowered blood pressure, increased socialization and exercise, improved coordination and balance, and decreased stress. Granted, positive patient outcomes can be dependent on the qualifications and experience of the AAT team. Specifically, the therapy team should complete adequate training, obtain national registration, and undergo yearly evaluation by a veterinarian and a professional therapy animal organization. The effectiveness of outcomes can be further complicated by the multidisciplinary nature of this intervention, along with the lack of standardized protocols and methods of evaluation. Therefore, frequent communication and collaboration are essential between the AAT team and the health care professionals or therapists involved in the patient's treatment plan (American Veterinary Medical Association, 2012b).

Precautions

Although research supports the positive benefits and the safety of AAT for patients with various health conditions, the potential risks, such as disease transmission, allergies, and bites, must be carefully taken into consideration (Tyberg & Frishman, 2008). The major concern for health care facilities is the transmission of infectious diseases. These potential risks can be decreased by using trained and registered AAT teams along with enforcing standard hand hygiene before and after every visit. Guidelines from the Centers for Disease Control recommend that animals used for AAT be clean, healthy, fully vaccinated, groomed, and free of parasites (Centers for Disease Control, 2003).

To prevent possible risks, a mechanism must be in place for regularly scheduled examinations and preventative care by a veterinarian to assess the physical and behavioral health and well-being of the animal. Results of these examinations must be shared with the appropriate animal regulatory agency and AAT organizations on an annual basis (American Veterinary Medical Association, 2012c).

A comprehensive review specifically examining the potential health risks of animals in the health care setting found that the potential benefits far outweighed the insignificant risks (Brodie, Biley, & Shewring, 2002).

USES

In addition to the types of interventions already mentioned, the variety of ways and settings in which AAT can be used are virtually limitless. One only has to be creative in the design of the intervention. The following is a partial list of additional ways AAT can be used and populations in which AAT has been studied (see Exhibit 15.2).

Cultural Applications

There is great diversity in culturally held attitudes about animals, especially pets, both among cultures and within them (Chandler, 2012). To understand the various attitudes about animals, it is important to consider the evolution of the domestication of animals and their role in society. Historically, only royalty and the wealthy were able to keep companion animals. Also significant is the influence of religious beliefs; for example, in some religions, cows are considered to be sacred and dogs are considered to be unclean.

Exhibit 15.2. *Populations in Which Animals and Animal-Assisted Therapy Have Been Studied*

Adult patients with heart failure (Cole et al., 2007)

Adult patients undergoing electroconvulsive therapy (Barker, Pandurangi, & Best, 2003)

Adult patients in a residential substance-abuse group therapy program (Wesley, Minatrea, & Watson, 2009)

Adults with fibromyalgia (Marcus et al., 2012b)

Children with acute pain (Braun, Stangler, Narveson, & Pettingell, 2009)

Children with attention-deficit/hyperactivity disorder (Cuypers, De Ridder, & Strandheim, 2011)

Children with autism (Bass, Duchowny, & Llabre, 2009; Pavlides, 2008)

Children with cancer (Gagnon et al., 2004)

Children with cerebral palsy (Zadnikar & Kastrin, 2011)

Children with special health care needs (Gasalberti, 2006)

Children with pervasive developmental disorders (Martin & Farnum, 2002)

Children undergoing dental procedures (Havener et al., 2001)

Elderly patients with schizophrenia (Barak et al., 2001)

Elderly patients with mental illness (Moretti et al., 2011)

Female abuse survivors (Porter-Wenzlaff, 2007)

Lonely elderly adults in long-term-care facilities (Banks & Banks, 2002)

Men with aphasia (Macauley, 2006)

Older adults with dementia (Richeson, 2003)

Patients with Alzheimer's disease and nutritional deficits (Edwards & Beck, 2002)

Patients in a rehabilitation facility using psychoactive medications (Lust, Ryan-Haddad, Coover, & Snell, 2007)

U.S. Army soldiers dealing with the stressors of living in a deployed environment (Fike, Najera, & Dougherty, 2012).

Before implementing AAT, it is vital to be aware of and consider the influence of cultural and personal attitudes about animals. Although one cannot stereotype people's views of animals based on their ethnic or cultural backgrounds, it is important to be aware of the possibility of cultural differences. For example, Koreans in their native country rarely have cats or dogs as pets because they have been viewed for a long time as a source of food (Chandler, 2012). In contrast, European Americans have integrated cats and dogs into their family system as pets for hundreds of years. Native Americans, on the other hand, may allow their cats and dogs to roam freely, and members of their community share in caring for the animals. Moreover, these animals may never be spayed or neutered, out of respect for the animals' purpose and spirit (Chandler, 2012).

The interest in AAT has grown around the world, following the United States. The Animals Asia Foundation introduced the Dr. Dog program in Hong Kong, China, the Philippines, Japan, India, and Taiwan, with more than 300 dogs visiting hospitals and schools. In Japan, the Companion Animal Partnership Program was developed by the Japan Animal Hospital Association in 1986. It is the most well-known and largest AAT program in Japan (ZENOAQ, 2009), with AAT teams visiting schools, nursing homes, and hospitals (Nagata, 2008). In fact, multiple studies examining the impact of AAT and AAA on older patients have been conducted in Japan (Kanamori et al., 2001; Kawamura, Niiyama, & Niiyama, 2009; Mano, Uchizono, & Nishimura, 2003).

In India, Saraswathi Kendra, in collaboration with the Blue Cross of India, pioneered the use of AAT for children with autism beginning in 1996; in 2001, Dr. Dog AAT programs were introduced in schools and nursing homes (Krishna, 2009). Also in India, Minal Kavishwar and therapy dog Kutty were the first registered therapy dog team. Kavishwar founded the Animal Angels Foundation of India, the first in the country to consist of mental health professionals who provide animal-assisted therapy for special-needs children in schools, hospitals, and psychiatric settings. This organization is also active in disaster response (Chandler, 2012). Perspectives on the use of AAT in Taiwan are included in Sidebar 15.1.

Sidebar 15.1. *Animal-Assisted Care in Long-Term-Care Facilities in Taiwan*

Jing-Jy Sellin Wang and Miaofen Yen, Tainan City, Taiwan

Within the Oriental culture, especially from the older generation's point of view, there are some taboos on the interaction between humans and animals; thus, compared to the West, using animals in the treatment of human health can be restricted. For example, although relationships with the cat can be very intimate in the West, many Taiwanese believe that cats have nine lives with negative meanings. Some superstitions say that cats can reduce a person's *yang spirit*. After one's death, the corpse would have negative resonance with the cat. Moreover, there are legends

(continued)

Sidebar 15.1. *Animal-Assisted Care in Long-Term-Care Facilities in Taiwan (continued)*

such as if a black cat jumps over a dead body, within 7 days it will be resurrected. Sometimes these legends make workers or older pateints in long-term-care facilities fearful. In addition, although the dog is very loyal, Taiwan is an island country, which may cause public environmental health problems due to the humidity, such as when an animal touches human skin. Having dogs is only suitable for the home. As a result, the most widely accepted animals in long-term-care facilities are fish and birds. System planning and targeted use of animal intervention can help the older subject, and professionals assist residents in long-term-care facilities through breeding fish and birds. This can modestly enhance residents' physiological, psychological, and spiritual well-being.

During her graduate studies, Jing-Yi Lee completed a thesis focused on the use of fish-assisted care in long-term-care facilities. In her study, 60 people with normal cognitive function were included. Older residents were selected from the same facility and randomly assigned to an experimental group and a control group of 30 individuals each.

Those in the experimental group were each given a small plastic fish tank containing water, plants, 12 guppies, and a fish feedbox to keep in their rooms. Institutional caregivers assisted residents with changing the water weekly, and residents had to feed the fish, observe them, and record their observations daily. Residents also participated in a weekly one-half hour group-sharing session. If caregivers found dead fish, they secretly replaced them with new fish when the resident was not in the room. However, if residents found dead fish by themselves, caregivers helped them to replace these with new fish immediately and record the incident. Those in the control group were each given a small plastic fish tank with water and plants to keep in their rooms. They were required to take care of and observe the plants, and also to record and share their observations. The residents of both groups lived on the same floor but in different rooms. After 3 months of intervention, the measures of the quality of life, self-esteem, vitality, and sense of self-control within the experimental group were better than in the control group. In addition, the level of depression was significantly lower in the experimental group than in the control group. Clearly, the experimental group had a meaningful experience of life and expectations in the weekly sharing. According to residents: "Now breeding [these] this fish is like raising children, so you have to take care [of] them very carefully, and some time you will worry that they eat not enough or the water is too dirty...." "Breeding a fish as treating a woman, need attentive care...." "I become very busy since I have breeding fish daily...." "Every day I look at my

(continued)

Sidebar 15.1. *Animal-Assisted Care in Long-Term-Care Facilities in Taiwan (continued)*

fish and worry about whether there is a dead fish or not, because it will infect [the] to other fish. Also I compare with other people to see if I keep them well...." "I am very happy when the fish give birth." A resident of the control group said, "I also want to have fish, because friends who breed fish become more active."

Another unpublished case study concerned bird-assisted care. An 80-year-old man with dementia was agitated and aggressive. The resident and caregivers received health services in the Dementia Care Clinic at the University Hospital, and the caregiver indicated that the subject had serious problem behaviors. Due to severe delusion, the resident did not sleep at night. After an interview, it was discovered that the resident had loved birds in the past. Therefore, the suggestion was given to the caregiver to purchase a birdcage and help the resident to breed a parrot. Because this resident was in a middle stage of dementia, his caregiver had to help in feeding the bird, changing the water, and cleaning up. The birdcage was hung at the resident's eye level, and he was encouraged to speak to the bird and to teach the bird to say "hello" and "thank you." Daily, after breakfast, the music of bird voices was played so that the subject could listen to this music with the bird. Caregivers were encouraged to write down their observations of interaction between the resident and bird and to note any changes in problem behaviors. After 3 months of the bird-assisted care intervention, it was reported that the subject's problem behaviors had improved and he had become less irritable. Due to the focus on the interactions with the bird during the day, the resident could fall asleep at night. Clearly, the resident's quality of life has been enhanced when he developed a close link with the bird. Thus, it was demonstrated that animal-assisted measures could be useful for older people or those with dementia and problem behaviors.

FUTURE RESEARCH

Although there has been great enthusiasm for AAT and a proliferation of therapy teams worldwide, these interventions often lack evidence to support their efficacy (Arkow, 2011). Most research to date supports AAT as making a significant contribution to quality of life for patients of all ages and a variety of physical and psychological health conditions; however, most studies tend to have small sample sizes and lack adequate control groups (Fine, 2010). Investigations are needed that use random assignment to an AAT intervention group and a standard care group to determine which intervention led to the better outcome. Explorations are also needed to examine the physiological mechanisms contributing to the positive effects of AAT on specific conditions, as well as the duration and frequency of AAT needed to provide maximum improvements. For example, because cardiovascular disease is the leading cause of death in the United States, the role of AAT within cardiovascular disease prevention programs needs to be examined. Additional research is needed to help identify which patients would most benefit from AAT.

Studies are needed to examine the relationships among the AAT team, patients, and staff in creating a healing environment that can be transformational for both subjects and staff in various health care settings (Zborowsky & Kreitzer, 2008). Further research is needed in settings such as schools, homeless shelters, outpatient clinics, and community health agencies. Additional work is necessary to examine the ethical use, potential fatigue, and health care needs of animals used for AAT. Given that animals have no voice in this intervention, it is imperative that their human companions ensure their physical and emotional well-being (Altschiller, 2011).

Nurses can take the lead in advocating for the appropriate use of AAT in their health care and school settings. Additional resources to assist in the implementation of AAT are listed in Exhibit 15.3.

Exhibit 15.3. *Additional Resources*

Bouchard, F., Landry, M., Belles-Isles, M., & Gagnon, J. (2004). A magical dream: A pilot project in animal-assisted therapy in pediatric oncology. *Canadian Oncology Nursing Journal, 14*(1), 14–17.

Breitenbach, E., Stumpf, E., & Lorenzov, E. (2009). Dolphin-assisted therapy: Changes in interaction and communication between children with severe disabilities and their caregivers. *Anthrozoos, 22*(3), 277–289.

Burch, M. (2010). *Citizen canine: Ten essential skills every well-mannered dog should know.* Freehold, NJ: Kennel Club Books.

Cangelosi, P., & Embrey, C. (2006). The healing power of dogs: Cocoa's story. *Journal of Psychosocial Nursing, 44*(1), 17–20.

Chu, C., Liu, C., Sun, C., & Lin, J. (2009). The effect of animal-assisted activity on inpatients with schizophrenia. *Journal of Psychosocial Nursing, 47*(12), 42–48.

DeCourcey, M., Russell, A., & Keister, K. (2010). Animal-assisted therapy: Evaluation and implementation of a complementary therapy to

(continued)

Exhibit 15.3. *Additional Resources (continued)*

improve the psychological and physiological health of critically ill patients. *Dimensions of Critical Care Nursing, 29*(5), 211–214.

Eaglin, V. (2008). Attitudes and perceptions of nurses in training and psychiatry and pediatric residents towards animal-assisted interventions. *Hawaii Medical Journal, 67*(2), 45–47.

Ernst, L. (2012, October). Animal-assisted therapy: Using animals to promote healing. *Nursing 2012, 42*(10), 54–58.

Geisler, A. (2004). Companion animals in palliative care: Stories from the bedside. *American Journal of Hospice & Palliative Care, 21*(4), 285–288.

Halm, M. (2008). The healing power of the human-animal connection. *American Journal of Critical Care, 17*(4), 373–376.

Horowitz, S. (2008). The human-animal bond: Health implications across the lifespan. *Alternative and Complementary Therapies, 14*(5), 251–256.

Johnson, R., Odendaal, J., & Meadows, R. (2002). Animal-assisted interventions research. *Western Journal of Nursing Research, 24*(4), 422–440.

Kilmer, K. (2008, May). Get involved in pet therapy programs. *Healthcare Traveler, 15*(11), 8–10.

Lally, R. (2007). The sounds of healing. *ONS Connect, 22*(2), 8–12.

Lavoie-Vaughan, N. (2003). Pet project: Four-legged caregivers benefit patients and staff. *Nursing Spectrum Midwest Edition, 4*(4), 8–10.

Lind, N. (2009). *Animal-assisted therapy activities to motivate and inspire.* Lombard, IL: PYOW.

McKenney, C., & Johnson, R. (2008). Unleash the healing power of pet therapy. *American Nurse Today, 3*(5), 29–31.

Mullet, S. (2008). A helping paw. *RN, 71*(7), 39–42. Retrieved January 14, 2009, from http://www.rnweb.com

Niksa, E. (2007). The use of animal-assisted therapy in psychiatric nursing. *Journal of Psychosocial Nursing, 45*(6), 56–58.

Perry, D., Rubinstein, D., & Austin, J. (2012). Animal-assisted group therapy in mental health settings. *Alternative and Complementary Therapies, 18*(4), 181–185.

Pichot, T. (2012). *Animal-assisted brief therapy.* New York, NY: Routledge.

Rossetti, J., & King, C. (2010). Use of animal-assisted therapy with psychiatric patients: A literature review. *Journal of Psychosocial Nursing, 48*(11), 44–48.

Schetchikova, N. (2008, August). Animal attraction. *American Chiropractic Association News, 4*(8), 26–27.

WEBSITES

American Hippotherapy Association

The mission of the American Hippotherapy Association is to educate and promote excellence in the field of equine-assisted therapy. This organization promotes the use of the movement of a horse as a treatment strategy in physical, occupational, and speech therapy sessions for people living with disabilities.
(www.americanhippotherapyassociation.org)

American Veterinary Medical Association

Established in 1863, members of the American Veterinary Medical Association (AVMA) recognize and promote the importance of the human–animal bond through clinical practice, service, and research. The policy section of this website includes guidelines for animal-assisted activity, animal-assisted therapy, and resident animal programs, including key definitions, guiding principles, preventive medical and behavioral strategies, and wellness guidelines.
(www.avma.org/KB/Policies/Pages/default.aspx)

CENSHARE: Center to Study Human–Animal Relationships and Environments

CENSHARE is a diverse group of people from the University of Minnesota and surrounding community dedicated to studying and improving human–animal relationships and environments. Its mission and vision include education, research, and service. CENSHARE is a nonprofit organization relying on external sponsorship to continue its activities.
(www.censhare.umn.edu)

Equine-Assisted Growth and Learning Association (EAGALA)

EAGALA is dedicated to improving the mental health of individuals, families, and groups around the world by setting the standard of excellence in equine-assisted psychotherapy and equine-assisted learning, also known as horse therapy or equine therapy.
(www.eagala.org)

Human–Animal Bond Research Initiative Foundation

The Human–Animal Bond Research Initiative (HABRI) Foundation is a national nonprofit foundation dedicated to promoting the positive role animals play in the health and well-being of people, families,

and communities. This foundation works to educate, inform, advocate, and support research and funding for human–animal related initiatives. The HABRI center is an online hub that archives evidence on the benefits of the human–animal bond and is maintained by Purdue University under the direction of Dr. Alan Beck. The information focuses on human and animal health, animal-assisted therapy, and public policy.
(www.habri.org/pet_charity.html)

Paws 4 Therapy

Paws 4 Therapy specializes in bringing AAT to the acute care hospital setting. Patty Kaplan, RN, BSN, founded Paws 4 Therapy in 2001 and is the director of AAT at Edward Hospital in Naperville, Illinois. In 2005 her AAT program was featured by the Joint Commission on Accreditation of Healthcare Organizations (JCAHO) as a "best practice."
(www.paws4therapy.com)

Pet Partners (Formerly Delta Society)

In 1977, the Delta Foundation was created in Portland, Oregon, under the direction of Michael McCulloch, MD. In 1981, the name was changed to Delta Society; and in 2012 the name Delta Society was changed to Pet Partners in order to clearly reflect its mission, which is to improve human health through positive interactions with therapy, service, and companion animals. Pet Partners volunteers visit hospitals and hospices with their animals to provide comfort to people in need. The Pet Partners Program is the first comprehensive standardized training in animal-assisted activities and therapy for volunteers and health care professionals.
(www.petpartners.org)

Reading Education Assistance Dogs (R.E.A.D.)

The mission of the R.E.A.D. program is to improve the literacy skills of children through the assistance of a registered therapy team as literacy mentors. The R.E.A.D. program improves a child's reading and communication skills by employing a powerful method—reading to an animal. This program began in 1999 in Salt Lake City, Utah, by the Intermountain Therapy Animals organization. Today, more than 3,000 therapy teams have been trained and registered with the R.E.A.D. program and work throughout the United States, Canada, Italy, Finland, France, Slovenia, South Africa, Spain, Sweden, and the United Kingdom.
(www.therapyanimals.org/Read_Team_Steps.html)

Therapet: Animal-Assisted Therapy

The mission of the Therapet Foundation is to use specially trained and certified animals to promote health, hope, and healing. Therapet assists with the establishment of AAT programs throughout the United States and provides education for health care professionals, along with AAT training and evaluation of animal and human volunteers. (www.therapet.org)

TherapyDogOrganizations.net

This website contains a list of therapy dog organizations in the United States and Canada (listed by state or province) that support therapy dog work by guiding teams through training, evaluation, registration, and placement in facilities desiring therapy dog visits. (www.therapydogorganizations.net)

Therapy Dogs International

Therapy Dogs International (TDI) is the oldest registry for therapy dogs in the United States. In 2012, there were 24,750 dog/handler teams registered with TDI. Founded in 1976 by Elaine Smith—an American registered nurse who observed the benefits of pets in the health care setting during a visit to England—TDI is dedicated to the regulation, testing, selection, and registration of qualified dogs and handlers for the purpose of visitations to hospitals, nursing homes, and facilities, or any place where therapy dogs are needed. Since the 1995 bombing of the Murrah Federal Building in Oklahoma City, Oklahoma, TDI has provided Disaster Stress Relief Dog teams in such places as New York City—during the September 11, 2001, attack on the World Trade Center—and New Orleans, Louisiana, during hurricane Katrina in 2005. (www.tdi-dog.org)

ACKNOWLEDGMENT

The author gratefully thanks her therapy dog, Libby, for showing her the true value of AAT.

REFERENCES

Altschiller, D. (2011). *Animal-assisted therapy.* Santa Barbara, CA: Greenwood.
American Kennel Club. (2011). *AKC canine good citizen program.* Retrieved from *http://akc.org*

American Veterinary Medical Association. (2012a). *U.S. pet ownership & demographics sourcebook*. Retrieved from https://www.avma.org/KB/Resources/Statistics/Pages/Market-research-statistics-US-Pet-Ownership-Demographics-Sourcebook.aspx

American Veterinary Medical Association. (2012b). *Guidelines for animal-assisted activity, animal-assisted therapy and resident animal programs*. Retrieved from https://www.avma.org/KB/Policies/Pages/Guidelines-for-Animal-Assisted-Activity-Animal-Assisted-Therapy-and-Resident-Animal-Programs.aspx

American Veterinary Medical Association. (2012c). *Wellness guidelines for animals in animal-assisted activity, animal-assisted therapy, and resident animal programs*. Retrieved from https://www.avma.org/KB/Policies/Pages/Wellness-Guidelines-for-Animals-in-Animal-Assisted-Activity-Animal-Assisted-Therapy-and-Resident-Animal-Programs.aspx

Arkow, P. (2011). *Animal-assisted therapy and activities: A study and research resource guide for the use of companion animals in animal-assisted interventions* (10th ed.). Self-published.

Banks, M., & Banks, W. (2002). The effects of animal-assisted therapy on loneliness in an elderly population in long-term care facilities. *Journal of Gerontology, 57*(7), 428–432.

Barak, Y., Savorai, O., Mavashev, S., & Beni, A. (2001). Animal-assisted therapy for elderly schizophrenic patients: A one-year controlled trial. *American Journal of Geriatric Psychiatry, 9*(4), 439–442.

Barker, S., Pandurangi, A., & Best, A. (2003). Effects of animal-assisted therapy on patients' anxiety, fear, and depression before ECT. *Journal of ECT, 19*(1), 38–44.

Bass, M., Duchowny, C., & Llabre, M. (2009). The effect of therapeutic horseback riding on social functioning in children with autism. *Journal of Autism & Developmental Disorders, 39*, 1261–1267.

Beck, C., Gonzales, F., Sells, C., Jones, C., Reer, T., Wasilewski, S., & Zhu, Y. (2012, April–June). The effects of animal-assisted therapy on wounded warriors in an occupational therapy life skills program. *Army Medical Department Journal*, pp. 38–45.

Becker, M. (2002). *The healing power of pets: Harnessing the amazing ability of pets to make and keep people happy and healthy*. New York, NY: Hyperion.

Braun, C., Stangler, T., Narveson, J., & Pettingell, S. (2009). Animal-assisted therapy as a pain relief intervention for children. *Complementary Therapies in Clinical Practice, 15*, 105–109.

Brodie, S., Biley, F., & Shewring, M. (2002). An exploration of the potential risks associated with using pet therapy in healthcare settings. *Journal of Clinical Nursing, 11*(4), 444–456.

Centers for Disease Control. (2003). Guidelines for environmental infection control in healthcare facilities. *MMWR Recommendations & Reports, 52*(RR-10), 1–42.

Chandler, C. (2012). *Animal assisted therapy in counseling*. New York, NY: Routledge.

Cole, K., Gawlinski, A., Steers, N., & Kotlerman, J. (2007). Animal-assisted therapy in patients hospitalized with heart failure. *American Journal of Critical Care, 16*(6), 575–585.

Cuypers, K., De Ridder, K., & Strandheim, A. (2011). The effect of therapeutic horseback riding on 5 children with attention deficit hyperactivity disorder: A pilot study. *Journal of Alternative and Complementary Medicine, 17*, 901–908.

Delta Society. (1996). *Standards of practice for animal-assisted activities and animal-assisted therapy*. Renton, WA: Author.

Edwards, N., & Beck, A. (2002). Animal assisted therapy and nutrition in Alzheimer's disease. *Western Journal of Nursing Research, 24*(6), 697–612.

Fike, L., Najera, C., & Dougherty, D. (2012, April–June). Occupational therapists as dog handlers: The collective experience with animal-assisted therapy in Iraq. *Army Medical Department Journal,* 51–54.

Filan, S., & Llewellyn-Jones, R. (2006). Animal-assisted therapy for dementia: A review of the literature. *Intelligence Psychogeriatric, 18*(4), 597–611.

Fine, A. (2010). *Handbook on animal-assisted therapy: Theoretical foundations and guidelines for practice* (3rd ed.). San Diego, CA: Academic Press.

Fine, A., & Beck, A. (2010). Understanding our kinship with animals: Input for health care professionals interested in the human/animal bond. In A. Fine (Ed.), *Handbook on animal-assisted therapy: Theoretical foundations and guidelines for practice* (pp. 3–15). San Diego, CA: Academic Press.

Fontaine, K. (2011). *Complementary & alternative therapies for nursing practice.* Upper Saddle River, NJ: Pearson.

Friedmann, E., Katcher, A., Lynch, J., & Thomas, S. (1980). Animal companions and one-year survival of patients after discharge from a coronary care unit. *Public Health Reports, 95*(4), 307–312.

Friedmann, E., & Thomas, S. (1995). Pet ownership, social support, and one-year survival after acute myocardial infarction in the Cardiac Arrhythmia Suppression Trial (CAST). *American Journal of Cardiology, 76,* 1213–1217.

Friedmann, E., & Thomas, S. (2003). Relationship between pet ownership and heart rate variability in patients with healed myocardial infarcts. *American Journal of Cardiology, 91,* 718–721.

Gagnon, J., Bouchard, F., Landry, M., Belles-Isles, M., Fortier, M., & Fillion, L. (2004). Implementing a hospital-based therapy program for children with cancer: A descriptive study. *Canadian Oncology Nursing Journal, 14,* 217–222.

Gasalberti, D. (2006). Alternative therapies for children and youth with special health care needs. *Journal of Pediatric Health Care, 20*(2), 133–136.

Granger, B., & Kogan, L. (2006). Characteristics of animal-assisted therapy/activity in specialized settings. In A. Fine (Ed.), *Handbook on animal-assisted therapy: Theoretical foundations and guidelines for practice* (pp. 263–285). New York, NY: Academic Press.

Hart, L. (2000). Methods, standards, guidelines, and considerations in selecting animals for animal-assisted therapy. In A. Fine (Ed.), *Handbook on animal-assisted therapy: Theoretical foundations and guidelines for practice* (pp. 81–97). New York, NY: Academic Press.

Havener, L., Gentes, L., Thaler, B., Megel, M., Baun, M., Driscoll, F., . . . Agrawal, S. (2001). The effects of a companion animal on distress in children undergoing dental procedures. *Issues in Comprehensive Pediatric Nursing, 24*(2), 137–152.

Kanamori, M., Suzuki, M., Yamamoto, K., Kanda, M., Matsui, Y., Kojima, E., . . . Oshiro, H. (2001). A day care program and evaluation of animal-assisted therapy for the elderly with senile dementia. *American Journal of Alzheimer's Disease & Other Dementias, 16*(4), 234–239.

Kawamura, N., Niiyama, M., & Niiyama, H. (2009). Animal-assisted activity experiences of institutionalized Japanese older adults. *Journal of Psychosocial Nursing, 47*(1), 41–47.

Kirton, A., Wirrell, E., Zhang, J., & Hamiwka, L. (2004). Seizure alerting and response behaviors in dogs living with epileptic children. *Neurology, 62*(12), 2303–2305.

Krishna, N. (2009). *Dr. Dog—A programme for children with autism.* Retrieved from the Institute for Remedial Intervention Services website: http://www.autismindia.com

Laun, L. (2003). Benefits of pet therapy in dementia. *Home Healthcare Nurse, 21*(1), 49–52.

Lindsay, S. (2000). *Handbook of applied dog training and behavior: Adaptation and learning.* Ames, IA: Iowa State.

Lust, E., Ryan-Haddad, A., Coover, K., & Snell, J. (2007). Measuring clinical outcomes of animal-assisted therapy: Impact on resident medication usage. *Consultant Pharmacist, 22*(7), 580–585.

Macauley, B. (2006). Animal-assisted therapy for persons with aphasia: A pilot study. *Journal of Rehabilitation Research & Development, 43*(3), 357–366.

Mano, M., Uchizono, M., & Nishimura, T. (2003). A trial of dog-assisted therapy for elderly people with Alzheimer's disease. *Journal of Japanese Society for Dementia Care, 2,* 150–157.

Marcus, D., Bernstein, C., Constantin, J., Kunkel, F., Breuer, P., & Hanlon, R. (2012a). Animal-assisted therapy at an outpatient pain management clinic. *Pain Medicine, 13* (1), 45–57.

Marcus, D., Bernstein, C., Constantin, J., Kunkel, F., Breuer, P., & Hanlon, R. (2012b). Impact of animal-assisted therapy for outpatients with fibromyalgia. *Pain Medicine.* doi:10.1111/j.1526-4637.2012.01522.x

Martin, F., & Farnum, J. (2002). Animal-assisted therapy for children with pervasive developmental disorders. *Western Journal of Nursing Research, 24*(6), 657–670.

Matuszek, S. (2010). Animal-facilitated therapy in various patient populations: Systematic literature review. *Holistic Nursing Practice, 24* (4), 187–203.

McCabe, B., Baun, M., Speich, D., & Agrawal, S. (2002). Resident dog in the Alzheimer's special care unit. *Western Journal of Nursing Research, 24*(6), 684–696.

Moretti, F., DeRonchi, D., Bernabel, V., Marchetti, L., Ferrari, B., Forlani, C., . . . Atti, A. (2011). Pet therapy in elderly patients with mental illness. *Psychogeriatrics, 11,* 125–129.

Nagata, K. (2008). Seniors benefiting from animal therapy. Retrieved from the *Japan Times* online: http://www.japantimes.co

Nightingale, F. (1992). *Notes on nursing.* Philadelphia, PA: J. B. Lippincott. (Original work published 1859)

Odendaal, J. (2000). Animal-assisted therapy: Magic or medicine? *Journal of Psychosomatic Research, 49,* 275–280.

Pavlides, M. (2008). *Animal-assisted interventions for individuals with autism.* Philadelphia, PA: Jessica Kingsley.

Porter-Wenzlaff, L. (2007). Finding their voice: Developing emotional, cognitive, and behavioral congruence in female abuse survivors through equine facilitated therapy. *Explore, 3*(5), 529–534.

Richeson, N. (2003). Effects of animal-assisted therapy on agitated behaviors and social interactions of older adults with dementia. *American Journal of Alzheimers Disorders and Other Dementias, 18*(6), 353–358.

Rivera, M. (2010). *On dogs and dying: Inspirational stories from hospice hounds.* West Lafayette, IN: Purdue University Press.

Sobo, E., Eng, B., & Kassity-Krich, N. (2006). Canine visitation (pet) therapy: Pilot data on decreases in child pain perception. *Journal of Holistic Nursing, 24*(1), 51–57.

Therapy Dogs International. (2012). *Mission statement and history.* Retrieved from http://www.tdi-dog.org

Tyberg, A., & Frishman, W. (2008). Animal-assisted therapy. In M. Weintraub, R. Mamtani, & M. Micozzi (Eds.), *Complementary and integrative medicine in pain management* (pp. 115–123). New York, NY: Springer Publishing Company.

U.S. Department of Justice. (2010). *Civil Rights Division, Americans with Disabilities Act, 2010 Revised Requirements: Service animals.* Retrieved from http://www.ada.gov/service_animals_2010.htm

Veterans Moving Forward. (2012). *Mission, vision and goals.* Retrieved from www.vetsfwd.org/site/overview.php

Vizek, V., Arambasic, L., Kerestes, G., Kuterovac, G., & Vlahovic-Stetic, V. (2001). Pet ownership in childhood and socio-emotional characteristics, work values and professional choices in early adulthood. *Anthrozoos, 14*(4), 224–231.

Wesley, M., Minatrea, N., & Watson, J. (2009). Animal-assisted therapy in the treatment of substance dependence. *Anthrozoos, 22*(2), 137–148.

Wolff, A., & Frishman, W. (2005). Animal-assisted therapy and cardiovascular disease. In W. Frishman, M. Weintraub, & M. Micozzi (Eds.), *Complementary and integrative therapies for cardiovascular disease* (pp. 362–368). St. Louis, MO: Elsevier Mosby.

Zadnikar, M., & Kastrin, A. (2011). Effects of hippotherapy and therapeutic horseback riding on postural control or balance in children with cerebral palsy: A meta-analysis. *Developmental Medicine & Child Neurology, 53*, 684–691.

Zborowsky, T., & Kreitzer, M. (2008). Creating optimal healing environments in a health care setting. *Minnesota Medicine, 91*(3), 35–38.

ZENOAQ. (2009). *Therapy animals in Japan.* Retrieved from http://www.zenoaq.jp/html

Part III: Manipulative and Body-Based Therapies

*T*he National Center for Complementary and Alternative Medicine (NCCAM) defines this group of therapies as "practices (that) focus primarily on the structures and systems of the body, including bones and joints, soft tissues, and circulatory and lymphatic systems" (2012, p. 2). Therapies that are found in this category on the National Institutes of Health website include spinal manipulation such as done by chiropractors and osteopaths, Feldenkrais method, Alexander technique, and massage. Massage and chiropractic medicine are among the most commonly used complementary therapies. Both of these therapies have also been used with children. A recent addition to the list of movement therapies often classified with body-based therapies is pilates, which has become very popular for both health club and home use.

Both spinal manipulation and massage have been used for centuries in the treatment of illness and the promotion of health. Massage has had a long history in nursing and was included as a nursing intervention in many of the early nursing texts. Massage has also been part of ancient health care systems in many countries: Japan, China, Greece, Egypt, and Rome (NCCAM, 2012).

Although a number of the therapies in this category are administered by specially trained therapists such as chiropractors and massage therapists, a number of the procedures can be and are administered by nurses, particularly certain types of massage and relaxation therapies. These are the techniques included in this part of the book. Massage can range from simple hand or foot massage to back rubs or full-body massages—the latter provided by nurses who have been trained as massage therapists. A large number of relaxation therapies exist and nurses choose from among these to fit the needs and likes of patients.

Exercise has been included in this portion because of its importance in health promotion as well as in recovery from illness. A large body of research exists supporting the importance of regular exercise on body, mind, and spirit. A regular exercise program should be part of the individual nurse's routine.

Tai Chi, although it could be classified as an energy therapy, has been placed in this section because it involves movement. Tai Chi classes are common in community settings and long-term care. One outcome from Tai Chi, decreased falls in older patients, has growing investigation generating new knowledge for practice.

Nurses will find more uses for manipulative and body-based therapies as exploration grows and as these treatments are used with more conditions and populations, particularly with children. Nurses also need to be aware of therapies or nuances of these therapies that exist in other health care systems and cultures so they can either include and accommodate preferences or use of such practices in the plan of care, or caution patients about their use because some may be contraindicated with some illnesses or conditions.

REFERENCE

National Center for Complementary and Alternative Medicine. (2012). *What is complementary and alternative medicine?* Retrieved from http://nccam.nih.gov/health/whatiscam

Chapter 16: Massage

MELODEE HARRIS

Massage is a widely used complementary therapy that has been employed by nurses since the time of Florence Nightingale. Early nurse specialists in massage traced the history of massage in textbooks such as *The Theory and Practice of Massage* (Goodall-Copestake, 1919); *Massage: An Elementary Text-book for Nurses* (Macafee, 1917); *Fundamentals of Massage for Students of Nursing* (Jensen, 1932); and *A Textbook of Massage for Nurses and Beginners* (Rawlins, 1933). The authors devoted extensive histories of massage "to teach the student appreciation for the subject" (Jensen, 1932, p. v). Macafee (1917) wrote, "The history of massage is as old as that of man. . . ." (p. 5). Both Eastern and Western cultures are a part of the history of the traditional nursing practice of massage.

In 3000 BCE, the Chinese documented the use of massage in *Cong Fau of Tao-Tse*. There is evidence in *Sa-Tsai-Tou-Hoei*, written in 1000 BCE and published in the 16th century, that the Japanese also used massage (Calvert, 2002; Jensen, 1932). Goodall-Copestake (1919) records how massage is associated with ancient Hindu writings. The Japanese translated massage or shampooing as *amma*. Natives from the Sandwich Islands used *lomi-lomi*; the Maoris of New Zealand used the term *romi-romi*; and the natives of Tong Island used *toogi-toogi* to mean massage (Kellog, 1895, p. 12). The French word *masser* or *to shampoo* was applied to massage (Goodall-Copestake, 1919, p. 1; Jensen, 1932, p. 20).

The Greeks and Romans influenced the use of massage in Western civilizations. Hippocrates, the Father of Medicine, incorporated massage into the practice of medicine. In 380 BEC Hippocrates wrote, "A physician must be experienced in . . . rubbing" (Goodall-Copestake, 1919, p. 2). Galen used massage principles with gladiator students in Pergamos (Jensen, 1932;

Rawlins, 1933). In 1813, Per. Henrik Ling of Sweden developed Swedish massage movements at the Royal Central Institute of Stockholm. In 1860, Dr. Johan Mezger of Amsterdam used massage on King Frederick VII (then crown prince) of Denmark, and his success promoted the popularity of massage across Scandinavia, the Netherlands, and Germany (Jensen, 1932).

Although throughout history it has been known as an art and a complementary/alternative therapy, the practice of massage continues to build on a robust foundation, and evidence-based practices related to massage are evolving. In the Western world, massage may be used to treat a disease or syndrome diagnosed by a health care provider. Eastern or Asian massage is recommended by Eastern medical providers to treat disharmony and imbalance in the human body (Massage Therapy Body of Knowledge [MTBOK], 2010; Wieting & Cugalj, 2011). Western massage may use effleurage, petrissage, tapotement, or deep friction (Wieting & Cugalj, 2011). Eastern massage practices include Shiatsu and may combine several techniques (Wieting & Cugalj, 2011). Today, across all cultures, massage is a holistic intervention that uses the natural healing process to connect the body, mind, and spirit.

DEFINITION

Massage is a part of almost every civilization. The definition and meaning of massage is influenced and interpreted by culture and the healing philosophy of the predominant health care discipline.

The term *massage* is derived from the Greek word *massein,* which means to knead (Calvert, 2002). The Arabic word *mass* or *mas'h*, to press softly, also means massage (Goodall-Copestake, 1919, p. 1). The definition of massage varies by discipline. Nursing was among the first disciplines to use massage. Physicians, physical therapists, massage therapists, and even cosmetologists use massage.

Physicians term massage as medical massage. The Greeks and Romans influenced physicians to use massage. Hippocrates used the word *friction* for massage in the treatment of sprains (Jensen, 1932). Norstroëm (1896) claimed that the use of massage came from "bonesetters." Today massage is used widely by doctors of osteopathic medicine.

Massage is within the scope of practice of physical therapy, and therapists use it across many settings (American Physical Therapy Association, 2011). Physical therapists use massage in sports medicine to reduce pain, rehabilitate, and boost physical performance for athletes (Brummitt, 2008).

According to the Massage Therapy Body of Knowledge (MTBOK) Task Force, massage therapists have a broad interpretation of massage. Massage, body massage, body rub, somatic therapy, and other similar terms are equivalent to massage therapy. The terms *massage therapy* and *bodywork* are often used interchangeably. The use of bodywork by massage therapists also includes a more holistic approach to enhance awareness of the mind–body–spirit connection. Clinical massage entails more extensive assessment and techniques focused on symptoms to mean treatment, orthopedic, and medical massage (MTBOK Task Force, 2010, p. 40).

Licensed nurse massage therapists use nursing theory and the nursing process with massage techniques (National Association of Nurse Massage Therapists, 2012). Bedside nurses are taught to use effleurage or slow-stroke back massage that does not require a separate license or training beyond nursing school. More than any other health care discipline, nurses have adopted massage into their curricula. In 1932, The National League of Nursing Education recommended 15 hours of lecture and training in massage for nursing curriculum (Ruffin, 2011, p. 67). Today, the National Council of State Boards of Nursing (NCSBN) includes complementary and alternative therapies in the NCLEX-RN® (National Council Licensure Examination) examinations. The NCSBN specifically mentions massage therapy in the 2013 NCLEX-RN test plan (NCSBN, 2012, p. 20). Swedish massage movements such as effleurage or slow-stroke back massage continue to be taught in schools of nursing.

Overall, *massage* is a broad term. Attempts to operationalize a definition that includes art, science, and also covers interpretations from culture and discipline are challenging. The American Massage Therapy Association defines *massage* as "manual soft tissue manipulation, and includes holding, causing movement, and/or applying pressure to the body" (Fletcher, 2009, p. 59). Simply put, "massage is a therapeutic manipulation of the soft tissues of the body with the goal of achieving normalization of those tissues" (Wieting & Cugalj, 2011, para. 5).

SCIENTIFIC BASIS

Although massage is both an art and a science, the early nurse massage specialists recognized massage as a science. Rawlins (1933) stated, "Massage is a science, not a fad of the times" (p. 19). Jensen (1932) defined *massage* as "the scientific manipulation of body tissue as a therapeutic measure" (p. 2).

Florence Nightingale based the use of nonpharmacological interventions such as massage on the Environmental Adaptation Theory. Nightingale believed that nurses should promote the best possible environment that would allow natural laws to improve the healing process (Dossey, Selanders, Beck, & Attewell, 2005).

Today, perhaps due to the relative lack of its study by rigorous research methods, massage is often thought of as more of an art than a science. Nurse researcher Dr. Tiffany Fields established the first center in the world devoted to the science of touch and massage. The Touch Research Institute was established in 1992 at the University of Miami School of

Medicine (Touch Research Institute, n.d.). Dr. Field was one of the first to study the effects of massage on weight gain in preterm infants (Field, 2002) and build the capacity for nursing science on massage.

Massage is used by nurses to promote health and wellness. It is used to increase circulation, relieve pain, induce sleep, reduce anxiety or depression, and improve quality of life (Rose, 2010). Massage produces therapeutic effects on multiple body systems: integumentary, musculoskeletal, cardiovascular, lymph, and nervous. Manipulating the skin and underlying muscle makes the skin supple. Massage increases or enhances movement in the musculoskeletal system by reducing swelling, loosening and stretching contracted tendons, and aiding in the reduction of soft-tissue adhesions. Friction to the cutaneous and subcutaneous tissues releases histamines that in turn produce vasodilation of vessels and enhance venous return (Snyder & Taniguki, 2010).

Massage is a proposed mechanism for relaxation to reduce psychological and physiological stress (Harris & Richards, 2010). Stress is also an individual subjective experience. When the body interprets a physiological or psychological response as stressful, the sympathetic nervous system stimulates the hypothalamic–pituitary–adrenal (HPA) axis in the brain. There is a release of stress hormones such as cortisol and epinephrine. Tactile stimulation in the body tissues causes neurohormonal responses throughout the nervous system. Mechanoreceptors cause impulses to travel from the peripheral nervous system, up the ascending spinal cord to the neuro cortex. The stimulus is then interpreted in the higher brain resulting in a neurological or biochemical response (Lawton, 2003). Massage activates the parasympathetic nervous system to decrease heart rate, blood pressure, and respirations that result in relaxation (Moraska, Pollini, Boulanger, Brooks, & Teitlebaum, 2010).

Studies show that massage produces physiological and psychological indicators for the relaxation response (Harris & Richards, 2010). Using foot massage with cardiac patients, Hattan, King, and Griffiths (2002) found that subjects receiving this therapy reported feeling much calmer. In a quasi-experimental study ($n = 24$), Holland and Pokorny (2001) showed a statistically significant difference ($p = 0.05$) in vital signs before and after the slow-stroke massage intervention. The decrease in vital signs indicates that massage may mediate the stress response (Harris & Richards, 2010).

Reduction of pain, a frequent desired outcome of massage, is closely related to the relaxation response. Through the relaxation response, massage relieves pain by stimulating the large-diameter nerve fibers that have an inhibitory input on T-cells (Furlan, Imamura, Dryden & Irvin, 2008). According to Wang and Keck, "massaging the hands and feet stimulates the mechanoreceptors that activate the nonpainful nerve fibers, preventing pain transmission from reaching consciousness" (2004, p. 59). Studies have validated that patients were more comfortable after the administration of massage (Frey Law et al., 2008; Wang & Keck, 2004).

Flowing, light touch, Kneading deep, vigorous pressure pt.)

In addition, research is emerging on how massage impacts the psycho-neuroimmunological functions of the body and mind. There was higher natural killer (NK) cytotoxicity and higher daily weight in preterm infants who received massage in a randomized placebo-controlled trial (Ang et al., 2012). Billhult, Lindholm, Gunnarsson, and Stener-Victoria (2008) explored the effect of massage on CD4 + and CD8 + T-cells in women with cancer. Findings revealed that massage had no effect on these indices.

Massage is a holistic therapy that promotes overall health, including emotional well-being (Currin & Meister, 2008); decreases pain and anxiety during labor (Chang, Wang, & Chen, 2002); and increases quality of life (Williams et al., 2005).

INTERVENTION

Various strokes are used to produce friction and pressure on cutaneous and subcutaneous tissues. The type of stroke and the amount of pressure chosen depend on the desired outcomes and the body part being massaged.

There are a number of types of massage: _Swedish_ (a massage using long, flowing strokes), _Esalen_ (a meditative massage using light touch), _deep tissue or neuromuscular_ (an intense kneading of the body), _sports massage_ (a vigorous massage to loosen and ease sore muscles), _Shiatsu_ (a Japanese pressure-point technique to relieve stress), and _reflexology_ (a deep foot massage that relates to parts of the body). The different types of massage incorporate a variety of strokes, varying levels of pressure, and a multitude of procedures. Massage strokes can be administered to the entire body or to specific areas of the body, such as the back, feet, or hands.

The environment in which massage is administered is important. The room must be warm enough for the person to be comfortable because shivering could negate the effects of the massage. In addition, privacy needs to be ensured. Adding music and aromatherapy to massage sessions has been thought to increase the effectiveness of massage. Before administering massage, the nurse should explain the intervention, obtain a history, and secure the permission of the patient.

Massage Strokes in Nursing

In 1895, Dr. J. H. Kellog from Battle Creek, Michigan, wrote _The Art of Massage_ to teach nurses and other practitioners how to use massage techniques (Calvert, 2002; Kellog, 1895). Although early in nursing history massage was prescribed by physicians, nurses responded by showing leadership to specialize in massage.

Commonly used strokes in administering massage include effleurage, friction, pressure, petrissage, vibration, and percussion.

Effleurage

Effleurage is a slow, rhythmic stroking, with light skin contact. Effleurage may be applied with varying degrees of pressure, depending on the part of the body being massaged and the outcome desired. The palmar surface of the hands is used for larger surfaces, the thumbs and fingers for smaller areas. On large surfaces, long, gliding strokes about 10 inches to 20 inches in length are applied.

Friction Movements

In *friction movements,* moderate, constant pressure to one area is made with the thumbs or fingers. The fingers may be held in one place or moved in a small circumscribed area.

Pressure Stroke

The *pressure stroke* is similar to the friction stroke, except pressure strokes are made with the whole hand.

Petrissage

Petrissage, or kneading, involves lifting a large fold of skin and the underlying muscle and holding the tissue between the thumb and fingers. The tissues are pushed against the bone, then raised and squeezed in circular movements. The grasp on the tissues is alternately loosened and tightened. Tissues are supported by one hand while being kneaded with the other. Variations include pinching, rolling, wringing, and kneading with fists or fingers. Petrissage is limited to tissues having a significant muscle mass.

Vibration Strokes

Vibration strokes can be administered with either the entire hand or with the fingers. Rapid, continuous strokes are used. Because administering vibration strokes requires a significant amount of energy, mechanical vibrators are sometimes used.

Percussion Strokes

For *percussion strokes,* the wrist acts as a fulcrum for the hand, with the hand hitting the tissue. Strokes are made with a rapid tempo over a large body area. Tapping and clapping are variants of percussion strokes.

Slow-Stroke Back Massage

Slow-stroke back massage, or *effleurage*, is a technique taught in nursing schools. See Exhibit 16.1 for a description of how to perform slow-stroke back massage.

Hand Massage

Techniques for performing hand massage are outlined in Exhibit 16.2. The techniques are easy to use with many populations, including older adults (Kolcaba, Schirm, & Steiner, 2006; Snyder, Eagan, & Burns, 1995) as well as infants and children (Field, 2002). A suggested period for administering massage is 2½ minutes per hand. The length of time is individualized for each patient, based on response.

Exhibit 16.1. *Technique for Slow-Stroke Back Massage*

1. **Environment**
   - The room should be at a comfortable temperature.
   - The lights should be dimmed.
   - Noise should be eliminated.
   - The nurse should keep talking at a minimum.

2. **The Patient**
   - Ask the patient whether there is a need to use the bathroom or whether there is any way the nurse can assist to promote relaxation before beginning the massage.
   - The patient should be assisted to a comfortable position.
   - Clothing should be removed so the back is exposed.
   - Modesty should be respected.

3. **The Slow-Stroke Back Massage**
   - Palms of the hands and fingers are used (effleurage).
   - The nurse warms her hands.
   - The nurse applies nonallergenic lotion to her hands.
   - Palms of the hands are placed in the sacral area on each side of the spine.
   - Gentle pressure is applied.
   - Long, slow, rhythmic, circular strokes are used to move upward on each side of the spine toward the base of the neck.
   - Then long, slow, rhythmic, circular strokes are used to move downward on each side of the spine toward the sacral area.

(continued)

Exhibit 16.1. *Technique for Slow-Stroke Back Massage (continued)*

- The masseur applies 12 to 15 strokes per minute to perform a rhythmic movement.
- The massage should continue until completion without removing the hands from the back.

4. **Completion**
   - Remove hands from the spine.
   - Replace clothing to the back.
   - Replace bedcovers.
   - Instruct the patient to rise slowly.
   - Instruct the patient to stay hydrated.
   - Quietly leave the room.

Protocol adapted from Harris, Richards, and Grando (2012).

Exhibit 16.2. *Techniques for Hand Massage*

Each hand is massaged for 2½ minutes. Do not massage if hand is injured, reddened, or swollen. Protocols from 5 minutes to 10 minutes for each hand have also been recommended (Kolcaba et al, 2006; Remington, 2002).

1. **Back of hand**
   - Short, medium-length, straight strokes are done from the wrist to the fingertips; moderate pressure is used (effleurage).
   - Large, half-circle, stretching strokes are made from the center to the side of the hand, using moderate pressure.
   - Small, circular strokes are made over the entire hand, using light pressure (make small o's with the thumb).
   - Featherlike, straight strokes are made from the wrist to the fingertips, using very light pressure.

2. **Palm of hand**
   - Short, medium-length, straight strokes are made from the wrist to the fingertips, using moderate pressure (effleurage).
   - Gentle milking and lifting of the tissue of the entire palm of the hand is done using moderate pressure.
   - Small circular strokes are made over the entire palm, using moderate pressure (making little o's with index finger).

(continued)

Exhibit 16.2. *Techniques for Hand Massage (continued)*

- Large, half-circle, stretching strokes are used, from the center of the palm to the sides, using moderate pressure.

3. **Fingers**
   - Gently squeeze each finger from the base to the tip on both sides and the front and back, using light pressure.
   - Gentle range-of-motion of finger.
   - Gentle pressure on nail bed.

4. **Completion**
   - Place client's hand on yours and cover it with your other hand. Gently draw your top hand toward you several times. Turn the client's hand over and gently draw your other hand toward you several times.

MEASUREMENT OF OUTCOMES

Both physiological and psychological outcomes have been used to measure the effectiveness of massage. Indices of relaxation—heart rate, blood pressure, respiration rate, skin temperature, cortisol level, and muscle tension—have been measured in many studies. Anxiety inventories and scales to determine pain level and quality-of-sleep as well as quality-of-life indices have been used to determine the efficacy of massage. Protocols for the duration of massage are needed. Typically, massage is dosed at 30-minute or 60-minute intervals because this is the duration of time used by massage therapists. The results of a randomized controlled trial ($n = 125$) used a 60-minute, once-weekly dose of massage in an 8-week protocol for osteoarthritis of the knee (Perlman et al., 2012, p. e30248). This was an optimal standard for future dose-finding studies. More research is needed to guide implementation and standardize massage protocols for other conditions. It is important that both short- and long-term effects of massage be measured.

PRECAUTIONS

Ernst (2003) reviewed the literature to determine adverse reactions to massage. Although a number of negative reactions were noted, the majority of these were associated with exotic types of massage and not with the Swedish massage technique. Another review of the literature (Batavia, 2004) indicated the following contraindications to performing massage including: arteritis, esophageal varicies, unstable hypotension, advanced respiratory failure, postmyocardial infarction, aneurysm, emboli, arrhythmia, anticoagulant therapy/disease, heart failure, phlebitis, varicose veins, deep vein thrombosis, atherosclerosis, tumor, and cancer.

The patient's history of massage gathered by the nurse prior to the intervention provides information about past use of massage and any adverse responses. It is also important to find out the person's overall response to touch. Some people may be averse to being touched because of past negative experiences. Others may be hypersensitive to touch. One method for overcoming this sensitivity is beginning with light touch and slowly increasing the pressure. The area to be massaged is assessed for redness, bruises, edema, or rashes prior to performing massage.

Age-related changes are important considerations for massage. Older adults experience more fragile skin and may take anticoagulants, which could cause bruising with massage. Osteoporosis and corticosteroids also place the older adult at risk for fracture. Arthritis, Parkinson's disease, and stroke may limit mobility. The nurse may need to modify massage techniques, positioning, and protocols when considering age-related changes and comorbidities (Rose, 2010).

Massage therapists and nurses have been reluctant to use massage with cancer patients (Gecsedi, 2002) because of the belief that the therapy may initiate or accelerate metastases. Guidelines are being developed to govern the use of massage with persons with cancer. A physician's order is needed for body region and technique to be used. Factors considered are the location of the tumor, the stage of the cancer, and the location of any metastatic lesions. Pressure in the immediate area of the cancer is to be avoided. A pilot study ($n = 12$) comparing reflexology and Swedish massage to reduce physiological stress and pain and improve mood was conducted on nursing home residents with cancer (Hodgson & Lafferty, 2012). The results revealed that both techniques were feasible and produced measurable improvements on cortisol levels, pain, and mood. The study supports the need to develop guidelines for older adults with cancer in the nursing home.

Because blood pressure may be lowered during massage, monitoring for light-headedness is suggested following the initial massage sessions, particularly in older adults. If light-headedness does occur, allowing the person to remain recumbent for several minutes at the conclusion of the massage may help to decrease the likelihood of hypotension and falls. Monitoring of blood pressure and pulse rate are required in persons with cardiac conditions, to determine whether adverse effects are being experienced.

USES

Exhibit 16.3 is a list of selected conditions for which massage is used. Evidence related to relaxation, pain, and sleep is discussed next.

Exhibit 16.3. *Uses of Massage*

Agitation (Remington, 2002)

Comfort (Kolcaba et al., 2006)

Decrease aggressive behaviors (Garner et al., 2008)

Facilitate communication (Kolcaba et al., 2006)

Increase psychological well-being (Hattan et al., 2002)

Increase weight in preterm infants (Field, 2002)

Lessen anxiety (Currin & Meister, 2008)

Lessen fatigue (Currin & Meister, 2008)

Lessen pain (Chang et al., 2002; Wang & Keck, 2004)

Promote relaxation/reduce stress (Harris & Richards, 2010)

Promote sleep (Harris et al., 2012; Richards, 1998)

Relaxation

Nurses use massage as an intervention to relieve physiological and psychological stress and promote relaxation (Harris & Richards, 2010). In a review of 22 studies in which massage had been used, Richards, Gibson, and Overton-McCoy (2000) found that the most commonly reported outcome was a reduction in anxiety.

Mok and Woo (2004) collected data on psychological indicators for decreased anxiety after a 10-minute slow-stroke back massage on hospitalized Chinese older patients diagnosed with stroke ($n = 102$). The results showed statistically significant results at the $p = 0.05$ level for relaxation using the Spielberger Self-Evaluation Questionnaire to provide evidence for the decrease in psychological indicators for stress. Another study (Chen et al., 2012) revealed statistically significant decreases—after back massage—in systolic blood pressure ($p < 0.01$), diastolic blood pressure ($p < 0.01$), pulse ($p < 0.01$), and respiratory rates ($p < 0.01$), as well as a statistically significant difference in anxiety ($p = 0.02$) in participants ($n = 64$) with severe congestive heart failure.

Several studies using hand massage reported a decrease in psychological indicators for stress (Hickes-Moore & Robinson, 2008; Kolcaba et al., 2006; Remington, 2002). Two randomized controlled trials on hand massage (Hickes-Moore & Robinson, 2008; Remington, 2002) used the Cohen Mansfield Agitation Index (CMAI) to test the effects of hand massage on reducing agitation. Hickes-Moore and Robinson (2008) and Remington (2002) reported statistically significant decreases in agitation 1 hour after hand massage in older participants. Kolcaba et al. (2006) showed statistically significant results for comfort using hand massage in the nursing home environment.

Pain

Reduction of pain is another condition for which massage is often used. Numerous studies have found that massage resulted in a reduction of pain. In a review of research on the use of massage and aromatherapy in persons with cancer, Wang and Keck (2004) reported a lessening of pain in postoperative patients, and Mok and Woo (2004) found that massage lessened pain in patients with strokes.

Sleep

The results from a study by Richards (1998) using polysomnography as an objective measure for sleep in hospitalized men ($n = 69$) compared a slow-stroke back massage intervention group between participants using relaxing music and a control group. The data did not show statistically significant results; however, a power analysis indicated a larger sample size was needed. A randomized controlled trial of massage on participants ($n = 57$) after coronary artery bypass graft surgery showed decreased fatigue and more effective sleep (Nerbass, Feltrim, de Souza, Ykeda, & Lorenzi-Filho, 2010). Another randomized controlled pilot study (Harris et al., 2012) with persons with dementia in the nursing home ($n = 40$) used actigraphy to objectively measure sleep in participants receiving a 3-minute, slow-stroke back massage compared with a usual-care control condition. There were no statistically significant differences between participants in the slow-stroke back massage intervention group and the control group. Although a larger sample size was needed, participants provided evidence in subjective comments for clinical significance for the use of slow-stroke back massage for relaxation and sleep in this population.

CULTURAL ASPECTS

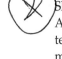

Shiatsu, a pressure-point type of massage, is popular in Japan and other Asian countries. Its underlying purpose is to rebalance the energy system in the body through pressure on specific points. Although Shiatsu may not be comforting during administration, relaxation is often felt at the conclusion. Shiatsu may be used to help alleviate other conditions. Taniguki (2008) found Shiatsu therapy to be highly efficacious in managing constipation in six elderly patients (from 81 years old to 93 years old) who were on bed rest and receiving home care.

In countries such as Japan, acupuncture and moxibustion are often used in addition to massage by massage therapists who also often have a license to practice acupuncture and moxibustion. Therefore, in some research studies, due to the cultural implications, massage cannot be separated from acupuncture and moxibustion (Hirakawa et al., 2005).

In a multicultural qualitative study (Kilstoff & Chenoweth, 1998), hand massage was conducted on Chinese-, Italian-, Vietnamese-, Arab-, French-, and English-speaking participants ($n = 39$; 16 dyads of persons with dementia and caregivers; 7 day-care staff) in a dementia care patient setting. The results showed reduction in stress, decreased agitation, increased alertness, improved self-hygiene, and improved sleep. Family caregivers also reported less distress, improved sleep, and feelings of calm.

Massage is widely used around the world as illustrated in the accounts of nursing students (see Sidebar 16.1).

Sidebar 16.1. *Accounts of Massage of International Nursing Students at Carr College of Nursing, Harding University, Searcy, Arkansas*

Larissa Pinczuk, Canada

As a missionary who lived in [the] Ukraine, I have travelled a lot and learned about many cultural practices and traditions. Among numerous home remedies and treatments that I have seen, the use of massage therapy seemed quite common, especially in care for the elderly. Some older people who cannot afford, or are afraid to seek, health care [often] turn to less-costly options, such as using massage as a method for pain relief. In everyday living, it is also used in the home to relieve anxiety and correct bad posture. Some people even attend extracurricular massage courses to gain the professional skills that could better help their sick loved ones at home.

Esi Fosua Yeboah, Ghana

The use of massage therapy in Ghana and the United States is similar. In Ghana, it is used for relaxation, increasing circulation, decreasing pain, and inducing sleep. It is also used for treatment of fibromyalgia and depression. The following comment was written in 2011 in a blog (www.massageprofessionals.com/profiles/blogs/initiating-our-association-in-africa) by Yaw Bateng, who has established a massage therapy school in Ghana: "the profession of massage has not been given attention in Africa, most especially in Ghana."

(continued)

Sidebar 16.1. *Accounts of Massage of International Nursing Students at Carr College of Nursing, Harding University, Searcy, Arkansas (continued)*

Azel Peralta, Philippines

In the Southeast Asian islands of the Philippines, one massage technique is called "hilot." This means *healer* or *to rub*. "Manghihilots," those who practice the hilot technique, usually learn their art through teachings and practices that have been passed down through the generations. Hilot is not something learned through schooling. People in the Philippine villages visit Manghihilots to look for a cure instead of traveling many miles to the cities to see a doctor. Hilot is a holistic art of healing and is used to correct imbalances in the body such as fluid, energy, fractures, sprains, and dislocations. Hilot is also used for inducing labor of pregnant women. Natural banana leaves and coconut oil, which are staples of these islands, are used in the process of locating the problem areas and diagnosing health problems. Techniques can range from a combination of a deep-tissue massage to manipulate muscle tissue, bones, and joints to using only a stroking or rubbing motion of the fingers.

Sivchhun Hun, Cambodia

Massage therapy is a big part of the lives of Cambodian people. It is used here for various reasons, including the benefits of relaxation. My parents have a massage therapist visit them at home daily around evening time. They believe that by receiving massage therapy before their bedtime it helps them to relax, to sleep better at night, and to feel better when they wake up in the morning.

FUTURE RESEARCH

There is a lack of rigorous research on complementary therapies such as massage. Specific techniques, questions related to who should administer the massage, specific protocols, dose-finding studies, qualitative research, and studies to support the clinical significance of massage are all areas for further investigation to build the nursing science in massage. One challenge in conducting research on massage is having a comparable control group. McNamara, Burnham, Smith, and Carroll (2003) compared massage and standard care in patients undergoing a diagnostic test.

Reflexology and Swedish massage (Hodgson & Lafferty, 2012) were compared on nursing home residents with cancer. A randomized controlled trial ($n = 125$) that compared structural and relaxation massage for low back pain used blinding to test the effectiveness of treatment for low back pain (Cherkin et al., 2012). More studies are needed that compare massage techniques for developing evidence-based practices. The results of a randomized controlled trial ($n = 125$; Perlman et al., 2012) showed that a 60-minute, once-weekly dose of massage was an optimal standard for future dose-finding studies in persons with osteoarthritis of the knee.

The following are suggestions for research that is needed so that practitioners may have more direction in using massage in clinical settings:

- Well-designed studies using blinding, randomization, and attention control groups with large sample sizes are needed.
- Few investigators have explored the impact massage has on psychoneuroimmunological indices. Studies on the use of massage with patients having HIV infection and cancer would guide nurses in its use with these groups.
- Dose-finding studies for administering massage and the number of sessions that produce the best results need to be established. There is great variation in these two parameters in published studies. Because of time constraints in practice settings, this information would be very helpful to busy practitioners.
- What, if any, is the effect of the gender of the therapist administering massage on the outcomes obtained? Few studies have reported on the significance of the gender of the therapist in relation to that of the patient.

REFERENCES

American Massage Therapy Association. Retrieved January 5, 2005, from http://www.amtamassage.org/about/definition.html

American Physical Therapy Association. (2011). *Today's physical therapists: A comprehensive review of a 21st century health care profession.* Alexandria, VA: Author.

Ang, J. Y., Lua, J. L., Mathur, A., Thomas, R., Asmar, B. I., Savasan, S., . . . Shankaran, S. (2012). A randomized placebo-controlled trial of massage therapy on the immune system of preterm infants. *Pediatrics, 130*(6), e1548–e1549. doi:10.1542/peds.2012-1096

Batavia, M. (2004). Contraindications for therapeutic massage: Do sources agree? *Journal of Bodywork and Movement Therapies, 8,* 48–57. doi:10.1016/S1360-8592(03)0008-6

Billhult, A., Lindhom, C., Gunnarsson, R., & Stener-Victoria, E. (2008). The effect of massage on cellular immunity, endocrine and psychological factors in women with breast cancer—A randomized controlled clinical trial. *Autonomic Neuroscience Basic and Clinical, 140,* 88–95. doi:10.1016/j.autneu.2008.03.006

Brummitt, J. (2008). The role of massage in sports performance and rehabilitation: Current evidence and future direction. *North American Journal of Sports Physical Therapy, 3,* 7–21.

Calvert, R. N. (2002). *The history of massage.* Rochester, VT: Healing Arts Press.

Chang, M. Y., Wang, S. Y., & Chen, C. H. (2002). Effects of massage on pain and anxiety during labour: A randomized controlled trial in Taiwan. *Journal of Advanced Nursing, 38,* 68–73.

Chen, W.-L., Liu, G.-J., Yeh, S.-H., Chiang, M.-C., Fu, M.-Y., & Hsieh, Y.-K. (2013). Effect of back massage intervention on anxiety, comfort, and physiologic responses in patients with congestive heart failure. *Journal of Alternative and Complementary Medicine, 19,* 464–470. doi:10.1089/acm.2011.0873

Cherkin, D. C., Sherman, K. J., Kahn, J., Wellman, R., Cook, A. J., Erro, J., . . . Deyo, R. A. (2012). A comparison of the effects of 2 types of massage and usual care on chronic low back pain. *Annals of Internal Medicine, 155*(1), 1–9.

Currin, J., & Meister, E. A. (2008). A hospital-based intervention using massage to reduce distress among oncology patients. *Cancer Nursing, 3,* 214–221. doi:10.1097/01. NCC.0000305725.65345.f3

Dossey, B. M., Selanders, L. C., Beck, D., & Attewell, A. (2005). *Florence Nightingale today: Healing, leadership, global action.* Silver Spring, MD: American Nurses Association.

Ernst, E. (2003). The safety of massage therapy. *Rheumatology, 42,* 1101–1106. doi:10.1093/ rheumatology/keg306

Field, T. (2002). Preterm infant massage therapy studies: An American approach. *Seminars in Neonatology, 7,* 487–494.

Fletcher, B. (2009). A bridge between the mind and body: The effects of massage on body image state. *Undergraduate Review, 5,* 58–63. Retrieved from http://vc.bridgew .edu/undergrad_rev/vol5/iss1/13

Frey Law, L. A., Evans, S., Kundston, J., Nus, S., Scholl, K., & Sluka, K. A. (2008). Massage reduces pain perception and hyperalgesia in experimental muscle pain: A randomized, controlled trial. *Journal of Pain, 9,* 714–721. doi:10.1016/ j.jpain.2008.03.009

Furlan, A. D., Imamura, M., Dryden, T., & Irvin, E. (2008). Massage for low-back pain. *Cochrane Database of Systematic Reviews, 4* Art. No.: CD001929. doi:10.1002/14651858. CD001929.pub2

Garner, B., Phillips, L. J., Schmidt, H. M., Markulev, C., O'Connor, J., Wood, S. J., . . . McGorry, P. D. (2008). Pilot study evaluating the effect of massage therapy on stress, anxiety, and aggression in a young adult psychiatric inpatient unit. *Australian & New Zealand Journal of Psychiatry, 42*(5), 414–422. doi:10.1080/00048670801961131

Gecsedi, R. A. (2002). Massage therapy for patients with cancer. *Clinical Journal of Oncology Nursing, 6,* 52–54. doi:10.1188/02.CJON.52-54

Goodall-Copestake, B. M. (1919). *The theory and practice of massage* (2nd ed.). New York, NY: Paul B. Hoeber.

Harris, M., & Richards, K. C. (2010). The physiological and psychological effects of slow-stroke back massage and hand massage on relaxation in the elderly. *Journal of Clinical Nursing, 19,* 917–926.

Harris, M., Richards, K. C., & Grando, V. T. (2012). The effects of slow-stroke back massage on minutes of nighttime sleep on persons with dementia in the nursing home. *Journal of Holistic Nursing, 30*(4), 255–263. doi:10.1177/08980101112455948

Hattan, J., King, L., & Griffiths, P. (2002). The impact of foot massage and guided relaxation following cardiac surgery: A randomized controlled trial. *Journal of Advanced Nursing, 37,* 199–207.

Hicks-Moore, S., & Robinson, B. (2008). Favorite music and hand massage. *Dementia, 7*(1), 95–108. doi:10.1177/1471301207085369

Hirakawa, Y., Masuda, Y., Kimata, T., Uemura, K., Kuzuya, M., & Iguchi, A. (2005). Effects of home massage rehabilitation for the bed-ridden elderly: A pilot trial with a three-month follow up. *Clinical Rehabilitation, 19,* 20–27. doi:10.1191/ 0269215505cr7950a

Hodgson, N. A., & Lafferty, D. (2012). Reflexology versus Swedish massage to reduce physiological stress and pain and improve mood in nursing home residents with cancer: A pilot study. *Evidence-Based Complementary and Alternative Medicine, 2012,* 1–5. doi:10.1155/2012/456897

Holland, B., & Pokorny, M. E. (2001). Slow stroke back massage on patients in a rehabilitation setting. *Rehabilitation Nursing, 26,* 182–186.

Jensen, K. L. (1932). *Fundamentals of massage for students of nursing.* New York, NY: Macmillan.

Kellog, J. H. (1895). *The art of massage.* Battle Creek, MI: The Good Health Publishing Co.

Kilstoff, K, & Chenoweth, L. (1998). New approaches to health and well-being for dementia day-care clients, family careers and day-care staff. *International Journal of Nursing Practice, 4*(2), 70–83. doi:10.1046/j.1440-172X.1998.00059.x

Kolcaba, K., Schirm, V., & Steiner, R. (2006). Effects of hand massage on comfort of nursing home residents. *Geriatric Nursing, 27,* 85–91.

Lawton, G. (2003). Toward a neurophysiological understanding of manual therapy neuro-manual therapy. Retrieved January 2, 2013, from http://www.americanmanualmedicine.com

Macafee, N. E. (1917). *Massage, an elementary text-book for nurses.* Pittsburgh, PA: Reed & Witting.

Massage Therapy Body of Knowledge (MTBOK). (2010). *Massage therapy body of knowledge* (MTBOK) version 1.0.

McNamara, M. E., Burnham, D. C., Smith, C., & Carroll, D. L. (2003). The effects of back massage before diagnostic cardiac catheterization. *Alternative Therapies in Health and Medicine, 9*(1), 50–57.

Mok, E., & Woo, C. P. (2004). The effects of slow-stroke massage on anxiety and shoulder pain in elderly stroke patients. *Complementary Therapies in Nursing & Midwifery, 10,* 209–216.

Moraska, A., Pollini, R. A., Boulanger, K., Brooks, M. Z., & Teitlebaum, L. (2010). Physiological adjustments to stress measures following massage therapy: A review of the literature. *eCAM, 7,* 409–418. doi:10.1093/ecam/nen029

National Association of Nurse Massage Therapists. (2012). *About us philosophy.* Retrieved January 1, 2013, from http://www.nanmt.org

National Council of State Boards of Nursing (NCSBN). (2012). *National Council of State Boards of Nursing 2013 NCLEX-RN® detailed test plan item writer/item reviewer/nurse educator version.* Chicago, IL: Author.

Nerbass, F. B., Feltrim, M. I. Z., de Souza, S. A., Ykeda, D. S., & Lorenzi-Filho, G. (2010). Effects of massage therapy on sleep quality after coronary artery bypass graft surgery. *Clinicals, 65,* 1105–1110. doi:10.1590/S1807-59322010001100008

Norstroëm, G. M. (1868/1896). *The handbook of massage.* New York, NY. (No publisher listed.)

Perlman, A. I., Ali, A., Njike, V. Y., Hom, D., Davidi, A., Gould-Fogeite, S., . . . Katz, D. L. (2012). Massage therapy for osteoarthritis of the knee: A randomized dose-finding trial. *PLoS ONE, 7*(2), e30248. doi:10.1371/journal.pone.0030248

Rawlins, M. (1933). *A textbook of massage for nurses and beginners* (2nd ed.). St. Louis, MO: The C. V. Mosby.

Remington, R. (2002). Calming music and hand massage with agitated elderly. *Nursing Research, 51*(5), 317–323.

Richards, K. C. (1998). Effect of a back massage and relaxation intervention on sleep in critically ill patients. *American Journal of Critical Care, 7,* 288–299.

Richards, K. C., Gibson, R., & Overton-McCoy, A. L. (2000). Effects of massage in acute and critical care. *AACN Clinical Issues, 11,* 77–96.

Rose, M. K. (2010). *Comfort touch.* Philadelphia, PA: Wolters Kluwer/Lippincott Williams & Wilkins.

Ruffin, P. T. (2011). A history of massage in nurse training school curricula (1860–1945). *Journal of Holistic Nursing, 29*, 61–67. doi:10.1177/0898010110377355

Snyder, M., Egan, E. C., & Burns, K. R. (1995). Efficacy of hand massage in decreasing agitation behaviors associated with care activities in persons with dementia. *Geriatric Nursing, 16*(2), 60–63.

Snyder, M., & Taniguki, S. (2010). Massage. In M. Snyder & R. Lindquist (Eds.), *Complementary and alternative therapies in nursing* (6th ed., pp. 337–448). New York, NY: Springer Publishing Company.

Taniguki, S. (2008). Use of Shiatsu with home care patients (Unpublished manuscript).

Touch Research Institute. (n.d.). *Touch Research Institute*. Retrieved from http://www6.miami.edu/touch-research

Wang, H. L., & Keck, J. F. (2004). Foot and hand massage as an intervention for postoperative pain. *Pain Management Nursing, 5*, 59–65.

Wieting, J. M., & Cugalj, A. P. (2011). *Massage, traction, and manipulation*. Retrieved December 29, 2012, from http://emedicine.medscape.com

Williams, A. L., Selwyn, P. A., Liberti, L., Molde, S., Njike, V. Y., McCorkle, R., . . . Katz, D. L. (2005). A randomized controlled trial of meditation and massage effects on quality of life in people with late-stage disease: A pilot study. *Journal of Palliative Medicine, 8*, 939–952.

Chapter 17: Tai Chi

KUEI-MIN CHEN

*T*ime pressure is emerging as a contemporary malaise. Lack of time is the major barrier to exercising regularly. Failure to exercise may lead to mental strain, nervous breakdown, or inefficiency in daily work (Strazdins & Loughrey, 2008). Good health is essential; how to acquire and maintain a healthy mind and body are vital concerns. It is commonly recognized that exercise and other forms of physical activity have a wide range of health benefits, both physiological and psychological, for all age groups (Warburton, Nicol, & Bredin, 2006). However, it is not easy to find an exercise that suits people of all ages.

Tai Chi is one intervention that is receiving increasing attention among many professionals: nurses, physicians, occupational therapists, physical therapists, and recreational therapists. It is a manipulative and body-based therapy that can heighten individuals' awareness of their bodies and take advantage of their body structure for expressing feelings and ideas. Gradually, people become more aware of their total being, and harmony is enhanced.

DEFINITION

Tai Chi, which means *supreme ultimate*, is a traditional Chinese martial art (Koh, 1981) and a mind–body exercise. It involves a series of fluid, continuous, graceful, dancelike postures, and the performance of movements known as forms (Yang, 2010). The graceful body movements engage continuous body and trunk rotation, flexion/extension of the hips and knees, postural alignment, and the coordination of the arms—integrated by

273

mental concentration, the balanced shifting of body weight, muscle relaxation, and breath control. Movements are performed in a slow, rhythmic, and well-controlled manner (Clark, 2011).

There are several styles of Tai Chi that are currently practiced: Chen (quick and slow large movements), Yang (slow large movements), Wu (midpaced, compact movements), and Sun (quick, compact movements) (Jou, 1983). Each style has a characteristic protocol that differs from the other styles in the postures or forms included, the order in which they appear, the pace at which movements are executed, and the level of difficulty; however, the basic principles are the same (Yang, 1991). For example, one significant difference between the Chen and Yang styles is that Yang movements are relaxed, evenly paced, and graceful. Yang is the most popular Tai Chi practiced by older adults (Jou, 1983). In comparison, the Chen style is characterized by alternating slow, gentle movements with quick and vigorous ones, and restrained and controlled actions, which reflect a more martial origin (Yang, 1991). Most Tai Chi movements were named after animals, such as "white crane spreads its wings" and "grasp the bird's tail" (Koh, 1981).

There are a few simplified forms of the ancient Tai Chi. For example, the Simplified Tai-Chi Exercise Program (STEP), developed by Chen, Chen, and Huang (2006), encompasses three phases: warm-up, Tai Chi exercises, and cool-down. In the warm-up phase, nine exercises are designed to loosen the body from head to toe; the second phase includes 12 easy-to-learn and easy-to-perform Tai Chi movements; three activities during the cool-down phase help the body to return to a preintervention state of rest. STEP differs from traditional Tai Chi styles in that it incorporates fewer leg movements, fewer knee bends, and less-complicated hand gestures. It was specifically designed for older adults suffering from chronic illness (Chen et al., 2006).

SCIENTIFIC BASIS

Tai Chi practice is closely linked to Chinese medical theory, in which the vital life energy, chi (or *qi*), is thought to circulate throughout the body in discrete channels called meridians. Using correct postures and adequate relaxation, the principle of Tai Chi is to promote the free flow of chi throughout the body, which improves the health of an individual. The movements of Tai Chi are regulated by the timing of deep breathing and the movement of the diaphragm. It offers a balanced exercise to the muscles and joints of various parts of the body (Clark, 2011). In addition, a peaceful state of mind and spiritual dedication to each movement during the exercise ensure that the central nervous system (CNS) is given sufficient training and is consequently toned up with time as the exercise continues. A strong CNS is essential for a healthy body and the various organs depend largely on its soundness (Clark, 2011).

INTERVENTION

In Eastern countries such as Taiwan, it is common and popular for older adults to practice Tai Chi as a group, in the early morning, in parks or on the athletic grounds of elementary schools. Tai Chi practice groups are usually led by masters who are pleased to share its essence with others. People who are interested in Tai Chi are welcome to join the groups and learn the movements from these masters. In Western countries, there is a growing interest in the practice of Tai Chi. Various Tai Chi clubs are available to the public through community centers, health clinics, or private organizations. General information is widespread through websites, books, and videos. Tai Chi is a convenient exercise that can be practiced in any place, at any time, and without any equipment.

Technique

As mentioned earlier, although various styles of Tai Chi are currently practiced, the underlying practice principles are the same. Five essential principles of movement are (Schaller, 1996):

- Hand and leg movements should be synchronous.
- The emphasis should be on a soft, relaxed, rather than on a hard, tense position.
- Moves should be practiced with a quiet and open mind.
- The soles of the feet should be rooted to the ground, with the knees bent in a low stance and the primary focus of awareness within the lower abdomen.
- The physical force should be rooted in the feet, passed up through the legs as weight is shifted, and distributed by the pivoting of the waist.

In the physical performance, an individual must relax and think of nothing else before starting. The movements should be slow and rhythmic with natural breathing. Every action becomes easy and smooth, the waist turns freely, and the feelings of comfort and relaxation are gradually developed (Clark, 2011). In the spiritual aspect, Tai Chi is an exercise that produces harmony of body and mind. Each movement should be guided by thought instead of physical strength. For instance, to lift up the hands, an individual must first have the necessary mental concentration, and then the hands can be raised slowly in a proper manner. Hence, the breathing will become deeper and the body will be strengthened (Clark, 2011).

Guidelines

The steps for performing the movement called "around the platter" are presented in Exhibit 17.1.

Various videotapes on Tai Chi are also available through local video rental stores. The following DVDs and/or books are useful for learning Tai Chi:

- *Element: Tai Chi for Beginners* (Barnes & Ambandos, 2009) is a DVD filmed on a tranquil location overlooking the Pacific Ocean. It features two practices that offer personal one-on-one instruction and allow you to experience the many layers of benefits this martial art has to offer.
- *Tai Chi Chuan Classical Yang Style: The Complete Form Qigong* (Yang, 2010) is an in-depth guide for beginners to learn Tai Chi Chuan properly. It offers a general plan for practicing Tai Chi Chuan, and then goes into great depth to present enough content for proper learning. Each movement is presented in a series of large photographs with clear same-page instructions for each Tai Chi posture.
- *The Complete Illustrated Guide to Tai Chi: A Step-by-Step Approach to the Ancient Chinese Movement* (Clark, 2011) contains a complete introduction to the principles and practices of Tai Chi and is accompanied by clear and instructive photography throughout. It includes sections on

Exhibit 17.1. *Procedure for Performing "Around the Platter"*

1. Hands are held at chest level, wrists slightly bent and elbows close to sides. Fingers are spread apart. Legs are slightly apart and bent with the left in front of the right. Weight is equally distributed between legs.

2. Begin to rock forward, shifting weight to the left leg with hands moving to the left. (Imagine a round platter at the chest level, and the hands circling around the platter from left to right.)

3. As most of the weight shifts to the left leg and the hands are directly in front of the body, the left heel comes off the ground. As the hands move right of midline, the weight begins to shift to the right leg. When the hands (held at chest level) have completed a full circle, most of the weight is on the right leg and the right toe is off the ground.

4. This movement can be repeated six to nine times and then repeated again going from right to left.

Adapted from Stone (1994).

the basic principles of movement and the body, how Tai Chi can help to heal, life energies, meridians, the seven major chakras, and step-by-step guides to the complete movement sequence.

■ *Complete Tai-Chi: The Definitive Guide to Physical and Emotional Self-Improvement* (Huang, 2011) includes a detailed guide to the 36 postures (with more than 250 illustrative photographs) of the Wu-style Tai Chi, which stresses the development of internal energy for self-healing and has gained enormous popularity as a healing exercise.

■ *Seated Tai Chi and Qigong: Guided Therapeutic Exercises to Manage Stress and Balance Mind, Body, and Spirit* (Quarta & Vallie, 2012) emphasizes that Tai Chi and Qigong are the perfect antidote to the stresses of modern life and a great way to stay healthy. This illustrated guidebook provides an explanatory introduction to these forms of exercise and shows how to build up a program from easy to more challenging steps.

WEBSITES

Additional information can be found through the following useful websites:

■ www.supply.com/lee/tcclinks.html provides links to more than 100 other websites on Tai Chi and related topics.
■ sunflower.signet.com.sg/~limttk/index.htm is a valuable site with complete historical and background information on Tai Chi.

Measurement of Outcomes

According to Plummer (1983), mind concentration and breathing control are two of the major tenets of Tai Chi practice. When practicing Tai Chi with a peaceful, focused mind and incorporating smooth breathing into each movement, a person will experience physical and psychological relaxation, which leads to enhanced well-being in both states (Plummer, 1983). With this conceptual framework in mind, the measurement of the effects of Tai Chi should include both physical and psychological well-being. Based on the literature, which will be discussed in detail later, more studies have been done to measure the physical outcomes of Tai Chi practice (such as cardiovascular functioning) with little emphasis on psychological well-being outcomes (such as mood states).

Precautions

Tai Chi is unique for its slow graceful movements with low impact, low velocity, and minimal orthopedic complications, and is a suitable conditioning exercise for older adults (Chen, Yen, Fetzer, Lo, & Lam, 2008).

Although many research studies have shown the benefits of Tai Chi, there are some contraindications to its practice, such as an acute stage of angina, ventricular arrhythmia, or myocardial ischemia. The instructor and the student have to be aware of these contraindications, and an initial assessment is necessary to determine an individual's exercise tolerance and other limitations (Forge, 1997). While learning Tai Chi, a novice should be periodically evaluated in terms of progress, program adherence, cognitive response, muscular strength, balance, and level of flexibility at fairly regular (e.g., every 4 weeks) intervals for the first 60 days to 90 days of participation in such a program. If progress is considered satisfactory, 6-month evaluations thereafter are recommended (Forge, 1997). It is strongly suggested that one learn Tai Chi from an experienced master who is able to teach the movements based on individual needs and physical tolerance. Advice on choosing a class is found in Exhibit 17.2.

Exhibit 17.2. *Selecting a Tai Chi Class*

1. If possible, find a studio or organization that specializes in Tai Chi.

2. Find an experienced teacher (6–10 years of experience) who demonstrates and verbally explains the movements. Ask to observe a class before joining.

3. Find a class with fewer than 20 students.

4. Avoid purchasing any special clothing or equipment.

Adapted from Downs (1992).

USES

Tai Chi is especially appropriate for older adults or for patients with chronic diseases because of its low intensity, steady rhythm, and low physical and mental tension (Greenspan, Wolf, Kelley, & O'Grady, 2007). It has been shown to enhance cardiovascular and respiratory functions, improve health-related fitness, and promote positive health status (Hackney & Earhart, 2008; Wang, 2012). In addition, practicing Tai Chi has been effective in lowering blood pressure (Figueroa, Demeersman, & Manning, 2012; Hackney & Earhart, 2008; Pan, Yan, Guo, & Yan, 2013). Studies also indicated that Tai Chi increases postural stability, enhances balance (Nguyen & Kruse, 2012; Wang, 2011; Wang, 2012), and improves muscle strength and endurance (Song, Roberts,

Lee, Lam, & Bae, 2010; Wang, 2011, 2012), which leads to a reduction in the risk of falls (Merom et al., 2012; Voukelatos, Cumming, Lord, & Rissel, 2007; Wolf et al., 2006). Tai Chi also plays an important role in symptom control of chronic illnesses such as osteoarthritis (Song et al.; Wang, 2011, 2012).

In addition, studies have indicated that Tai Chi practice may also provide psychological benefits, such as enhanced positive mood states (Taylor-Piliae, Haskell, Stotts, & Froelicher, 2006; Wang, 2011, 2012), and quality of sleep (Caldwell, Emery, Harrison, & Greeson, 2011; Hosseini, Esfirizi, Marandi, & Rezaei, 2011; Nguyen & Kruse, 2012).

Researchers have suggested that Tai Chi could be incorporated into community programs or senior center activities to promote the well-being of community-dwelling older adults. It could also be included as one of the activities in nursing homes or in rehabilitation programs in hospital settings (Chen, Hsu, Chen, Tseng, 2007; Hung & Chen, 2007). Furthermore, Tai Chi has been applied in other populations. For example, Tai Chi improves the pulmonary function of asthmatic children (Caldwell, Harrison, Adams, & Triplett, 2009; Chang, Yang, Chen, & Chiang, 2008) and enhances balance, gait, and mobility of people with Parkinson disease (Hackney & Earhart, 2008). Tai Chi has also been practiced in many countries, including the United States, the United Kingdom, Australia, Hong Kong, Singapore, and Taiwan. How Tai Chi is used in the United Kingdom is discussed in Sidebar 17.1.

Sidebar 17.1. *Use of Tai Chi in the United Kingdom*

Graeme D. Smith, Edinburgh, United Kingdom

Although part of traditional Chinese medicine (TCM), Tai Chi appears to be increasingly used in the United Kingdom for health-related benefits and stress relief. To date, there is little UK-based research to support the popularity of this activity. Anecdotally, Tai Chi seems to be used mostly by older people for physical and mental health benefits. The National Health Service (NHS) in the United Kingdom notes that appropriate use of Tai Chi may prevent falls and improve overall psychological well-being in older adults. The basis of these claims may come from the improved balance control and flexibility those who practice Tai Chi may achieve. However, as with other forms of complementary and alternative medicine, high-quality rigorous research is required to substantiate these claims. Unfortunately, to date such research is lacking.

(continued)

> **Sidebar 17.1.** *Use of Tai Chi in the United Kingdom (continued)*
>
> Private health care providers in the United Kingdom also promote Tai Chi as a very low-impact, feel-good form of exercise. There would appear to be no real safety issues associated with using Tai Chi, although people who are pregnant, have a hernia, back pain, or severe osteoporosis are encouraged to speak to their family doctor before they start Tai Chi. Also from a safety perspective, individuals are encouraged to find out about a Tai Chi instructor's qualifications and experience before they enroll in a program. At present, there is no statutory regulation of Tai Chi in the United Kingdom. Several Tai Chi bodies do exist, including the Tai Chi Union for Great Britain. This is the largest collective of independent Tai Chi instructors in the United Kingdom. They aim to unite Tai Chi practitioners, and promote Tai Chi in all its aspects—health, aesthetic meditation, self-defense, and general improvement of standards. Tai Chi UK is another existing organization that claims Tai Chi can be "the ultimate holistic experience." Development of such groups is a clear indication of Tai Chi's increasing popularity in the United Kingdom.

FUTURE RESEARCH

Overall, practicing Tai Chi appropriately has various benefits, as evidenced in the literature, and it is highly recommended for the appropriate populations. More studies about the effects of Tai Chi from a nursing perspective are needed in order to provide guidance to nurses in its use with various populations (Chen & Liu, 2004). Some questions for further research include:

- Which populations can most benefit from practicing Tai Chi and are there conditions that would preclude its use?
- What is the nature of change in the well-being status of older adults who practice Tai Chi?
- What are the differences on well-being outcomes of beginners (people who are just starting to learn Tai Chi movements), practitioners (people who have practiced Tai Chi regularly for more than a year), and masters (people who have practiced Tai Chi regularly for more than a decade and are licensed by the National Tai Chi Association to be instructors)?

REFERENCES

Barnes, S., & Ambandos, A. (2009). *Element: Tai chi for beginners* (DVD). Toronto, Canada: HarperCollins.

Caldwell, K., Emery, L., Harrison, M., & Greeson, J. (2011). Changes in mindfulness, well-being, and sleep quality in college students through taijiquan courses: A cohort control study. *Alternative and Complementary Medicine, 17*, 931–938.

Caldwell, K., Harrison, M., Adams, M., & Triplett, N. T. (2009). Effects of pilates and taiji quan training on self-efficacy, sleep quality, mood, and physical performance of college students. *Journal of Bodywork and Movement Therapies, 13*, 155–163.

Chang, Y. F., Yang, Y. H., Chen, C. C., & Chiang, B. L. (2008). Tai chi chuan training improves the pulmonary function of asthmatic children. *Journal of Microbiology, Immunology, and Infection, 41*, 88–95.

Chen, C. H., Yen, M., Fetzer, S., Lo, L. H., & Lam, P. (2008). The effects of tai chi exercise on elders with osteoarthritis: A longitudinal study. *Asian Nursing Research, 2*, 235–241.

Chen, K. M., Chen, W. T., & Huang, M. F. (2006). Development of the simplified tai-chi exercise program (STEP) for the frail older adults. *Complementary Therapies in Medicine, 14*, 200–206.

Chen, K. M., Hsu, Y. C., Chen, W. T., & Tseng, H. F. (2007). Well-being of institutionalized elders after yang style tai chi practice. *Journal of Clinical Nursing, 16*, 845–852.

Chen, K. M., & Liu, T. H. (2004). The state of the art: Research-based use of tai chi in the elderly populations. *Journal of Long-Term Care, 8*, 223–235.

Clark, A. (2011). *The complete illustrated guide to tai chi: A step-by-step approach to the ancient Chinese movement.* Toronto, Canada: HarperCollins.

Downs, L. B. (1992). Tai chi. *Modern Maturity, 35*, 60–64.

Figueroa, M. A., Demeersman, R. E., & Manning, J. (2012). The autonomic and rate pressure product responses of tai chi practitioners. *North American Journal of Medical Sciences, 4*, 270–275.

Forge, R. L. (1997). Mind–body fitness: Encouraging prospects for primary and secondary prevention. *Journal of Cardiovascular Nursing, 11*, 53–65.

Greenspan, A. I., Wolf, S. L., Kelley, M. E., & O'Grady, M. (2007). Tai chi and perceived health status in older adults who are transitionally frail: A randomized controlled trial. *Physical Therapy, 87*, 525–535.

Hackney, M. E., & Earhart, G. M. (2008). Tai chi improves balance and mobility in people with Parkinson disease. *Gait & Posture, 28*, 456–460.

Hosseini, H., Esfirizi, M. F., Marandi, S. M., & Rezaei, A. (2011). The effect of tai chi exercise on the sleep quality of the elderly residents in Isfahan, Sadeghieh, elderly home. *Iranian Journal of Nursing and Midwifery Research, 16*, 55–60.

Huang, A. (2011). *Complete tai-chi: The definitive guide to physical and emotional self-improvement.* North Clarendon, VT: Tuttle.

Hung, S. M., & Chen, K. M. (2007). Effects of the Simplified Tai-Chi Exercise Program in promoting the health of the urban elderly. *Journal of Evidence-Based Nursing, 3*(3), 225–235.

Jou, T. H. (1983). *The tao of tai chi chuan: Way to rejuvenation* (3rd ed.). Piscataway, NJ: Tai Chi Foundation.

Koh, T. C. (1981). Tai chi chuan. *American Journal of Chinese Medicine, 9*, 15–22.

Merom, D., Pye, V., Macniven, R., van der Ploeg, H., Milat, A., Sherrington, C., . . . Bauman, A. (2012). Prevalence and correlates of participation in fall prevention exercise/physical activity by older adults. *Preventive Medicine, 55*(6), 613–617.

Nguyen, M. H., & Kruse, A. (2012). A randomized controlled trial of tai chi for balance, sleep quality and cognitive performance in elderly Vietnamese. *Clinical Interventions in Aging, 7*, 185–190.

Pan, L., Yan, J., Guo, Y., & Yan, J. (2013). Effects of tai chi training on exercise capacity and quality of life in patients with chronic heart failure: A meta-analysis. *European Journal of Heart Failure, 15*(3), 316–323. doi:10.1093/eurjhf/hfs170

Plummer, J. P. (1983). Acupuncture and tai chi chuan (Chinese shadow boxing): Body/mind therapies affecting homeostasis. In Y. Lau & J. P. Fowler (Eds.), *The scientific basis of traditional Chinese medicine: Selected papers* (pp. 22–36). Hong Kong, PRC: Medical Society.

Quarta, C. W., & Vallie, M. M. (2012). *Seated tai chi and qigong: Guided therapeutic exercises to manage stress and balance mind, body and spirit.* London, UK: Singing Dragon.

Schaller, K. J. (1996). Tai chi chih: An exercise option for older adults. *Journal of Gerontological Nursing, 22*(10), 12–17.

Song, R., Roberts, B. L., Lee, E. O., Lam, P., & Bae, S. C. (2010). A randomized study of the effects of tai chi on muscle strength, bone mineral density, and fear of falling in women with osteoarthritis. *Journal of Alternative and Complementary Medicine, 16,* 227–233.

Stone, J. F. (1994). *Tai chi chih: Joy through movement.* Fort Yates, ND: Good Karma.

Strazdins, L., & Loughrey, B. (2008). Too busy: Why time is a health and environmental problem. *New South Wales Public Health Bulletin, 18,* 219–221.

Taylor-Piliae, R. E., Haskell, W. L., Stotts, N. A., & Froelicher, E. S. (2006). Improvement in balance, strength, and flexibility after 12 weeks of tai chi exercise in ethnic Chinese adults with cardiovascular disease risk factors. *Alternative Therapies in Health and Medicine, 12*(2), 50–58.

Voukelatos, A., Cumming, R. G., Lord, S. R., & Rissel, C. (2007). A randomized, controlled trial of tai chi for the prevention of falls: The Central Sydney tai chi trial. *Journal of the American Geriatrics Society, 55,* 1185–1191.

Wang, C. (2011). Tai chi and rheumatic diseases. *Rheumatic Diseases Clinics of North America, 37,* 19-32.

Wang, C. (2012). Role of tai chi in the treatment of rheumatologic diseases. *Current Rheumatology Reports, 14,* 598–603.

Warburton, D. E. R., Nicol, C. W., & Bredin, S. S. D. (2006). Prescribing exercise as preventive therapy. *Canadian Medical Association Journal, 174,* 961–974.

Wolf, S. L., O'Grady, M., Easley, K. A., Guo, Y., Kressig, R. W., & Kutner, M. (2006). The influence of intense tai chi training on physical performance and hemodynamic outcomes in transitionally frail, older adults. *Journals of Gerontology. Series A, Biological Sciences and Medical Sciences, 61,* 184–189.

Yang, J. M. (2010). *Tai chi chuan classical yang style: The complete form qigong.* Wolfeboro, NH: Yang's Martial Arts Association.

Yang, Z. (1991). *Yang style taijiquan* (2nd ed.). Beijing, China: Morning Glory.

Chapter 18: Relaxation Therapies

Elizabeth L. Pestka, Susan M. Bee, and Michele M. Evans

Many people's lives are very stressful so it is important to have techniques to help lower stress levels to maintain health. Complementary therapies can be used to decrease stress by reducing muscle tension in the body. Relaxation therapies have been shown to manage stress, offer pain relief, and promote health. A great many relaxation therapies exist. The ones discussed in this chapter range from the simple and easily implemented diaphragmatic breathing (DB) to more complex methods such as progressive muscle relaxation (PMR) and autogenic training (AT). Using a combination of these therapies is common because they provide a variety in terms of time to learn and to use.

DEFINITIONS

Relaxation therapies help reduce the tension that exists in muscles and this often generalizes to other areas of the body, including the mind. Learning to relax can reduce the destructive effects and symptoms of stress-induced illnesses and improve a person's quality of life. Teaching patients relaxation techniques allows them to become more active partners in their health care.

DB, or relaxed deep breathing, uses the diaphragm when taking a breath. The purpose of relaxed breathing is to slow breathing and to reduce the use of shoulder, neck, and upper chest muscles to breathe more efficiently, which improves oxygenation to the entire body.

PMR is the tensing and releasing of successive muscle groups. This treatment was introduced by Jacobson (1938) and is still used widely today. A person's attention is drawn to discriminating between the feelings experienced when a muscle group is relaxed and when it is tensed.

Autogenic training (AT) is a relaxation method that uses both imagery and body awareness to reduce stress and muscle tension. This technique was developed and published by the German neurologist Schultz (Schultz & Luthe, 1959) and addresses autonomic sensations that lead to muscle relaxation. *watch waves, breath slow*

SCIENTIFIC BASIS

The aim of relaxation therapies is to reduce stress and the accompanying effects that stress has on the body. Real and perceived events and thoughts can create stress that activates the sympathetic nervous system. This begins a cascade of physical and chemical reactions. The heart pounds and blood pressure rises, respirations become shallow, pupils dilate, and the muscles tense as the body prepares to cope with the stressor. This is often called the fight-or-flight response. The parasympathetic nervous system is known as the rest and digest or rest and restore response. When one response is activated, the other is quiet. Prolonged activation of the sympathetic nervous system over time can have deleterious effects on the body. The desired outcome of relaxation strategies is the mitigation of persisting high levels of stress and activation of the parasympathetic nervous system.

When a person breathes, the body takes in oxygen and releases carbon dioxide. If the body detects an imbalance in these two gases, it signals for changes in breathing that may lead to fast, shallow breathing called hyperventilation, often in response to stressful events or pain. Diaphragmatic breathing (DB) is a relaxation technique that uses the diaphragm to breathe deeply and improve oxygenation to the entire body. It is a learned skill, and practice is required for optimal benefit. Research from Schmidt, Joyner, Tonyan, Reid, and Hooten (2012) provides evidence that using DB for 10 minutes three times per day significantly reduces self-rating of anxiety, depression, fatigue, sleep quality, and pain.

Jacobson (1938) reported that PMR decreased the body's oxygen consumption, metabolic rate, respiratory rate, muscle tension, premature ventricular contractions, and systolic and diastolic blood pressure, and increased alpha brain waves. Subsequent studies, including that of Zhao et al. (2012), have validated Jacobson's findings with results indicating a decrease in self-reported anxiety and depression, and an increase in quality of life for persons with endometriosis.

AT reduces excessive autonomic arousal and, in addition, it is effective in raising dysfunctionally low levels of autonomic functions such as

PMR — Progressive muscle relaxation

autogenic training

a low heart rate. It is known as a self-regulatory model. AT may not only affect sympathetic tone but may also activate the parasympathetic system as well. The increase in parasympathetic dominance results in peripheral vasodilation and increased feelings of warmth and heaviness in the body. An example of evidence supporting the use of AT is a study by Miu, Heilman, and Miclea (2009) that found heart rate volume and vagal control of the heart were positively impacted by use of this therapy.

INTERVENTIONS

Relaxation means more than simply having peace of mind or resting. It means eliminating tension from the body and mind. Learning relaxation skills requires the person to focus on the mind–body connection, such as when muscles are tensed, and practice ways to relax the muscles to improve overall health and wellness.

Techniques

Diaphragmatic Breathing Technique

DB can be used before and during stressful situations, such as a painful procedure, or for overall health enhancement. It is a relatively simple relaxation technique that can be used in any health care setting and does not require extensive training of the instructor or the patient. The instructions for DB are found in Exhibit 18.1. Emphasis needs to be placed on the person practicing DB throughout the day until it becomes a natural way of breathing. For best effect, an individual should practice this technique frequently when neither anxious nor short of breath. Access naturalhealthperspective.com/resilience/deep-breathing.html for succinct information on DB.

Exhibit 18.1. *Instructions for Diaphragmatic (Deep) Breathing*

Sit comfortably with feet flat on the floor.

Loosen tight clothing around abdomen and waist.

Hands may be placed in lap or at sides.

Breathe in slowly (through nose if possible) allowing abdomen to expand with inhalation.

Exhale at normal rate.

Pursed-lip breathing—which creates a very small opening between lips through which to breathe out—may be used.

Progressive Muscle Relaxation Technique

Numerous techniques for muscle relaxation have been developed since Jacobson published his technique in 1938. Often the procedures include attention to breathing (Schaffer & Yucha, 2004). The instructor assists the individual in identifying a place that is quiet and restful in which to practice relaxation. A comfortable chair that provides support for the body is recommended. Clothing should be loose and not restrictive; shoes, glasses, and contact lenses should be removed. The person may wish to use the bathroom before practicing muscle relaxation.

The PMR therapy developed by Bernstein and Borkovec (1973) is widely used. They combined the 108 muscles and muscle groups of Jacobson's original technique into the initial tensing and relaxing of 16 muscle groups. Subsequently, the number of groups was reduced to seven and then four (Exhibit 18.2). Although Bernstein and Borkovec included instructions for tensing muscles of the feet, those are not included in Exhibit 18.2 because spasms in the foot may result when tensing these muscles. The ultimate goal is to achieve muscle relaxation throughout the body without initially having to tense the muscles. Through practice, the individual acquires a mental image of how the muscles feel when they are relaxed and is able to relax them using this image.

Education on the scientific basis for the use of PMR is provided during the first session. Stressors, the impact of stress on the body, and the signs and symptoms of high levels of stress are discussed. Descriptions and demonstrations for achieving tension of each muscle group are given, and participants then practice tensing each of the muscle groups.

After progressing through all the muscle groups, the instructor asks the patient to identify whether tension remains in any of them. The instructor observes the patient to assess for general relaxation focusing on slowed, deeper breathing; arms relaxed and shoulders forward; and feet apart with toes pointing out. At the conclusion of the session, 2 or 3 minutes are provided for the patient to enjoy the feelings associated with relaxation. Terminating relaxation is done gradually. The instructor counts backward from four to one. The individual is given the opportunity to ask questions or discuss the feelings experienced.

Bernstein and Borkovec proposed using 10 sessions to teach PMR. However, in many studies instruction has been limited to fewer sessions with positive results. A critical factor in determining the number of teaching sessions needed is ensuring that people have mastered relaxing the muscle groups and have integrated PMR into their lifestyles.

An essential factor in the effectiveness of PMR and other relaxation techniques is daily practice. At least one 15-minute practice session a day is recommended. Schaffer and Yucha (2004) suggest two 10-minute sessions.

Exhibit 18.2. *Guidelines for Progressive Muscle Relaxation for 14 Muscle Groups*

General Information

Instruct persons to tense a specific muscle group when they hear "tense" and to release the tension when they hear "relax." Tension is held for 7 seconds. Draw attention to the feeling of tension and relaxation. When muscles are relaxed, attention is drawn to the differences between the two states.

Tensing Specific Muscle Groups

Dominant hand and forearm: Make a tight fist and hold it.

Dominant upper arm: Push elbow down against the arm of the chair.

Repeat instructions for the nondominant arm.

Forehead: Lift eyebrows as high as possible.

Central face (cheeks, nose, eyes): Squint eyes and wrinkle nose.

Lower face and jaw: Clench teeth and widen mouth.

Neck: Pull chin down toward chest but do not touch chest.

Chest, shoulders, and upper back: Take deep breath and hold it, pull shoulder blades back.

Abdomen: Pull stomach in and try to protect it.

Dominant thigh: Lift leg and hold it straight out.

Dominant calf: Point toes toward ceiling.

Repeat instructions for the nondominant side.

Adapted from Bernstein and Borkovec (1973).

Helping patients find a time of day to practice relaxation is an important component of instruction. Often an audiotape of the instructions is provided for home practice. Persons are also instructed to use the relaxation technique anytime they feel tense or before an event that may cause them to become anxious and tense. Refer to www.guidetopsychology.com/pmr .htm for comprehensive instructions on PMR.

Autogenic Training

Autogenic training (AT) is a relaxation method that is self-generated or self-guided using relaxation phases. A health care provider familiar with the therapy can recommend the therapy and provide assistance with learning the method. AT is gaining in worldwide use and is intended to create a feeling of warmth and heaviness throughout the body while experiencing a profound state of physical relaxation, bodily health, and mental health. AT is most effective when done in a quiet place, with the person wearing loose clothing and not wearing shoes. Practice should be done at a time when the individual has not recently eaten a large meal. The person focuses intently on inner experiences, with exclusion of external events. When the session finishes, people relax with their eyes closed for a few seconds and then get up slowly. Instructions for self-guided AT are given in Exhibit 18.3. Refer to www.guidetopsychology .com/autogen.htm for an example of in-depth instructions on phases to be used for relaxation. To maintain proficiency, practicing at least once a day is recommended.

Exhibit 18.3 *Instructions for Self-Guided Autogenic Training*

AT consists of a warm-up period of breathing and progressively learning six phases of relaxation that all together may take several months to fully master. On completion, a person will progress through and include:

Warm-up: Focused breathing on slowly exhaling

Phase I: Heaviness—arms and legs are heavy

Phase II: Warmth—arms and legs are warm

Phase III: A calm heart—heartbeat is calm

Phase IV: Breathing—breathing is steady

Phase V: Stomach—stomach is soft and warm

Phase VI: Cool forehead—forehead is cool

Completion: Feel supremely calm

Measurement of Outcomes

Although findings from many studies have shown positive outcomes from the use of relaxation techniques, positive results have not been reported in all the research in which these therapies were explored. Reasons for the differences in outcomes may relate to the wide variation in the types of relaxation techniques, the length and type of instruction, the degree of mastery of the therapy, and irregular or sporadic use of the procedures.

A variety of outcomes have been used to measure the efficacy of relaxation techniques. Physiological measurements that are often used include respiratory rate, heart rate, and blood pressure. Electromyogram readings are occasionally taken to determine the degree of tension in the specific muscle groups. Practitioners need to be alert to underlying pathology or medications that may interfere with reduction in physiological parameters.

Anxiety is the most frequently used subjective measure. The State-Trait Anxiety Inventory (STAI) of Spielberger, Gorsuch, Luschene, Vagg, and Jacobs (1983) has been widely used. People's self-reports about feelings of relaxation have been included in many studies because satisfaction is a good indicator of whether an individual will continue to use an intervention. Reports of reduction of pain, symptoms of depression, increases in comfort, and improved sleep are other results that have been used to measure the effects of these techniques.

autogenic

Precautions

Although muscle relaxation techniques have been used with multiple populations and have been proven to be an effective therapy for nurses to use, some cautions should be observed. It is important for practitioners to know whether patients practice the relaxation techniques on a regular basis because this may affect the pharmacokinetics of medications. Adjustment in doses of medication for hypertension, diabetes, and seizures may be indicated.

Relaxation of muscles may produce a hypotensive state. People are instructed to remain seated for a few minutes after practice. Movement in place and gradual resumption of activities helps in raising the blood pressure. Taking a person's blood pressure at the conclusion of teaching sessions helps in identifying those who are prone to hypotensive states after muscle relaxation, and AT as the relaxation therapy may have caused hypotension.

Some individuals with chronic pain have reported a heightened awareness of pain following the tensing and relaxing of muscles. Concentrating on tensing and relaxing of muscles may draw attention to the pain rather than to the muscle sensation. A good assessment of patients is needed to determine whether negative outcomes are occurring.

Children younger than school age lack the discipline to do AT. Also those with limited mental ability, acute central nervous system disorders, or uncontrolled psychosis may be unable to process the in-depth instructions (Linden, 2007). In some patients, AT may produce the side effects of anxiety, sadness, resurfaced memories and suppressed thoughts, or reawakened pain sensation from old illnesses or injuries. These effects may stem from disinhibition of various cortical processes due to the autogenic formulas and the focus on body sensations (Lehrer, 2009).

USES

Promoting an understanding of the anticipated positive benefits of the therapies is critical. Relaxation therapies have been used to achieve a variety of outcomes in diverse populations. Exhibit 18.4 lists conditions and populations, including the country in which the research was conducted,

Exhibit 18.4. *Selected Studies Supporting Use of Therapies*

Therapy	Health Condition	Study Authors	Country of Study
DB	Chronic pain and fibromyalgia	Busch et al. (2012) Schmidt et al. (2008) Schmidt et al. (2012)	Germany USA USA
DB	Anxiety	Chen et al. (2012)	Taiwan
DB	Type 2 diabetes mellitus	Hedge et al. (2012)	India
DB	Breast cancer	Dhillon et al. (2009)	USA
DB	Coronary heart disease	Chung et al. (2010)	Taiwan
DB	Chronic obstructive pulmonary disease	Yamaguti et al. (2012)	Brazil
DB	Gastroesophageal reflux disease	Eherer et al. (2012)	Austria
DB	Dysfunctional voiding (with children)	Zivhovic et al. (2012)	Serbia
DB and PMR	Multiple sclerosis	Artemiadis et al. (2012)	Greece
PMR	Hypertension	Kaushik, Kaushik, Mahajan, and Rajesh (2006) Sheu et al. (2003) Yung et al. (2001)	India Taiwan China
PMR	Cancer (decrease nausea & vomiting, pain, & depression)	Campos de Carvalho, Titareli Merizio Martins, and Benedita dos Santos (2007) Kweekeboom et al. (2008) Sloman (2002)	Brazil USA Australia
PMR	Chronic obstructive pulmonary disease	Chang et al. (2004)	USA
PMR	Asthma	Nickel et al. (2006)	Germany
PMR	Osteoarthritis	Baird and Sands (2004)	USA
PMR	Insomnia	Richardson (2003)	USA
PMR	Headache	Fichtel and Larrson (2001)	Sweden

Handwritten margin notes: Diaphramic Breathing; Progressive muscle relaxation

(continued)

Exhibit 18.4 *Selected Studies Supporting Use of Therapies (continued)*

Therapy	Health Condition	Study Authors	Country of Study
PMR	Stress	Pawlow and Jones (2002)	USA
PMR	Postoperative pain	dePaula, deCarvalho, and dos Santos (2002)	Brazil
		Good, Anderson, Stanton-Hicks, Grass, and Makii (2002)	USA
PMR	Ectopic pregnancy	Pan, Zhang, and Li (2012)	China
PMR	Endometriosis	Zhao et al. (2012)	China
PMR	Acute schizophrenia	Chen et al. (2009)	Taiwan
AT	Cancer (stress)	Hidderly and Holt (2004)	United Kingdom
AT	Chest pain	Asbury, Kanji, Ernst, Barbir, and Collins (2009)	United Kingdom
AT	Multiple sclerosis	Sutherland, Andersen, and Morris (2005)	Australia
AT	Posttraumatic stress disorder	Mitani et al. (2006)	Japan
AT	Anxiety disorder	Miu et al. (2009)	Netherlands
AT	Insomnia	Bowden et al. (2012)	United Kingdom
AT	Chronic subjective dizziness	Goto, Tsutsumi, Kabeya, and Ogawa (2012)	Japan
AT	Breastfeeding	Vidas, Folnegovic-Smalc, Catipovic, and Kisic (2011)	Croatia
AT	Irritable bowel syndrome	Shinozaki et al. (2010)	Japan

AT, autogenic training; DB, diaphragmatic breathing; PMR, progressive muscle relaxation.

Autogenic [handwritten marginal annotation]

showing widespread use of these therapies. Use of DB, PMR, and AT in reduction of anxiety and stress, relief of pain, and health promotion are discussed. Sidebar 18.1 describes how these relaxation therapies are used in the Republic of Singapore.

Reduction of Anxiety and Stress

As noted in Exhibit 18.4, these therapies have been effective in reducing the stress associated with a number of conditions. DB training significantly lowered anxiety measures in an experimental group of 51 participants in

Sidebar 18.1 *Use of Relaxation Therapies in Republic of Singapore*

Siok-Bee Tan, Republic of Singapore

In Singapore, relaxation techniques may be taught by nurses, psychologists, therapists, or other health professionals. A substantial number of practitioners do not use these strategies. At present, most nurses working in Singapore hospitals who use relaxation techniques favor deep DB. A minority of nurses, due to inadequate training, use PMR and AT. Because these techniques require additional time, they are not feasible in fast-paced hospitals. Nevertheless, in the mental health institutions, relaxation techniques are more widely used. In outpatient areas relaxation therapies can also be better used. For example, nurses who assist in the Chronic Disease Management Workshop teach both DB and PMR.

Siok-Bee Tan, PhD, MN, RN, APN, an advanced practice nurse in Singapore, uses a combination of medical, nursing, and therapy models in clinical care. By using various relaxation therapies, she specializes in helping patients who have intractable pain and chronic neurological conditions. Techniques are important for success of the relaxation procedures but it is also crucial to first ensure rapport is established. For example, in the practice of AT, the key is to access the subconscious mind with relaxation and this requires considerable time and discipline to learn. In a culture where patients mostly prescribe medication and surgery, it is a challenge to get patients to adopt the therapy for relaxation. With rapport, patients have the trust to commit their time to practice and in turn be able to bypass the critical factor of the conscious mind to access the subconscious mind and register the positive suggestions. Dr. Tan has successfully empowered many patients in using the healing powers of the mind as they go into a trance state during AT.

It would be prudent to enable a greater number of nurses to complete training in this area, not only for the financial savings it might provide by shortening hospital stays but also for the benefits it gives to patients by equipping them with tools to manage anxiety and concerns at home. However, there is a need for a shift in the hospital culture for relaxation techniques to be fully used. Relaxation therapies must be viewed as advancement in pain and anxiety care and must be given an opportunity to be implemented by health professionals. The hospital culture in Singapore is focused on medication or surgery. However, there is some hope because mind–body medicine is slowly gaining entry into the mainly medically dominated treatment. Patient care would be optimal if more health care professionals were willing to use complementary techniques as part of the recovery regime. If this occurs, patients, doctors, nurses, and all other practitioners would benefit enormously.

China (Chen, Huang, & Chen, 2012). Sloman (2002) reported that with the use of PMR there was a reduction in depression and anxiety in patients with advanced stages of cancer. Following AT, a group of patients with posttraumatic stress disorder in a study by Mitani, Fujita, Sakamoto, and Shirakawa (2006) showed a significant decline in cardiac sympathetic nervous activity and a significant increase in cardiac parasympathetic nervous activity indicating a reduction in anxiety. Miu et al. (2009) found that AT increased heart rate variability and facilitated vagal control of the heart, reducing symptoms of anxiety. Relaxation techniques can be used both to decrease and prevent stress, which is a risk factor for many health conditions.

Pain

Relaxation therapies have been used extensively in the management of many types of pain. Muscle tension increases the perception of pain, so lessening anxiety and tension may help in reducing it. Schmidt, Hooten, Kerkvliet, Reid, and Joyner (2008) reported that three 10-minute sessions each day of DB in patients with chronic pain were associated with significant changes in a number of areas of physiological and psychological functioning. Results indicated significant improvements in fatigue, pain management, self-efficacy, and changes in pain severity. Mean pain severity scores changed from 4.56 to 3.78 ($p < .05$) on a 0 to 10 rating scale. Further supporting research by Schmidt et al. (2012) with patients with fibromyalgia found that the use of three 10-minute daily sessions of DB showed significant improvements in pain severity, fatigue, pain self-efficacy, cold pressor tolerance, and heart rate variability in measurements 2 weeks apart. Using a treatment of listening twice a day to an audiotaped PMR script resulted in a significant reduction in pain and improvement in mobility in a group of patients with osteoarthritis (Baird & Sands, 2004). In a study by Kweekeboom, Hau, Wanta, and Bumpus (2008), cancer patients positively reported their perception of the effectiveness of PMR on reducing the intensity of their pain even more than their pain scores indicated. They identified benefitting from active involvement in their pain management. AT was used with 21 patients with irritable bowel syndrome with results indicating a significant decrease in the rating of bodily pain (Shinozaki et al., 2010).

Health Promotion

Nursing has been at the forefront in teaching patients about health-promotion practices. Reducing and managing stress is an important preventative health strategy and these therapies can be used for reducing risks for numerous conditions. Although relaxation therapies may not reduce heart rate and blood pressure in those who have readings within the normal range, use of these techniques on a regular basis by healthy persons may help to prevent the development of hypertension. PMR was found to decrease both systolic and diastolic blood pressure and heart rate in those with essential hypertension; these indices decreased more as they continued to practice (Sheu, Irvin, Lin, & Mar, 2003; Yung, French, & Leung, 2001). Sleep is essential for overall health; Bowden, Lorenc, and Robinson (2012) found that use of AT resulted in significant improvement in sleep-onset latency and stated that study participants (153) with insomnia reported feeling more refreshed and energized. Those with type II diabetes mellitus responded positively to DB, with significant reductions in fasting and postprandial plasma glucose and glycated hemoglobin levels (Hedge et al., 2012). This therapy may have the potential as a preventive measure for a condition that is increasing in the United States.

FUTURE RESEARCH

Relaxation therapies discussed in this chapter have been used singly and in combination with other therapies to reduce and prevent stress. A scientific body of knowledge is emerging to guide the use of these techniques in practice, but more research is necessary. The following are several areas in which studies are needed:

- Many of the studies have been completed with relatively small samples. Larger sample sizes will provide greater support for these interventions.
- A combination of therapies has been used in a number of studies. Some research used excellent designs to compare the efficacy of each technique. However, numerous other studies fail to differentiate the effects from each therapy. Attention to study design in relaxation therapy studies is needed because time is involved in teaching multiple procedures, and patients may be overwhelmed with too many interventions and expectations.
- Sheu and colleagues (2003) found continuing improvement following a 1-month period of practice. In the majority of studies, however, the effects of relaxation therapies have been evaluated immediately following administration of the intervention. Longitudinal studies are needed to determine long-term effects.
- As the focus of health care becomes more individualized, it is important to identify relaxation therapies most likely to be effective for people based on their genetic information, cultural background, and lifestyle preferences. Studies connecting phenotype with genotype will be informative.
- Targeting the establishment of specific intervention methods and most effective treatment doses for maximum effects will support integration into clinical practice.

■ More research concentrating on using these therapies for health promotion and disease prevention in primary care settings may help to improve delivery of health care.

REFERENCES

Artemiadis, A., Vervainioti, A., Alexopoulos, E., Rombos, A., Anagnostouli, M., & Darviri, C. (2012). Stress management and multiple sclerosis: A randomized controlled trial. *Archives of Clinical Neuropsychology, 27*, 406–416.

Asbury, E., Kanji, N., Ernst, E., Barbir, M., & Collins, P. (2009). Autogenic training to manage symptomatology in women with chest pain and normal coronary arteries. *Menopause, 16*(1), 1–6.

Baird, C., & Sands, L. (2004). A pilot study of the effectiveness of guided imagery with progressive muscle relaxation to reduce chronic pain and mobility difficulties of osteoarthritis. *Pain Management Nursing, 5*(3), 97–104.

Bernstein, D., & Borkovec, T. (1973). *Progressive relaxation training.* Champaign, IL: Research Press.

Bowden, A., Lorenc, A., & Robinson, N. (2012). Autogenic training as a behavioural approach to insomnia: A prospective cohort study. *Primary Health Care Research & Development, 13*(2), 175–185.

Busch, V., Magert, W., Kern, U., Haas, J., Hajak, G., & Eichhammer, P. (2012). The effect of deep slow breathing on pain perception, autonomic activity, and mood processing–an experimental study. *Pain Medicine, 13*, 215–228.

Campos de Carvalho, E., Titareli Merizio Martins, F., & Benedita dos Santos, C. (2007). A pilot study of a relaxation technique for management of nausea and vomiting in patients receiving cancer chemotherapy. *Cancer Nursing, 30*(2), 163–167.

Chang, B., Jones, D., Hendricks, A., Boehmer, U., Locastro, J., & Slawsky, M. (2004). Relaxation response for Veterans Affairs patients with congestive heart failure: Results from a qualitative study within a clinical trial. *Preventive Cardiology, 7*(2), 64–70.

Chen, W., Chu, H., Lu, R., Chou, Y., Chen, C., Chang, Y., . . . Chou, K. (2009). Efficacy of progressive muscle relaxation training in reducing anxiety in patients with acute schizophrenia. *Journal of Clinical Nursing, 18*, 2187–2196.

Chen, Y., Huang, X., & Chen, C. (2012, July–August). *Performance of 10-minutes of diaphragmatic breathing relaxation training in relieving in outpatients and accompanied relatives.* Paper presented at Sigma Theta Tau 23rd International Nursing Research Congress, Brisbane, Australia.

Chung, L., Tsai, P., Liu, B., Chou, K., Lin, W., Shyu, Y., & Wang, M. (2010). Home based deep breathing for depression in patients with coronary heart disease: A randomized controlled trial. *International Journal of Nursing Studies, 47*, 1346–1353.

dePaula, A., deCarvalho, E., & dos Santos, C. (2002). The use of the "progressive relaxation" technique for pain relief in gynecology and obstetrics. *Revista Latino-Americana de Enfermagen, 10*, 654–659.

Dhillon, W., Abd Al-Noor, N., Gill, A., Gupta, N., DeBari, V., Guron, G., & Maroules, M. (2009). Impact of deep breathing and relaxation exercises on health related quality of life in breast cancer patients receiving chemotherapy. *Cancer Research, 69* (Suppl. 3) 680S–680S.

Eherer, A., Netolitzky, F., Hogenauer, C., Puschnig, G., Hinterleitner, T., Schneidl, S., . . . Hoffmann, K. (2012). Positive effect of abdominal breathing exercise on gastro-esophageal reflux disease: A randomized, controlled study. *American Journal of Gastroenterology, 107*(3), 372–378.

Fichtel, A., & Larrson, B. (2001). Does relaxation treatment have differential effects on migraine and tension-type headache in adolescents? *Headache, 41,* 290–296.

Good, M., Anderson, G., Stanton-Hicks, M., Grass, J., & Makii, M. (2002). Relaxation and music reduce pain after gynecologic surgery. *Pain Management Nursing, 3,* 61–70.

Goto, F., Tsutsumi, T., Kabeya, M., & Ogawa, K. (2012). Outcomes of autogenic train-ing for patients with chronic subjective dizziness. *Journal of Psychosomatic Research, 72*(5), 410–411.

Hedge, S., Adhikari, P., Subbalakshmi, N., Nandini, M., Rao, G., & D'Souza, V. (2012). Diaphragmatic breathing exercise as a therapeutic intervention for control of oxidative stress in type 2 diabetes mellitus. *Complementary Therapies in Clinical Practice, 18,* 151–153.

Hidderly, M., & Holt, M. (2004). A pilot randomized trial assessing the effects of auto-genic training in early stage cancer patients in relation to psychological status and immune system responses. *European Journal of Oncology Nursing, 8,* 61–65.

Jacobson, E. (1938). *Progressive relaxation.* Chicago: University of Chicago Press.

Kaushik, R., Kaushik, R., Mahajan, S., & Rajesh, V. (2006). Effects of mental relaxation and slow breathing in essential hypertension. *Complementary Therapies in Medicine, 14,* 120–126.

Kwekkeboom, K., Hau, H., Wanta, B., & Bumpus, M. (2008). Patients' perceptions of the effectiveness of guided imagery and progressive muscle relaxation interventions used for cancer pain. *Complementary Therapies in Clinical Practice, 14,* 185–194.

Lehrer, P. (2009). *Mosby's complementary and alternative medicine: A research-based approach* (3rd ed., L. Freeman, Ed.). St. Louis, MO: Mosby Elsevier.

Linden, W. (2007). *Autogenic training.* New York, NY: Guilford Press.

Mitani, S., Fujita, M., Sakamoto, S., & Shirakawa, T. (2006). Effect of autogenic training on cardiac autonomic nervous activity in high-risk fire service workers for post-traumatic stress disorder. *Journal of Psychosomatic Research, 60,* 439–444.

Miu, A. C., Heilman, R. M., & Miclea, M. (2009). Reduced heart rate variability and vagal tone in anxiety; trait versus state, and the effects of autogenic training. *Autonomic Neuroscience-Basic and & Clinical, 145*(1/2), 99–103.

Nickel, C., Lahmann, C., Muehlbacher, M., Gil, F., Kaplan, P., Buschmann, W., . . . Nickel, M. (2006). Pregnant women with bronchial asthma benefit from progres-sive muscle relaxation: A randomized, prospective, controlled trial. *Psychotherapy and Psychometrics, 75,* 237–243.

Pan, L., Zhang, J., & Li, L. (2012). Effects of progressive muscle relaxation training on anxiety and quality of life of inpatients with ectopic pregnancy receiving metho-trexate treatment. *Research in Nursing & Health, 35,* 376–382.

Pawlow, L., & Jones, G. (2002). The impact of abbreviated progressive muscle relax-ation on salivary cortisol. *Biological Psychology, 60,* 1–16.

Richardson, S. (2003). Effects of relaxation and imagery on the sleep of critically ill adults. *Dimensions of Critical Care Nursing, 22,* 182–190.

Schaffer, S. D., & Yucha, C. B. (2004). Relaxation & pain management: The relaxation response can play a role in managing chronic and acute pain. *American Journal of Nursing, 104*(8), 75–82.

Schmidt, J., Hooten, W., Kerkvliet, J., Reid, K., & Joyner, M. (2008). Psychological and physiological correlates of a brief intervention to enhance self-regulation in chronic pain [Abstract]. *The Journal of Pain, 9*(4), 55.

Schmidt, J., Joyner, M., Tonyan, H., Reid, K., & Hooten, W. (2012). Psychological and physiological correlates of a brief intervention to enhance self-regulation in patients with fibromyalgia. *Journal of Musculoskeletal Pain, 20*(3), 211–221.

Schultz, J. H., & Luthe, W. (1959). *Autogenic training: A psycho-physiological approach in psychotherapy.* New York, NY: Grune and Statton.

Sheu, S., Irvin, B. L., Lin, H. S., & Mar, C. L. (2003). Effects of progressive muscle relaxation on blood pressure and psychosocial status of clients with essential hypertension. *Holistic Nursing Practice, 17*(1), 41–47.

Shinozaki, M., Kanazawa, M., Kano, M., Endo, Y., Nakaya, N., Hongo, M., & Fukudo, S. (2010). Effect of autogenic training on general improvement in patients with irritable bowel syndrome: A randomized controlled trial. *Applied Psychophysiology & Biofeedback, 35*(3), 189–198.

Sloman, R. (2002). Relaxation and imagery for anxiety and depression control in community patients with advanced cancer. *Cancer Nursing, 25*, 432–435.

Spielberger, C., Gorsuch, R., Luschene, R., Vagg, P., & Jacobs, G. (1983). *Manual for STAI.* Palo Alto, CA: Consulting Psychological Press.

Sutherland, G., Andersen, M., & Morris, T. (2005). Relaxation and health-related quality of life in multiple sclerosis: The example of autogenic training. *Journal of Behavioral Medicine, 28*(3), 249–256.

Vidas, M., Folnegovic-Smalc, V., Catipovic, M., & Kisic, M. (2011). The application of autogenic training in counseling center for mother and child in order to promote breastfeeding. *Collegium Antropologicum, 35*(3), 723–731.

Yamaguti, W., Claudino, R., Neto, A., Chammas, M., Gomes, A., Salge, J., . . . Carvalho, C. (2012). Diaphragmatic breathing training program improves abdominal motion during natural breathing in patients with chronic obstructive pulmonary disease: A randomized controlled trial. *Archives of Physical Medicine and Rehabilitation, 93*, 571–577.

Yung, P., French, P., & Leung, B. (2001). Relaxation training as complementary therapy for mild hypertension control and the implications of evidence-based medicine. *Complementary Therapies in Nursing & Midwifery, 7*, 59–65.

Zhao, L., Wu, H., Zhou, X., Wang, Q., Zhu, W., & Chen, J. (2012). Effects of progressive muscular relaxation training on anxiety, depression and quality of life of endometriosis patients under gonadotrophin-releasing hormone agonist therapy. *European Journal of Obstetrics & Gynecology and Reproductive Biology, 162*, 211–215.

Zivkovic,V., Lazovic, M., Vlajkovic, M., Slavkovic, A., Dimitrijevic, L., Stonkovic, I., & Vacic, N. (2012). Diaphragmatic breathing exercises and pelvic floor retraining in children with dysfunctional voiding. *European Journal of Physical Rehabilitation Medicine, 48*(3), 413–421.

Chapter 19: Exercise

DIANE TREAT-JACOBSON, ULF G. BRONÄS,
AND DERECK SALISBURY

*E*xercise is well recognized as a lifelong endeavor essential for energetic, active, and healthy living. In large, longitudinal studies in the United States and elsewhere it has been established that morbidity and mortality are reduced in physically fit individuals, compared with sedentary individuals (Samitz, Egger, & Zwahlen, 2011). Although the research supporting the benefits of exercise is substantial, it is often overlooked in the practice of conventional Western medicine.

Exercise, either alone or as an alternative or complementary therapy, has been linked to many positive physiological and psychological responses, from reduction in the stress response to an increased sense of well-being (Ehrman, Gordon, Visich, & Keteyian, 2008). Surprisingly, despite the tremendous benefits of exercise, it is an activity largely ignored by the general population. Indeed, in 1996 the U.S. Surgeon General issued a report identifying millions of inactive Americans as being at risk for a wide range of chronic diseases and ailments, including coronary heart disease (CHD), adult-onset diabetes, colon cancer, hip fractures, hypertension, and obesity. Since then, there have been numerous updates to that report. The U.S. Department of Health and Human Services (USDHHS) publication *Healthy People 2020* (USDHHS-PAAC, 2008) continues to specify several objectives for improving health, including physical activity and exercise. These include reducing the percentage of adults who do not participate in any physical activity; increasing the percentage of adults who engage in moderate physical activity on most days of the week; and increasing the percentage of adults participating in vigorous exercise, as well as exercises to improve strength and flexibility. The physical activity objectives in *Healthy People 2020* reflect the strong state of science supporting the health benefit of exercise as indicated by the Physical Activity Guidelines Advisory Committee (USDHHS-PAAC, 2008). There are additional objectives related to physical activity and exercise habits of children and adolescents, including goals to increase participation in daily school physical education classes, increase physical activity in childcare settings, and reduce television and computer usage. The alarmingly low percentage of children participating in physical activity in school and outside of school (less than 27%) is reportedly contributing to the nation's growing childhood obesity problem (National Research Council, 2011).

In 2007, the American Heart Association (AHA) and the American College of Sports Medicine (ACSM) issued several updates (Haskell et al., 2007; Nelson et al., 2007; Williams et al., 2007) to the Surgeon General's 1996 guidelines. This was followed in 2008 by a report and revised guidelines from the USDHHS Physical Activity Advisory Committee (USDHHS-PAAC, 2008), and again in 2011 by the ACSM (Garber et al., 2011). These updated guidelines are based on new data from several large-scale trials completed since the 1996 report. It is important to recognize the role of exercise as a component of good health. Exercise *must* be an integral part of one's personal lifestyle if it is to have optimum effects. During the past few decades, there has been an increase in the popularity of non-Western styles of exercise and physical activity, such as Qigong and the related movements in yoga and Tai Chi. These forms of exercise and physical activity also build on meditative moments and, as such, may provide a more enjoyable form of physical activity for older adults than walking exercise.

Maintaining physical fitness should be enjoyable and rewarding for persons of all ages and can contribute significantly to extending longevity and improving quality of life. Nurses' knowledge of exercise and its application in multiple populations will assist in the delivery of expert nursing care. This chapter discusses the definition, physiological basis, and application of exercise as a nursing intervention in a variety of populations, along with specific cultural applications.

DEFINITION

Physical activity is defined as "any bodily movement produced by skeletal muscles that results in caloric expenditure" (American College of Sports Medicine, 2006). Definitions of exercise are complex and vary according to scientific discipline; however, they all incorporate physical activity into their descriptions. Exercise is commonly considered to be a planned, recurring subset of physical activity that results in physical fitness, a term used to describe cardiorespiratory fitness, muscle strength, body composition, and flexibility related to the ability of a person to perform physical activity (Thompson et al., 2003).

Exercise is commonly classified according to the rate of energy expenditure, which is expressed in either absolute terms as metabolic equivalents (METs) or in relative terms according to what percentage of maximal heart rate or maximal oxygen consumption is achieved (Astrand, Rodahl, Dahl, & Stromme, 2004; Thompson et al., 2003). Exercise is aerobic when the energy demand by the working muscles is supplied by aerobic ATP (adenosine triphosphate) production as allowed by inspired oxygen and mitochondrial enzymatic capacity (Astrand et al., 2004). In general, aerobic exercise increases demand on the respiratory, cardiovascular, and musculoskeletal systems. Sustained periods of work require aerobic metabolism of energy at a level compatible with the body's oxygen supply capabilities (i.e., oxygen uptake equals oxygen requirements of the tissues). Anaerobic exercise is exercise during which the energy demand exceeds what the body is able to produce through the aerobic process or when the body is performing short bursts of high intensity exercise (Astrand et al., 2004).

SCIENTIFIC BASIS

Better understanding of exercise physiology and the body's response to various stages of physical activity will assist in the development of exercise programs appropriate for the individual and the goal of the exercise. The response of the body to exercise occurs in stages. The initial response to acute exercise is a withdrawal of parasympathetic stimulation of the heart through the vagus nerve. This results in a rapid increase in heart rate (HR) and cardiac output. The sympathetic stimulation occurs more slowly and becomes a dominant factor once HR is above approximately 100 beats per minute. Sympathetic stimulation is fully completed after approximately 10 seconds to 20 seconds, during which time a large sympathetic outburst occurs and the heart overshoots the rate needed, but then returns to the rate required for increased activity.

The brain stimulates the initial cardiovascular response together with impulses from muscles being exercised, and these impulses are sent to the brain; an increase in HR is initiated and the blood flow is shunted toward the exercising muscles (Astrand et al., 2004). During this phase, there is a sluggish adjustment of respiration and circulation, resulting in an O_2 deficit; the initial energy needed by the exercising tissue is mainly fueled by the anaerobic metabolism of creatine phosphate and anaerobic glycolysis (glucose) (Jones & Poole, 2005).

As exercise continues, oxygen consumption (VO_2) increases in a linear fashion in relation to the intensity of exercise. The increase in VO_2 is caused by an increase in oxygen extraction by the working muscles and an increase in cardiac output. Oxygen extraction by the working muscle tissues is approximately 80% to 85%, or a threefold increase from rest, in sedentary and moderately active individuals. This is caused by an increase in the number of open capillaries, thereby reducing diffusion distances and increasing capillary blood volume (Fletcher et al., 2001). Cardiac output is increased to meet the increased O_2 demands of the working muscle. The increase in cardiac output is caused by increased stroke volume, which is due to an increase in ventricular filling pressure brought on by increased venous return and decreased peripheral resistance offered by the exercising muscles. Together with the withdrawal of parasympathetic stimulation and increases in sympathetic stimulation, the increase in HR further accentuates the increase in cardiac output as well as increased myocardial contractility (from positive inotropic sympathetic impulses to the heart) (Astrand et al., 2004). In normal individuals, cardiac output can increase four to five times, allowing for increased delivery of O_2 to exercising muscle beds and facilitating removal of lactate, CO_2, and heat. Respiration increases to deliver O_2 and to allow for elimination of CO_2. Blood pressure increases as a result of increased cardiac output and the sympathetic vasoconstriction of vessels in the nonexercising muscles, viscera, and skin. During this "steady state" exercise phase, O_2 uptake equals O_2 tissue requirement, aerobic metabolism of glucose and fatty acids occurs, and there is no accumulation of lactic acid.

As exercise becomes more strenuous, there is a shift toward anaerobic metabolism of glucose, resulting in increased production of lactic acid. The anaerobic threshold is a point during exercise at which ventilation abruptly increases despite linear increases in work rate. As exercise goes beyond steady state, the O_2 supply does not meet the oxygen requirement, and energy is provided through anaerobic glycolysis and creatine phosphate breakdown. This increases proton release and phosphate accumulation, increasing acidosis (Robergs, Ghiasvand, & Parker, 2004; Westerblad, Allen, & Lannergren, 2002). Shortly beyond the anaerobic threshold, fatigue and dyspnea ensue and work ceases, coinciding with a significant drop in blood glucose levels. Exercise at a level that allows for aerobic metabolism and reduces the need for anaerobic metabolism and reliance on glucose metabolism as the primary fuel may delay onset of these biochemical changes.

Following cessation of exercise, there is a period of rapid decline in oxygen uptake followed by a slow decline toward resting levels. This slow phase of oxygen uptake return is termed excess postexercise oxygen consumption (LaForgia, Withers, & Gore, 2006). During this period, the body attempts to resynthesize used creatine phosphate, remove lactate, restore muscle and blood oxygen stores, decrease body temperature, return to resting levels of HR and BP (blood pressure), and lower circulating catecholamines (Astrand et al., 2004). It is important to facilitate this phase of exercise by performing a 5- to 10-minute cool-down.

INTERVENTION

Healthy People 2020 is a continuing set of initiatives for the United States to achieve by the year 2020 through the use of the National Physical Activity Plan (NPAP). The NPAP aims to create a national culture that supports incorporation of physical activity throughout everyday life, with the objective of improving health, fitness, and quality of life. Updated guidelines from the ACSM and USDHHS-PAAC, affirming the Surgeon General's 1996 report, specifically state that exercise is considered to be beneficial to health, with a class 1A (highest) evidence base, and that physical activity:

1. Decreases risk of premature death
2. Decreases risk of premature death from heart disease
3. Decreases risk of acquiring type 2 diabetes
4. Decreases risk of incurring high blood pressure
5. Decreases high blood pressure in hypertensive individuals
6. Decreases risk of acquiring colon cancer
7. Decreases feelings of uneasiness and despair

The updated report further confirms that exercise also

1. Aids in weight control
2. Helps in the strengthening and maintenance of muscles, joints, and bones
3. Assists older adults with balance and mobility
4. Fosters feelings of psychological well-being

In addition to these benefits, the ACSM (Garber et al., 2011) and the USDHHS-PAAC (USDHHS-PAAC, 2008) have published scientific statements summarizing evidence confirming physical activity as a significant factor in both primary and secondary prevention of cardiovascular disease. There is a relationship between lack of physical activity and development of coronary artery disease and increased cardiovascular mortality (USDHHS-PAAC, 2008; Garber et al., 2011). Further, there is evidence that individuals who engage in regular exercise as part of their recovery postmyocardial infarction have improved rates of survival (Kwan & Balady, 2012).

Given that the benefits apply to all age groups across a broad spectrum of health and disease, it is important for nurses to recognize opportunities to promote exercise as a nursing intervention. There are countless activities included under the umbrella of exercise. Finding the activity that fits an individual's capabilities and that meets the purposes for which exercise is prescribed is key to the success of the intervention. When prescribing an intervention, it is important to take into account the recommended or advisable exercise intensity for the patient population being served.

Evidence suggests that exercise is more likely to be initiated if the individual: (a) recognizes the need to exercise; (b) perceives the exercise to be beneficial and enjoyable; (c) understands that the exercise has minimal negative aspects, such as expense, time burden, or negative peer pressure; (d) feels capable and safe engaging in the exercise; and (e) has ready access to the activity and can easily fit it into the daily schedule (USDHSS-PAAC, 2008).

Technique

An aerobic exercise session should involve three phases: warming up, aerobic exercise, and cooling down. These phases are designed to allow the body an opportunity to sustain internal equilibrium by gradually adjusting its physiological processes to the stress of exercise and thus maintaining homeostasis. It should be noted that the new guidelines have explicitly stated that, to achieve optimal health benefits, the exercise should be in addition to activities of daily living that are not of moderate intensity or lasting 10 minutes or longer. Further, although resistance training will not be discussed in depth here, the new guidelines recommend that resistance training should be performed on at least 2 nonconsecutive days per week, and should involve 8 to 10 of the major muscle groups and one set of 8 to 12 repetitions at a resistance that causes significant fatigue (ACSM, 2009; USDHHS-PAAC, 2008; Garber et al., 2011).

Warm-Up Phase

The goal of the warm-up is to allow the body time to adapt to the rigors of aerobic exercise. Warming up results in an increase in muscle temperature, a higher need for oxygen to meet the increased demands of the exercising muscles, dilatation of capillaries resulting in increased circulation, adjustments within the neural respiratory center to the demands of exercise, and a shifting of blood flow centrally from the periphery, resulting in increased venous return (Bishop, 2003). In addition, a good warm up increases flexibility and decreases or prevents arrhythmias and ischemic electrocardiographic changes.

Warming-up exercises should be done for 10 minutes, involve all major body parts, and achieve a heart rate within 20 beats per minute of the target HR for the subsequent aerobic exercise. In addition, a good warm-up should incorporate stretching exercises. Stretching exercises are done at a slow, steady pace and help maintain a full range of motion in body joints while strengthening tendons, ligaments, and muscles.

Aerobic Exercise Phase

The aerobic phase of exercise is also known as the stimulus phase. It consists of four essential components: intensity (which is usually measured as the relative percentage of maximal aerobic capacity), frequency, duration, and mode of exercise. The combination of these components determines the effectiveness of the exercise and is known as the activity dose. The mode of exercise should involve rhythmic, continuous movement of large muscle groups—walking, jogging, cycling, swimming, or cross-country skiing. The frequency should be 5 days per week, with a duration of at least 30 minutes for health benefits, 60 minutes for prevention of weight gain, and 60 minutes to 90 minutes for aiding in weight loss and preventing weight regain following weight loss. The new guidelines explicitly state that achieving weight loss by exercise alone is difficult and therefore recommends that a weight-loss regimen should be a combination of calorie restriction and increased physical activity.

The updated guidelines further reaffirm that the duration of exercise is cumulative and can be achieved by exercising three times for a minimum of 10 minutes. The intensity can be either moderate or vigorous. If the exercise performed is vigorous, the duration can be shortened to 20 minutes. Moreover, the 2011 guidelines clarify that the moderate and vigorous exercise can be combined to achieve the recommended activity dose per week (Garber et al., 2011). To simplify this concept, the new guidelines recommend using the activity dose of MET × minutes to meet the minimum physical activity recommendations of approximately 500 MET-minutes per week, with a recommended weekly target of 500 MET-minutes to 1,000 MET-minutes per week. To find the specific MET that each activity requires, the reader is encouraged to visit the University of South Carolina's Prevention Research Center website (prevention.sph .sc.edu/tools/compendium.htm). For individual determination of intensity, the HR range can be used. For most people, physical fitness improvements may be gained with an intensity of exercise sufficient to achieve 55% to 75% of maximal HR. However, the updated guidelines recommend using the MET-minutes method for determination of activity dose (USDHHS-PAAC, 2008; Haskell et al., 2007).

As physical fitness improves, it may be necessary to increase one of the components to gain additional benefits (USDHHS-PAAC, 2008; Garber et al., 2011; Haskell et al., 2007). It should be emphasized that it is the accumulated amount of daily moderate physical activity and exercise that is important. Although those who perform 30 minutes of accumulated moderate physical activity show significant health benefits compared to sedentary individuals, people who perform more than 60 minutes show additional health benefits, including prevention of weight gain. A balance needs to be achieved to obtain maximal benefit with the least risk and discomfort. Adjustment of intensity is important not only for safety reasons, but also for comfort and enjoyment of the activity. If exercise can be kept at a comfortable level, the individual is more likely to continue to perform the activity. As tolerance develops, any or all of the exercise components can be increased to meet the person's aerobic capacity. For example, if an individual is comfortable with the intensity of the exercise, the duration and frequency can be increased to further improve training effect.

Cool-Down

Immediately following the endurance exercises, the person should engage in a cooling-down period. The cool-down allows the body to return to its normal resting state. This allows the HR and BP to return to resting levels and attenuates any postexercise hypotension by improving venous return. The cool-down also improves heat dissipation and elimination of blood lactate and provides a means to combat any potential postexercise rise in catecholamines. The body needs 5 minutes to 10 minutes to adjust to a slower pace. Cooling-down exercises may include walking slowly, deep breathing, and stretching.

Maintenance

The maintenance phase begins after 6 months of regular training, with the goal of maintaining achieved improvements in physical fitness (USDHHS-PAAC, 2008). Maintaining the exercise program is the key to the effectiveness of the intervention. Setting both short- and long-term goals helps improve adherence. The individual can experience a sense of accomplishment on meeting short-term goals while still striving for overall goals. Keeping a record or graph supplies a visual demonstration of progress and may provide insight into adjustments to the exercise program that may assist in achievement of goals.

Reversibility and Detraining

Once participation in exercise has ceased, there is a rapid return to preexercise levels of physical fitness. Most of the rapid decline occurs during the first 5 weeks following cessation of exercise and is usually complete within 12 weeks (Mujika & Padilla, 2001). With disuse, the muscle tissues atrophy. Additionally, the decreased caloric expenditure leads to a positive energy balance, which can result in increased accumulation of adipose tissue.

Specific Technique: Walking

One of the strategies identified by *Healthy People 2020* to improve health and quality of life through daily physical activity is an increase in "trips made by walking." Walking has declined rapidly in the United States and has reached the point at which 75% of all trips of 1 mile or less are made by car. Walking is an easy and enjoyable activity that has significant health benefits. Moreover, it is an exercise in which people of all age groups and varying levels of ability can engage to improve endurance. A major advantage is that walking requires no special equipment, facilities, or new skills. It is also safer and easier to maintain than many other forms of exercise. Intensity, duration, and frequency are easily regulated and adjusted to accommodate a wide range of physical capabilities and limitations. The initial intensity should be outlined at the start of the program and is dependent on baseline level of conditioning, physical or disease-related limitations or precautions, and outcome goals.

A walking program can be approached in two ways. The exercise can be completed in one or more daily sessions. For example, a previously sedentary individual may wish to begin an exercise program consisting of 10-minute walks and progressively increase the time or intensity as physical fitness increases. The more traditional alternative is to engage in one longer session at least five times per week; the recommended frequency for optimal benefits is 60 minutes to 90 minutes of enjoyable moderate physical activity 5 days of the week (USDHHS-PAAC, 2008; Haskell et al., 2007). These sessions would include a warm-up session of 5 minutes to 10 minutes, an aerobic period that could start at 10 minutes to 15 minutes and be gradually increased to 30 minutes to 60 minutes to 90 minutes, and a cool-down period of 5 minutes to 10 minutes (USDHHS-PAAC, 2008; Haskell et al., 2007). The American Heart Association–sponsored website startwalkingnow.org contains many resources for individuals interested in starting a walking program. Tips for fitness walking are presented in Exhibit 19.1.

Exhibit 19.1. *Tips for Fitness Walking*

- Warm up by performing a few stretches.
- Think tall as you walk. Stand straight with your head level and your shoulders relaxed.
- Your heel will hit the surface first. Use smooth movements rolling from heel to toe.
- Keep your hands free and let your arms swing naturally in opposition to your legs.
- When you're ready to pick up the pace, quicken your step and lengthen your stride, but don't compromise your upright posture or smooth, comfortable movements.
- To increase your intensity, burn more calories, and tone your upper body, bend your arms at the elbows and pump your arms. Keep your elbows close to your body.
- Breathe in and out naturally, rhythmically, and deeply.
- Use the talk test to check your intensity, or take your pulse to see whether you are within your target heart rate.
- Cool down during the last 3 minutes to 5 minutes by gradually slowing your pace to a stroll.

Source: American Heart Association (2013).

Exercising individuals should monitor the response of their bodies to the activity, to ensure that the intensity is appropriate. This can be done in several ways.

Monitor Target Heart Rate

To gain improvements in physical fitness, the target HR for a previously sedentary individual should be between 50% and 75% of the maximal HR, which is calculated by subtracting one's age from 220 (AHA, 2012). The HR should be assessed one third to half-way through the exercise session and immediately after stopping exercise. Exercise intensity can be increased or decreased based on this measurement.

The Talk Test

The talk test can replace target HR monitoring when an individual is exercising at a moderate intensity (Loose et al., 2012). If the exercise prevents the individual from talking comfortably, the intensity should be decreased. A variation of this technique is to whistle; if the individual is unable to whistle, the intensity is too great and should be decreased.

Rating of Perceived Exertion

Rating of perceived exertion (RPE) is a scale that describes the sense of effort during the exercise. This scale can be ranked from 1 to 10, with 1 being no effort and 10 being maximal effort (Groslambert & Mahon, 2006).

CONDITIONS AND POPULATIONS IN WHICH THE INTERVENTION HAS BEEN USED

Several populations for whom exercise is particularly beneficial include children, older adults, those with affective disorders, individuals with heart disease, and those with peripheral arterial disease. The application and demonstrated effects of exercise intervention in each of these populations are discussed below.

Overweight Children and Adolescents

The number of overweight children and adolescents is rapidly increasing. Of particular concern are the increasing rates of type 2 diabetes mellitus and metabolic syndrome diagnosed in overweight children and adolescents, problems that used to be primarily limited to adults. Lack of physical activity and excess caloric intake cause central obesity, which, in turn, is believed to promote development of these conditions (National Research Council, 2011). Treatment includes dietary modification and initiation of physical activity. Increased physical activity has been shown to improve insulin sensitivity, BP, cholesterol, and vascular function, and prevent further weight gain (National Research Council, 2011). The current recommendations are essentially the same as for healthy adults: 60 minutes to 90 minutes of enjoyable, moderate physical activity 5 days a week. An additional goal is to achieve less than 2 hours per day of consecutive sedentary activity, and at least 90 minutes of physical activity to achieve weight loss and prevent weight regain (USDHHS-PAAC, 2008).

Older Adults

The fastest growing segment of the population in the United States is individuals over the age of 65. The benefit of exercise as a therapy to prevent or delay functional decline and disease and improve quality of life is demonstrated by the numerous favorable changes occurring in response to exercise. Improvements in cardiovascular function have been shown to help lower risk factors for disease and reduce the need for assisted living (Cress et al., 2005). Older adults are especially prone to the "hazards of immobility" that affect many of the body's systems. Exercise results in increased bone strength (Kohrt, Bloomfield, Little, Nelson, & Yingling, 2004) and increased total body calcium as well as improved coordination, which may result in a reduction in falls (Chodzko-Zajko et al., 2009). Exercise has also been shown to improve body functioning, overall well-being, and quality of life in older adults (Chodzko-Zajko et al., 2009).

It is particularly important to tailor or customize exercise programs for older adults, who may have specific limitations. Exercise needs to be initiated at lower levels and increased gradually. The ACSM guidelines recommend using similar guidelines for people over the age of 65 as mentioned above, with one important modification—use of the Rating of Perceived Exertion (0–10) instead of the MET level for determination of intensity. Specifically, a moderate intensity is considered an RPE of 5 to 6 out of 10 and vigorous intensity is considered a 7 to 8 out of 10 (Chodzko-Zajko et al., 2009). Previously sedentary older individuals may be more comfortable initiating an exercise program with some supervision, which allows them to become accustomed to this new level of activity in a safe environment. Group exercise may be especially appealing to older persons. The new guidelines recommend—with the specific inclusion of resistance training 2 (or more) nonconsecutive days per week—using 8 to 10 major muscle groups and one set of 10 to 15 repetitions at a moderate intensity as based on the RPE scale (5–6 out of 10). Moreover, the updated guidelines recommend that older individuals should perform flexibility and balance (e.g., dancing) exercises a minimum of 10 minutes, three times per week, to prevent age-related loss of range of motion (and, hence, prevent falls; Chodzko-Zajko et al., 2009; USDHHS-PAAC, 2008).

Affective Disorders

Exercise is an effective although underused intervention for individuals with affective disorders. There is considerable evidence supporting the positive effects of exercise in combating depression and anxiety (Carek, Laibstain, & Carek, 2011; Herring, Puetz, O'Connor, & Dishman, 2012; Mason & Holt, 2012; Rimer et al., 2012). There are fewer, if any, side effects when compared with pharmacotherapy, and exercise is often more cost-effective than psychotherapy and pharmacotherapy. Although most studies have evaluated the effects of aerobic activity as the intervention, anaerobic activity has also been shown to be beneficial in alleviating depression (Levinger et al., 2011; Martins et al., 2011). This suggests that improvement in mood is associated with exercise in general, rather than increased aerobic capacity.

Heart Disease

Cardiac (exercise) rehabilitation is a common intervention prescribed for those with CHD, providing a safe environment for the initiation of an exercise program (Heran et al., 2011). Programs usually have several phases and are tailored to the specific needs, limitations, and characteristics of individual patients, helping them resume active and productive lives (Kwan & Balady, 2012). Exercise has multiple protective mechanisms that contribute to reduction of CHD risk, including antiatherosclerotic, antiarrhythmic, anti-ischemic, and antithrombotic effects (Leon & Bronas, 2009; Leon et al., 2005).

Exercise training has been shown to improve symptom-limited exercise capacity in CHD patients, primarily as a result of peripheral hemodynamic adaptations. Patients with CHD have a low skeletal muscle oxidative capacity, which is significantly improved with training, despite relatively low workloads and exercise intensities, consistent with other nonheart disease populations (Dorosz, 2009). Prior to training, patients with CHD are often unable to perform activities of daily living (ADL) without symptoms. Exercise-trained CHD patients function further above the ischemic threshold in performing ADL and thus require a lower percentage of maximal effort to perform activities. This increases stamina and endurance and helps to maintain independence (Dorosz, 2009). Even patients with heart failure, who typically have very poor cardiac function, have found that cardiac rehabilitation improves their exercise tolerance (Downing & Balady, 2011; Keteyian, Pina, Hibner, & Fleg, 2010).

Peripheral Artery Disease

Peripheral artery disease (PAD), a prevalent atherosclerotic occlu-
sive disease, limits functional capacity and is related to decreased
quality of life. Individuals with PAD typically experience exercise-
induced ischemic pain in the lower extremities, known as claudication.
Exercise training is one of the most effective interventions available for
the treatment of claudication due to PAD (Hamburg & Balady, 2011).
Exercise training has been shown to improve walking distance up to
200% (Watson, Ellis, & Leng, 2008). Prior to program initiation, an exercise prescription should be generated based on a graded exercise test
and patients should start training at the intensity at which the onset
of claudication occurs (Bronas et al., 2009). During a typical session,
patients will exercise at a moderate pace until they experience moderate to severe claudication. At that point they will rest until the pain
subsides. This exercise/rest pattern is repeated throughout the exercise
session. The most effective exercise programs for the treatment of claudication include the following components: the patient should exercise
to the point of almost maximal claudication; the exercise session should
be at least 30 minutes in length, with at least three sessions per week;
and the exercise program should continue for at least 6 months, with
intermittent walking as the most effective mode of exercise (Anderson
et al., 2013).

MEASUREMENT OF EFFECTIVENESS

The appropriate measure of the effectiveness of an exercise intervention
depends on the specific exercise prescribed and the goals of the intervention. Changes in atherosclerotic risk factors (i.e., cholesterol levels, triglyc-
erides, insulin sensitivity, waist circumference, BP, and body mass index)
may be measured if cardiovascular health is the primary outcome of the
exercise program. If cardiovascular fitness is the targeted outcome, an aerobic exercise program would be prescribed and improvements in the cardiovascular system such as increased cardiac output, VO_2, and improved
local circulation would be used to determine the effectiveness of the intervention (Fletcher et al., 2001). Cardiovascular response to submaximal
exercise may provide further information and may be even more beneficial in assessing the impact on quality of life, as most ADL are performed
at submaximal intensity. Exercise prescribed to improve function may use
parameters such as improved joint mobility, prevention or reduction of
osteoporosis, and improved strength in determining exercise effectiveness.

Assessment may also include changes in physical functioning and
disability, ability to perform ADL, changes in symptoms and activity tolerance, and other variables that reflect the individual's ability to function

in daily life. Lower intensity programs, which may not demonstrate great changes in maximal exercise capacity, might produce sufficient changes in these outcome variables to make a difference in the individual's quality of life. Such programs would be especially appropriate in older and very sedentary individuals, for whom low-intensity exercise can produce a modest increase in fitness and more significant improvements in function. Development and implementation of programs designed to meet the specific needs of patients can help maximize functional and quality-of-life outcomes.

PRECAUTIONS

Before initiating an exercise program, preparticipation screening procedures are recommended. These include such questionnaires as the Physical Activity Readiness Questionnaire (PAR-Q), designed to identify potential patients in need of medical advice prior to exercising (Adams, 1999). If a patient is identified as having potential or actual medical concerns, it is advisable that a graded exercise test be performed. The ACSM recommends that a graded exercise test be performed for any individual with more than two risk factors for CHD. This is done to rule out any potential contraindications to exercise and to provide a tool for determining initial exercise intensity (ACSM, 2006; Fletcher et al., 2001).

To avoid injury, it is important to begin an exercise program slowly, to follow safety guidelines, and to exercise consistently, several times per week. Potential exercise-related injuries include muscle and joint pain, cramps, blisters, shin splints, low back pain, tendonitis, and other sprains or muscle strains. The most commonly reported adverse event of exercise is musculoskeletal injury; approximately 25% of adults between 20 and 85 years of age reported an injury occurring at least once during 1 year (Hootman et al., 2002). It is possible that some of these are misclassified as injuries instead of muscle soreness due to a rapid increase in volume or intensity of training without proper knowledge of the principles of training.

The AHA (2013) has listed general guidelines to help ensure exercise safety. These include: (a) stretching the muscles and tendons prior to beginning exercise; (b) wearing appropriate footwear; (c) exercising on a surface with some give to it, especially during high-impact activities; and (d) learning the exercise properly and continuing good form even with increased speed or intensity. Should exercise-related injuries occur, they can usually be treated with one or a combination of therapies, including rest, ice, compression, and elevation (AHA, 2013).

Previously sedentary older individuals and those with chronic disease, especially heart disease, should consult a physician prior to initiating an exercise program to ensure that an appropriate exercise prescription is given. The warning signs of heart disease should be spelled out prior to initiation of an exercise program, especially to those in high-risk categories.

CULTURAL APPLICATIONS

The benefits of exercise and physical activity appear to be equal across gender and race; however, this topic remains poorly studied and recommendations are primarily based on assumptions that findings in one population will carry over to another population. It should be mentioned that there exist cultural preferences, including religious and ethnic preferences, in the use of exercise and physical activity. Although there has been little systematic investigation regarding these preferences, their potential influence should be considered when prescribing exercise and physical activity. For example, with certain ethnicities, it may be beneficial to modify an exercise program to allow exercise with a garment that covers the body.

The use of alternate exercise techniques has gained popularity during the past few decades, especially among older adults. These forms of physical activity include meditative forms of movement in the practice of Qigong and its specific forms such as Tai Chi and yoga (discussed in separate chapters in this book). Within these alternate forms of physical activity, numerous styles and movements have been reported, but the overarching theme of this form of physical activity remains the same. Although the evidence base for this type of exercise is less than for structured Western-style exercise (e.g., walking), it appears that these alternate forms of physical activity may provide health benefits, especially in improving balance and lowering fear of falling. However, it should be noted that most reported studies have been small and have employed a large variation of these techniques.

Other cultures have also been able to incorporate daily physical activity as part of their usual routine either by necessity or by choice. For example, European countries have facilitated walking and cycling as modes of transportation by incorporating walkways and bicycle lanes in city planning. It should be noted here that these forms of transportation are also culturally accepted as the primary modes of transportation, whereas in the United States this is commonly not the case. Exercise in Sweden, as one exemplar of activity incorporated into European lifestyle, is presented in Sidebar 19.1.

There is a clear need for future city planning to incorporate safe, accessible, and enjoyable walkways and bicycle lanes for the American population to be able to incorporate daily physical activity into their lives and gain the health benefits associated with increased physical activity

Sidebar 19.1. *Exercise in Sweden*

Ulf G. Bronäs, Stockholm, Sweden

In Sweden (as in most of Europe), major cities are built to facilitate walking and cycling as the primary modes of transportation to and from work, school, day care, grocery shopping, and places of entertainment. Walkways and bicycle lanes are incorporated in the city planning and allow for easy access for most people. It is common for parents to bring their children to day care by walking or using a specialized bicycle child seat assembled on the back of the bicycle. Once the child is older, the family will bike together to day care or school. Parents will drop their children off at day care or school and continue biking either to work or to a mass-transit station. More than 60% of Swedes use public transportation to and from work, which facilitates both walking and bicycling. These modes of transportation are culturally accepted and used as primary methods of transportation in Sweden and throughout Europe. It is often said that to experience Europe, one must walk the cities. The cities are built to promote walking; it is the most convenient (and least expensive) form of transportation. Availability of multiple walkways and bicycle lanes is evident in the cities, allowing the population the option of incorporating daily physical activity into their lives.

levels. This will help change the cultural perspective of physical activity in this country and support walking and/or bicycling as a preferred mode of transportation.

FUTURE RESEARCH

There are many gaps in our knowledge related to exercise, its measurement, the benefits, and methods to improve exercise adherence. Specific areas of needed research include:

- Investigations of cultural and ethnic differences in physical activity and response to exercise
- Investigations of the benefit of exercise in persons with disabilities, including mental and physical disabilities
- Development of strategies to increase lifelong physical activity and exercise
- Determining how electronic or social media can improve short- and long-term adherence.

WEBSITES

General Guidelines and Information

- Centers for Disease Control and Prevention (CDC)
  (www.cdc.gov/physicalactivity)
- President's Council on Physical Fitness and Sports
  (www.fitness.gov)
- U.S. Department of Health and Human Services, Physical Activity
  Guidelines
  (www.health.gov/paguidelines)

Guidelines and Information Pertaining to Individuals and Families

- CDC
  (www.cdc.gov/physicalactivity/index.html)
- Exercise and Physical Activity: Your Everyday Guide from the National
  Institute on Aging
  (nihseniorhealth.gov/exerciseforolderadults/healthbenefits/01.html)
- National Institutes of Health
  (nihseniorhealth.gov/exercise/toc.html)
- Office of the Surgeon General
  (www.surgeongeneral.gov/obesityprevention/index.html)
- President's Council on Physical Fitness and Sports
  (www.presidentschallenge.org)

School

- CDC, Division of Adolescent and School Health
  (www.cdc.gov/HealthyYouth/physicalactivity)

Communities

- Federal Highway Administration
  (www.fhwa.dot.gov/environment/bicycle_pedestrian)
- National Institutes of Health
  (www.nhlbi.nih.gov/health/public/heart/obesity/wecan)
- National Park Service
  (www.nps.gov/ncrc/programs/rtca/helpfultools/ht_publications
  .html)

Worksite

- CDC, Healthier Worksite Initiative
  (www.cdc.gov/nccdphp/dnpao/hwi/index.htm)

REFERENCES

Adams, R. (1999). Revised physical activity readiness questionnaire. *Canadian Family Physician, 45,* 992.

American College of Sports Medicine. (2006). *Guidelines for graded exercise testing and exercise prescription* (7th ed.). Baltimore, MD: Lippincott, Williams & Willkins.

American College of Sports Medicine. (2009). American College of Sports Medicine position stand. Progression models in resistance training for healthy adults. *Medicine and Science in Sports and Exercise, 41*(3), 687–708. doi:10.1249/MSS.0b013e3181915670; 10.1249/MSS.0b013e3181915670

American Heart Association. (2012). *Target heart rates.* Retrieved April 26, 2013, from http://www.heart.org/HEARTORG/GettingHealthy/PhysicalActivity/Target-Heart-Rates_UCM_434341_Article.jsp

American Heart Association. (2013). *Start walking now.* Retrieved April 26, 2013, from http://www.startwalkingnow.org/home.jsp

Anderson, J. L., Halperin, J. L., Albert, N. M., Bozkurt, B., Brindis, R. G., Curtis, L. H., . . . Shen, W. K. (2013). Management of patients with peripheral artery disease (compilation of 2005 and 2011 ACCF/AHA guideline recommendations): A report of the American College of Cardiology Foundation/American Heart Association Task Force on Practice Guidelines. *Circulation, 127*(13), 1425-1443. doi:10.1161/CIR.0b013e31828b82aa; 10.1161/CIR.0b013e31828b82aa

Astrand, P., Rodahl, K., Dahl, K., & Stromme, B. (2004). *Textbook of work physiology* (4th ed.). Champaign, IL: Human Kinetics.

Bishop, D. (2003). Warm up I: Potential mechanisms and the effects of passive warm up on exercise performance. *Sports Medicine (Auckland, N.Z.), 33*(6), 439–454.

Bronas, U. G., Hirsch, A. T., Murphy, T., Badenhop, D., Collins, T. C., Ehrman, J. K., . . . Regensteiner, J. G. (2009). Design of the multicenter standardized supervised exercise training intervention for the claudication: Exercise vs endoluminal revascularization (CLEVER) study. *Vascular Medicine, 14*(4), 313–321.

Carek, P. J., Laibstain, S. E., & Carek, S. M. (2011). Exercise for the treatment of depression and anxiety. *International Journal of Psychiatry in Medicine, 41*(1), 15–28.

Chodzko-Zajko, W., Proctor, D., Fiatarone Singh, M., Minson, C., Nigg, C., Salem, G., . . . Skinner, J. (2009). American College of Sports Medicine position stand. Exercise and physical activity for older adults. *Medicine and Science in Sports and Exercise, 41*(7), 1510–1530. doi:10.1249/MSS.0b013e3181a0c95c

Cress, M. E., Buchner, D. M., Prohaska, T., Rimmer, J., Brown, M., Macera, C., . . . Chodzko-Zajko, W. (2005). Best practices for physical activity programs and behavior counseling in older adult populations. *Journal of Aging & Physical Activity, 13*(1), 61–74.

Dorosz, J. (2009). Updates in cardiac rehabilitation. *Physical Medicine & Rehabilitation Clinics of North America, 20*(4), 719–736.

Downing, J., & Balady, G. J. (2011). The role of exercise training in heart failure. *Journal of the American College of Cardiology, 58*(6), 561–569. doi:10.1016/j.jacc.2011.04.020; 10.1016/j.jacc.2011.04.020

Ehrman, J. K., Gordon, P. M., Visich, P. S., & Keteyian, S. J. (Eds.). (2008). *Clinical exercise physiology* (2nd ed.). Champaign. IL: Human Kinetics.

Fletcher, G. F., Balady, G. J., Amsterdam, E. A., Chaitman, B., Eckel, R., Fleg, J., . . . Bazarre, T. (2001). Exercise standards for testing and training: A statement for healthcare professionals from the American Heart Association. *Circulation, 104,* 1694–1740.

Garber, C. E., Blissmer, B., Deschenes, M. R., Franklin, B. A., Lamonte, M. J., Lee, I. M., . . . Swain, D. P. (2011). American College of Sports Medicine position stand. Quantity and quality of exercise for developing and maintaining cardiorespiratory, musculoskeletal, and neuromotor fitness in apparently healthy adults: Guidance for prescribing exercise. *Medicine and Science in Sports and Exercise, 43*(7), 1334–1359. doi:10.1249/MSS.0b013e318213fefb

Groslambert, A., & Mahon, A. D. (2006). Perceived exertion: Influence of age and cognitive development. *Sports Medicine (Auckland, N.Z.), 36*(11), 911–928.

Hamburg, N. M., & Balady, G. J. (2011). Exercise rehabilitation in peripheral artery disease: Functional impact and mechanisms of benefits. *Circulation, 123*(1), 87–97. doi:10.1161/CIRCULATIONAHA.109.881888

Haskell, W. L., Lee, I. M., Pate, R. R., Powell, K. E., Blair, S. N., Franklin, B. A., . . . Bauman, A. (2007). Physical activity and public health: Updated recommendation for adults from the American College of Sports Medicine and the American Heart Association. *Circulation, 116,* 1081–1093.

Heran, B. S., Chen, J. M., Ebrahim, S., Moxham, T., Oldridge, N., Rees, K., & Taylor, R. S. (2011). Exercise-based cardiac rehabilitation for coronary heart disease. *Cochrane Database of Systematic Reviews (Online), (7):CD001800.* doi:10.1002/14651858. CD001800.pub2

Herring, M. P., Puetz, T. W., O'Connor, P. J., & Dishman, R. K. (2012). Effect of exercise training on depressive symptoms among patients with a chronic illness: A systematic review and meta-analysis of randomized controlled trials. *Archives of Internal Medicine, 172*(2), 101–111. doi:10.1001/archinternmed.2011.696

Hootman, J. M., Macera, C. A., Ainsworth, B. E., Addy, C. L., Martin, M., & Blair, S. N. (2002). Epidemiology of musculoskeletal injuries among sedentary and physically active adults. *Medicine and Science in Sports and Exercise, 34*(5), 838–844.

Jones, A. M., & Poole, D. C. (2005). Oxygen uptake dynamics: From muscle to mouth—An introduction to the symposium. *Medicine and Science in Sports and Exercise, 37*(9), 1542–1550.

Keteyian, S. J., Pina, I. L., Hibner, B. A., & Fleg, J. L. (2010). Clinical role of exercise training in the management of patients with chronic heart failure. *Journal of Cardiopulmonary Rehabilitation and Prevention, 30*(2), 67–76. doi:10.1097/HCR.0b013e3181d0c1c1

Kohrt, W. M., Bloomfield, S. A., Little, K. D., Nelson, M. E., & Yingling, V. R. (2004). American College of Sports Medicine position stand: Physical activity and bone health. *Medicine & Science in Sports & Exercise, 36*(11), 1985–1996.

Kwan, G., & Balady, G. J. (2012). Cardiac rehabilitation 2012: Advancing the field through emerging science. *Circulation, 125*(7), e369–373. doi:10.1161/CIRCULATIONAHA.112.093310

LaForgia, J., Withers, R. T., & Gore, C. J. (2006). Effects of exercise intensity and duration on the excess post-exercise oxygen consumption. *Journal of Sports Sciences, 24*(12), 1247–1264. doi:10.1080/02640410600552064

Leon, A. S., & Bronas, U. G. (2009). Pathophysiology of coronary heart disease and biological mechanisms for the cardioprotective effects of regular aerobic exercise. *American Journal of Lifestyle Medicine, 3*(5), 379–385.

Leon, A. S., Franklin, B. A., Costa, F., Balady, G. J., Berra, K. A., Stewart, K. J., . . . Lauer, M. S. (2005). Cardiac rehabilitation and secondary prevention of coronary heart disease. *Circulation, 111,* 369–376.

Levinger, I., Selig, S., Goodman, C., Jerums, G., Stewart, A., & Hare, D. L. (2011). Resistance training improves depressive symptoms in individuals at high risk for type 2 diabetes. *Journal of Strength & Conditioning Research, 25*(8), 2328–2333.

Loose, B. D., Christiansen, A. M., Smolczyk, J. E., Roberts, K. L., Budziszewska, A., Hollatz, C. G., & Norman, J. F. (2012). Consistency of the counting talk test for exercise prescription. *Journal of Strength and Conditioning Research/National Strength & Conditioning Association, 26*(6), 1701–1707. doi:10.1519/JSC.0b013e318234e84c

Martins, R., Coelho, E., Silva, M., Pindus, D., Cumming, S., Teixeira, A., & Verissimo, M. (2011). Effects of strength and aerobic-based training on functional fitness, mood and the relationship between fatness and mood in older adults. *Journal of Sports Medicine & Physical Fitness, 51*(3), 489–496.

Mason, O. J., & Holt, R. (2012). Mental health and physical activity interventions: A review of the qualitative literature. *Journal of Mental Health (Abingdon, England), 21*(3), 274–284. doi:10.3109/09638237.2011.648344

Mujika, I., & Padilla, S. (2001). Cardiorespiratory and metabolic characteristics of detraining in humans. *Medicine and Science in Sports and Exercise, 33*(3), 413–421.

National Research Council. (2011). *Early childhood obesity prevention policies.* Washington, DC: National Academies Press.

Nelson, M. E., Rejeski, J. E., Blair, S. N., Duncan, P. W., Judge, J. O., King, A. C., . . . Casteneda-Sceppa, C. (2007). Physical activity and public health in older adults: Recommendation from the American College of Sports Medicine and the American Heart Association. *Circulation, 116,* 1094–1105.

Rimer, J., Dwan, K., Lawlor, D. A., Greig, C. A., McMurdo, M., Morley, W., & Mead, G. E. (2012). Exercise for depression. *Cochrane Database of Systematic Reviews (Online), 7,* CD004366. doi:10.1002/14651858.CD004366.pub5

Robergs, R., Ghiasvand, F., & Parker, D. (2004). Biochemistry of exercise-induced metabolic acidosis. *American Journal of Physiology. Regulatory, Integrative, and Comparative Physiology, 287,* R502–R516.

Samitz, G., Egger, M., & Zwahlen, M. (2011). Domains of physical activity and all-cause mortality: Systematic review and dose-response meta-analysis of cohort studies. *International Journal of Epidemiology, 40*(5), 1382–1400. doi:10.1093/ije/dyr112

Thompson, P. D., Buchner, D., Pina, I. L., Balady, G. J., Williams, M. A., Marcus, B. H., . . . Wenger, N. K. (2003). Exercise and physical activity in the prevention and treatment of atherosclerotic cardiovascular disease: American Heart Association scientific statement. *Circulation, 107,* 3109–3116.

U.S. Department of Health and Human Services, Physical Activity Advisory Committee. (2008). *Physical activity guidelines advisory committee report, 2008.* Washington, DC: USDHHS/PAAC. Retrieved from http://www.health.gov/paguidelines/guidelines/default.aspx

U.S. Surgeon General. (1996). *Report on physical activity and health.* Retrieved February 3, 2009, from http://www.cde.800/nccdphd/sgr/mm.htm

Watson, L., Ellis, B., & Leng, G. C. (2008). Exercise for intermittent claudication. *Cochrane Database of Systematic Reviews (Online), (4):CD000990.* doi:10.1002/14651858.CD000990.pub2

Westerblad, H., Allen, D., & Lannergren, J. (2002). Muscle fatigue: Lactic acid or inorganic phosphate the major cause? *News in Physiological Science, 17*, 17–21.

Williams, M. A., Haskell, W. L., Ades, P. A., Amsterdam, E. A., Bittner, V., Franklin, B. A., ... Stewart, K. J (2007). Resistance exercise in individuals with and without cardiovascular disease: 2007 update: A scientific statement from the American Heart Association council on clinical cardiology and council on nutrition physical activity and metabolism. *Circulation, 116*, 572–584.

Part IV: Natural Products

The National Center for Complementary and Alternative Medicine (NCCAM; 2012) includes herbal preparations (also called botanicals), vitamins, minerals, dietary supplements or nutraceuticals, essential oils, and live microorganisms (usually bacteria) in a category of therapies entitled *natural products*. This group also includes the growing area of probiotics. People from even the earliest times have used herbal preparations to improve health or cure illnesses. Hildegard of Bingen, a Benedictine nun, wrote treatises in the 12th century detailing a large number of natural products such as herbs that could be used in healing (*Encyclopedia of World Biography*, 2004). Herbal product compounds for traditional Chinese medicine were documented in the Chinese *Materia Medica* as early as 400 BCE (Beijing Digital Museum of Traditional Chinese Medicine, 2012).

Although the use of herbal preparations decreased in the 20th century as new medicines evolved, there has been resurgence in the public's use of natural products. The 2007 National Health Interview Survey included questions on the use of complementary therapies (Barnes, Bloom, & Nahin, 2008). The report noted that 17.7% of those surveyed used one or more nonvitamin/nonmineral natural products. This was true for both adults and children. Commonly used products included fish oil/omega 3s (37% of adults) and echinacea (37.2% of children) (Barnes et al., 2008).

Use of natural products in healing continues to be a part of the practices in many non-Western health care systems. For example, herbal preparations are a prominent part of Native American healing practices and traditional Chinese medicine; such preparations from natural products are also used in other parts of the world as illustrated in the international sidebars included with the chapters.

The majority of the products in this category are available over the counter, so health care professionals are not actively involved in their implementation. As noted earlier, natural products are an integral part of health practices in other cultures. Because a number of these products may interact with prescribed medications or other treatments, it is critical that the health care team be aware of a patient's use of natural products. Thus, inquiry about their use needs to be a part of all patient assessments. Information to inform practitioners about the effects of these therapies and cautions in their use is available online in the Natural Standard comprehensive database (National Standard Database, 2013).

One therapy that is becoming more commonly used by nurses is aromatherapy. Although not specifically mentioned by NCCAM, the essential oils used in aromatherapy are natural products. Essential oils may be consumed; however, the greater use, and the area in which nurses more often use aromatherapy, is external—either by application to the skin or inhalation. The essential oils used in aromatherapy need to be differentiated from the artificial oils found in many popular bath-and-body shops.

Research on natural products, especially herbal preparations, has only recently begun in the United States. However, a considerable body of research has been developed in other countries such as Germany. The German *Commission E Monographs* is akin to the *Physician's Desk Reference (PDR)* in the United States; specific monographs containing reliable information related to herbal preparations are included on the American Botanical Council website (cms.herbalgram.org/commissione/index.html).

REFERENCES

Barnes, P.M., Bloom, B., & Nahin, R. (2008, December 10). *Complementary and alternative medicine use among adults and children: United States, 2007* (CDC National Health Statistics Report #12). Retrieved from http://www.cdc.gov/nchs/data/nhsr/nhsr012.pdf

Beijing Digital Museum of Traditional Chinese Medicine. (2012) *Classic literature of traditional Chinese medicine.* Retrieved from http://en.tcm-china.info/culturehistory/literature/75830.shtml

Encyclopedia of World Biography (EWB). (2004). Hildegard of Bingen. Retrieved from http://www.encyclopedia.com/doc/1G2-3404708047.html

National Center for Complementary and Alternative Medicine. (2012). *What is complementary and alternative medicine?* Retrieved from http://nccam.nih.gov/health/whatiscam

National Standard Database. (2013). *National standard: The authority on integrative medicine.* Retrieved from http://www.naturalstandard.com

Chapter 20: Aromatherapy

Linda L. Halcón

Aromatherapy is a relatively recent addition to nursing care in the United States, although it is growing in popularity within health care settings worldwide. Aromatherapy is offered by nurses in many countries, including Switzerland, Germany, Australia, Canada, Japan, Korea, and the United Kingdom, and it has been a medical specialty in France for many years. This modality is particularly well suited to nursing, because it incorporates the therapeutic value of sensory experience (i.e., smell) and often includes the use of touch in the delivery of care. It also builds on a rich heritage of botanical therapies within nursing practice (Libster, 2002, 2012).

Aromatherapy has been part of herbal or botanical medicine for millenia. There is evidence of plant distillation and the use of essential oils and other aromatic plant products dating back 5,000 years. In ancient Egypt and the Middle East, plant oils were used in embalming, incense, perfumery, and healing. Therapeutic applications of essential oils were recorded as part of Greek and Roman medicine, and essential oils have been used in Ayurvedic medicine and in traditional Chinese medicine for more than 1,000 years. With the expansion of trade and improvements in distillation methods, essential oils became common elements of herbal medicine and perfumery in Europe during the Middle Ages (Keville & Green, 2009). In the late 1800s, scientists noted the association between environmental exposure to plant essential oils and the prevention of disease, and microbiologists conducted studies showing the in vitro activity of certain plant oils against microorganisms (Battaglia, 2003). More recent studies confirm the antimicrobial properties of essential oils (Solorzano-Santos & Miranda-Novales, 2012).

The development of clinical aromatherapy within the context of modern Western health science began in France just prior to World War I, when chemist Maurice Gattefossé was healed of a near-gangrenous wound with lavender essential oil. He subsequently championed its use for infections and battle wounds. Physician Jean Valnet and nurse Marguerite Maury followed Gattefossé in promoting the therapeutic value of essential oils in Europe, and, in the 1930s, interest in the anti-infective value of essential oils began to appear in the European and Australian medical literature (Price & Price, 2011). The use of essential oils continued sporadically as a nonconventional treatment modality in the West until the recent explosion of interest in botanical medicines, when its use became more visible and widespread. In their groundbreaking survey research on the use of complementary and alternative therapies in the United States, Eisenberg et al. (1998) reported that 5.6% of 2,055 adults surveyed used aromatherapy. More recent large surveys estimating the overall prevalence of complementary therapies have not included aromatherapy as a separate modality (Barnes, Bloom, & Nahin, 2008; Tindle, Davis, Phillips, & Eisenberg, 2005). Surveys of special populations, however, suggest its continuing and increasing use by the public (Crawford, Cincotta, Lim, & Powell, 2006; Sinha & Efron, 2005).

DEFINITION

There are many operant definitions of aromatherapy, and some of them contribute to common misconceptions. The word *aromatherapy* can lead people to believe that it simply involves smelling scents but this is incorrect. It is important to remember that the widespread use of synthetic scents in household and personal products is not considered aromatherapy. Styles (1997) defined aromatherapy as the use of essential oils for therapeutic purposes that encompass mind, body, and spirit—a broad definition that is consistent with holistic nursing practice. The National Cancer Institute defines aromatherapy as the "therapeutic use of essential oils from flowers, herbs, and trees for the improvement of physical, emotional, and spiritual well-being" (National Cancer Institute [NCI], 2012). Buckle defined clinical aromatherapy in nursing as the use of essential oils for expected and measurable health outcomes (Buckle, 2000). Because aromatherapy clinical research is still in its early developmental stages in the United States, the evidence base for using aromatherapy in nursing practice sometimes may be difficult to establish; however, there are findings for and against the use of a number of essential oils, and it is important to evaluate the available scientific data for aromatherapy practice.

Essential oils are obtained from a variety of plants worldwide, but not all plants produce essential oils. For those that do, the essential oils may be found in the plants' flowers, leaves, stems, bark, roots, seeds, resin, or peels. Most essential oils are obtained by steam distillation of a specific plant material. Steam-distilled essential oils are concentrated substances made up of the oil-soluble, lower-molecular-weight chemical constituents found in the source-plant material. Essential oils from citrus fruit peels are usually obtained by expression (similar to grating or grinding). Carbon dioxide extraction is increasingly accepted by scientists and practitioners as an acceptable method for obtaining essential oils; however, other types of solvent extraction generally are not preferred for clinical use. Expressed and CO_2 extracted essential oils contain a broader range of the chemicals present in the plant material; thus, they may have different therapeutic properties. Essential oils do not necessarily have the same medicinal properties as the plants from which they are derived because they do not contain the whole spectrum of chemicals present in the whole plant.

Nurses have an important role in helping patients to differentiate among the range of botanical products that are easily available. Misunderstanding the origin and makeup of these products can result in unnecessary risk. The most commonly used botanical products can be viewed as a continuum (Exhibit 20.1). On one end of the continuum are *whole herbs*, referring to unprocessed material from whole plants or parts of plants (Exhibit 20.1, far-right box). This is the oldest and most common form of botanical medicines worldwide. *Tinctures* and *ointments* are different from the whole plant and are also different from essential oils (Exhibit 20.1, second box from right). They are often confused with each other, and it is important that nurses understand the difference in order to provide advice on their relative safety. Tinctures contain chemicals obtained from the plant material using alcohol as a solvent, and they include both water-soluble and oil-soluble chemicals. Tinctures are often taken orally or sublingually, with the dose and timing depending on the practitioner and the purpose. They are not as concentrated as essential oils. Ointments are made using vegetable oil (e.g., olive oil) rather than alcohol as the solvent. Plant-based tinctures and ointments are widely available. *Flower essences* (Exhibit 20.1, second box from left) are also often confused with essential oils. Essences contain little if any of the original plant material, but they are thought to contain the vibrations or frequencies of the plants they are made from. It is the frequency that is considered the source of their therapeutic action, not the physical chemistry. *Homeopathy* (Exhibit 20.1, far-left box) was developed in Europe and was very popular in the United States in the late 1800s and early

Exhibit 20.1. *A Simple Continuum of Plant Medicines*

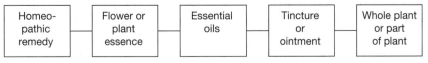

| Homeo-pathic remedy | Flower or plant essence | Essential oils | Tincture or ointment | Whole plant or part of plant |

Source: Halcón (2013).

1900s (Dooley, 2002). It declined in popularity as biomedicine became the dominant paradigm. Homeopathic remedies contain no molecules of the materials from which they are made. They are thought to work subtly on a vibrational level to promote balance and healing. Homeopathic remedies may be prescribed by a homeopathic physician or may be obtained over the counter. Homeopathy is becoming more popular in the United States once again; thus, nurses may benefit from understanding its basic concepts and differentiating it from other natural products.

SCIENTIFIC BASIS

Essential oils processed by any of the above methods are highly volatile, complex mixtures of organic chemicals consisting of terpenes and terpenic compounds. The chemistry of an essential oil largely determines its therapeutic properties. There are 60 to 300 separate chemicals in each essential oil, and the proportions of the constituents for a particular plant species vary depending on a host of genetic and environmental factors. Knowing the plant species, the chemotype, the part of the plant used, the country of origin, and the method of extraction can provide an indication of an essential oil's chemical constituents using readily available aromatherapy textbooks.

The pharmacological activity of essential oils begins on entry into the body through the olfactory, respiratory, gastrointestinal, or integumentary systems. All body systems can be affected once the chemical molecules making up essential oils reach the circulatory and nervous systems. A proportion of the compounds within an essential oil finds its way into the body, however applied (Tisserand & Balacs, 1995), although the degree and rate of absorption vary depending on the route of administration. Inhaled aromas have the fastest effect, although compounds have been detected in the blood following massage (Cross, Russell, Southwell, & Roberts, 2008).

When inhaled, the many different molecules in each essential oil act as olfactory stimulants that travel via the nose to the olfactory bulb, and from there impulses travel to the brain. The amygdala and the hippocampus are of particular importance in the processing of aromas. The amygdala governs emotional responses. The hippocampus is involved in the formation and retrieval of explicit memories. The limbic system interacts with the cerebral cortex, contributing to the relationship between thoughts and feelings; it is directly connected to those parts of the brain that control heart rate, blood pressure, breathing, stress levels, and hormone levels (Kiecolt-Glaser et al., 2008). Although inhalation of essential oils is largely thought to affect the mind and body through the process of olfaction, some molecules from any inhaled vapor travel to the lungs, where they can have an effect on breathing and may be absorbed into the circulatory system. Tisserand and Balacs (1995) gave the example of the effect of *Lavandula angustifolia* (true lavender), thought to reduce the effect of external emotional stimuli by increasing gamma-aminobutyric acid (GABA), which in turn inhibits neurons in the amygdala, producing a sedative effect similar to that of diazepam (Tisserand, 1988). More recent work supports physiological bases for the neurological actions of essential oils (Bagetta et al., 2010; Komiya, Takeuchi, & Harada, 2006).

It is estimated that, at most, about 10% of an essential oil may be absorbed through the skin upon topical application (Cross et al., 2008; Tisserand, 2010), and there is controversy about skin penetration among essential oil researchers. Essential oils seem to be absorbed through the skin by diffusion, with the epidermis and fat layer acting as a reservoir before the components of the essential oils reach the dermis and the bloodstream. In some instances, topically applied essential oil preparations were used to enhance the dermal penetration of pharmaceuticals (Nielsen, 2006; Williams & Barry, 1989). There is some debate among essential oil experts about the rate and extent of penetration and absorption; however, there is evidence that penetration can vary depending on the condition of the skin, the age of the patient, and the carrier or vehicle for the essential oil. In addition, massage can enhance dermal penetration through heat and friction, and occlusion can enhance penetration. Essential oils are excreted from the body through the kidneys, respiration, and insensate loss.

INTERVENTION

The choice of application method depends on the condition being treated or the desired effect, the nurse's knowledge and practice parameters, the available or desired time for the action to occur, the targeted outcome, the chemical components of the essential oil, and the preferences and psychological needs of the patient.

Although essential oils are not always pleasant smelling, inhalation is one of the simplest and most direct application procedures. With this method, 1 drop to 5 drops of an essential oil can be placed on a tissue or floated on hot water in a bowl and then inhaled for 5 minutes to 10 minutes. Other inhalation techniques include the use of diffusers, burners, nebulizers, and vaporizers that can be operated by heat, battery, or electricity and may or may not include the use of water. Larger, portable aroma-inhalation systems are available commercially to provide controlled release of essential oils into rooms of any size.

Inhalation effects as well as skin effects are experienced when essential oils are used in a bath. Baths have been found especially helpful to promote relaxation and sleep in care settings and in the home. Lavender (*L. angustifolia*) is the essential oil most commonly used for these purposes, not only because it promotes relaxation but also because it is generally well tolerated on the skin. For bath-use techniques, see Exhibit 20.2.

Exhibit 20.2. *Therapeutic Bath with Essential Oils*

Four drops to six drops of the essential oil may be dissolved first in a teaspoon of whole milk, rubbing alcohol, or carrier oil (cold-pressed) and then placed in the bath water. Because essential oils are not soluble in water, they would float on the top of the water if they were used without a dispersant, and this could result in an uneven and possibly too concentrated treatment. An essential-oil bath should last about 10 minutes to 15 minutes. Essential oils also may be dissolved in salts (e.g., Epsom salts), which may be soothing to muscles and joints. One such recipe for bath salts consists of 1 tablespoon of baking soda, 2 tablespoons of Epsom salts, and 3 tablespoons of sea salt with 4 drops to 6 drops of essential oils mixed throughout. Salts should be added to the bath water just before immersion and after agitating the water to disperse them.

Compresses can be a useful method for applying essential oils to treat skin conditions or minor injuries. To prepare a compress, add 4 drops to 6 drops of essential oil to warm water. Soak a soft cotton cloth in the mixture, wring it out, and apply the cloth to the affected area, contusion, or abrasion. Cover the compress with plastic wrap to retain moisture, place a towel over the plastic wrap, and keep it in place for as long as desired (up to 4 hours). The use of very warm water can enhance the absorption of some of the components of essential oils (Buckle, 2003).

Massage also can facilitate absorption of essential oils through the skin and can reduce the patient's perceived stress, thus enhancing the healing process and possibly communication as well. To create a mixture for massage, dilute 1 drop to 2 drops of an essential oil in a teaspoon (5 mL) of cold-pressed vegetable oil, organic and scent-free cream, or gel. Mixtures for massage are generally 1% to 5% essential oil concentration (Tisserand & Balacs, 1995), using very low concentrations when massaging large areas of the body.

Essential oils should not be used undiluted on mucous membranes; even on intact skin they are generally used in concentrations seldom exceeding 10%. When used to treat conditions such as vaginal infections, essential-oil preparations can be created or purchased as pessaries or suppositories. Only essential oils high in alcohols, such as tea tree, are appropriate in pessaries; alcohols are less likely to cause skin irritation. If essential oils are applied via tampons, they should be changed regularly (Buckle, 2003). Oral thrush (candidiasis) in adults also can be treated with diluted essential oils by the swish-and-spit method, taking care not to swallow (Jandourek, Vaishampayan, & Vazquez, 1998). Recent studies suggest that essential oils in a mouthwash solution can help prevent dental caries and treat periodontal disease (Bagg, Jackson, Sweeney, Ramage, & Davies, 2006; Carvalhinho, Costa, Coelho, Martins, & Sampaio, 2012).

General Guidelines for Use of Essential Oils

Nurses should be aware of general safety guidelines for patient education and in practice. These include:

- Store essential oils away from open flames; they are volatile and highly flammable.
- Store essential oils in a cool place away from sunlight; use amber- or dark blue-colored glass containers. Close the container immediately after use. Essential oils can oxidize in the presence of heat, light, and oxygen, changing their chemistry and thus their actions in unpredictable ways.
- Be aware that essential oils can stain clothing and textiles and that undiluted essential oils can degrade some plastics. Take appropriate precautions.
- Keep essential oils away from children and pets unless you are well-versed in clinical aromatherapy. The literature contains cases of adverse reactions or deaths related to improper applications or accidental ingestion in young children and pets (Halicioglu, Astarcioglu, Yaprak, & Aydinlioglu, 2011).
- Use essential oils from reputable suppliers. Seek the advice of a trained aromatherapist or the recommendation of a knowledgeable clinical provider. If using essential oils in clinical or research settings, test results verifying the chemical constituency should be obtained.
- Special care is needed when using essential oils with or around persons who have a history of severe asthma or multiple allergies. Be sure to ask.
- Despite the relative safety of essential oils when used properly, sensitization and skin irritation can occur with topical application. In these cases, any residual essential oil solution should be removed with oil or whole milk, rinsed with water, and its use should be discontinued. Most such reactions resolve without treatment; however, a health care provider should be consulted if discomfort/itching is severe or persists.
- If an essential oil gets into the eyes, rinse it out with milk or carrier oil first and then with water.

Measurement of Outcomes

Selection of suitable methods to assess aromatherapy effects will depend on the problem for which essential oils are used and the targeted outcomes of treatment. For example, if lavender is used to promote sleep, measures might include physiological markers, changes in sleep patterns, or comparison of signs and symptoms of insomnia between a treated group and another group that is similar in all ways other than the treatment. For psychological conditions such as depression or anxiety, many reliable survey instruments are available and they can be further validated by adding physiological measures such as cortisol levels or skin temperature. For infectious disease outcomes, standard laboratory tests can be used to measure the effect of treatment on microbial load. Other useful measures could include digital photography, pain scales, quality-of-life scales, tests of cognitive performance, or electroencephalogram results. Using established measurement tools where possible is helpful in facilitating interpretation and comparing the effects of essential oils with those of other approaches.

Precautions

Aromatherapy is a very safe complementary therapy if it is used with knowledge and within accepted guidelines. Many essential oils have been tested by the food and beverage industry for use as flavorings and preservatives, and much research has been carried out by the perfume and tobacco industries. Most of the essential oils commonly used in clinical aromatherapy have been given GRAS (generally regarded as safe) status. However, nurses should not administer essential oils orally, as this is outside a nurse's scope of practice, and poisonings have been documented (Jacobs & Hornfeldt, 1994; Janes, Price, & Thomas, 2005). A list of contraindicated essential oils can be found in training manuals; both novices and more experienced practitioners should consult these lists. Most essential oils should not be used during early pregnancy and should be used cautiously in later pregnancy. Nurses need to be aware of essential oils that can cause photosensitivity, such as bergamot (*Citrus bergamia*) and other citrus oils (Clark & Wilkinson, 1998; Keljova, Jirova, Bendova, Gajdos, & Kolarova, 2010), and they should provide appropriate patient education and protection when these are used.

Essential oils are very concentrated and potent compounds, and in most cases they must be diluted in carrier oils for topical use. Tea tree (*Melaleuca alternifolia*) and lavender (*Lavandula angustifolia*) are among the few exceptions to this rule. These essential oils can be used full strength on minor cuts, abrasions, and small burns.

Some essential oils are known to be carcinogenic and others are contraindicated in persons with specific conditions. Essential oils can potentiate or decrease the effects of medications (Tisserand & Balacs, 1995). Extra care is needed when using essential oils with patients receiving chemotherapy because they may affect the absorption rate of cancer-treating and other drugs (Fox, Gerber, DuPlessis, & Hamman, 2011; Jain, Aqil, Ahad, Ali, & Khar, 2008; Lim, Liu, & Chan, 2009; Paduch, Kandefer-Szerszen,

Trytek, & Fiedurek, 2007; Williams & Barry, 1989). In short, it cannot be assumed that all essential oils are safe in all situations simply because they are *natural*.

Product identity confusion is another potential threat to safety. As noted above, essential oils should not be confused with herbal extracts, which are completely different chemical mixtures, and they cannot be used interchangeably. Besides their chemical dissimilarities, herbal extracts and teas are usually taken internally, whereas essential oils generally are not. Nurses share responsibility for ensuring product integrity when essential oils are used in clinical practice. Chemical testing of those essential oils used in patient care should be incorporated into ongoing quality assurance/quality control programs.

Nurses using essential oils regularly should protect themselves from unintended effects. Because essential oils are volatile, their molecules will be inhaled by those applying them as well as by patients. It has been demonstrated that hand dermatitis may be associated with long-term unprotected use of lotions and other products containing essential oils (Crawford, Katz, Ellis, & James, 2004; Uter et al., 2010).

Perhaps one of the greatest risks in aromatherapy is using an incorrect essential oil for a particular health outcome. This could stem from a nurse's lack of knowledge of plant taxonomy. Many essential oils have familiar common names such as lavender, rose, and rosemary, but it is important to know the full botanical name. For example, "lavender" is a common name that covers *three different kinds* of lavender *and* a number of hybrid plants. The genus of lavender is *Lavandula*, and all lavenders begin with this word. *Lavandula angustifolia* is one of the most widely used and researched essential oils and is recognized as a relaxant. The other two species used in aromatherapy have very different properties. *Lavandula latifolia* (spike lavender) is a stimulant and expectorant; *Lavandula stoechas* is antimicrobial and not safe to use for long periods of time. The picture is sometimes further complicated by hybrid species such *Lavandula x intermedia*. Nurses who use aromatherapy clinically must know the full botanical name of an essential oil they intend to use. The botanical names of commonly used essential oils are found in Exhibit 20.3.

Credentialing

Currently there is no recognized national certification examination for aromatherapists and no governing body. The Aromatherapy Registration Council, a nonprofit entity that was established in 2000, administers a national exam and can provide the public with a list of registered aromatherapy practitioners. Nurses and health professionals wishing to use aromatherapy in their practice should check with their licensing bodies; nurses should check with their state board of nursing. Many states allow nurses to use aromatherapy in their practice if they have received specialized

Exhibit 20.3. *Common and Botanical Names of Essential Oils Frequently Used in Aromatherapy*

Common Name	Botanical Name
Chamomile, German	*Matricaria recutita*
Chamomile, Roman	*Chamaemelum nobile*
Eucalyptus	*Eucalyptus globulus, Eucalyptus radiata*
Ginger	*Zingiber officinale*
Lavender, true	*Lavandula officinalis* or *Lavandula angustifolia*
Lemon	*Citrus limon*
Orange	*Citrus sinensis*
Peppermint	*Mentha piperita*
Rose	*Rosa damascene*
Rosemary	*Rosmarinus officinalis*
Tea tree	*Melaleuca alternifolia*

education. There are many different courses available and health professionals should choose one that is relevant to their own clinical practice. Two large aromatherapy professional organizations in the United States are the National Association of Holistic Aromatherapy (www.naha.org) and the Alliance of International Aromatherapists (www.alliance-aromatherapists.org). There are no requirements in the United States at this time for a person administering aromatherapy to be certified or accredited; however, Canadian nurses have established criteria for practice. The length of training programs in aromatherapy may range from one weekend to several years. Generally, it is not necessary to be a health professional to enroll in these educational programs. Despite the lack of uniform credentialing, it is no longer unusual for hospitals and other clinical settings to include aromatherapy services, and nurses often spearhead the changes. Thus they must insist that policies and procedures include good quality assurance and quality control.

USES

Many health outcomes that fall within the domain of nursing practice can be addressed with essential oils, either alone or combined with other approaches. Essential oils can affect people psychologically and physically. They can increase or decrease sympathetic activity in individuals, affecting blood pressure, plasma adrenaline, and plasma catecholamine levels (Haze, Sakai, & Gozu, 2002; Menezes, Barreto, Antoniolli, Santos, &

de Sousa, 2010). The effect of essential oil odors can be relaxing or stimulating, depending on a person's previous experiences, likes and dislikes, and the chemistry of the essential oil used; therefore, it is important to explore patient preference and the purpose for which the oil is being used when selecting essential oils for therapeutic purposes.

Essential oils are used therapeutically to address a broad range of symptoms and body systems, and there are many aromatherapy texts describing their use and recommending particular essential oils for specific conditions. It would be difficult to identify evidence other than case studies or historical anecdotes for some of these uses, and this has hindered the adoption of aromatherapy in clinical settings. The main current applications of essential oils in conventional health care settings are to help address pain, anxiety, nausea, sleeplessness, or agitation, and to prevent or treat infections. Nurse midwives have long incorporated essential oils into their practices, notably to reduce pain and aid relaxation during and after childbirth (Allaire, Moos, & Wells, 2000; Burns, Blamey, Ersser, Barnetson, & Lloyd, 2000; Conrad & Adams, 2012; Imura, Misao, & Ushijima, 2006; Sheikhan et al., 2012). In long-term-care and hospital settings, essential oils are increasingly used to help reduce anxiety and agitation in patients with or without dementia (Bowles, Griffiths, Quirk, & Croot, 2002; Gray & Clair, 2002; Kritsidima, Newton, & Asimakopoulou, 2009; Lin, Chan, Ng, & Lam, 2007; Morris, 2008; Woelk & Schlafke, 2010), promote sleep and reduce nighttime sedation (Lewith, Godfrey, & Prescott, 2005), and promote wound healing (Culliton & Halcón, 2011; Kerr, 2002; Lusby, Coombes, & Wilkinson, 2006).

Aromatherapy has been used to address acute or chronic pain (Davies, Harding, & Baranowski, 2002; Gedney, Glover, & Fillingim, 2004; Ghelardini, Galeotti, Salvatore, & Mazzanti, 1999; Kim et al., 2007), fatigue and nausea (Lua & Zakaria, 2012; Tate, 1997), infection control (Bassol & Juliani, 2012; Gravett, 2001; Paule, 2001; Thompson et al., 2011), and mood and cognition (Imura et al., 2006; Kiecolt-Glaser et al., 2008; Morris, 2002; Moss, Rouse, Wesnes, & Moss, 2010). The literature includes other studies reporting the use of essential oils in the treatment of head lice (Barker & Altman, 2010; Choi, Yang, Lee, Clark, & Ahn, 2010; Gonzalez Audino, Vassena, Zerba, & Picollo, 2007), and as an aid to smoking cessation (Rose & Behm, 1994) and drug withdrawal (Kunz, Schultz, Lewitzky, Driessen, & Rau, 2007; Lemme, 2009).

There is considerable and growing international literature on the use of plant essential oils against pathogenic microorganisms. The efficacy of essential oils in the treatment and prevention of infectious diseases has important implications for patient health as well as institutional disinfection and hygiene (Edwards-Jones, Buck, Shawcross, Dawson, & Dunn, 2004; Harkenthal, Reichling, Geiss, & Saller, 1999), especially with the increase in resistance bacteria (Hammer, Carson, & Riley, 2008). Methicillin-resistant *Staphylococcus aureus* and other microorganisms have been found to be sensitive to tea tree oil (*Melaleuca alternifolia*) (Bagg et al., 2006; Carson,

Hammer, Messager, & Riley, 2005; Halcón & Milkus, 2004). Preliminary work suggests that essential oils may also be effective in other difficult-to-treat infections and wounds (Culliton & Halcón, 2011; Sherry, Sivananthan, Warnke, & Eslick, 2003).

Aromatherapy is one of the complementary therapies most used for children and adolescents (Simpson & Roman, 2001). Despite the many aromatherapy products on the market for babies, it is recommended that essential oils be used cautiously, if at all, in infants, except for specific purposes. Many accidental poisonings of young children have been reported, illustrating the importance of keeping essential oils out of reach in bottles with integral drop dispensers and the necessity of knowing the safety profile of each essential oil (Tisserand & Balacs, 1995). Essential oils are used in pediatric oncology settings for nausea and fatigue. They have also been used to treat head lice and acne (Enshaieh, Jooya, Siadat, & Iraji, 2007), and to help with infantile colic (fennel seed) (Alexandrovich, Rakovitskaya, Kolmo, Sidorova, & Shushunov, 2003). Nurses who are knowledgeable about essential oils can introduce them in pediatric practice and remain within safety guidelines.

CULTURAL ASPECTS

There are regional, cultural, and religious traditions and preferences for the types of essential oils used therapeutically. For example, Ayurvedic practices include many essential oils that are produced in the Indian subcontinent, including those from sandalwood, jasmine, and other floral or spicy aromatic plants. The Middle East and Africa are the sources of such oils as frankincense, myrrh, ylang ylang, ravensara, and others. In Europe and much of the United States, essential oil production focuses on herbs or flowers that grow and thrive in temperate climates, such as peppermint, lavender, and basil. Citrus oils are produced in countries with warmer climates. However, the lines are not as distinct as in earlier times when the procurement of essential oils was limited to native and local plants. Plants are routinely transported and grown in nonnative regions, and the essential oils most commonly used for therapeutic purposes are now readily available throughout the world, obtainable through global trade and Internet sales.

Cultural plant-healing traditions often have been altered and adopted by newcomers. The case of Australian tea tree oil provides an example of adaptation of cultural and regional health practices over time. *Melaleuca alternifolia* grows in one area of Australia as a native plant, and it was used as an herbal anti-infective medicine by Aboriginal peoples for centuries. More than 200 species of the genus *Melaleuca* are native to Australia and New Zealand, and only a few have been explored for modern medicinal uses as essential oils (Weiss, 1997). *Melaleuca alternifolia* is one of many plants referred to as "tea tree" in Australia and New Zealand; hence the importance of relying on Latin names for identification. The healing properties of this plant were noted by European explorers and settlers, and at some point the foliage was distilled to produce a very concentrated antiseptic substance—tea tree oil. Since the early 1900s there has been intermittent interest in tea tree oil on the part of the medical community. This interest has expanded in recent years, partly through partnerships between the Australian government and the private agricultural sector to expand tea tree oil's economic impact. Both public and private funding was provided for excellent scientific research on the antimicrobial properties of tea tree oil, subsequently added to by health care researchers and scientists around the world. Extensive information can be found at the website of the Tea Tree Oil Research Group, University of Western Australia (www.marshallcentre.uwa.edu.au/research/tea-tree-oil). Tea tree is now an important plantation crop, and the antimicrobial properties of tea tree oil (*M. alternifolia*) are somewhat known in Western biomedical health care settings, but more widely so by the public. Affordable, pure essential oil or health products with tea tree oil as a major ingredient are available worldwide, benefiting the Australian agricultural sector and health care. For a description of aromatherapy and issues relevant to its use in nursing practice in Australia, see Sidebar 20.1.

Sidebar 20.1. *Aromatherapy in Nursing Practice in Australia*

Trisha Dunning, Deakin University, Victoria, Australia

Anecdotally, aromatherapy is one of the most popular complementary therapies Australian nurses use, often combined with massage. National population data about the use of complementary and alternative medicine (CAM) suggest about 70% of nurses use CAM, including aromatherapy; however, there are no national data about how many nurses are qualified aromatherapists, the number who work as aromatherapists in private practice, or how many incorporate aromatherapy in their nursing practice. One reason for the lack of such data is that aromatherapy is a self-regulated practice, unlike nursing. Currently, traditional Chinese medicine (TCM) is the only CAM regulated by the Australian Health Practitioner Regulation Agency.

Most Australians who use aromatherapy do so on a self-selected basis, and many may not understand the risks and benefits of essential oils or how to use them appropriately. In addition, aromatherapy products are often purchased from pharmacies, health food shops, local community markets, and supermarkets where expert advice is not available and there is no guarantee of quality. Significantly, the public often confuses fragrances and essential oils, largely due to marketing of fragrance products in beauty and home care.

Education

Many CAM professional groups—including the International Aromatherapy and Aromatic Medicine Association, the organization most aromatherapists in Australia (including nurses) belong to—have specific requirements for membership. Membership rules include: completing accredited courses, ensuring knowledge is current, and holding professional indemnity. Aromatherapy training is delivered at certificate and diploma level by various private education providers and can often be completed online. Many of these courses lead to qualifications in beauty therapy rather than clinical aromatherapy. Some university CAM courses include information about aromatherapy. The quality of these courses varies in course content, teaching quality, amount and quality of supervised clinical practice, and assessment criteria.

Clinical Applications

Aromatherapy is used in a variety of clinical settings in Australia; however, it may not always be truly integrated into care plans and the outcomes are not always monitored systematically. Key areas of practice in which aromatherapy is used include palliative and cardiovascular care, to manage stress and pain, promote relaxation, and improve emotional well-being. Essential oils are mostly used externally in vaporizers and massage or applied to furnishings and clothing or used in baths.

Until recently, aromatherapy was commonly used in older care facilities to address odor, reduce stress, promote sleep, and reduce the need for sedatives. One program, Creative Ways to Care, was developed to assist caregivers in home care for relatives with dementia. The program had been widely implemented in older care settings. However, CAM use (including aromatherapy) in such facilities has declined since the Aged Care Funding Instrument (ACFI) was introduced and residents now have to pay for CAM therapies. The introduction of the ACFI has also affected the enrollment in CAM courses.

Quality, Safety, and Evidence

A number of factors affect aromatherapy safety and quality:

1. The individual (reason for using essential oils knowledge, health status, concomitant use of other CAM, and conventional medicines)
2. The practitioner (knowledge, competence)
3. Essential oils and carrier substances (labels, quality, purity, storage conditions, and manufacturing processes)
4. Application method (internal or external use)
5. Environment (where aromatherapy is delivered)

6. Evidence base for use (articulated in policies and procedures or guidelines)
7. Regulation of products and practitioners (essential oils are regulated in Australia as medicines under the Therapeutic Goods Act [1989] and must meet a range of other regulations such as labeling and packaging).

The growing interest in discovery of new plant medicines that have health applications or profit possibilities has fueled expanded research on essential oils. It is important to note, however, that much of this research is aimed at improved food preservation and the resultant prevention of food-borne illness of insects and parasites (Samarasekera, Weerasinghe, & Hemalal, 2008; Singh et al., 2008). As new essential oils are produced and tested for their health and environmental applications (Baik et al., 2008; Dongmo et al., 2008), their production can provide international trade opportunities and improved agricultural sustainability in addition to usually very affordable natural medicines.

FUTURE RESEARCH

Aromatherapy researchers face several unique challenges. First, it is exceedingly difficult to conduct aromatherapy randomized controlled trials—the gold standard for quantitative research—because of the difficulty in blinding research subjects and staff to odor. Some researchers have attempted to use specialized masks to eliminate smell for participants, whereas others have used alternate and supposedly nontherapeutic smells for control groups. These approaches can improve study methods but still have limitations.

Another research challenge is presented by the essential oils themselves due to their natural chemical variation. Pure and genuine essential oils cannot be truly standardized because each batch varies depending on growing conditions, plant stresses, harvesting and processing differences, and even storage factors. When using essential oils in research or clinical practice, it is essential to obtain chemical testing and verify that the specific batch used meets the standard ranges of the major constituents. Yet another research challenge is the use of blends versus single essential oils. There is evidence of synergistic and antagonistic effects when different oils are combined, making it more difficult to identify therapeutic elements. Finally, many studies test essential oil mixtures applied topically via massage, making it difficult to separate the effect of massage from that of the essential oil. Nurses should be aware of these research challenges when evaluating the evidence base for aromatherapy in practice.

There is a large body of unpublished research on the therapeutic effects of essential oils, much of it proprietary and conducted by the food, cosmetics, and flavoring industries. There is also a large volume of scientific research published in languages other than English, notably from Japan, China, India, and various countries in Europe. Despite a growing body of research in English-speaking countries, there remains a dearth of studies in English and a great need for additional research. Work is needed to test the efficacy of essential oils already in common use and to extend the practice of aromatherapy in clinical settings where, for some conditions and individuals, it may be a cost-effective alternative or adjunct therapy with fewer side effects than pharmaceuticals and other biomedical treatments.

WEBSITES

The following are websites that nurses may find helpful in identifying more information about essential oils:

Alliance of International Aromatherapists
(www.alliance-aromatherapists.org)

Aromatherapy Registration Council
(www.aromatherapycouncil.org)

National Association of Holistic Aromatherapists
(www.naha.org)

REFERENCES

Alexandrovich, I., Rakovitskaya, O., Kolmo, E., Sidorova, T., & Shushunov, S. (2003). The effect of fennel (*Foeniculum vulgare*) seed oil emulsion in infantile colic: A randomized, placebo-controlled study. *Alternative Therapies, 9*(4), 58–61.

Allaire, A., Moos, M., & Wells, S. (2000). Complementary and alternative medicine in pregnancy: A survey of North Carolina certified nurse-midwives. *Obstetrics & Gynecology, 95*(1), 19–23.

Bagetta, G., Morrone, L., Rombola, L., Amantea, D., Russo, R., Berliocchi, L., . . . Corasaniti, M. (2010). Neuropharmacology of the essential oil bergamot. *Fitoterapia, 81*(6), 453–461.

Bagg, J., Jackson, M., Sweeney, M., Ramage, G., & Davies, A. (2006). Susceptibility to *Melaleuca alternifolia* (tea tree) oil of yeasts isolated from the mouths of patients with advanced cancer. *Oral Oncology, 42*(5), 487–492.

Baik, J., Kim, S., Lee, J., Oh, T., Kim J., Lee, N., & Hyun, C. (2008). Chemical composition and biological activities of essential oils extracted from Korean endemic citrus species. *Journal of Microbiology and Biotechnology, 18*(1), 74–79.

Barker, S. C., & Altman, P. M. (2010). A randomised, assessor blind, parallel group comparative efficacy trial of three products for the treatment of head lice in children—Melaleuca oil and lavender oil, pyrethrins and piperonyl butoxide, and a "suffocation" product. *BMC Dermatology, 10*(1), 6.

Barnes, P. M., Bloom, B., & Nahin, R. (2008). Complementary and alternative medicine use among adults and children: United States 2007. *National Health Statistics Report (NHSR)*, (12), 1–23.

Bassol, I. H. N., & Juliani, H. R. (2012). Essential oils in combination and their antimicrobial properties. *Molecules, 17*(4), 3989–4006. doi:10.3390/molecules17043989

Battaglia, S. (2003). *The complete guide to aromatherapy* (2nd ed.). Brisbane, Australia: International Centre of Holistic Aromatherapy.

Bowles, E. J., Griffiths, M., Quirk, L., & Croot, K. (2002). Effects of essential oils and touch on resistance to nursing care procedures and other dementia-related behaviours in a residential care facility. *International Journal of Aromatherapy, 12*(1), 22–29.

Buckle, J. (2000). The "M" technique. *Massage and Bodywork, 15*, 52–64.

Buckle, J. (2003). *Clinical aromatherapy: Essential oils in practice* (2nd ed.). New York, NY: Churchill Livingstone.

Burns, E. E., Blamey, C., Ersser, S. J., Barnetson, L., & Lloyd, A. J. (2000). An investigation into the use of aromatherapy in intrapartum midwifery practice. *Journal of Alternative and Complementary Therapies, 6*(2), 141–147.

Carson, C., Hammer, K., Messager, S., & Riley, T. (2005). Tea tree oil: A potential alternative for the management of methicillin-resistant *Staphylococcus aureus* (MRSA). *Australian Infection Control, 10*(1), 32–34.

Carvalhinho, S., Costa, A. M., Coelho, A. C., Martins, E., & Sampaio, A. (2012). Susceptibilities of *Candida albicans* mouth isolates to antifungal agents, essential oils and mouth rinses. *Mycopathologia, 174*(1), 69–76.

Choi, H.-Y., Yang, Y.-C., Lee, S. H., Clark, J. M., & Ahn, Y.-J. (2010). Efficacy of spray formulations containing binary mixtures of clove and eucalyptus oils against susceptible and pyrethroid/malathion-resistant head lice (Anoplura: Pediculae). *Journal of Medical Entomology, 47*(3), 387–391.

Clark, S., & Wilkinson, S. (1998). Phototoxic contact dermatitis from 5-methoxypsoralen in aromatherapy oil. *Contact Dermatitis, 38*(5), 289–290.

Conrad, P., & Adams, C. (2012). The effects of clinical aromatherapy for anxiety and depression in the high risk postpartum woman—A pilot study. *Complementary Therapies in Clinical Practice, 18*(3), 164–168.

Crawford, G., Cincotta, D., Lim, A., & Powell, C. (2006). A cross-sectional survey of complementary and alternative medicine use by children and adolescents attending the University Hospital of Wales. *BMC Complementary and Alternative Medicine, 6*(16), 1–10.

Crawford, G., Katz, K., Ellis, E., & James, W. (2004). Use of aromatherapy products and increased risk of hand dermatitis in massage therapists. *Archives of Dermatology, 140*(8), 991–996.

Cross, S., Russell, M., Southwell, I., & Roberts, M. (2008). Human skin penetration of the major components of Australian tea tree oil applied in its pure form and as a 20% solution *in vitro*. *European Journal of Pharmaceutics & Biopharmaceutics, 69*(1), 214–222.

Culliton, P., & Halcón, L. (2011). Chronic wound treatment with topical tea tree oil. *Alternative Therapies in Health and Medicine, 17*(2), 46–47.

Davies, S. J., Harding, L. M., & Baranowski, A. P. (2002). A novel treatment of postherpetic neuralgia using peppermint oil. *Clinical Journal of Pain, 18*(3), 200–202.

Dongmo, P., Tchoumbougnang, F., Sonwa, E., Kenfack, S., Zollo, P., & Menut, C. (2008). Antioxidant and anti-inflammatory potential of essential oils of some *Zanthoxylum* (Rutaceae) of Cameroon. *International Journal of Essential Oil Therapeutics, 2*(2), 82–88.

Dooley, T. R. (2002). *Homeopathy: Beyond flat earth medicine* (2nd ed). San Diego, CA: Timing Publications.

Edwards-Jones, V., Buck, R., Shawcross, S., Dawson, M., & Dunn, K. (2004). The effect of essential oils on methicillin-resistant *Staphylococcus aureus* using a dressing model. *Burns, 30*(8), 772–777.

Eisenberg, D. M., Davis, R. B., Ettner, S. L., Appel, S., Wilken, S., Van Rompay, M. I., & Kessler, R. C. (1998). Trends in alternative medicine in the USA, 1990–1997: Results of a follow-up national survey. *Journal of the American Medical Association, 280*(18), 1569–1575.

Enshaieh, S., Jooya, A., Siadat, A., & Iraji, F. (2007). The efficacy of 5% topical tea tree oil gel in mild to moderate acne vulgaris: A randomized, double-blind placebo-controlled study. *Indian Journal of Dermatology, Venereology and Leprology, 73*(1), 22–25.

Fox, L. T., Gerber, M., DuPlessis, J., & Hamman, J. H. (2011). Transdermal drug delivery enhancement by compounds of natural origin. *Molecules, 16*(12), 10507–10540.

Gedney, J. J., Glover, T. L., & Fillingim, R. B. (2004). Sensory and affective pain discrimination after inhalation of essential oils. *Psychosomatic Medicine, 66*(4), 599–606.

Ghelardini, C., Galeotti, N., Salvatore, G., & Mazzanti, G. (1999). Local anaesthetic activity of the essential oil of *Lavandula angustifolia*. *Planta Medica, 65*(8), 700–703.

Gonzalez Audino, P., Vassena, C., Zerba, E., & Picollo, M. (2007). Effectiveness of lotions based on essential oils from aromatic plants against permethrin resistant *Pediculus humanus capitis*. *Archives of Dermatological Research, 299*(8), 389–392.

Gravett, P. (2001). Aromatherapy treatment for patients with Hickman Line infection following high-dose chemotherapy. *International Journal of Aromatherapy, 11*(1), 18–19.

Gray, S., & Clair, A. (2002). Influence of aromatherapy on medication administration to residential-care residents with dementia and behavioral challenges. *American Journal of Alzheimer's Disease and Other Dementias, 17*(3), 173–196.

Halcón, L. (2013). Aromatherapy in pregnancy and childbirth. In M. Avery (Ed.), *Supporting a physiologic approach to pregnancy and birth*. Ames, IA: Wiley Blackwell.

Halcón, L., & Milkus, K. (2004). *Staphylococcus aureus* and wounds: A review of tea tree oil (*Melaleuca alternifolia*) as a promising antibiotic. *American Journal of Infection Control, 32*(7), 402–408.

Halicioglu, O., Astarcioglu, G., Yaprak, I., & Aydinlioglu, H. (2011). Toxicity of salvia officinalis in a newborn and a child: An alarming report. *Pediatric Neurology, 45*(4), 259–260.

Hammer, K. A., Carson, C. F., & Riley, T. V. (2008). Frequencies of resistance to *Melaleuca alternifolia* (tea tree) oil and rifampicin in *Staphylococcus aureus, Staphylococcus epidermidis* and *Enterococcus faecalis*. *International Journal of Antimicrobial Agents, 32*(2), 170–173.

Harkenthal, M., Reichling, J., Geiss, H., & Saller, R. (1999). Comparative study on the *in vitro* antibacterial activity of Australian tea tree oil, cajuput oil, niaouli oil, manuka oil, kanuka oil, and eucalyptus oil. *Pharmazie, 54*(6), 460–463.

Haze, S., Sakai, K., & Gozu, Y. (2002). Effects of fragrance inhalation on sympathetic activity in normal adults. *Japanese Journal of Pharmacology, 90*(3), 247–253.

Imura, M., Misao, H., & Ushijima, H. (2006). The psychological effects of aromatherapy-massage in healthy postpartum mothers. *Journal of Midwifery & Women's Health, 51*(2), e21–e27.

Jacobs, M., & Hornfeldt, C. (1994). Melaleuca oil poisoning. *Clinical Toxicology, 32*(4), 461–464.

Jain, R., Aqil, M., Ahad, A., Ali, A., & Khar, R. K. (2008). Basil oil is a promising skin penetration enhancer for transdermal delivery of labetolol hydrochloride. *Drug Development and Industrial Pharmacy, 34*(4), 384–389.

Jandourek, A., Vaishampayan, J., & Vazquez, J. (1998). Efficacy of melaleuca oral solution for the treatment of fluconazole refractory oral candidiasis in AIDS patients. *AIDS, 12*(9), 1033–1037.

Janes, S. E. J., Price, C. S. G., & Thomas, D. (2005). Essential oil poisoning: N-acetylcysteine for eugenol-induced hepatic failure and analysis of a national database. *European Journal of Pediatrics, 164*(8), 520–522.

Keljova, K., Jirova, D., Bendova, H., Gajdos, P., & Kolarova, H. (2010). Phototoxicity of essential oils intended for cosmetic use. *Toxicology in Vitro, 24*(8), 2084–2089.

Kerr, J. (2002). Research project—Using essential oils in wound care for the elderly. *Aromatherapy Today, 23*, 14–19.

Keville, K., & Green, M. (2009). *Aromatherapy: A complete guide to the healing art* (2nd ed.). Berkeley, CA: Crossing Press.

Kiecolt-Glaser, J., Graham, J., Malarkey, W., Porter, K., Lemeshow, S., & Glaser, R. (2008). Olfactory influences on mood and autonomic, endocrine, and immune function. *Psychoneuroendocrinology, 33*(3), 328–339.

Kim, J. T., Ren, C. J., Fielding, G. A., Pitti, A., Kasumi, T., Wajda, M., . . . Bekker, A. (2007). Treatment with lavender aromatherapy in the post-anesthesia care unit reduces opioid requirements of morbidly obese patients undergoing laparoscopic adjustable gastric banding. *Obesity Surgery, 17*(7), 920–925.

Komiya, M., Takeuchi, T., & Harada, E. (2006). Lemon oil vapor causes an anti-stress effect via modulating 5-HT and DA activities in mice. *Behavioural Brain Research, 172*(2), 240–249.

Kritsidima, M., Newton, T., & Asimakopoulou, K. (2009). The effects of lavender scent on dental patient anxiety levels: A cluster randomised-controlled trial. *Community Dentistry and Oral Epidemiology, 38*(1), 83–87.

Kunz, S., Schultz, M., Lewitzky, M., Driessen, M., & Rau, H. (2007). Ear acupuncture for alcohol withdrawal in comparison with aromatherapy: A randomized-controlled trial. *Alcoholism: Clinical and Experimental Research, 31*(3), 436–442.

Lemme, P. (2009). The use of essential oils in psychiatric medication withdrawal. *International Journal of Clinical Aromatherapy, 6*(2), 15–23.

Lewith, G. T., Godfrey, A. D., & Prescott, P. (2005). A single-blinded, randomized pilot study evaluating the aroma of *Lavandula angustifolia* as a treatment for mild insomnia. *Journal of Alternative and Complementary Medicine, 11*(4), 631–637.

Libster, M. (2002). *Delmar's integrative herb guide for nurses*. Victoria, Australia: Delmar Thompson Learning.

Libster, M. (2012). *The nurse herbalist: Integrative insights for holistic practice*. Naperville, IL: Golden Apple Publications.

Lim, P. F. C., Liu, X. Y., & Chan, S. Y. (2009). A review on terpenes as skin penetration enhancers in transdermal drug delivery. *Journal of Essential Oil Research, 21*(5), 423–428.

Lin, P., Chan, W., Ng, B., & Lam, L. (2007). Efficacy of aromatherapy (*Lavender angustifolia*) as an intervention for agitated behaviours in Chinese older persons with dementia: A cross-over randomized trial. *International Journal of Geriatric Psychiatry, 22*(5), 205–210.

Lua, P. L., & Zakaria, N. S. (2012). A brief review of current scientific evidence involving aromatherapy use for nausea and vomiting. *Journal of Alternative and Complementary Medicine, 18*(6), 534–540.

Lusby, P. E., Coombes, A. L., & Wilkinson, J. M. (2006). A comparison of wound healing following treatment with *Lavandula x allardii* honey or essential oil. *Phytotherapy Research, 20*(9), 755–757.

Menezes, I. A. C., Barreto, C. M. N., Antoniolli, A. R., Santos, M. R. V., & de Sousa, D. P. (2010). Hypotensive activity of terpenes found in essential oils. *Zeitschrift für Naturforschung C: A Journal of Biosciences, 65*(9), 562–566.

Morris, N. (2002). The effects of lavender (*Lavandula angustifolium*) baths on psychological well-being: Two exploratory randomized control trials. *Complementary Therapies in Medicine, 10*(4), 223–228.

Morris, N. (2008). The effects of lavender (*Lavandula angustifolia*) essential oil baths on stress and anxiety. *International Journal of Clinical Aromatherapy, 5*(1), 3–7.

Moss, L., Rouse, M., Wesnes, K. A., & Moss, M. (2010). Differential effects of the aromas of *Salvia* species on memory and mood. *Human Psychopharmacology: Clinical & Experimental, 25*(5), 388–396.

National Cancer Institute (NCI), National Institutes of Health. (2012). *Aromatherapy and essential oils*. Retrieved from http://www.cancer.gov/cancertopics/pdq/cam/aromatherapy/patient/page1

Nielsen, J. (2006). Natural oils affect the human skin integrity and the percutaneous penetration of benzoic acid-dose dependency. *Basic & Clinical Pharmacology & Toxicology, 98*(6), 575–581.

Paduch, R., Kandefer-Szerszen, M., Trytek, M., & Fiedurek, J. (2007). Terpenes: Substances useful in human healthcare. *Archivum Immunologiae et Therapaie Experimentalis, 55*(5), 315–327.

Paule, A. (2001). Antimicrobial properties of essential oil constituents. *International Journal of Aromatherapy, 11*(3), 126–133.

Price, S., & Price L. (2011). *Aromatherapy for health professionals* (4th ed.). Edinburgh, Scotland: Churchill Livingstone.

Rose, J., & Behm, F. (1994). Inhalation of vapor from black pepper extract reduces smoking withdrawal symptoms. *Drug and Alcohol Dependence, 34*(3), 225–229.

Samarasekera, R., Weerasinghe, I., & Hemalal, K. (2008). Insecticidal activity of menthol derivatives against mosquitoes. *Pest Management Science, 64*(3), 290–295.

Sheikhan, F., Jahdi, F., Khoei, E. M., Shamsalizadeh, N., Sheikhan, M., & Haghani, H. (2012). Episiotomy pain relief: Use of lavender oil essence in primiparous Iranian women. *Complementary Therapies in Clinical Practice, 18*(1), 66–70.

Sherry, E., Sivananthan, S., Warnke, P., & Eslick, G. (2003). Topical phytochemicals used to salvage the gangrenous lower limbs of type 1 diabetic patients. *Diabetes Research and Clinical Practice, 62*(1), 65–66.

Simpson, N., & Roman, K. (2001). Complementary medicine use in children: Extent and reasons. A population based study. *British Journal of General Practice, 51*(472), 914–916.

Singh, G., Kiran, S., Marimuthu, P., de Lampasona, M., de Heluani, C., & Catalan, C. (2008). Chemistry, biocidal and antioxidant activities of essential oil and oleoresins from *Piper cubeba* (seed). *International Journal of Essential Oil Therapeutics, 2*(2), 50–59.

Sinha, D., & Efron, D. (2005). Complementary and alternative medicine use in children: Extent and reasons. A population based study. *British Journal of General Practice, 51*(472), 914–916.

Solorzano-Santos, F., & Miranda-Novales, M. (2012). Essential oils from aromatic herbs as antimicrobial agents. *Current Opinion in Biotechnology, 23*(2), 136–141.

Styles, J. (1997). The use of aromatherapy in hospitalized children with HIV. *Complementary Therapies in Nursing & Midwifery, 3*(1), 16–20.

Tate, S. (1997). Peppermint oil, a treatment for postoperative nausea. *Journal of Advanced Nursing, 26*(3), 543–549.

Thompson, P., Jensen, T., Hammer, K., Carson, C., Molgaard, P., & Riley, T. (2011). Survey of the antimicrobial activity of commercially available Australian tea tree (*Melaleuca alternifolia*) essential oil products *in vitro*. *Journal of Alternative and Complementary Medicine, 17*(9), 835–841.

Tindle, H., Davis, R., Phillips, R., & Eisenberg, D. (2005). Trends in the use of complementary and alternative medicine by U.S. adults: 1997–2002. *Alternative Therapies in Health and Medicine, 11*(1), 42–49.

Tisserand, R. (1988). Lavender beats benzodiazepines. *International Journal of Aromatherapy, 1*(2), 102.

Tisserand, R. (2010, May). *Essential oil therapeutics*. Paper presented at the Workshop for Plant Extracts International, Hopkins, MN.

Tisserand, R., & Balacs, T. (1995). *Essential oil safety*. London, UK: Churchill Livingstone.

Uter, W., Schmidt, E., Geier, J., Lessmann, H., Schnuch, A., & Frosch, P. (2010). Contact allergy to essential oils: Current patch test results (2000-2008) from the Information Network of Departments of Dermatology (IVDK). *Contact Dermatitis, 63*(5), 277–283.

Weiss, E. (1997). *Essential oil crops*. Cambridge, UK: CAB International.

Williams, A., & Barry, B. (1989). Essential oils as novel skin penetration enhancers. *International Journal of Pharmaceutics, 57*(2), R7–R9.

Woelk, H., & Schlafke, S. (2010). A multi-center, double-blind, randomised study of the lavender oil preparation silexan in comparison to lorazepam for generalized anxiety disorder. *Phytomedicine, 17*(2), 94–99.

Chapter 21: Herbal Medicines

GREGORY A. PLOTNIKOFF

Herbs, and related natural products such as spices, are the oldest and most widely used form of medicine in the world. The use of herbs for the treatment of disease and the promotion of well-being can be traced back in many cultures at least 2,500 years. For example, in the 5th century BCE, Hippocrates recommended leaves and bark of the willow tree (genus *Salix*) for pain and inflammation. However, herbal medicines are not restricted to historical use. Today, in addition to the well-known examples of aspirin from the willow tree, digoxin from the foxglove plant *Digitalis purpurea*, and paclitaxel from the pacific yew tree *Taxus brevifolia*, both over-the-counter and prescription plant-derived medications are frequently used, including anticholinergic agents, anticoagulants, antihypertensives, and antineoplastic agents. And just a small percentage of the world's plant species provide medicines. There are likely many more waiting to be discovered. The most recently celebrated example is that of a potent antimalarial medication. Chinese scientists led by Dr. Youyou Tu discovered and isolated artemisinin from sweet wormwood (*Artemesia annua* L), a plant used for medicinal purposes in China for more than 2,000 years. For her work, Dr. Tu was honored with the very prestigious Lasker-DeBakey Clinical Research Award in 2011 (Miller & Su, 2011).

The most comprehensive and reliable data on the use of herbal medicine in the United States comes from the 2007 National Health Interview Survey (NHIS), a survey of 23,300 adults and 9,400 adults on behalf of a child in their household. Use of natural products, including herbs, for medicinal purposes was documented in 17.7% of the U.S. population (Barnes, Bloom, & Nahin, 2008).

The high prevalence of use in all regions of the United States and across all ages, genders, ethnicities, and medical diagnoses means that health professionals must address herbal medicine use in all patient encounters (Arcury et al., 2006; Cherniack et al., 2008). In the 2002 NHIS study, 55% of adults believed that use of complementary and alternative medicines (CAM) would support health when used in combination with conventional medical treatments (Barnes, Powell-Griner, McFann, & Nahin, 2004). This is significant. Use of herbal medicines may not be disclosed unless specifically requested by the nurse, pharmacist, or physician. Even in 2008, as many as 62.5% of regular herbal medicine users also used prescription medicines; however, only 33% routinely reported their use to their care provider (Archer & Boyle, 2008). The 2004 Council for Responsible Nutrition survey of 1,000 randomly selected U.S. adults documented that 90% looked to health care professionals, including nurses, for guidance in herbal medicine use (Ward & Blumenthal, 2005). Thus, herbal medicine warrants significant attention by all nurses.

DEFINITION

Herbal medicines, or plant-based therapies, continue to occupy a place of central importance in the world's many healing traditions. These include the use of single herbs in many Western traditions and multiple-herb combinations in traditional Asian medical systems. Frequently, herbs are part of an overarching belief system that may involve spiritual or metaphysical components. Herbal medicines are often included in the work of shamans and other traditional healers who serve as intermediaries with the spirit world. Herbal medicines are also a tool in traditional Asian medicine and are used, like acupuncture, to open blocked channels (meridians) for the free flow of *qi* (life spirit or force).

Herbal medicines, also known as botanicals or phytotherapies, are one component of the range of natural products sold in the United States as dietary supplements. These include fungi-based products (mycotherapies); essential oils (aromatherapies); and vitamin, mineral, and nutritional therapies (nutraceuticals). Since the passage of the Dietary Supplement Health and Education Act of 1994 (DSHEA, U.S. Congress, 1994), these biological modifiers have been available over the counter as dietary supplements. Though neither food nor drug, these substances are still regulated by the Food and Drug Administration (FDA), but with less stringent requirements. Unlike foods and drugs, dietary supplements can be sold based on evidence of safety in the possession of the manufacturer and can only be removed from the market if the FDA can prove them unsafe under ordinary conditions of use.

Under DSHEA, herbal medicines can be sold for "stimulating, maintaining, supporting, regulating and promoting health" rather than for treating disease. As dietary supplements rather than drugs, herbal medicines cannot claim to restore normal (or correct abnormal) function. Additionally, herbs cannot claim to "diagnose, treat, prevent, cure, or mitigate" (U.S. Congress, 1994). Herbal medicine companies can assert that their product supports cardiovascular health but not that it lowers cholesterol. To do so would suggest that the product is intended for treating a disease (hypercholesterolemia) and is therefore subject to FDA pharmaceutical regulations.

This has raised questions about what constitutes a disease. The FDA originally defined a disease as any deviation, impairment, or interruption of the normal structure or function of any part, organ, or system of the body that is manifested by a characteristic set of one or more signs and symptoms. This definition generated many concerns. "Normal structure" appeared to be normed to a 30-year-old man and therefore did not account for gender or aging. For example, are menopause and menstrual cramps diseases? With no signs or symptoms, is hypercholes terolemia a disease or a risk factor? After significant public outcry, the FDA adopted the definition of disease found in the Nutrition Labeling and Health Act of 1989. Disease is currently considered damage to an organ, part, structure, or system of the body such that it does not function properly (e.g., cardiovascular disease) or a state of health leading to such (e.g., hypertension).

SCIENTIFIC BASIS

Significant research has been done using Western biomedical/scientific models on numerous single herbal agents. Beginning in 1978, the German government's *Bundesgesunheitsamt* (Federal Health Agency) began evaluating the safety and efficacy of phytomedicines. The health professionals charged with doing so, known as the Commission E, met until 1994 and evaluated 300 herbal medicines, of which they recognized 190 as suitable for medicinal use. The complete reports have been translated and are available from the American Botanical Council (2000).

Beginning in 1996, significant meta-analyses and review articles of single herb products began appearing on a regular basis in leading Western medical journals. These are readily accessible via the National Library of Medicine's PubMed website (www.ncbi.nlm.nih.gov/PubMed). Compiling data from similar studies for analysis (meta-analysis) is complicated by the fact that many studies published to date have left out important information, including naming the specific plant species studied (e.g., echinacea versus *Echinacea purpurea, E. pallida,* or *E. angustifolia*); the parts used (stems, leaves, or roots); the form (pressed juice, powdered whole extract, aqueous extract, ethanol extract, or aqueous-ethanol extract); and the formulation (stated proportions of water to alcohol or specifically extracted fractions and concentrations).

Standardization of herbal medicines is crucial both for scientific study and consumer protection. Standardization is equated with reproducibility, guaranteed potency, quality of active ingredients, and documentable effectiveness. However, with herbal medicines, standardization presents several problems. First, the active ingredient may not be known. Second, there may be more than one active ingredient. Third, both content and activity of an herbal medicine may be related to the means of extraction and processing. This significantly complicates both research and counseling for health professionals and consumers.

A growing number of health care professionals are studying the effects of these substances. With an increase in the FDA's involvement, we can look forward to a more reliable herb market. Expanded knowledge of herbal indications may augment the safety and efficacy of herbal therapies for patients.

INTERVENTION

Technique

Herbal medicines and dietary supplements need to be addressed in clinical settings in the same manner one addresses pharmaceutical agents. Every health professional needs to be aware of the wide use of herbal medicines and other dietary supplements. Efficient and effective patient advocacy means including questions on alternative therapies as a standard part of each patient interview. Reasonable questions include: "Are you using any herbs? Vitamins? Dietary supplements?" Follow-up questions could cover: "What dose? What source? What directions are you following? Why are you taking it?" Asking about the source of information can be quite helpful, as in, "Are you working with any other health professionals?" As with all good interviewing, listening for understanding rather than agreement or disagreement enhances the therapeutic alliance. In addition to knowing the type of herb used, the dose of each herb, and the intended purpose of each herb, gathering information regarding the duration of herb use will also be helpful in assessing patients and providing the best possible care.

Unfortunately, professionals often do not ask such questions and up to 69% of CAM-using patients do not volunteer such information (Graham et al., 2005). This "don't ask, don't tell" policy makes no sense in patient care. All health professionals need to create a safe environment that is conducive to patients' open sharing of important information, such as herbal use or use of other complementary/alternative therapies without fear of ridicule or other negative responses. "Ask, then, ask again" is a practice policy foundational to safe and effective patient care.

Precautions

A common misconception regarding herbal medicines is that herbs have no side effects because they are natural. However, herbs do indeed have side effects and may be toxic or poisonous if not used appropriately. Consider the toxicity of such widely used natural products as coffee, cocaine, and tobacco. Another dilemma is patient use of herbs in lieu of their prescribed medications. Although herbs may be a good option in particular cases and conditions, the decision to decline medications should be based on fully informed judgments in partnership with a health professional.

Interviewing for herbal medicine use is crucial for identifying those patients at risk for interactions with prescription medications or for excessive bleeding in surgery. Patients with special risks of drug interactions include those taking the following pharmaceutical agents: anticoagulants, hypoglycemics, antidepressants, sedative-hypnotics, antihypertensives, and medications with narrow therapeutic windows such as digoxin and theophylline. The significance of having knowledge of the ingestion of herbal medicines is illustrated in the list of known interactions of St. John's wort with commonly prescribed agents (see Exhibit 21.1).

Pregnancy, lactation, breastfeeding, and child care are special topics in herbal medicine use. For these situations, the most authoritative references are cited in Exhibit 21.2. In the absence of clinical trial data, use is guided by historical experience or breast milk analysis. Herbs that increase breast milk production, such as fenugreek, are frequently recommended by the International Board of Certified Lactation Consultants (IBCLC).

Exhibit 21.1. *Effect of St. John's Wort on Bioavailability of Selected Medications*

St. John's wort decreases the bioavailability of:
Calcium channel blockers Coumadin Cyclosporine Digoxin Irinotecan Oral contraceptives Protease inhibitors Simvastatin Tacrolimus Theophylline

Note: The effect can remain strong for weeks after stopping ingestion.

Exhibit 21.2. *Suggested Additional Reading for Pregnancy, Breastfeeding, Lactation, and Child Care*

Hale, T. W. (2004). *Medications and mother's milk: A manual of lactational pharmacology* (11th ed.). Amarillo, TX: Pharmasoft Medical Publishers.

Humphrey, S. (2004). *The nursing mother's herbal.* Minneapolis, MN: Fairview Press.

Kemper, K. J. (2002). *The holistic pediatrician* (2nd ed.). New York, NY: Perennial Currents.

Romm, A. J. (2003). *The natural pregnancy book.* Berkeley, CA: Ten Speed Press.

Exhibit 21.3. *Five Key Patient Teaching Points*

1. Just because it is natural does not mean it is safe.
2. Just because it is safe does not mean it is effective.
3. Labels may not equal contents.
4. Self-diagnosis and self-treatment can result in self-malpractice.
5. Herbs are never a replacement for an emergency room.

Nursing skills include the ability to counsel. Exhibit 21.3 lists key teaching points regarding herbal medicines. Herbal therapies are only safe if herbs are prepared in the right way and used for the precise indication, in the correct amounts, for the exact duration, and with appropriate monitoring. Potential herb–herb and herb–drug interactions should be considered when patients are using herbal products. The lack of national standards in the collection and preparation of herbal products complicates this field in the United States. Because many herbs have potential or actual risks that need to be recognized, it is important for health providers to have reliable and accessible sources of information to prevent adverse herb-related reactions and also to identify and manage complications of herbal therapies; Exhibit 21.4 cites selected reputable herbal references.

All serious adverse reactions should be reported to the FDA through the MedWatch program at 1-800-332-1088 or at www.fda.gov medwatch. An example of a complication associated with herbal therapy is illustrated in the case of the use of *Ma huang* (Ephedra), marketed in the United States until recently as a major ingredient in formulations for weight reduction. Because use of this herb had been linked to numerous adverse cardiovascular events, including stroke, myocardial infarction, and sudden death (Haller & Benowitz, 2000), the FDA banned sales of this herb in April 2004.

Exhibit 21.4. *Websites and Additional Resources*

American Botanical Council
(www.herbalgram.org)

American Nutraceutical Association
(www.americanutra.com)

Blumenthal, M., Goldberg, A., & Brinckmann, J. (Eds.). (2000). *Herbal medicine—The expanded Commission E Monographs.* Austin, TX: American Botanical Council.

FDA Center for Food Safety and Applied Nutrition—a link to report adverse events
(www.cfsan.fda.gov/~dms/aems.html)

HerbalGram magazine—published quarterly by the American Botanical Council and the Herb Research Foundation
(www.herbalgram.org)

Herb Research Foundation
(www.herbs.org)

Micromedex Alternative Medicine Database—an authoritative, full-text drug-information resource; includes alternative medicine and is one of the most comprehensive resources for herbal medicine.
(www.library.ucsf.edu/db/micromedex.html)

National Center for Complementary and Alternative Medicine
(www.nccam.nih.gov)

Springhouse. (2005). *Nursing Herbal Medicine Handbook* (3rd ed.). Philadelphia, PA: Lippincott, Williams, & Wilkins.

Tarascon Pocket Pharmacopoeia—contains a section on herbal and alternative therapies and has a PDA version that may be downloaded for a free trial.
(www.tarascon.com)

USES

Given the volume and variety of products, herbal medicine knowledge relevant for nursing practice cannot be summarized quickly. This chapter addresses three of the most important herbs from an evidence-based perspective. The reader will note that there is a significant range in scientific data available on each and the theoretical risks should be acknowledged and carefully considered both by patients and health professionals. Further, the clinical knowledge related to combining herbal products with prescription and nonprescription drugs is only in the developmental stages; much remains to be known about interactions and side effects.

Chronic illness (such as cancer or autoimmune disease or chronic pain), surgery, and use of prescription medications are three situations in which herbal medicine reviews by nurses are important. Echinacea does stimulate the immune system, but this is not necessarily a positive effect. Ginkgo biloba's pharmacological activity places people at risk in surgery. St. John's wort is effective for depression but can render many prescription medications ineffective or even toxic as previously noted. Readers should be aware that many herbs have a sufficient evidence base and potential as alternatives to Western medicine. However, herbal medicine in the United States is a very broad and multicultural phenomenon; it is difficult to know all products used by or all products of potential benefit to patients. Readers should be aware that there are reputable clinical resources readily accessible for assistance in informed decision making (e.g., see Exhibits 21.2 and 21.4).

The recent legalization of marijuana (*Cannabis sativa*) for distribution through approved dispensaries in 16 states and the District of Columbia deserves special attention. Medicinal marijuana is the first herbal medicine to require a prescription in the United States. Even before such changes in state laws, several prescription forms of cannabinoids existed in the United States and Canada. Dronabinol and Nabilone were used for treatment of nausea and vomiting associated with chemotherapy or anorexia with weight loss in patients with AIDS. However, since 1970, marijuana as an herbal medicine has been considered a Schedule 1 substance and therefore illegal and without medical value. This understanding has been challenged by the discovery of what has been termed the endocannabinoid system. The presence of cannabinoid receptors CB1 and CB2 in the central nervous system (CNS) and elsewhere suggests the possibility of many promising pharmaceutical applications (Bostwick, 2012; Bostwick, Reisfield, & DuPont, 2013).

The most frequent medical use of the leaves and flowering tops of the marijuana plant is for pain and muscle spasticity (Borgelt, Franson, Nussbaum, & Wang, 2013). Safety concerns for all patients include dizziness, impaired memory and cognition, increased risk of schizophrenia in adolescents, as well as accidental ingestions by children and pets. A cannabis withdrawal syndrome has also been described (Crippa et al., 2013). Cannabis use disorders (CUD) exist, especially among persons with a diagnosis of substance abuse and bipolar illness personality disorders. Nurses and all health professionals will increasingly need to screen patients for appropriate medical use (Lev-Ran, Le Foll, McKenzie, George, & Rehm, 2013).

Echinacea (Echinacea angustifolia, E. pallida, E. purpurea)

Echinacea is the most commonly used herbal medicine in the United States, used by people of all ages, genders, and ethnicities. This includes

19.8% of herbal medicine-using adults and 37.2% of herbal medicine-using children (Barnes et al., 2008). North American gardens commonly contain Echinacea, also known as the purple coneflower. It was traditionally used by Native Americans and early settlers as a remedy for infections and for healing wounds. Several components, particularly the alkamides and caffeic acid derivatives, have clear pharmacological activity (Barnes, Anderson, Gibbons, & Phillipson, 2005). In vitro research suggests an immunostimulatory effect principally by macrophage, polymorphonuclear leukocyte, and natural killer cell activation (Barrett, 2003). Monocyte secretion of tumor necrosis factor-alpha (TNF-α) is particularly stimulated (Senchina et al., 2005).

Echinacea is promoted in the United States for the prevention and treatment of the common cold. In Europe, it is used topically for wound healing and intravenously for immunostimulation. Several methodologically valid clinical studies have been published in recent years with unimpressive results, suggesting that Echinacea is not effective for the treatment or prevention of upper respiratory illness for adults. A 2006 meta-analysis by the prestigious Cochrane Collaborative stated that the Echinacea products used in clinical trials differed greatly, finding that preparations based on the aerial parts of *Echinacea purpurea* may be effective for the early treatment of colds (Linde, Barrett, Wolkart, Bauer, & Melchart, 2006). A follow-up meta-analysis of 14 randomized, controlled trials documented that Echinacea decreased the odds of developing a common cold by 58% and reduced the duration of symptoms by 1.4 days (Shah, Sander, White, Rinaldi, & Coleman, 2007). The most recent randomized, controlled placebo study of Echinacea followed 755 healthy participants for 4 months. The intervention used alcohol extract from freshly harvested *E. purpurea* leaves/roots. The active Echinacea intervention significantly reduced the total number of cold episodes (149 vs. 188), cumulated episode days (672 vs. 850), and episodes with any pain medication use (58 vs. 88), all $p < 0.05$. Recurrent infections also appeared to be reduced, 65 episodes in 28 participants taking Echinacea and 100 episodes in 43 participants taking placebo, $p < 0.05$ (Jawad, Schoop, Suter, Klein, & Eccles, 2012).

Echinacea has a good safety profile but has been associated (very infrequently) with gastric upset, rashes, and severe allergic reactions. It is not recommended for those with allergies to members of the Asteraceae family (formerly termed *Compositae*), which includes ragweed, daisies, thistles, and chamomile. More important, nonspecific immunostimulation may exacerbate preexisting autoimmune disease or precipitate autoimmune disease in genetically predisposed persons (Lee & Werth, 2004). TNF-α and interleukin-1 are proinflammatory cytokines, and recent evidence demonstrates that anti-TNF and anti–interleukin-1 therapies are effective for autoimmune diseases, including Crohn's disease and rheumatoid arthritis. Echinacea cannot be recommended for people with other chronic immunologic diseases, including multiple sclerosis, lupus, and HIV.

There are no verifiable reports of drug–herb interactions with any Echinacea product. *E. purpurea* products have a low potential for generating any cytochrome P450 drug–herb interactions (Freeman & Spelman, 2008, Hermann & von Richter, 2012). The LD_{50} of intravenously administered Echinacea juice is 50 mL/kg in mice and rats. Regular oral administration to mice at levels greater than proposed human therapeutic doses has failed to demonstrate toxic effects (Mengs, Clare, & Poiley, 1991).

Ginkgo (Ginkgo biloba)

Ginkgo is the number-one-selling herb in Europe for improvement of blood flow and enhancement of cognition. Clinically, ginkgo is used for circulatory problems such as peripheral artery disease (Pittler & Ernst, 2005), impotence (Sikora, 1989), and cerebral insufficiency (Kleijnen & Knipschild, 1992). The German government's Commission E also approved its use for dementia syndromes with memory deficits, disturbances in concentration, depressive emotional conditions, dizziness, tinnitus, and headaches.

The *Cochrane Review* in 2007 stated that ginkgo appears safe with no excess side effects, compared with placebo. Benefits were seen at doses of 200 mg a day beginning at 12 weeks. However, they noted that, because of variability in trial design and quality, the evidence for predictable and clinically significant benefit is unconvincing (Birks & Grimley Evans, 2007). A follow-up systematic review noted that in all studies with active controls, ginkgo was at least as effective as the pharmaceutical intervention (May et al., 2009). An additional review found that of seven studies with relatively high external validity and good overall quality, five showed a positive result in more than 50% of parameters measured (Bornhöft, Maxion-Bergemann, & Matthiessen, 2008).

European studies published in 1994 and 1996 demonstrated ginkgo's effectiveness in slowing or reversing dementia (Hofferberth, 1994; Kanowski, Herrmann, Stephan, Wierich, & Horr, 1996). A study published in 1997 affirmed these findings for patients with Alzheimer's disease and multi-infarct dementia in an American trial with 309 subjects (LeBars et al., 1997). Most recently, a double-blind, randomized, placebo-controlled trial of *Gingko biloba* (as EGB761) at 240 mg daily for 24 weeks in 410 participants with mild to moderate dementia and neuropsychiatric symptoms suggests efficacy. The study demonstrated safety and clinically significant findings ($p < 0.001$) in favor of EBG761 for cognition by a short cognitive performance test (Syndrom-Kurztest [SKT] test battery, Erzigkeit, 1992) and neuropsychiatric symptoms (by the Neuropsychiatric Inventory). Additionally, EGB761 administration improved functional measures and quality of life of patients (Herrschaft et al., 2012).

Recently, intriguing data have been published that suggest possible use of ginkgo in Parkinson's disease (Ahmad et al., 2005; Kim, Lee, Lee, & Kim, 2004) and diabetic retinopathy (Huang, Jeng, Kao, Yu, & Liu, 2004).

Additionally, there is interest in its use for cell phone users (Ilhan et al., 2004) and stressed adults (Walesiuk, Trofimiuk, & Braszko, 2005). However, larger trials are still needed to confirm such therapeutic benefit. Additionally, there is no convincing evidence that ginkgo enhances cognitive function in healthy young people (Canter & Ernst, 2007). *Gingko biloba* (as EGB761) does not appear beneficial for prevention of chemotherapy-associated cognitive changes (Barton et al., 2013) or for improvement of cognitive function in multiple sclerosis (Lovera et al., 2012).

Ginkgo's leaf extracts are used in Europe both orally and intravenously for treatment of Alzheimer's dementia, multi-infarct dementia, peripheral vascular disease, and vertigo (Kaufmann, 2002; Li, Ma, Scherban, & Tam, 2002). Ginkgo's active ingredients are terpene trilactones (6%; specifically, ginkgolides and bilobalide) and flavanoid glycosides (24%), which are the bases for standardized leaf extracts. Ginkgo's mechanism of action is believed to be its in vitro antioxidative, antiplatelet, antihypoxic, antiedemic, hemorrheologic, and microcirculatory actions (Mahadevan & Park, 2008). It is more effective than beta-carotene and Vitamin E as an oxidative scavenger and inhibitor of lipid peroxidation of cellular membranes (Pietschmann, Kuklinski, & Otterstein, 1992) and stimulates the release of nitric oxide (Chen, Salwinski, & Lee, 1997). Ginkgo is also a potent antagonist of platelet-activating factor (Engelsen, Nielson, & Winther, 2002) and thus inhibits platelet aggregation and promotes clot breakdown. Ginkgo in the CNS inhibits production of proinflammatory cytokines and upregulates anti-inflammatory cytokines (Jiao, Rui, Li, Yang, & Qiu, 2005). These properties may result in neuroprotective and ischemia reperfusion–protective effects (Oyama, Chikahisa, Ueha, Kanemaru, & Noda, 1996; Sener et al., 2005; Shen & Zhou, 1995).

Side effects with ginkgo are uncommon. They include gastrointestinal discomfort, headache, and dizziness. Because of its antiplatelet effect, however, it has been reported widely as a risk of significant bleeding when used with anticoagulants and other antiplatelet agents (Bebbington, Kulkarni, & Roberts, 2005; Matthews, 1998; Rosenblatt & Mindel, 1997; Rowin & Lewis, 1996). The most recent studies on ginkgo and platelet activity in vivo do not support concerns for perioperative bleeding or potentiation of anticoagulant or antiplatelet drugs (Beckert, Concannon, Henry, Smith, & Puckett, 2007; Bone, 2008). At this time, most surgeons request that ginkgo be discontinued 10 days prior to surgery and not restarted until the surgical wound has healed sufficiently to allow for aspirin use.

St. John's Wort (Hypericum perforatum)

St. John's wort, one of the world's top-selling herbs, has been used for centuries in Europe as a sedative and as a balm for skin injuries. Since 1996, it has been widely promoted in the United States as a wonder drug for depression or as "nature's Prozac." Today, it is often used to treat mild to moderate depression, anxiety, and sleep disorders. A task force of the American Psychiatric Association has noted promising research results in depression and recommended further study (Freeman et al, 2010). One study with 100 postmenopausal women demonstrated significant reductions in hot flash duration and severity (Abdali, Khajehei, & Tavatabaee, 2010).

In vitro studies have shown that *Hypericum* extract inhibits the neuronal uptake of the neurotransmitters serotonin, noradrenaline, dopamine, gamma-aminobutyric acid (GABA), and L-glutamate (Muller, Rolli, Schafer, & Hafner, 1997). No in vivo monoamine-oxidase [MAO]-inhibiting activity has been demonstrated with *Hypericum*.

Three significant reviews appeared in 2008 that demonstrated positive effects for *Hypericum* (Carpenter, Crigger, Kugler, & Loya, 2008; Kasper et al., 2008; Linde, Berner, & Kriston, 2008). In the *Cochrane Review* meta-analysis of 29 trials with 5,489 patients, 18 comparisons with placebo and 17 comparisons with prescription antidepressants were included. For nine large trials, the response-rate compared with placebo was 1.28 (95% confidence interval [CI]: 1.10, 1.49) and for nine smaller trials, the response-rate ratio was 1.87 (95% CI: 1.22, 2.87). The review team concluded that St. John's wort extracts are superior to placebo and similarly effective as standard prescription antidepressants with fewer side effects (Linde et al., 2008).

There is no one active ingredient in St. John's wort. Bioactive components include the napthodianthones hypericin and pseudohypericin and the phloroglucinols hyperforin and adhyperforin. Ginkgo also contains many flavonoids (Butterweck & Schmidt, 2007).

As previously noted in Exhibit 21.1, St. John's wort decreases the bioavailability of numerous agents. However, the most serious toxicity associated with St. John's wort is the negative interactions with prescription drugs. St. John's wort is a potent inducer of both P-glycoprotein and cytochrome P450 (CYP) 3A4, the hepatic enzyme involved in the metabolism of more than 50% of all prescription drugs (Zhou & Lai, 2008). Significant interactions include anticancer agents (imatinib and irinotecan), anti-HIV drugs (indinavir, lamivudine, and nevirapine), anti-inflammatory drugs (ibuprofen and fexofenadine), antibiotics/antifungals (erythromycin and voriconazole), cardiac medications (digoxin, ivabradine, warfarin, verapamil, nifedipine, atorvastatin, pravastatin, and talinolol), CNS agents (amitriptyline, buspirone, phenytoin, methadone, midazolam, alprazolam, and sertraline), diabetes medications (tolbutamide and gliclazide), and immunosuppressants (cyclosporine and tacrolimus), as well as oral contraceptives, proton pump inhibitors, and theophylline (Di, Li, Xue, & Zhou, 2008). Hence, the use of St. John's wort can be life threatening for people requiring prescription medications. Because of its long half-life, the herb should be discontinued at least 5 days prior to initiation of any of the above medications, and close monitoring of drug levels may be indicated. Additional theoretical concerns include the risk of photosensitivity or the precipitation of a serotonergic crisis in interaction with other prescription antidepressants.

CULTURAL APPLICATIONS

The practice of Western herbalism parallels that of Western pharmaceutical interventions. One herb with a defined pharmacological activity can be applied to a given patient with a given medical diagnosis. Successful treatment is understood as relief or eradication of the offending symptoms. Herbal medicines differ from pharmaceuticals in that—unlike plant-derived medications such as digoxin—single active agents are not identified, isolated, purified, and concentrated for human use. There is a presumed synergy of multiple bioactive components. Rigorous scientific studies are thus much more difficult to conduct than for pharmaceuticals.

In sharp contrast to the North American experience, Asian herbal traditions use formulas containing multiple herbs that are customized for the patient and often for unmeasurable constitutional states and unquantifiable outcomes. Up to 12 ingredients can exist in these formulas. Ingredients can include plants, mushrooms, and minerals. In Chinese formulas, animal parts are often included.

Of particular interest may be Japan's Kampo tradition as described in Sidebar 21.1. Today, in Japan, medical students are routinely taught to prescribe 148 ancient, multi-herb formulas that are approved by

---

Sidebar 21.1. *Kampo, Japan's Traditional Medicine*

Kenji Watanabe, Keio University Center for Kampo Medicine, Shinjuku-ku, Japan

Kampo, Japan's traditional medicine, is widely practiced, approved by the government's regulatory agencies, and covered by the national health plan. Unlike North American medical schools, Japanese medical students are taught to prescribe ancient, multiherb formulas. Both physicians and nurses are expected to know common uses and common side effects of these formulas.

Kampo literally means "way of the Han dynasty," the governmental period of ancient China from 220 BCE to 200 CE. During this time, many key medical texts were prepared. Japanese healers reinterpreted these to fit Japanese culture and historical experience. For this reason, Kampo today has many similarities to traditional Chinese medicine (TCM). However, there are several key points of differentiation. First, the Kampo

(continued)

Sidebar 21.1. *Kampo, Japan's Traditional Medicine (continued)*

physical examination focuses on the abdomen. Tongue and pulse diagnoses are considered but the abdominal examination, termed *fukushin*, is prioritized. Second, although many formulas are shared, Kampo uses may be quite different. Third, Kampo diagnostic and therapeutic approaches are standardized and easily work in conjunction with Western diagnoses and treatment plans. There is a robust scientific literature, especially in the basic sciences, to support rational herbal medicine prescribing.

Kampo herbal formulas are widely prescribed in both university and community hospitals across Japan. The Japanese Society of Oriental Medicine (JSOM) has annual meetings that attract many thousands of practitioners. Kampo is well understood in Japan.

Kampo's popularity and documented safety have promoted increasing international interest. As a result, JSOM has produced an introductory text in English. An excellent English translation of the works of revered Kampo master Keisetsu Otsuka has recently been published, and the International Society for Japanese Kampo Medicine (ISJKM) now holds international meetings in English (www.isjkm.com). Furthermore, in 2013, the journal *Evidence-Based Complementary and Alternative Medicine* hosted a special issue on the collaboration of Japanese Kampo medicine and Western medicine. Additionally, the World Health Organization (WHO) is developing a common platform for Western medicine and traditional medicine via the *International Classification of Diseases* (ICD). Under the revision from *ICD-10* to *ICD-11* (currently *ICD-11* beta is on the web apps.who.int/classifications/icd11/browse/f/en) traditional Asian medicine, including Kampo, will be incorporated. This will enhance mutual communication between Western medicine and Kampo internationally.

Recent Articles of Great Interest to English-Speaking Audiences

- Cameron, S., Reissenweber, H., & Watanabe, K. (2012). Asian medicine: Japan's paradigm [letter]. *Nature, 482*(7835), 35.
- Gepshtein, Y., Plotnikiff, G. A., & Watanabe, K. (2008). Kampo in women's health: Japan's traditional approach to premenstrual symptoms. *Journal of Alternative Complementary Medicine, 14*(4), 427–435.
- Ilto, A., Munakata, K., Imazu, Y., & Watanabe, K. (2012). First nationwide survey of Japanese physicians on the use of traditional Japanese medicine (Kampo) in cancer treatment. *Evidence Based Complementary Alternative Medicine* (eCAM), 1–8. Retrieved from http://www.ncbi.nlm.nih.gov/pmc/articles/PMC3526010

(continued)

Sidebar 21.1. *Kampo, Japan's Traditional Medicine (continued)*

■ Iwase, S., Yamaguchi, T., Miyajo, T., Terawaki, K., Inui, Q., & Uesono, Y. (2012). The clinical use of Kampo medicines (traditional Japanese herbal treatments) for controlling cancer patients' symptoms in Japan: A national cross-sectional survey. *BMC Complementary and Alternative Medicine*. Retrieved from http://www.biomedcentral.com/1472-6882/12/222

■ Watanabe, K., Matsuura, K., Gao, P., Hottenbacher, L., Tokunaga, H., Nishimura, K., . . . Witt, C. M. (2011). Traditional Japanese Kampo medicine: Clinical research between modernity and traditional medicine-the state of research and methodological suggestions for the future. *Evidence Based Complementary Alternative Medicine, 8*(1), 1–19.

Japan's equivalent of the FDA and covered by their national health plan. Approximately 70% of all physicians do prescribe these multi herb formulas, including nearly 100% of Japanese gynecologists. Diagnosis is made by physical exam of tongue, pulse, and abdomen. Diagnoses can be very subjective, such as *katakori* (literally, frozen shoulder, but patients have full range of motion) and *hiesho* (cold condition with normal body temperatures). There is no 1:1 correlation between a condition such as *hiesho* and a formula. Several formulas exist and are used for multiple conditions. The correct formula is based on the patient's history, physical exam, and response to initial treatment (Plotnikoff, Watanabe, & Yashiro, 2008).

FUTURE RESEARCH

Before even Western single-herb medicines can be more widely accepted by the conventional allopathic medical system, more randomized, double-blind, placebo-controlled trials are needed in the United States. The National Institutes of Health National Center for Complementary and Alternative Medicine (NCCAM) has funded and will continue to fund such clinical trials of herbal therapies. Promising understudied areas of research for herbal therapies include:

■ Perimenopausal hot-flash management
■ Prevention of chemotherapy side effects, including peripheral neuropathy
■ Chronic pain
■ Disabling fatigue
■ Refractory insomnia

Additionally, significant efforts are needed to identify the most promising herbal supports for radiation therapy, irritable bowel and inflammatory bowel, gastroparesis, as well as asthma and heart disease.

Western medicine has yet to explore the potential benefits from the world's many healing traditions that use customized combinations of herbs. To research these will require a new paradigm, one that accounts for potential synergy and counterbalancing activities of multiple ingredients. Although intriguing preliminary data exist for many dietary supplements, the historic paucity of funding mechanisms in these areas has meant that scientific support for the use of many commercial products lags significantly behind consumer marketing efforts.

REFERENCES

Abdali, K., Khajehei, M., & Tavatabaee, H. R. (2010). Effect of St. John's wort on severity, frequency and duration of hot flashes in premenopausal, perimenopausal and postmenopausal women: A randomized, double-blind, placebo controlled study. *Menopause, 17*(2), 326–331.

Ahmad, M., Saleem, S., Ahmad, A., Yousuf, S., Ansari, M. A., Khan, M. B., . . . Islam, F. (2005). Ginkgo biloba affords dose-dependent protection against 6-hydroxydopamine-induced parkinsonism in rats: Neurobehavioral, neuro-chemical and immunohisto-chemical evidence. *Journal of Neurochemistry, 93,* 94–104.

American Botanical Council. (2000). *Herbal medicine: Expanded commission E monographs.* Austin, TX: American Botanical Council.

Archer, E. L., & Boyle, D. K. (2008). Herb and supplement use among the retail population of an independent, urban herb store. *Journal of Holistic Nursing, 26,* 27–35.

Arcury, T. A., Suerken, C. K., Brzywacz, J. G., Bell, R. A., Lang, W., & Quandt, S. A. (2006). Complementary and alternative medicine use among older adults: Ethnic variation. *Ethnic Diseases, 16,* 723–731.

Barnes, J., Anderson, L. A., Gibbons, S., & Phillipson, J. D. (2005). *Echinacea* species (*Echinacea angustifolica* [DC.] Hell., *Echinacea pallida* [Nutt.] Nutt., *Echinacea purpurea* [L.] Moench): A review of their chemistry, pharmacology and clinical properties. *Journal of Pharmacy and Pharmacology, 57,* 929–954.

Barnes, P. M., Bloom, B., & Nahin, R. (2008, December 10). Complementary and alternative medicine use among adults and children: United States, 2007. *CDC National Health Statistics Report #12.*

Barnes, P. M., Powell-Griner, E., McFann, K., & Nahin, R. I. (2004). Complementary and alternative medicine use among adults: United States, 2002. *Advance Data, 343,* 1–19.

Barrett, B. (2003). Medicinal properties of echinacea: A critical review. *Phytomedicine, 10,* 66–86.

Barton, D. L., Burger, K., Novotny, P. J., Fitch, T. R., Kohli, S., Soori, G., . . . Loprinzi, C. L. (2013). The use of Gingko biloba for the prevention of chemotherapy-related cognitive dysfunction in women receiving adjuvant treatment for breast cancer, N00C9. *Support Care Cancer, 21*(4), 1185–1192.

Bebbington, A., Kulkarni, R., & Roberts, P. (2005). Ginkgo biloba: Persistent bleeding after total hip arthroplasty caused by herbal self-medication. *Journal of Arthroplasty, 20,* 125–126.

Beckert, B. W., Concannon, M. J., Henry, S. L., Smith, D. S., & Puckett, C. L. (2007). The effect of herbal medicines on platelet function: An in vivo experiment and review of the literature. *Plastic and Reconstructive Surgery, 120,* 2044–2050.

Birks, J., & Grimley Evans, J. (2007, April 18). Ginkgo biloba for cognitive impairment and dementia. *Cochrane Database of Systematic Reviews.* doi:10.1002/14651858. CD003120.pub2

Blumenthal, M., Busse, W. R., Goldberg, A., et al. (1998). *The complete German Commission E monographs.* Austin, TX: American Botanical Council.

Bone, K. M. (2008). Potential interaction of ginkgo biloba leaf with antiplatelet or anticoagulant drugs: What is the evidence? *Molecular Nutrition and Food Research, 52,* 764–771.

Borgelt, L. M., Franson, K. L., Nussbaum, A. M., & Wang, G. S. (2013). The pharmacologic and clinical effects of medical cannabis. *Pharmacotherapy, 33*(2), 195–209.

Bornhöft, G., Maxion-Bergemann, S., & Matthiessen, P. F. (2008). Die Rolle der externen Validität bei der Beurteilung klinischer Studien zur Demenzbehandlung mit Ginkgo-biloba-Extrakten [External validity of clinical trials for treatment of dementia with ginkgo biloba extracts]. *Zeitschrift für Gerontologie und Geriatrie, 41,* 298–312.

Bostwick, J. M. (2012). Blurred boundaries: The therapeutics and politics of medical marijuana. *Mayo Clinic Proceedings, 87*(2), 172–186.

Bostwick, J. M., Reisfield, G. M., DuPont, R. L. (2013) Clinical decisions. Medicinal use of marijuana. *New England Journal of Medicine, 368*(9), 866–868.

Butterweck, V., & Schmidt, M. (2007). St. John's wort: Role of active compounds for its mechanism of action and efficacy. *Wiener medizinische Wochenschrift, 157,* 356–361.

Canter, P. H., & Ernst, E. (2007). Ginkgo biloba is not a smart drug: An updated systematic review of randomized clinical trials testing the nootropic effects of G. biloba extracts in healthy people. *Human Psychopharmacology, 22,* 265–278.

Carpenter, C., Crigger, N., Kugler, R., & Loya, A. (2008). Hypericum and nurses: A comprehensive literature review on the efficacy of St. John's wort in the treatment of depression. *Journal of Holistic Nursing, 26,* 200–207.

Chen, X., Salwinski, S., & Lee, T. J. (1997). Extracts of Ginkgo biloba and ginsenosides exert cerebral vasorelaxation via a nitric oxide pathway. *Clinical Experimental Pharmacology and Physiology, 24,* 958–959.

Cherniack, E. P., Ceron-Fuentes, J., Florez, H., Sandals, L., Rodriguez, O., & Palacios, J. C. (2008). Influence of race and ethnicity on alternative medicine as a self-treatment for common medical conditions in a population of multi-ethnic urban elderly. *Complementary Therapies in Clinical Practice, 14,* 116–123.

Crippa, J. A., Hallak, J. E., Machado-de-Sousa, J. P., Queiroz, R. H., Bergamaschi, M., Chagas, M. H., & Zuardi, A. W. (2013). Canabidiol for the treatment of cannabis withdrawal syndrome: A case report. *Journal of Clinical Pharmacology and Therapeutics, 38*(2), 162–164.

Di, Y. M., Li, C. G., Xue, C. C., & Zhou, S. F. (2008). Clinical drugs that interact with St. John's wort and implication in drug development. *Current Pharmacology Design, 14,* 1723–1742.

Engelsen, J., Nielson, J. D., & Winther, K. (2002). Effect of coenzyme Q10 and ginkgo biloba on warfarin dosage in stable, long-term warfarin treated outpatients: A randomized double blind placebo-crossover trial. *Thrombosis & Haemostatis, 87*(6), 1075–1076.

Erzigkeit, H. (1992). SKT manual. A short cognitive performance test for assessing memory and attention. Concise version. Castrop-Rauxel: Geromed.

Freeman, C., & Spelman, K. (2008). A critical evaluation of drug interactions with Echinacea spp. *Molecular Nutrition and Food Research, 52,* 789–798.

Freeman, M. P., Fava, M., Lake, J., Trivedi, M. H., Wisner, K. L., & Mischoulon, D. (2010). Complementary and alternative medicine in major depressive disorder: The American Psychiatric Association Task Force Report. *Journal of Clinical Psychiatry, 71*(6), 669–681.

Graham, R. E., Ahn, A. C., Davis, R. B., O'Connor, B. B., Eisenberg, D. M., & Phillips, R. S. (2005). Use of complementary and alternative medical therapies among racial and ethnic minority adults: Results from the 2002 National Health Interview Survey. *Journal of the National Medical Association, 97*, 535–545.

Haller, C. A., & Benowitz, N. L. (2000). Adverse cardiovascular and central nervous system events associated with dietary supplements containing ephedra alkaloids. *New England Journal of Medicine, 343*(25), 1833–1838.

Hermann, R., & von Richter, O. (2012). Clinical evidence of herbal drugs as perpetrators of pharmacokinetic drug interactions. *Planta Medica, 78*(13), 1458–1477.

Herrschaft, H., Nacu, A., Likhachev, S., Sholomov, I., Hoerr, R., & Schlaefke, S. (2012). Gingko biloba extract EGB761 in dementia with neuropsychiatric features: A randomized, placebo-controlled trial to confirm the efficacy and safety of a daily dose of 240 mg. *Journal of Psychiatric Research, 46*(6), 716–723.

Hofferberth, B. (1994). The efficacy of Egb 761 in patients with senile dementia of the Alzheimer's type: A double-blind, placebo-controlled study on different levels of investigation. *Human Psychopharmacology, 9*, 215–222.

Huang, S. Y., Jeng, C., Kao, S. C., Yu, J. J., & Liu, D. Z. (2004). Improved haemorrheological properties by ginkgo biloba extract EGb 761 in type 2 diabetes mellitus complicated with retinopathy. *Clinical Nutrition, 23*, 615–621.

Ilhan, A., Gurel, A., Armutcu, F., Kamisli, S., Iraz, M., Akyol, O., & Ozen, S. (2004). Ginkgo biloba prevents mobile phone-induced oxidative stress in rat brain. *Clinica Chimica Acta, 340*, 153–162.

Jawad, M., Schoop, R., Suter, A., Klein, P., & Eccles, R. (2012). Safety and efficacy profile of Echinacea purpurea to prevent common cold episodes: A randomized, double-blind, placebo-controlled trial. *Evidence Based Complementary and Alternative Medicine*, http://dx.doi.org/10.1155/2012/841315

Jiao, Y. B., Rui, Y. C., Li, T. J., Yang, P. Y., & Qiu, Y. (2005). Expression of pro-inflammatory and anti-inflammatory cytokines in brain of atherosclerotic rats and effects of ginkgo biloba extract. *Acta Pharmacologica Sinica, 26*, 835–839.

Kanowski, S., Herrmann, W. M., Stephan, K., Wierich, W., & Horr, R. (1996). Proof of efficacy of the ginkgo biloba extract Egb 761 in outpatients suffering from mild to moderate primary degenerative dementia of the Alzheimer's type of multi-infarct dementia. *Pharmacopsychiatry, 29*, 47–56.

Kasper, S., Gastpar, M., Müller, W. E., Volz, H. P., Dienel, A., Kieser, M., & Möller, H. J. (2008). Efficacy of St. John's wort extract WS 5570 in acute treatment of mild depression: A reanalysis of data from controlled clinical trials. *European Archives of Psychiatry and Clinical Neuroscience, 258*, 59–63.

Kaufmann, H. (2002). Treatment of patients with orthostatic hypotension and syncope. *Clinical Neuropharmacology, 25*(3), 133–141.

Kim, M. S., Lee, J. I., Lee, W. Y., & Kim, S. E. (2004). Neuroprotective effect of ginkgo biloba L. extract in a rat model of Parkinson's disease. *Phytotherapy Research, 18*, 663–666.

Kleijnen, J., & Knipschild, P. (1992). Ginkgo biloba for cerebral insufficiency. *British Journal of Pharmacology, 34*, 352.

LeBars, P. L., Katz, M. M., Berman, N., Itil, T. M., Freedman, A. M., & Schatzberg, A. F. (1997). A placebo-controlled, double-blind, randomized trial of an extract of ginkgo biloba for dementia. *Journal of the American Medical Association, 278*, 1327–1332.

Lee, A. N., & Werth, V. P. (2004). Activation of autoimmunity following use of immuno-stimulatory herbal supplements. *Archives of Dermatology, 140*, 723–727.

Lev-Ran, S., Le Foll, B., McKenzie, K., George, T. P., & Rehm, J. (2013). Cannabis use and cannabis use disorders among individuals with mental illness. *Comprehensive Psychiatry, 54*(6), 589–598.

Li, X. F., Ma, M., Scherban, K., & Tam, Y. K. (2002). Liquid chromatography-electrospray mass spectrometric studies of ginkgolides and bilobalide using simultaneous monitoring of proton, ammonium, and sodium adducts. *Analyst, 127*, 641–646.

Linde, K., Barrett, B., Wölkart, K. Bauer, R., & Melchart, D., (2006). Echinacea for preventing and treating the common cold. *Cochrane Database of Systematic Reviews, 1*, CD000530.

Linde, K., Berner, M. M., & Kriston, L. (2008). St. John's wort for major depression. *Cochrane Database of Systematic Reviews, 4*, CD000448.

Lovera, J. F., Kim, E., Heriza, E., Fitzpatrick, M., Hunziker, J., Turner, A. P., . . . Bourdette, D. (2012). Gingko biloba does not improve cognitive function in MS: A randomized placebo-controlled trial. *Neurology, 79*(12), 1278–1284.

Mahadevan, S., & Park, Y. (2008). Multifaceted therapeutic benefits of ginkgo biloba L.: Chemistry, efficacy, safety and uses. *Journal of Food Science, 73*(1), R14–R19.

Matthews, M. K., Jr. (1998). Association of ginkgo biloba with intracerebral hemorrhage. *Neurology, 50*, 1933–1934.

May, B. H., Lit, M., Xue, C. C., Yang, A. W., Zhang, A. L., Owens, M. D., & Story, D. F. (2009). Herbal medicine for dementia: A systematic review. *Phytotherapy Research, 23*, 447–459.

Mengs, U., Clare, C. B., & Poiley, J. A. (1991). Toxicity of Echinacea purpurea. Acute, subacute and genotoxicity studies. *Arzneitmittel-Frosch, 41*, 1076–1081.

Miller, L. H., & Su, X. (2011) Artemisinin: Discovery from the Chinese herbal garden. *Cell, 146*(6), 855–858.

Muller, W. E., Rolli, M., Schafer, C., & Hafner, U. (1997). Effects of hypericum extract (L160) in biochemical models of antidepressant activity. *Pharmopsychiatry, 30*(Suppl. 2), S102–S107.

Oyama, Y., Chikahisa, L., Ueha, T., Kanemaru, K., & Noda, K. (1996). Ginkgo biloba extract protects brain neurons against oxidative stress induced by hydrogen peroxide. *Brain Research, 712*, 349–352.

Pietschmann, A., Kuklinski, B., & Otterstein, A. (1992). Protection from UV-light-induced oxidative stress by nutritional radical scavengers. *Zeitschrift fur die Gesamte Innere Medizin und Ihre Grenzgebite, 47*(11), 518–522.

Pittler, M. H., & Ernst, E. (2005). Complementary therapies for peripheral artery disease: Systematic review. *Atherosclerosis, 18*, 1–7.

Plotnikoff, G. A, Watanabe, K., & Yashiro, F. (2008). Kampo: From old wisdom comes new knowledge. *HerbalGram, 78*, 46–56.

Rosenblatt, M., & Mindel, J. (1997). Spontaneous hyphema associated with ingestion of ginkgo biloba extract. *New England Journal of Medicine, 336*, 1108.

Rowin, J., & Lewis, S. L. (1996). Spontaneous bilateral subdural hematomas associated with chronic ginkgo biloba ingestion have also occurred. *Neurology, 46*, 1775–1776.

Senchina, D. S., McDann, D. A., Asp, J. M., Johnson, J. A., Cunnick, J. E., Kaiser, M. S., & Kohut, M. L. (2005). Changes in immunomodulatory properties of Echinacea spp. root infusions and tinctures stored at 4 degrees C for four days. *Clinica Chimica Acta, 355*, 67–82.

Sener, G., Sener, E., Sehirli, O., Ogune, A. V., Cetinel, S., Gedik, N., & Sakarcan, A. (2005). Ginkgo biloba extract ameliorates ischemia reperfusion-induced renal injury in rats. *Pharmacology Research, 52*(3), 216–222.

Shah, S. A., Sander, S., White, C. M., Rinaldi, M., & Coleman, C. I. (2007). Evaluation of echinacea for the prevention and treatment of the common cold: A meta-analysis. *Lancet Infectious Disease, 7,* 473–480.

Shen, J. G., & Zhou, D. Y. (1995). Efficiency of ginkgo biloba extract (Egb 761) in antioxidant protection against myocardial ischemia and re-perfusion injury. *Biochemical Molecular Biological Institute, 35,* 125–134.

Sikora, K. (1989). Complementary medicine and cancer treatment. *Practitioner, 233*(1476), 1285–1286.

U.S. Congress, House of Representatives, Committee on Government Reform. (1999, March 25). *Dietary Supplement Health and Education Act: Is the FDA trying to change the intent of Congress?* Washington, DC: U.S. Government Printing Office.

U.S. Congress (1994). 103rd Congress. Dietary Supplement Health and Education Act of 1994. Pub. L. 103-417. 108 Stat/4325-4335. In Library of Congress, Washington, D.C.

U.S. Congress, Senate Committee on Labor and Human Resources. (1989, November 13). *Nutrition Labeling and Education Act of 1989* [S.1425]. Washington, DC: U.S. Government Printing Office.

Walesiuk, A., Trofimiuk, E., & Braszko, J. J. (2005). Ginkgo biloba extract diminishes stress-induced memory deficits in rats. *Pharmacology Reporter, 57,* 176–187.

Ward, E., & Blumenthal, M. (2005). Americans confident in dietary supplements according to CRN survey. *HerbalGram, 66,* 64–65.

Zhou, S. F., & Lai, X. (2008). An update on clinical drug interactions with the herbal antidepressant St. John's wort. *Current Drug Metabolism, 9*(5), 394–409.

Chapter 22: Functional Foods and Nutraceuticals

Melissa H. Frisvold

*I*n the 21st century, the focus of the relationship between eating habits and health is changing from an emphasis on health maintenance through recommended dietary allowances of nutrients, vitamins, and minerals to an emphasis on the use of foods to provide better health, increase vitality, and aid in preventing disease and many chronic illnesses. The connection between food and health is not new. Indeed, the adage "Let food be your medicine and medicine your food" was adopted by Hippocrates (trans. 1932). Today, the philosophy that supports the paradigm of nutraceuticals as functional foods is once again at the forefront.

The U.S. consumer has become increasingly interested in the use of functional foods and nutraceuticals to improve health. There has been a paradigm shift from a reliance on prescription drugs to the realization that food can and should play an important role in health and well-being. This shift has created a market for functional foods and nutraceuticals (Bagchi, 2008). With the developing market of functional foods, it is estimated that in 2010 consumers in the United States spent approximately $126.31 per capita out of pocket on functional foods (Deloitte, 2012).

The vast array of nutraceutical products is staggering. Products range from single-ingredient nutrients such as calcium to drinks fortified with electrolytes and cereals fortified with iron (Haller, 2010). Many companies are using soy protein isolates in foods ranging from candy bars and salad dressings to infant formulas. Plant stanols and sterols are being added to margarinelike spreads in an effort to reduce total cholesterol and low-density lipoprotein (LDL) levels.

Coverage of all nutraceuticals is beyond the scope of this chapter. There has been a plethora of functional foods developed in recent times. An estimate is that more than 100 million people in the United States use nutraceuticals. This makes the nutraceutical industry an $86 billion industry (National Nutraceutical Center, 2012). In the interest of brevity, several selected products are covered in depth in this chapter. Because the use of nutraceuticals is so prevalent and because their use may impact health and wellness, it is important that nurses know about nutraceuticals and their potential benefits and risks.

DEFINITIONS

According to Haller (2010), the term *nutraceutical* is a portmanteau of the words *nutrition* and *pharmaceutics*. Originally coined by Dr. Stephen DeFelice, nutraceuticals are defined as "food, or parts of food, that provide medical or health benefits, including the prevention and treatment of disease" (National Nutraceutical Center, 2012). Nutraceutical categories include dietary supplements such as Ginkgo biloba, functional foods such as plant stanols, and medicinal foods such as health bars with added medication (National Nutraceutical Center, 2012). Nutraceuticals encompass any food part that may offer a benefit to health (Haller, 2010). These terms are often used interchangeably. The number and variety of nutraceuticals available in the United States are staggering, For example, many grocery stores carry cereals fortified with omega-3 fatty acids, Ginseng-enriched sports drinks, dairy products with various strains of probiotics, and orange juice that contains added calcium. The intent of the Dietary Supplement Health and Education Act, passed in 1994, was to protect the rights of consumers to have access to dietary supplements (and thus nutraceuticals and functional foods) to promote good health (Food and Drug Administration [FDA], 2012). Under the provisions of the law, dietary supplement ingredients are exempt from drug regulations; and thus premarketing approval, including demonstration of benefit and safety, is not required (Haller, 2010).

Functional foods are defined as manufactured foods for which scientifically valid claims can be made. They may be produced by food-processing technologies, traditional breeding, or by genetic engineering. Functional foods should safely deliver a long-term health benefit. Accordingly, a functional food may be one of the following:

- A known food to which a functional ingredient from another food is added
- A known food to which a functional ingredient new to the food supply is added
- An entirely new food that contains one or more functional ingredients (Pariza, 1999)

The Japanese, who were among the first to use functional foods, have highlighted three conditions that define a functional food:

- It is a food (not a capsule, tablet, or powder) derived from naturally occurring ingredients.
- It can and should be consumed as part of a daily diet.
- It has a particular function when ingested, serving to regulate a particular body process: enhancement of the biological defense mechanism, prevention of a specific disease, recovery from a specific disease, control of physical and mental conditions, and slowing of the aging process (PA Consulting Group, 1990).

According to these definitions, unmodified whole foods such as fruits and vegetables represent the simplest form of a functional food. For example, broccoli, carrots, or tomatoes would be considered functional foods because they contain high levels of physiologically active components such as beta-carotene, lycopene, and sulforaphane. Modified foods, including those that have been fortified with nutrients or enhanced with phytochemicals, are also within the realm of functional foods.

SCIENTIFIC BASIS

During the past century there have been many changes in the types of foods people eat. This reflects the application of scientific findings and technological innovations in the food industry. Although much research has been conducted on nutrition and health and disease, scientific exploration on the use of nutraceuticals has been more limited.

Interest in foodstuffs has generated investigation to link nutrient and food intake with improvements in health or prevention of disease. Studies in the epidemiological literature have been reviewed and suggest a possible association between a low consumption of fruits and vegetables and the incidence of certain diseases such as heart disease (He, Nowson, & MacGregor, 2006; He, Nowson, Lucas, & MacGregor, 2007), and a recent research article in the *Journal of the National Cancer Institute* (2013) suggests that vegetable consumption may reduce the risk of certain types of breast cancer (Rathner, 2013).

Much scientific study has been conducted on the role of the various products added to normal foods to enhance their ability to inhibit or prevent diseases. Many regard dietary intake as the best means of acquiring necessary nutrients (Kottke, 1998). For example, a report by the World Cancer Research Fund/American Institute for Cancer Research (2007) suggests that although there may be evidence to support that the consumption of some fruits and vegetables may protect against certain types of cancers, it is important to point out that these foods contain various micronutrients and therefore it is difficult to tease out that a certain element of the food alone is responsible for this protective effect. However, supplementation of nutrients is common. Therefore, the findings of scientific research focused on selected nutraceuticals are summarized below.

Dietary Plant Stanols and Sterols

The cholesterol-lowering potential of dietary plant stanols and sterols has been known for many years (Plat et al., 2012). Modifying plant stanols and sterols structurally makes them easily incorporated into fat-containing foods without losing their effectiveness in lowering cholesterol (Cater & Grundy, 1998). Dietary plant stanols and sterols inhibit the absorption of cholesterol in the small intestine, which in turn can lower LDL blood cholesterol (de Jong, Plat, & Mensink, 2003). In fact, it has been suggested that lifestyle modification, which includes dietary changes such as the inclusion of plant stanols and sterols, should be the primary treatment for lowering cholesterol (Turpeinen et al., 2012). Thus functional foods offer a safe and easily attainable method to decrease heart disease risk (Turpeinen et al., 2012). Currently, the recommended intake dose of plant stanols and plant sterols is 2g a day (Plat et al., 2012). However, it has been demonstrated in a limited number of clinical trials that a further reduction in LDL cholesterol may be achieved at doses as high as 9g a day but additional research is necessary before this can be recommended (Plat et al., 2012).

Plant sterols and their esters are generally recognized as safe (GRAS) food-grade substances, a designation indicating that there has been a history of safe intake of these products with no demonstrated harmful health effects found in the research (Wrick, 2005). Overall, the Nutrition Committee of the American Heart Association advises that stanols and sterol esters not be used as a preventive measure in the general population with normal cholesterol levels, in light of limited data regarding any potential risks. They may be used, however, for adults with hypercholesterolemia or adults requiring secondary prevention after an atherosclerotic event (Lichtenstein et al., 2006).

Glucosamine and Chondroitin Sulfate

Glucosamine, an amino sugar the body produces, and chondroitin sulfate, a complex carbohydrate found in and around cartilage cells, are natural substances (National Center for Complementary and Alternative Medicine, 2013). Glucosamine and chondroitin sulfate are two separate products; however, they are often sold together to diminish the pain and stiffness of osteoarthritis. Historically, German physicians were reported to be the first to use glucosamine in 1969 to diminish pain and increase mobility in patients with osteoarthritis (Natural Standard, 2013a). According to Kolata (2006), glucosamine and chondroitin sulfate are the most popular supplements in the United States. Natural Standard ranks glucosamine and chondroitin sulfate as grade A (strong scientific evidence) for osteoarthritis of the knee, and chondroitin sulfate without glucosamine as grade A for general osteoarthritis (2013b). The results of several studies in the literature, however, have been mixed. A National Institutes of Health trial conducted by Clegg, Red, and Harris (2006) on glucosamine and chondroitin and their potential use in arthritis (GAIT) was inconclusive. Meta-analyses by McAlindon, LaValley, Gulin, and Felson (2000) and by Towheed and Hochberg (1997) reviewed clinical trials of glucosamine and chondroitin in the treatment of osteoarthritis. McAlindon and colleagues included 13 double-blind, placebo-controlled trials of more than 4 weeks' duration, testing oral or parenteral glucosamine or chondroitin for treatment of hip or knee arthritis. All 13 studies were classified as positive, demonstrating substantial benefits in treating arthritis when compared with placebo. Towheed and Hochberg reviewed nine randomized, controlled studies of glucosamine in osteoarthritis. Glucosamine was superior when compared with placebo in seven randomized trials. Two of the randomized trials compared glucosamine with ibuprofen. In these two trials, glucosamine was superior in one and equivalent in the other. A recent meta-analysis in 2010 concluded that compared with placebo, glucosamine, chondroitin, or the combination of these two products did not reduce joint pain (Wandel et al., 2010).

Glucosamine continues to be a major market force in the United States with estimated sales in 2009 of $872 million (Brissette, 2011). Sales have slowed, however, when compared to other nutraceuticals, possibly due to research questioning its effectiveness.

Coenzyme Q10

Coenzyme Q10 (CoQ10) is a compound made naturally in the body. It is used by cells to produce energy needed for cell growth and maintenance. It is also used by the body as an antioxidant. Tissue levels of CoQ10 decrease with age. It has been suggested that CoQ10 may stimulate the immune system and increase resistance to disease; however, currently there are no well-designed clinical trials to support this claim (National Cancer Institute, 2013). Cardiovascular health continues to be the main area of study for use with this compound. Several controlled trials of CoQ10 have been performed for the indication of congestive heart failure, and the results have been varied (Khatta et al., 2000). There have also been suggested benefits to health from CoQ10 for statin-associated myalgias (Caso, Kelly, McNurland, & Lawson, 2007). A review article by Littarru and Tiano (2010) suggests there may be some potential benefit from CoQ10 for fatigue and performance issues with exercise, preeclampsia, and for men with a decreased sperm count (Littaru & Tiano, 2010). Further research is needed to verify these claims. Other therapeutic claims attributed to

CoQ10 involve hypertension, impaired immune status, adjuvant therapy for breast cancer, and various neurologic disorders. As always, caution must be exercised when suggesting supplementation with any nutraceutical during pregnancy.

Probiotics

Probiotics are microorganism supplements intended to improve health or treat a certain disease. Probiotics are also called friendly bacteria, and the normal digestive tract contains 400 types of probiotic bacteria (Natural Standard, 2013b). Yogurt is an example of a probiotic food source. Probiotics also come in other forms such as tablets or capsules. They have not been approved by the Food and Drug Administration (FDA) for any indication. Although the exact mechanism of action is unclear, there are several that are proposed: a lowering in intestinal pH and inhibition of pathogenic bacteria, a physical or chemical prevention of colonization of pathogenic bacteria, or an induction or enhancement of an immune response (The Medical Letter, 2013). The focus of research and the most promising results continue to be in disorders associated with the gastrointestinal tract. Based on the results of a few randomized controlled clinical trials, probiotics may be useful to treat *Clostridium difficile* (Johnson et al., 2012) and diarrhea, which is associated with antibiotic use (Kligler & Cohrssen, 2008). Probiotics have also been studied for potential use in women for bacterial vaginosis, vulvovaginal candidiasis, and urinary tract infections. The results have been conflicting. There is some evidence to support the use of probiotics for symptomatic and asymptomatic bacterial vaginosis but no evidence to support the use of probiotics for vulvovaginal candidiasis (Jurden, Buchanan, Kelsberg, & Safranek, 2012). A systematic review by Barrons and Tassone (2008) failed to find support for the use of probiotics in the treatment of bacterial vaginosis or urinary tract infections in women due to lack of standardization of probiotic strain and product stability.

Further studies are necessary because some of the initial work did demonstrate some promise, but these studies should focus on specific strains of probiotics. Finally, according to the Natural Standard Monograph (2013b) on probiotics, there is grade A evidence (strong evidence to support) for the use of probiotics for diarrhea and atopic dermatitis. There is grade B evidence to support probiotic use for immune enhancement, ulcerative colitis, dental caries, cirrhosis, and sinusitis. It is important to note that there are many different strains of probiotics and they are not all recommended for treatment of various health conditions; therefore, each condition should be carefully researched before recommendations for use are made.

Exhibit 22.1. *Guidelines: Nutraceutical Assessment Guide for Nurses*

- Screen for nutraceutical use as a routine part of the health assessment interview process. Because surgical complications can arise from nutritional supplement use, their dosage is often discontinued a few weeks before surgery.
- Acquire a working knowledge of functional foods and nutraceuticals that includes benefits/risks, costs, and possible drug interactions.
- Develop effective communication strategies to ensure that all members of a patient's health care team are aware of any nutraceutical use.
- Explore the reasons for the use of nutritional supplements and functional foods. Can the same benefits be achieved by using another product that is safer or less expensive?
- Consider the unique health care needs of various populations. It is important that pregnant women, children, older adults, and populations with certain medical conditions discuss any nutritional supplementation use with their health care provider prior to initiation.
- Provide educational resources for patients that are easy to access, timely, evidence based, and easy to understand.
- Remember to consult with and refer patients to nutritionists—knowledgeable and accessible resources in this promising and rapidly changing area of health and wellness.

INTERVENTION

Many people are using nutraceuticals. Hence, it is important that nurses include assessment of nutraceutical use when they obtain the health history of the patient. Exhibit 22.1 presents guidelines for nurses to use in assessing patients. In addition, Exhibit 22.2 lists reputable sites for information about nutraceuticals. Patients should be encouraged to be open about their use as part of their communication about their preferences and efforts toward good health; thus, the response of health providers should be open and nonjudgmental, despite the potential need to counsel changes or discontinuance of the nutraceutical based on the evidence or knowledge of the provider. The expertise of professionals of other disciplines may be called on as well through referral or consultation to ensure that the patient receives up-to-date information from the latest evidence regarding safety and efficacy of the product used.

Exhibit 22.2. *Websites*

American Dietetic Association
(www.eatright.org)

American Nutraceutical Association
(www.ana-jana.org)

International Food Safety Council
(www.ific.org/nutrition/functional/index.cfm)

Mayo Clinic
(www.mayoclinic.org)

National Institutes of Health—National Center for Complementary and Alternative Medicine
(nccam.nih.gov)

National Institutes of Health—National Library of Medicine
(www.ncbi.nlm.nih.gov)

National Institutes of Health—Office of Dietary Supplements
(dietary-supplements.info.nih.gov)

Natural Medicines Comprehensive Database
(www.naturaldatabase.com)

U.S. Department of Agriculture—Food and Nutrition Information Center
(www.nal.usda.gov)

U.S. Department of Health and Human Services—Office of Disease Prevention and Health Promotion
(www.healthfinder.gov)

U.S. Food and Drug Administration—Center for Food Safety and Applied Nutrition
(www.cfsan.fda.gov/~dms/supplmnt.html)

Measurement of Outcomes

Outcomes of therapy can be assessed in a number of ways, depending on the nutraceutical and the intent of the therapy. For example, blood levels of the nutrient or effect on the target organ (e.g., bone density, with the use of calcium) could be monitored over time. Also, it is important that potential side effects of the therapy be evaluated in periodic physical assessments and comprehensive histories. Positive or negative changes in subjective health, energy, and symptoms, or those subsequent to changes in nutraceutical use, can also be assessed in individuals as data for tolerance as part of cost–benefit evaluation. Good teaching of nutraceutical principles, intended purpose, and doses and effects of functional foods will result in informed use by clients and greater awareness of intended and adverse effects.

Precautions

As stated previously, it is of paramount importance that nutraceutical use be assessed as part of the health history and nutritional assessment. Safe use, including safe dosage, drug interactions, and side effects, must be carefully considered. MEDLINE offers a system for checking interactions among commonly used nutraceuticals and prescription drugs (MEDLINE, 2013).

A consistent concern cited in the literature is the lack of regulation of nutraceuticals. Dietary supplements fall under the jurisdiction of the FDA but do not have the same regulations as food and drug products (FDA, 2013). According to the Dietary Supplement Health and Education Act (DSHEA), the manufacturer is responsible to ensure that a product is safe before it is marketed and once the supplement reaches the market, the FDA is responsible to take action if issues with the product arise (FDA, 2012).

One safety mechanism in place to ensure the production of quality products for consumers is a voluntary dietary supplement verification program through the U.S. Pharmacopeial Convention (USP). If a product contains the USP-verified mark on its label, it demonstrates that the item has been tested and audited as a supplement that meets certain criteria for declared potency and amount, that it does not contain harmful levels of contaminants, and that it meets the FDA's good manufacturing practices (U.S. Pharmacopeial Convention, 2013).

USES

Nutraceuticals have been used to promote health and to prevent and treat illness. Nutraceuticals can be used to target deficiencies, establish optimal nutritional balance, or treat diseases. Because heart disease, cancer, and stroke are leading causes of death in the United States, greater access to nutraceuticals that have been shown to improve risk-factor profiles is desirable. Furthermore, people in the United States and worldwide could benefit from nutraceuticals when there are deficiencies of specific nutrients.

Children and Adolescents

There is a paucity of literature about nutraceutical use in the child and adolescent population. This is a population with unique nutritional needs because this is a time when growth and development occur at a rapid pace. Not only can nutrition during this time impact current health status, it may have implications for lifelong health as well.

Heart disease, once thought to be a disease of aging, is now recognized as starting in childhood. One recommended approach to this problem is through dietary interventions that treat dyslipidemia with a low-fat diet supplemented with water-soluble fiber, plant stanols, and plant sterols (Kwiterovich, 2008).

In 2001, the American Academy of Pediatrics (AAP) published a survey of its members on the beliefs and use of complementary and alternative therapies (CAM) in their respective practices. Based on the findings of this survey, in 2002, the AAP developed a task force to educate families, patients, and physicians about complementary therapies. One outcome of this task force was the recommendation to research the use of CAM therapies in the pediatric population. It is important to recognize that many families are using nutraceuticals such as nutritional supplements or functional foods with their children. For example, a study on CAM use in teenagers found that among teenagers who use complementary and alternative therapies, 75% use herbal products and other nutritional supplements (Kemper, Vohra, & Walls, 2008).

Women's Health and Nutritional Needs

Throughout their life span, women have unique nutritional needs that place them at risk for nutrition-related diseases and conditions. Nutrition has been shown to have a significant influence on the risk of chronic disease and on the maintenance of optimal health status. Although food should be the first choice in meeting such needs, nutritional supplementation may be necessary (American Dietetic Association, 2001). Following are some examples of increased nutritional needs across the life span of women:

- An increase in calcium during pregnancy and menopause is necessary.
- Folic acid requirements increase during pregnancy to prevent neural tube defects.
- Iron needs increase during menstruation and pregnancy.

Although acquiring these nutrients through food sources would be ideal, supplementation is often necessary. It is also important to remember that intake of certain nutrients above a certain level can be teratogenic (e.g., too much vitamin A in the first trimester of pregnancy) and, because many foods are often enriched with vitamins and minerals, it is possible to consume too much.

CULTURAL APPLICATIONS

The influence of culture on both the use and acceptance of functional foods is an important consideration. The attitudes of one's culture mold one's views about everything, including food (McCracken, 1986). A functional food may be more accepted if it is seen as consistent with traditional consumption (Wansink, 2002). A study by Mullie et al. (2009) found a correlation between culture and the intake of functional foods. For example, soy is widely used in Asian cultures and is considered to be a traditional food source, with customary soy intake being estimated at 30 grams to 50 grams per day (Cornwell, Cohick, & Raskin, 2004). Hence, the use of soy as a nutraceutical may be more widely and easily accepted by someone in an Asian culture because this food is already so widely used. In addition, how food itself is viewed within the context of culture may have a strong influence on the use of nutraceuticals and functional foods. The use of nutraceuticals in Eastern Europe is described in Sidebar 22.1.

Sidebar 22.1. *Nutraceuticals in Russia and Ukraine*

Olga Formogey, Russia and Ukraine

Use of herbal products and supplements is growing in countries such as Russia and Ukraine, ascending from small villages and towns in rural areas and becoming increasingly more popular in large cities. The health and wellness market in Eastern Europe is currently experiencing dynamic growth, with consumers in large cities following the global trend toward healthy food and lifestyles. Fortified and functional food and beverages are present in all food sectors in the Russian and Ukrainian markets. Probiotic dairy products, such as yogurt and kefir, have always been popular in Russia. Russians are very conscious of their body image. Yogurt, yogurt drinks, and kefir are popular food items because yogurt already has a healthy image among consumers. The most popular yogurts besides local products are Danone and Vimm-Bill-Dann. Activia yogurts by Danone are enriched with streptococcus and *lactobacillus bulgaricus* bacteria. Other popular fortified foods are milk enriched with vitamin D and calcium, and bread or wheat products containing folic acid.

(continued)

Sidebar 22.1. *Nutraceuticals in Russia and Ukraine (continued)*

In Russia, dietary supplements are defined as biologically active dietary supplements (BADS). The aging Russian population, along with the increasing prevalence of urban lifestyle-related diseases, has shifted the focus from nutrition issues to using dietary supplements and vitamins to reach and maintain optimal health. Consumers are becoming increasingly focused on nutrition and health and interested in the role that vitamins and dietary supplements play. Dietary supplements in Russia and Ukraine are distributed only through pharmacies and are controlled by the Ministry of Healthcare.

FUTURE RESEARCH

Although nutraceuticals have a longstanding historical usage, increased interest in these substances to promote health, prevent disease, and treat specific medical conditions is reflected in heightened attention to nutritional science and growing consumption. A consistent theme throughout this chapter has been the need for more research in this area. The book *Complementary and Alternative Medicine in the United States* (Institute of Medicine, 2005) summarizes succinctly what the goal for research in this arena should be: "In terms of medical therapies, a commitment to public welfare is the obligation to generate and provide to health care practitioners, policy makers, and the public access to the best information available on the efficacy of CAM therapies" (p. 169). Consistent with this sentiment, and because there is so much interest and hope in this area, interdisciplinary research teams may explore the following questions:

- Which of the current nutraceuticals should be incorporated in a normal diet on a regular basis to promote health?
- Are nutraceuticals cost-effective?
- What are the side effects associated with short- and long-term use of specific nutraceuticals?
- Can we increase research in the use of nutraceuticals in the pediatric population?
- What are innovative ways to educate health care providers about nutraceuticals?
- Can we discover more effective methods to educate the U.S. health care consumer about the benefits/risks of nutraceuticals?
- How does culture affect the use of functional foods?

ACKNOWLEDGMENT

The author wishes to acknowledge and thank Bridget Doyle for her contributions to this chapter in a previous edition.

REFERENCES

American Academy of Pediatrics. (2001). *Periodic Survey #49: Complementary and alternative medicine (CAM) therapies in pediatric practices.* Retrieved May 25, 2005, from http://www.aap.org/research/periodicsurvey/ps49bex.htm

American Dietetic Association. (2001). *Position paper: Nutrition and women's health.* Retrieved May 31, 2005, from http://www.eatright.org/Member/Policy Initiatives/index_21017.cfm

Anonymous. (2013). Probiotics revisted [review]. *The Medical Letter on Drugs & Therapeutics, 55*(1407), 3–4.

Bagchi, D. (2008). Preface. In D. Bagchi (Ed.), *Nutraceutical and functional food regulation in the United States* (pp. xi–xiv). Waltham, MA: Academic Press.

Barrons, R., & Tassone, D. (2008). Use of *Lactobacillus* probiotics for bacterial genitourinary infections in women: A review. *Clinical Therapeutics, 30*(3), 453–468.

Brissette, S. (2011). Glucosamine—The bubble is burst . . . maybe. . . . *Health World Net.* Retrieved from http://www.healthworldnet.com/articles/the-cutting-edge/glucosamine-the-bubble-is-burst...-maybe.html

Caso, G., Kelly, P., McNurland, M. A., & Lawson, W. E. (2007). Effect of coenzyme q10 on myopathic symptoms in patients treated with asthma. *American Journal of Cardiology, 99*(10), 1409.

Cater, N. B., & Grundy, S. M. (1998). Lowering serum cholesterol with plant sterols and stanols: Historical perspectives. In T. T. Nguyen (Ed.), *New developments in the dietary management of high cholesterol* (Postgraduate Medicine Special Report, pp. 6–14). Minneapolis, MN: McGraw-Hill.

Clegg, D., Red, D. J., & Harris, C. L. (2006). Glucosamine, chondroitin sulfate, and the two in combination for painful knee osteoarthritis. *New England Journal of Medicine, 354*(8), 795–808.

Cornwell, T., Cohick, W., & Raskin, I. (2004). Dietary phytoestrogens and health. *Phytochemistry, 65*, 995–1016.

de Jong, A., Plat, J., & Mensink, R. P. (2003). Metabolic effects of plant sterols and stanols [review]. *Journal of Nutritional Biochemistry, 14*(7), 362–369.

Deloitte Center for Health Solutions. (2012). *The hidden costs of U.S. healthcare: Consumer discretionary healthcare spending.* Retrieved from http://www.deloitte.com/assets/Dcom-UnitedStates/Local Assets/Documents/us_dchs_2012_hidden_costs112712.pdf

Food and Drug Administration. (2012). *Dietary supplement.* Retrieved from http://www.fda.gov/food/dietarysupplements

Haller, C. A. (2010). Nutraceuticals: Has there been any progress? *Clinical Pharmacology & Therapeutics, 87*(2), 137–141.

He, F. J., Nowson, C. A., Lucas, M., & MacGregor, G. A. (2007). Increased consumption of fruit and vegetables is related to a reduced risk of coronary heart disease: Meta-analysis of cohort studies. *Journal of Hypertension, 21*(9), 717–728.

He, F. J., Nowson, C. A., & MacGregor, G. A. (2006). Fruit and vegetable consumption and stroke: Meta-analysis of cohort studies. *Lancet 367*, 320–326.

Hippocrates. (1932). *Hippocrates* (W. H. S. Jones, Trans.). Cambridge, MA: Harvard University Press.

Institute of Medicine. (2005). *Complementary and alternative medicine in the United States.* Washington, DC: National Academies Press.

Johnson, S., Maziade, P. J., McFarland, L. V., Trick, W., Donskey, C., Currie, B., . . . Goldstein, E. J. (2012). Is primary prevention of Clostridium difficile infection possible with specific probiotics? *International Journal of Infectious Diseases, 16,* e786–e792.

Jurden, L., Buchanan, M., Kelsberg, G., & Safranek, S. (2012). Can probiotics safely prevent recurrent vaginitis? *Journal of Family Practice, 61,* 357–358.

Kemper, K. J., Vohra, S., & Walls, R. (2008). The use of complementary and alternative medicine in pediatrics. *Pediatrics, 122*(6), 1374–1386.

Khatta, M., Alexander, B. S., Krichten, C. M., Fisher, M. L., Freudenberger, R., Robinson, S. W., & Gottlieb, S. S. (2000). The effect of coenzyme Q10 in patients with congestive heart failure. *Annals of Internal Medicine, 132*(8), 636–640.

Kligler, B., & Cohrssen, A. (2008). Probiotics. *Complementary & Alternative Medicine, 78*(9), 1073–1078.

Kolata, G. (2006). Supplements fail to stop arthritis pain, study says. *New York Times.* Retrieved December 31, 2008, from http://www.nytimes.com/2006/02/23/health/23arthritis.html

Kottke, M. K. (1998). Scientific and regulatory aspects of nutraceutical products in the United States. *Drug Development and Industrial Pharmacy, 24*(12), 1177–1195.

Kwiterovich, P. (2008). Recognition and management of dyslipidemia in children and adolescents. *Journal of Clinical Endocrinology & Metabolism, 93*(11), 4200–4209.

Lichtenstein, A. H., Appel, L. J., Brands, M., Carnethon, M., Daniels, S., Franch, H. A., . . . Wylie-Rosett, J. (2006). AHA scientific statement diet and lifestyle recommendations revision 2006: A scientific statement from the American Heart Association nutrition committee. *Circulation, 114,* 82–96. doi:10.1161/CIRCULATIONAHA.106.17615103

Littarru, G. P., & Tiano, L. (2010). Clinical aspects of coenzyme Q10: An update. *Nutrition, 26,* 250–254.

McAlindon, T. E., LaValley, M. P., Gulin, J. P., & Felson, D. T. (2000). Glucosamine and chondroitin for treatment of osteoarthritis: A systematic quality assessment and meta-analysis. *Journal of the American Medical Association, 283*(11), 1483–1484.

McCracken, G. (1986). Culture and consumption: A theoretical account of the structure and movement of the cultural meaning of consumer goods. *Journal of Consumer Research, 13,* 71–84.

MEDLINE. (2013). *Drugs, supplements and herbal information.* Retrieved from http://www.nlm.nih.gov/medlineplus/druginformation.html

Mullie, P., Guelinckx, I., Clarys, P., Degrave, E., Hulens, M., & Vansant, G., (2009). Cultural, socioeconomic and nutritional determinants of functional food consumption patterns. *European Journal of Clinical Nutrition, 63,* 1290–1296.

National Cancer Institute. (2013). *Coenzyme Q10: Questions and answers, cancer facts.* Retrieved March 31, 2013, from http://www.cancer.gov/cancertopics/pdq/cam/coenzymeQ10/patient/page2

National Center for Complementary and Alternative Medicine. (2013). Glucosamine and chondroitin. Retrieved from http://nccam.nih.gov/health/chondroitin

National Nutraceutical Center. (2012). *What are nutraceuticals?* Retrieved from http://www.clemson.edu/NNC/what_are_nutra.html

Natural Standard. (2013a). *Herbs/supplements/glucosamine.* Retrieved from www.naturalstandard.com

Natural Standard. (2013b). *Probiotics.* Retrieved from www.naturalstandard.com

PA Consulting Group. (1990). *Functional foods: A new global added value market?* London, UK: PA Consulting Group.

Pariza, M. (1999). Functional foods: Technology, functionality and health benefits. *Nutrition Today, 34,* 150–151.

Plat, J., Mackay, D., Baumgartner, S., Clifton, P. M., Gylling, H., & Jones, P. J. J. (2012). Progress and prospective of plant sterol and plant stanol research: Report of the Maastricht meeting. *Atherosclerosis, 225,* 521–533.

Rathner, Z. (2013). Fruit and vegetable intake is associated with lower risk of ER-breast cancer [First published online January 24, 2013]. *Journal of the National Cancer Institute.* Retrieved from *JNCI: Journal of the National Cancer Institute.* doi:10.1093/jnci/djt009

Towheed, T. E., & Hochberg, M. C. (1997). A systematic review of randomized controlled trials of pharmacological therapy in osteoarthritis of the hip. *Journal of Rheumatology, 24,* 349–357.

Turpeinen, A. M., Ikonen, M., Kivimäki, A. S., Kautiainen, H., Vapaatalo, H., & Korpela, R. (2012). A spread containing bioactive milk peptides Ile–Pro–Pro and Val–Pro–Pro, and plant sterols has antihypertensive and cholesterol-lowering effects. *Food and Function, 3,* 621–627.

U.S. Pharmacopeial Convention. (2013). *USP verified dietary supplements.* Retrieved from http://www.usp.org/print/usp-verification-services/usp-verified-dietary-supplements/verification-process

Wandel, S., Juni, P., Tendal, B., Nuesch, E., Villiger, P. M., Welton, N. J., & Reichenbach, S. (2010). Effects of glucosamine, chondroitin, or placebo in patients with osteoarthritis of hip or knee: Network meta-analysis. *British Medical Journal, 341,* c4675. doi:10.1136/bmj.c4675

Wansink, B. (2002). Changing habits on the home front: Lost lessons from World War II research. *Journal of Public Policy Marketing, 21,* 90–99.

World Cancer Research Fund & American Institute for Cancer Research. (2007). Food, nutrition, physical activity, and the prevention of cancer: A global perspective. Washington, DC: American Institute for Cancer Research. Retrieved from http://www.dietandcancerreport.org/expert_report/report_contents/index.php

Wrick, K. L. (2005). The impact of regulations in the business of nutraceuticals in the United States: Yesterday, today and tomorrow. In C. M. Hasler (Ed.), *Regulation of functional foods & nutraceuticals: A global perspective* (pp. 3–36). Hoboken, NJ: Wiley-Blackwell.

Part V: Energy Therapies

The National Center for Complementary and Alternative Medicine (NCCAM) does not specify a distinct category for energy therapies but places them within "other CAM practices." Nursing has used energy therapies for many years. Krieger initiated investigations of therapeutic touch, an energy therapy, in the 1970s (Krieger, 1979). The diverse therapies included in this part of the book reveal nursing's interest in and use of energy therapies.

The concept of energy and its use is universal. Most cultures have a word to describe energy: *Qi* (pronounced *chee*) is a basic element of traditional Chinese medicine (TCM); *ki* is the Japanese word for energy; in India it is *prana*; the Dakota Indian word for energy is *ton*; and the Sioux Indian word is *waken*. Scientists and consumers express some skepticism about the efficacy of energy therapies because of the difficulty in determining how energy works and how the effects can be measured.

NCCAM (2012) delineates two types of energy: veritable (measurable) and putative (yet to be measured). Veritable energy therapies include magnet therapies and light therapy. Putative therapies include healing touch and Qigong. Much of TCM is based on the flow of energy throughout the body on meridians. Acupressure and reflexology, two therapies included in this portion of the book, are based on the flow of energy through meridians identified in TCM.

Healing touch encompasses a group of therapies used by nurses around the world. These techniques may or may not involve actual physical touching of the body. The nurse (or other therapist) seeks to bring energy into the patient or to balance energy within the person. Reiki, an energy therapy originating in Japan, is becoming more widely used in the United States.

Use of bioelectromagnetic therapies is increasing. These therapies, based on electromagnetic fields, include magnets, crystals, transcutaneous nerve stimulation (TENS), and pulsed fields. TENS has been used for several decades in pain management. Research on these therapies is increasing.

Light and sound therapies are included in the energy category. Light therapy has been used to treat seasonal affective disorder, which is more common in northern climates. Sound therapies include vibrational therapies and the voice.

Florence Nightingale noted the importance of the environment in the healing process (Nightingale, 1859/1936/1992). Instead of the sterile environs found in traditional health facilities, colors, shapes, plants, artwork, and so on, as part of healing and healing environments, are receiving considerable attention for their potential impact on healing. Energy therapies are used throughout the world and perspectives on their use in selected countries are noted in chapter sidebars.

Although difficulties are encountered in the measurement of outcomes from many of the therapies included in this section, intuitively many people recognize the existence of these energy forces that have an impact on health promotion and healing.

REFERENCES

Krieger, D. (1979). *The therapeutic touch: How to use your hands to help or to heal.* New York, NY: Simon & Schuster.

National Center for Complementary and Alternative Medicine. (2102). What is complementary and alternative medicine? Retrieved from http://nccam.nih.gov/health/whatiscam

Nightingale, F. (1992). *Notes on nursing.* Philadelphia, PA: Lippincott, Williams & Wilkins. (Original work published 1859, revised 1936.)

Chapter 23: Light Therapy

Niloufar Niakosari Hadidi

*T*his chapter provides a definition and overview of light therapy, its history, cultural applications, and scientific basis. It further expands on the use of light therapy to treat seasonal affective disorders and identifies other health conditions for which light therapy could be beneficial. Techniques that could be used by nurses educated in its practice, precautions, and recommendations for future research are provided.

DEFINITION

Light therapy is defined as daily exposure to full-spectrum or bright light to treat conditions such as seasonal affective disorder (SAD). This needs to be differentiated from phototherapy, which is used to treat conditions such as hyperbilirubinemia or psoriasis (Lam, 1998). This chapter focuses on a description of light therapy as used in the treatment of SAD.

Seasonal affective disorder (SAD) is a mood disorder that occurs more frequently in the dark winter months and disappears spontaneously in spring. However, it has been found to occur with less frequency in summer, and can occur repeatedly year after year. According to the *Diagnostic and Statistical Manual of Mental Disorders*, 5th edition (*DSM-5;* American Psychiatric Association, 2013), SAD is categorized as an indicator of major depression; patients with SAD experience episodes of major depression that tend to recur at specific times of the year (American Psychiatric Association, 2013).

These seasonal episodes may take the form of major depressive or bipolar disorders. Many symptoms of SAD are similar to symptoms of nonseasonal depressive episodes: low mood (often without prominent diurnal variation), loss of interest, anhedonia, anergia, poor motivation, low libido, anxiety, irritability, and social withdrawal (Eagles, 2004). More than one half of patients with SAD experience an increase in sleep duration with poor quality. Further, about the same numbers of patients experience increases in appetite and weight gain and have cravings for carbohydrates and chocolate (Eagles, 2004). Symptoms often start in autumn and winter, peak between December and February, and then subside during spring and summer.

Prevalence rates of SAD have been estimated to be between 0.4% and 5% in the general population with symptoms present for approximately 40% of the year; and these patients experience significant morbidity and impairment in psychosocial function (Kurlansik & Ibay, 2012; Westrin & Lam, 2007). SAD is reported to be more prevalent in women than in men and among younger age groups (MacCosbe, 2005). The exact causes of SAD are unknown; however, research has demonstrated that reduced sunlight may disrupt the circadian rhythm that is responsible for the body's internal clock (Edery, 2000). The disruption of this cycle may lead to depression.

History of Light Therapy

Since the beginning of time, people have realized the healing power of light. The history of light therapy goes back to ancient Egypt, where sunlight was used for medical treatments. Healing temples were built with colored crystals that were affixed on the surface of stone walls so that they were aligned with the sun's rays. People would lie down on benches and their bodies would be immersed with pure or colored lights (Curtis-King, 2008). Later, Hippocrates described the use of sunlight to cure various medical disorders. Although ancient Romans and Arab physicians had no scientific explanation for light therapy at the time, they knew that the healing power of light was helpful for medical treatments (Curtis-King, 2008).

In the early 1980s, researchers discovered that specialized bright light (20 times brighter than normal indoor light) was the most effective treatment for winter depression (Kripke, 1998a). Now research is confirming that this light is effective in improving the symptoms of nonseasonal depression as well (Kripke, 1998b). In fact, a systematic review of 62 reports on the efficacy of light therapy on nonseasonal depression found it to be effective and an excellent criterion to include in treatment of nonseasonal depression today (Even, Schroder, Friedman, & Rouillon, 2008). Light therapy has been reported to have a 70% positive response (Miller, 2005).

SCIENTIFIC BASIS

Research has demonstrated that individuals with SAD are positively affected by light (Flory, Ametepe, & Bowers, 2010; Golden et al., 2005; Gordijn, 't Mannetje, & Meesters, 2012; Meesters, Dekker, Schlangen, Bos, & Ruiter, 2011), sometimes as immediately as after even one light therapy session (Reeves et al., 2012). Light plays an important role in secretion of melatonin, as well as serotonin.

Melatonin is a natural hormone produced by the pineal gland, a pea-sized structure located at the center of the brain. Melatonin synthesis is stimulated by darkness. When light enters the retina, it stimulates the hypothalamus and inhibits the pineal gland from converting serotonin to melatonin (Miller, 2005). It is important to note that the impact of melatonin on circadian rhythms is compromised by cardiovascular and neuro-degenerative diseases as well as aging (Altun & Ugur-Altun, 2007).

Although studies suggest that administering melatonin supplements at night may help individuals with disrupted circadian rhythms, in a recent meta-analysis of the impact of melatonin on sleep, the authors suggested that melatonin results in only a 2% to 3% improvement in sleep efficiency (Brzezinski et al., 2005).

Lewy and colleagues (1995) report that taking melatonin supplements and exposure to bright light may change the circadian rhythm and melatonin secretion. The authors suggest that light therapy and melatonin administration could be helpful for winter depression, jet lag, and shift work.

INTERVENTION

Technique

The recommended device for provision of light therapy is a fluorescent light box that produces light intensities of greater than 2,500 lux (Westrin & Lam, 2007). Lux is a unit of illumination intensity that corrects for the photopic spectral sensitivity of the human eye. To better understand the concept of lux, indoor evening room light is usually less than 100 lux, whereas a brightly lit office is less than 500 lux. In contrast, outdoor light is much brighter: a cloudy, gray winter day is around 4,000 lux and a sunny day can be 50,000 lux to 100,000 lux or more (Westrin & Lam, 2007). The most effective dose has been reported to be 10,000 lux for 30 minutes daily; lower intensities (i.e., 2,500 lux) can also be effective, however, they require longer durations of 2 to 3 hours (Terman & Terman, 2005). It is recommended that broad-spectrum white light from fluorescent lamps in which the ultraviolet (UV) and infrared (IR) light are being filtered be used because UV and IR wavelengths are potentially damaging to the eyes (Howland, 2009). Although earlier studies indicated that bright light therapy did not benefit nondepressed individuals without history of SAD (Avery et al., 2001; Kasper et al., 1989), a recent study reported improved mood and vitality more than 1 month after using 1 hour of bright light exposure daily in healthy individuals. This effect was enhanced by the addition of physical exercise to light exposure (Partonen & Lönnqvist, 2000).

It is recommended that patients diagnosed with SAD start light therapy in the fall and continue until symptoms are resolved in the spring or summer (Kurlansik & Ibay, 2012). Light must enter the eyes for light therapy to be effective in the treatment of depressive conditions; however, the person should not be looking at the light directly. The result of several clinical trials has led to the recommended dose of 10,000 lux for 30 minutes soon after awakening in the morning (Terman & Terman, 2005).

The light enters the eye, and is transmitted with nerve impulses to the pineal gland, which controls melatonin secretion. Patients often report relief of depressive symptoms in 3 days to 4 days. The time of the day is also an important consideration in light therapy. Often, light therapy is administered in the early morning on arising. Using a pooled clustering technique of 332 patients from 14 research centers across 5 years, Terman and colleagues (1989) concluded that early-morning exposure was more effective in reducing depression than when administered at other times of the day.

Whereas the exact mechanism of light therapy is unknown but believed to be through an ocular process, extraocular transcranial photo-transduction in mammals results in changes in reproductive cycles and increased serotonin levels in the brain (Campbell, Murphy, & Suhner, 2001). Based on this information, Timonen and colleagues (2012) have hypothesized that light therapy may be effective if delivered in methods other than through eye mediation. They conducted a pilot study in 22 physically healthy patients with SAD in whom light therapy (6.0–8.5 lumens) was administered via earplugs in bilateral ear canals for 8 to 12 minutes per episode 5 days a week for 4 weeks. This study was conducted during the darkest part of the year in Finland. Seventy-seven percent of the subjects experienced full remission of SAD symptoms (Timonen et al., 2012). Ninety-two percent of the subjects achieved at least a 50% reduction in self-reported anxiety symptoms. These preliminary results in this pilot study challenge the existing model of light therapy mechanism of action, warranting further exploration.

It is often recommended that individuals with SAD should exercise outdoors during daylight as much as possible (Eagles, 2004). Social contact should be continued, and it is helpful to sufferers of SAD if family and friends have some knowledge of this condition and what to expect.

Studies have demonstrated, however, that only 12% to 41% of patients with SAD continue to use light therapy even after they have had successful use of the therapy in a previous winter (Rohan, Roecklein, Lacy, & Vacek, 2009; Schwartz, Brown, Wehr, & Rosenthal, 1996). Roecklein, Schumacher, Miller, and Ernecoff (2012) found that continued use of light therapy was more likely to occur if patients were confident that they would use the therapy even if it was inconvenient and if they had family and friends who were supportive of adherence to the therapy. This would suggest that if a provider enhances the behavioral change of therapy use through engaging family support and improved self-efficacy, patient adherence to light therapy may improve, increasing the likelihood of ongoing symptom relief.

Light Therapy or Antidepressant?

It has been suggested that the more individuals have visible symptoms of SAD, characterized by hypersomnia or excessive daytime sleepiness, carbohydrate carving, and weight gain, the more they would benefit from light therapy rather than from antidepressants (Eagles, 2004). Further, often people have a preference for natural light therapy over pharmacologic antidepressants (Eagles, 2004).

The use of light therapy for nonseasonal affective disorder as well as bipolar disorder has been reported in the literature. In a study on the impact of light therapy as an adjuvant treatment to antidepressants, the investigators randomized 30 bipolar and depressed patients into either the treatment group receiving antidepressant and light therapy or the control group receiving antidepressant and placebo. The result indicated that there was a significant improvement ($p < .05$) in mood in the treatment group, with individuals receiving light therapy in addition to antidepressant showing faster response as well (Benedetti et al., 2003).

Measurement of Outcomes

Several clinical, placebo-controlled studies have been done using light therapy to treat SAD. These studies confirm that light is not only as effective as other methods, it causes no long-term side effects. A meta-analysis of randomized controlled trials of bright light therapy for treatment of SAD suggests that light therapy is effective, with effect sizes equivalent to those of antidepressant pharmacology trials for SAD (Golden et al., 2005). However, it must be noted that the authors indicated that most of the studies that met their selection criteria for the meta-analysis did not meet the recognized criteria for rigorous clinical trials.

Studies on use of light therapy as a preventative measure for SAD suggest that a brief course of light therapy at the onset of symptoms is sufficient for prevention of relapse for the rest of the winter season (Westrin & Lam, 2007).

Another meta-analysis of literature (work published between January 1975 and July 2003) on phototherapy (either bright light or dawn simulation) suggested that bright light therapy is an effective treatment for SAD. Dawn simulation is a treatment that involves using a program that mimics natural springtime. The strategy is to set the time of sunrise signal earlier than outdoors in winter by using a relatively dim light, gradually increasing the light over 90 minutes from 0.001 lux to 300 lux while the patient sleeps with eyes dark-adapted (Terman & Terman, 2005). In their 6-year study, comparing bright light, dawn simulation, and brief light pulse as compared to a control group receiving high- and low-density negative air ionization while asleep, the investigators concluded that after 3 weeks of treatment, all three conditions were more effective than the control group (Terman & Terman, 2006).

Precautions/Side Effects

The major contradictions for the use of light therapy are retinal disease or diseases that may involve the retina, such as diabetes; it is also contraindicated for those taking photosensitizing medications, such as lithium, phenothiazine antipsychotics, melatonin, and St. John's wort (Reme, Rol, Grothmann, Kaase, & Terman, 1996). An ophthalmologic examination is often recommended for these high-risk patients before starting light therapy.

Adverse effects associated with light therapy are often attributed partially to factors such as parameters of light exposure, timing, dose (intensity, duration) and method of exposure (diffused, direct, focused). For example, if morning light is timed too early, patients experience premature awakening, with difficulty falling sleep again. If, on the other hand, evening light is scheduled too late, patients experience initial insomnia and hyperactivity (Terman & Terman, 2005).

Other common side effects reported are headache, eyestrain, agitation, or feeling nervous or tense (Kogan & Guilford, 1998; Lam, 1998). Less common but more serious side effects of mania and hypomania have been reported (Lam, 1998).

It is possible to buy a light-therapy box over the counter without a physician's prescription; however, one must know that not all light-therapy boxes being sold have been tested for safety and effectiveness. That is why it is crucial to consult with one's health care provider before buying one.

It is important to keep in mind that light therapy should be considered adjunctive therapy for patients with any diagnosable depressive or mood disorders. Primary assessment and treatment for these types of disorders should always be done by psychiatric professionals to ensure appropriate comprehensive treatment.

USES

In addition to the use of light therapy for SAD, other uses of light therapy have been reported. These include, for example, the treatment of chronic depression, antepartum depression, premenstrual depression, and sleep–wake cycle issues (Pail et al., 2011). Other uses of light therapy are for subsyndromal SAD (similar to SAD, except that patients do not meet the criteria for major depressive disorder), antepartum and postpartum major depressive disorder, premenstrual dysphoric disorder, bulimia nervosa, and attention deficit disorder (Terman & Terman, 2005).

Light therapy for treatment of sleep problems in older adults has been suggested by several studies. As humans age, sleep patterns change; most commonly, with advancing age, persons have difficulty falling sleep, staying asleep, have early-morning awakenings, and difficulty falling back to sleep (Montgomery & Dennis, 2002). Severe sleep disturbances may lead to depression and cognitive impairments (Ford & Kamerow, 1989). Lack of sleep can impair memory, disrupt metabolism, and hasten death (Davenport, 2002). In a study by Campbell and colleagues (1993) on 16 men and women between the ages of 62 and 81 with sleep disturbance who were exposed to bright light therapy, investigators found substantial positive changes in sleep quality as a result of light therapy use. Waking time within sleep was reduced by an hour, and sleep efficiency improved from 77.5% to 90% without altering time spent in bed.

A Committee on Chronotherapeutics that had been delegated by the International Society for Affective Disorders concluded that light therapy is effective for the treatment of patients with seasonal affective disorders, as well as those with major depressive disorders. Thus, light therapy can be provided as an adjunctive therapy or as an alternative therapy for patients who are unwilling or unable to take antidepressants (Dallaspezia et al., 2012; Martiny et al., 2012; Wirz-Justice et al., 2005). Antepartum and perinatal depression is a common condition requiring judicious intervention to treat the mother while minimizing any potential risks to the unborn child as well as nursing infants. Light therapy can be a nonpharmacologic approach to improve depressive symptoms in the pregnant or nursing mother with no known risk to the fetus or infant (Crowley & Youngstedt, 2012; Wirz-Justice et al., 2011).

AGE-RELATED IMPLICATIONS

It has been suggested that light therapy may be an effective therapy for improving sleep patterns of individuals with dementia (Mishima et al., 2007; Skjerve, Bjorvatn, & Holsten, 2004). To determine whether high-intensity ambient light in public areas of long-term-care facilities would improve sleep patterns and circadian rhythms of persons with dementia, Sloane and colleagues (2007) conducted a study in geriatric units on 66 older adults with dementia. Results suggested that bright light had a modest but measurable salutary effect on sleep in this population. Further, the investigators concluded that ambient light might be preferable to stationary devices such as light boxes for older people with dementia in long-term-care settings. However, a critical review of literature by Shinmi and colleagues on bright light therapy suggests that, due to methodological issues, the impact of bright light on sleep and behavior in dementia patients is inconclusive (Shinmi, Hae, & Sook, 2003).

Light therapy has been shown to be effective in additional older populations. Seniors living in long-term-care facilities had improved cognitive function indicators as well as improvement in anxiety scores when receiving light therapy (Royer et al., 2012). Further, 89 patients over the age of 60 with major depressive disorders demonstrated improved mood, increased sleep efficiency, and a steeper rise of evening melatonin when exposed to 3 weeks of bright light therapy (Lieverse et al., 2011).

Due to age-related changes of clouding of the lens and ocular media and cataract formation in some cases, exposure to blue and white light can cause discomfort (Reme, 1996).

CULTURAL APPLICATIONS

The ancient Chinese knew of the healing power of natural light. The Chinese principles of feng shui are not only based on the principle of the right placement of certain natural elements, but also on the use of light to bring a sense of balance and harmony to our lives with good "Chi" or "life-giving energy" (Curtis-King, 2008).

The traditional Chinese medicine (TCM) term Qi or "life force flow" implies that there are energetic pathways in the body, similar to the concepts underlying the application of acupuncture (Brooke, 2007). However, instead of needles, "colorpuncture" uses a pen torch that is fitted with interchangeable glass rods to focus light on specific points on the skin. With each treatment, a prescribed pattern of colors in a certain sequence is used to get to the root of the illness. It is believed in the framework of TCM that disease is an indication that the body is out of balance. Thus, the precise targeted light treatments can release emotional trauma and bring the body back to a balanced state (Brooke, 2007).

Light has been long used in health and creating healing environments for aesthetic and practical reasons in countries around the world. Well-used light in the ambient environment can boost mood and well-being. The "built" environment can capitalize on natural light. The use of light in architecture in Iran is described in Sidebar 23.1.

Sidebar 23.1. *Use of Light as an Architectural Asset in Iran*

Mansour Hadidi, Architect, Shiraz, Iran

Light (fire) was one of the four sacred elements in ancient Persia; the other three were Water, Earth (soil), Air (wind). Zoroastrians (followers of Persian prophet Zoroaster) believed that fire must never be extinguished in the temple. Zoroaster is thought to have lived in eastern Persia (today's Iran) in 600 BCE. Zoroastrians (Persians) probably were the first to introduce the idea of binary powers (as opposed to the Greeks who believed in multiple gods and goddesses). Ahura Mazda was the god of light and goodness; Angra Mainyu was the god of darkness and "evil spirit" who, at the end, was believed to be defeated by goodness. The words *Ahura* and *Mazda* mean light and wisdom, respectively.

Iran is a light-rich country, located between the 25° N at its southernmost and 39° N at its northernmost latitude. There is a broad range of temperatures and climate and elevations, water and desert areas, with some regions seeing no rain for half the year. Due to its global position, sunlight is a beautiful asset of the country. The elevation in mountainous regions also contributes to the intensity and effects of sunlight. The climate is temperate and there is plentiful sunshine on most days, especially in the arid desert areas.

Architects in Iran, even from early times, have understood the importance of light in the design and construction of buildings. Natural light, plentiful in Iran, plays an important role in the illumination of buildings. The beauty of natural light can be observed in homes, workspaces, hotels, hospitals, schools, mosques, and other buildings. Exposure to light can be uplifting and energizing. It can improve mood and vitality with potential effects on human productivity. Early-morning exposure has wakening effects and can be more effective.

Stained glass was used to soften the light where the heat from light was excessive. Architects used a balance between light and heat. Another approach was using indirect light. For example, in areas close to the desert, small patios were designed to bring in light while preventing direct sunshine, and heat as a result. An important consideration is the direction of windows in buildings. While southern exposures are the most popular for daytime living areas (such as living room and family room) due to receiving the highest amount of natural light during the day, northern windows are best for bedrooms and spaces that are used at night.

With the advent of electricity, air-conditioning, and heating appliances, architects had more freedom to design buildings with other factors in

(continued)

Sidebar 23.1. *Use of Light as an Architectural Asset in Iran* (continued)

mind. For example, although architects were aware that light could add to the beauty and illumination of a building, the view of the vista's surroundings became a higher priority. In old structures, reticular stone panels were often used to prevent excessive heat from sunshine. However, in modern buildings, large glass windows mostly cover the façade.

FUTURE RESEARCH

Future research should focus on light therapy as a preventive strategy for SAD, as well as for other conditions such as nonseasonal affective disorder, bipolar disorder, premenopausal syndrome, and premenstrual depression.

There have been successful preliminary studies focused on the impact of melatonin in treatment of severe postoperative delirium unresponsive to antipsychotics or benzodiazepines (Hanania & Kitain, 2002). It would be interesting to investigate whether light therapy would have a similar impact on reducing the incidence or severity of postoperative delirium.

REFERENCES

Altun, A., & Ugur-Altun, B. (2007). Melatonin: Therapeutic and clinical utilization. *International Journal of Clinical Practice, 61*(5), 835–845.

American Psychiatric Association, Task Force on *DSM-5*. (2013). *Diagnostic and statistical manual of mental disorders* (5th ed.). Washington, DC: American Psychiatric Press.

Avery, D. H., Eder, D. N., Bolte, M. A., Hellekson, C. J., Dunner, D. L., Vitiello, M. V., & Prinz, P. N. (2001). Dawn simulation and bright light in the treatment of SAD: A controlled study. *Biological Psychiatry, 50*(3), 205–216.

Benedetti, F., Colombo, C., Pontiggia, A., Bernasconi, A., Florita, M., & Smeraldi, E. (2003). Morning light treatment hastens the antidepressant effect of citalopram: A placebo-controlled trial. *Journal of Clinical Psychiatry, 64*(6), 648–653.

Brooke, P. (2007). *The power of light.* Retrieved April 10, 2013, from http://poweroflight.nfshost.com

Brzezinski, A., Vangel, M. G., Wurtman, R. J., Norrie, G., Zhdanova, I., Ben-Shushan, A., & Ford, I. (2005). Effects of exogenous melatonin on sleep: A meta-analysis. *Sleep Medicine Reviews, 9*(1), 41–50.

Campbell, S. S., Dawson, D., & Anderson, M. W. (1993). Alleviation of sleep maintenance insomnia with timed exposure to bright light. *Journal of American Geriatrics Society, 41*(8), 829–836.

Campbell, S. S., Murphy, P. J., & Suhner, A. G. (2001). Extraocular phototransduction and circadian timing systems in vertebrates. *Chronobiology International, 18,*137–172.

Crowley, S. K., & Youngstedt, S. D. (2012). Efficacy of light therapy for perinatal depression: A review. *Journal of Physiological Anthropology, 31,* 15. doi:10.1186/1880-6805-31-15

Curtis-King, L. (2008). The healing power of incoherent polarized light. *Light and Colour, 144,* 24–26.

Dallaspezia, S., Benedetti, F., Colombo, C., Barbini, B., Fulgosi, M.C., Garinelli, C., & Smeraldi, E. (2012). Optimized light therapy for non-seasonal major depressive disorder. *Journal of Affective Disorders, 138*(3), 337–342.

Davenport, R. J. (2002). Up all night. *Science of Aging Knowledge Environment, 30,* 104. Retrieved October 2008, from http://sageke.sciencemag.org/cgi/content/abstract/sageke;2002/30/nw104

Eagles, J. M. (2004). Light therapy and the management of winter depression. *Advances in Psychiatric Treatment, 10,* 233–240.

Edery, I., (2000). Circadian rhythms in a nutshell. *Physiological Genomics, 3,* 59–74.

Even, C., Schroder, C. M., Friedman, S., & Rouillon, F. (2008). Efficacy of light therapy in nonseasonal depression: A systematic review. *Journal of Affective Disorders, 108*(1), 11–24.

Flory, R., Ametepe, J., & Bowers, B. (2010). A randomized, placebo-controlled trial of bright light and high-density negative air ions for treatment of seasonal affective disorder. *Psychiatry Research, 177*(1/2), 101–108.

Ford, D. E., & Kamerow, D. B. (1989). Epidemiologic study of sleep disturbances and psychiatric disorders. *Journal of the American Medical Association, 262,* 1479–1484.

Golden, R. N., Gaynes, B. N., Ekstrom, R. D., Hamer, R. M., Jacobsen, F. M., Suppes, T., . . . Nemeroff, C. B. (2005). The efficacy of light therapy in the treatment of mood disorders: A review and meta-analysis of the evidence. *American Journal of Psychiatry, 162*(4), 656–662.

Gordijn, M.C., 't Mannetje, D., & Meesters, Y. (2012). The effects of blue-enriched light treatment compared to standard light treatment in seasonal affective disorder. *Journal of Affective Disorders, 136*(1/2), 72–80.

Hanania, M., & Kitain, E. (2002). Melatonin for treatment and prevention of postoperative delirium. *Anesthesia and Analgesia, 94,* 338–339.

Howland, R. H. (2009). An overview of seasonal affective disorder and its treatment options. *Physician and Sportsmedicine, 37*(4), 104.

Kasper, S., Rogers, S. L., Yancey, A., Schulz, P. M., Skwerer, R. G., & Rosenthal, N. E. (1989). Phototherapy in individuals with and without subsyndromal seasonal affective disorder. *Archives of General Psychiatry, 46*(9), 837.

Kogan, A.O., & Guilford, P.M. (1998). Side effects of short term 10,000 lux light therapy. *American Journal of Psychiatry, 155*(2), 293–294.

Kripke, D. F. (1998a). Light therapy and depression. *Journal of Affective Disorders, 62*(3), 221–223.

Kripke, D. F. (1998b). Light treatment for non-seasonal major depression: Are we ready? In R. W. Lam (Ed.), *Seasonal affective disorder and beyond* (pp. 159–172). Washington, DC: American Psychiatric Press.

Kurlansik, S. L., & Ibay, A. D. (2012). Seasonal affective disorder. *American Family Physician, 86*(11), 1037–1041.

Lam, R. W. (Ed.). (1998). *Seasonal affective disorder and beyond: Light treatment for SAD and non-SAD conditions.* Washington, DC: American Psychiatric Press.

Lewy, A. J., Sack, R. L., Blood, M. L., Bauer, V. K., Cutler, N. L., & Thomas, K. H. (1995). Melatonin marks circadian phase position and resets the endogenous circadian pacemaker in humans. *Ciba Foundation Symposium, 183,* 303–317.

Lieverse, R., Van Someren, E. J. W., Nielen, M. M. A., Uitdehaag, B. M. J., Smit, J. H., & Hoogendijk, W. J. G. (2011). Bright light treatment in elderly patients with nonseasonal major depressive disorders: A randomized, placebo-controlled trial. *Archives of General Psychiatry, 68*(1), 61–70.

MacCosbe, P. E. (2005). Recognizing SAD in the clinical setting: An interview with Paul E. MacCosbe, PharmD, FCP. *Medscape Nurses.* Retrieved April 13, 2013, from http://www.medscape.com/viewarticle/507103

Martiny, K., Refsgaard, E., Lund, V., Lunde, M., Sorensen, L., Thougaard, B., . . . Bech, P. (2012). A 9-week randomized trial comparing a chronotherapeutic intervention (wake and light therapy) to exercise in major depressive disorder patients treated with duloxetine. *Journal of Clinical Psychiatry, 73*(9), 1234–1242.

Meesters, Y., Dekker, V., Schlangen, L. J., Bos, E. H., & Ruiter, M. J. (2011). Low-intensity blue-enriched white light (750 lux) and standard bright light (10,000 lux) are equally effective in treating seasonal affective disorder. A randomized controlled study. *BMC Psychiatry, 11*, 17. doi:10.1186/1471-244X-11-17

Miller, A. L. (2005). Epidemiology, etiology, and natural treatment of seasonal affective disorder. *Alternative Medicine Review: A Journal of Clinical Therapeutics, 10*(1), 5–13.

Mishima, K., Okawa, M., Hishikawa, Y., Hozumi, S., Hori, H., & Takahashi, K. (2007). Morning bright light therapy for sleep and behavior disorders in elderly patients with dementia. *Acta Psychiatrica Scandinavica, 89*(1), 1–7.

Montgomery, P., & Dennis, J. A. (2002). Bright light therapy for sleep problems in adults aged 60+. Cochrane Database of Systematic Reviews 2002, Issue 2. Art. No.: CD003403. doi:10.1002/14651858.CD003403

Pail, G., Huf, W., Pjrek, E., Winker, D., Willeit, M., Praschak-Rieder, N., & Kasper, S. (2011). Bright light therapy in the treatment of mood disorders. *Neuropsychobiology, 64*(3), 152–162.

Partonen, T., & Lönnqvist, J. (2000). Bright light improves vitality and alleviates distress in healthy people. *Journal of Affective Disorders, 57*, 55–61.

Reeves, G. M., Nijjar, G. V., Langenberg, P., Johnson, M. A., Khabazghazvini, B., Sleemi, A., . . . Postolache, T. T. (2012). Improvement in depression scores after 1 hour of light therapy treatment in patients with seasonal affective disorder. *Journal of Nervous and Mental Disease, 200*(1), 51–55.

Reme, C. E., Rol, P., Grothmann, K., Kaase, H., & Terman, M. (1996). Bright light therapy in focus: Lamp emission spectra and ocular safety. *International Journal of Technology Assessment in Health Care, 4*, 403–413.

Roecklein, K. A., Schumacher, J. A., Miller, M. A., & Ernecoff, N. C. (2012). Cognitive and behavioral predictors of light therapy use. *PloS ONE (Electronic Resource), 7*(6), e39275.

Rohan, K. J., Roecklein, K. A., Lacy, T. J., & Vacek, P. M. (2009). Winter depression recurrence one year after cognitive–behavioral therapy, light therapy, or combination treatment. *Behavioral Therapy, 40*, 225–238.

Royer, M., Ballentine, N. H., Eslinger, P. J., Houser, K., Mistrick, R., Behr, R., & Rakos, K. (2012). Light therapy for seniors in long term care. *Journal of American Medical Directors Association, 13*(2), 100–102.

Schwartz, P. J., Brown, C., Wehr, T. A., & Rosenthal, N. E. (1996). Winter seasonal affective disorder: A follow up study of the first 59 patients of the National Institute of Mental Health seasonal studies program. *American Journal of Psychiatry, 153*, 1028–1036.

Shinmi, K., Hae, H. S., & Sook, J. Y. (2003). The effect of bright light on sleep and behavior in dementia: An analytic review. *Geriatric Nursing, 24*(4), 239–243.

Skjerve, A., Bjorvatn, B., & Holsten, F. (2004). Light therapy for behavioural and psychological symptoms of dementia. *International Journal of Geriatric Psychiatry, 19*(6), 516–522.

Sloane, P. D., Williams, C. S., Mitchell, C. M., Preisser, J. S., Wood, W., Barrick, A. L., . . . Zimmerman, S. (2007). High-intensity environmental light in dementia: Effect on sleep and activity. *Journal of the American Geriatrics Society, 55*(10), 1524–1533.

Terman, M., Terman, J. S., Quitkin, F. M., McGrath, P. J., Stewart, J. W., & Rafferty, B. (1989). Light therapy for seasonal affective disorder. A review of efficacy. *Neuropsychopharmacology, 2*(1), 1–22.

Terman, M., & Terman, J. S. (2005). Light therapy for seasonal and nonseasonal depression: Efficacy, protocol, safety and side effects. *CNS Spectrums, 10*(8), 647.

Terman, M., & Terman, J. (2006). Controlled trial of naturalistic dawn simulation and negative air ionization for seasonal affective disorder. *American Journal of Psychiatry, 163*(12), 2126–2133.

Timonen, M., Nissila, J., Liettu, A., Jokelainen, J., Jurvelin, H., Aunio, A., . . . Takala, T. (2012). Can transcranial brain-targeted bright light treatment via ear canals be effective in relieving symptoms in seasonal affective disorder? A pilot study. *Medical Hypotheses, 78*(4), 511–515.

Westrin, A., & Lam, R. W. (2007). Seasonal affective disorder: A clinical update. *Annals of Clinical Psychiatry, 19*(4), 239–246.

Wirz-Justice, A., Bader, A., Frison, U., Stieglitz, R. D., Alder, J., Bitzer, J., . . . Riecher-Rossler, A. (2011). A randomized, double-blind, placebo-controlled study of light therapy for antepartum depression. *Journal of Clinical Psychiatry, 72*(7), 986–993.

Wirz-Justice, A., Benedetti, F., Berger, M., Lam, R. W., Martiny, K., Terman, M., & Wu, J. C. (2005). Chronotherapeutics (light and wake therapy) in affective disorders. *Psychological Medicine, 35*(7), 939–944.

Chapter 24: Healing Touch

ALEXA W. UMBREIT

All cultures, both ancient and modern, have developed some form of touch therapy as part of people's desire to heal and care for one another. The oldest written evidence of the use of touch to enhance healing comes from Asia more than 5,000 years ago (Hover-Kramer, Mentgen, & Scandrett-Hibdon, 1996; Jackson & Keegan, 2009; Krieger, 1979). This therapeutic use of the hands has been passed on from generation to generation as a tool for healing. However, philosophical and cultural differences have influenced the way touch has been used throughout the world. The Eastern viewpoint has based its touch-healing practices on energy channels (called meridians), energy fields (auras), and energy centers (chakras). Expert practitioners in energetic touch therapies use their hands to influence this flow of energy to promote balance and healing. The Western viewpoint focuses on physiological changes that occur at the cellular level from touch therapies that are believed to influence healing. A blending of both Eastern and Western techniques has led to an explosion of a wide variety of touch therapies (Jackson & Keegan, 2009). Nursing has used touch throughout its history and today's nurses are integrating many touch techniques into their practice. One of these therapies is Healing Touch, which now boasts more than 50,000 persons who have been trained worldwide, with nearly 2,000 certified practitioners, and 200 certified instructors during the past 23 years (Healing Touch International, 2012a).

DEFINITION

Healing Touch (HT) is a type of complementary therapy that uses gentle touch and energy-based techniques to influence and support the human energy system within the body (energy centers) and surrounding the body (energy fields) supporting the body's natural ability to heal (Healing Touch International, 2012b; Healing Touch Program, 2012a). HT is classified as a presumptive energy or biofield therapy by the National Institutes of Health, National Center for Complementary and Alternative Medicine (NCCAM, 2012). Based on a holistic view of health and illness, HT focuses on creating an energetic balance of the whole body at the physical, emotional, mental, and spiritual levels rather than on dysfunctional parts of the body. Through this process of balancing the energy system and therefore opening up energy blockages, an environment is created that is conducive to self-healing. Through the interaction of the energy fields between practitioner and client, the use of the HT practitioner's hands, an intention focusing on the client's highest good, and a centering process, noninvasive HT techniques specific for the client's needs are used to create this energetic balance (Umbreit, 2000). Krieger (1979) describes the centering process as a meditation in which one eliminates all distractions and concentrates on that place of quietude within which one can feel truly integrated, unified, and focused. Finding this "place of quietude within" is achieved by many through deep belly breathing, prayer, meditation, or any other technique that slows one down, calms the mind, and accesses a deeper spirit of compassion and strength. To be centered is to be fully present with another person or situation, engaged with heart and mind, deeper feelings, and thoughts. The centered state of mind is maintained throughout the HT treatment.

Umbreit (2000) describes the role of the HT practitioner as observation, assessment, and repatterning of the client's energy field, which is disrupted when there is disease, illness, psychological stressors, and pain. Practitioners describe these disruptions in the energy field as blockages, leaks, imbalances, or congestion. The goal of the HT practitioner is to open up these blockages, seal the leaks, rebalance the energy field to symmetry, and release congestion.

HT evolved from the pioneering work of the therapeutic touch (TT) community that was started in 1970 by a nurse, Dr. Dolores Krieger, and Dora Kunz, a natural intuitive healer, who assisted many physicians with perplexing patient cases. Together they established TT, described as a "contemporary interpretation of several ancient healing practices . . . [consisting of learning] skills for consciously directing or sensitively modulating human energies" (Krieger, 1993, p. 11). The practice is based on the assumption that humans are complex energy fields and the potential exists to enhance the natural healing potential in another

(Therapeutic Touch, 2004). In health care, TT philosophy, practice, and research have become the base for many newer energetic modalities, including HT.

The HT curriculum, started in 1989 and endorsed by the American Holistic Nurses' Association (AHNA), involves a formal educational program that teaches techniques, including interventions described by Brugh Joy (1979) and Alice Bailey (1984), concepts presented by Rosalyn Bruyere (1989) and Barbara Brennan (1986), and original techniques developed by the founder of HT, Janet Mentgen, and her students (Scandrett-Hibdon, 1996). The six-level HT educational curriculum in energy-based practice moves from beginning to advanced practice, certification, and instructor level. Advanced practice requires at least 100 hours of workshop instruction plus a 1-year rigorous and comprehensive course of study involving an extensive reading program and a wide variety of complementary therapies, as well as work on case studies, mentoring, ethics, client–practitioner relationships, establishment of a practice, and integration of activities within the health community (Healing Touch International, 2012c). Emphasis is based on self-care and development of the student. After this, students may apply for certification. Instructor status requires more education and mentoring. The HT coursework is open to nurses, massage therapists, and other health care professionals, and to the lay person who desires an in-depth understanding and practice of healing work using touch and energy-based concepts (Healing Touch Program, 2012b; Schommer & Larrimore, 2010).

SCIENTIFIC BASIS

The nursing profession has long been described as dedicated to the art and science of human caring. Rogers (1990) and Watson (1985) have written extensively about caring as a central quality of the nursing profession, along with nursing's concern for the promotion of health and well-being, taking into account the individual's constant interaction with the environment. It was this concern that led nurse-theorist Rogers to develop her concepts of the nature of individuals as energy fields in constant interplay with the surrounding environment (Hover-Kramer et al., 1996). Rogers's theoretical framework postulates that all living things are composed of energy, and there is a continual exchange of energy among them as they strive toward the goal of balance and universal order. Using the hands, intention, and centering, the HT practitioner assesses the client's energy field and helps direct it to a more open, symmetrical pattern that enhances the client's ability to self-heal. The nursing diagnosis used for HT and other biofield therapies is defined as a "Disturbed Energy Field [state in which a] disruption of the flow of energy surrounding a person's being results in a disharmony of the body, mind, and/or spirit" (Carpenito, 2013, p. 252).

It is still not clear how energy field modalities, including HT, influ-ence the energy patterns of a recipient or how recipients use the energy to enhance their self-healing processes; however, the effects of energy-based healing interactions are measurable and significant (Hover-Kramer, 2002). The fields of physics, engineering, biology, and physiology continue to research this area of energy exchange in an attempt to explain what occurs during an energetic interaction (Feinstein & Eden, 2008; Forbes, Rust, & Becker, 2004; Oschman, 2000). Schwartz (2007) states that present-day physicists continue to further analyze Einstein's premise that everything is energy and organized in energy fields.

Oschman reports that various energy therapies actually stimulate tissue healing by the production of pulsating electromagnetic fields that induce currents to flow within the body's tissue. It is proposed that these currents are generated via the heartbeat and move throughout the cir-culatory system and the "living matrix," which Oschman describes as an informational nervous system of the body where electron movement occurs, producing these waves (Oschman, 2008). He states that the heart generates the body's largest electromagnetic field, which can be mea-sured in the space around the body using the superconducting quantum interference device (SQUID). The SQUID has been used to measure these biomagnetic fields emanating from the hands of energy field practitio-ners who use therapeutic touch, Qigong, yoga, and meditation. It has been found that low electromagnetic frequencies (a coherent pattern) can be emitted from a trained energy healer's hands at a rate needed for tissue healing, which has the possibility to convert a stalled healing process to active repair by restoring coherence to the tissue (Oschman, 2008). One may think of HT as a method in which the practitioner's focused healing intention is communicated to the subtle energy of the client's cells influencing the dynamic matter of the client's living matrix (Oschman, 2009).

Other instruments have been invented to directly measure the human energy field (e.g., Kirlian photography, gaseous discharge visualization, and polycontrast interference) but these instruments are not consistently accurate (Duerden, 2004). Eschiti (2007) states, "until science is able to pro-vide accurate, direct measurement of the human energy field, research will need to be conducted by measuring possible effects on the field in an indirect manner" (p. 10).

The concept of energy systems as part of the human interactive environment and healing has been part of many cultures for centuries. Ancient East Indian traditions speak of a universal energy (*prana*) that flows and activates the life force (*kundalini*) (Hover-Kramer et al., 1996). In China, Japan, and Thailand, the basic life energy is called *Chi*, *Qi*, or *Ki*. The Egyptians called it *ankh* and the Polynesians refer to it as *mana*. Many other cultures throughout the world have equivalent terms for describing human energies (Hover-Kramer, 2002). The common principle is that an imbalance in this energy force can result in illness.

It is unknown precisely how symptoms are managed by HT interventions. What have been observed are changes in outcomes being measured in the nursing research. It may be postulated that because energy fields are in constant interaction within and outside the physical body, internal mechanisms are stimulated by this movement of energy (Umbreit, 2000). However, any explanations given for energy healing remain theoretical, due to limited experimental data and difficulty using traditional scientific analysis because paradoxical findings often coexist (Engebretson & Wardell, 2002).

Studies specific to HT interventions have focused on managing the symptoms of pain, anxiety, and stress; decreasing the side effects of cancer treatments; promoting faster postprocedural recovery; improving mental health, including posttraumatic stress disorder (PTSD); using HT with the older adult to manage pain, improve appetite, sleep, behavior patterns, and functional abilities; increasing relaxation; and promoting a sense of well-being (Bulbrook, 2000; Cook, Guerrerio, & Slater, 2004; Dowd, Kolcaba, Steiner, & Fashinpaur, 2007; Geddes, 2002; Hardwick, 2012; Hutchison, 1999; Jain et al., 2012; Krucoff et al., 2001, 2005; MacIntyre et al., 2008; Maville, Bowen, & Benham, 2008; Megel, Anderson, Lu, & Strybol, 2012; Post-White et al., 2003; Scandrett-Hibdon, Hardy, & Mentgen, 1999; Seskevich, Crater, Lane, & Krucoff, 2004; Silva, 1996; Umbreit, 2000; Wang & Hermann, 2006; Wardell, 2000; Wardell, Rintala, Tan, & Duan, 2006; Wardell & Weymouth, 2004; Wilkinson et al., 2002).

In pediatrics, several small research studies have been completed (Kemper, Fletcher, Hamilton, & McLean, 2012; McDonough-Means, Edde, & Bell, 2009; Speel, 2012; Verret, 2000; Wong, Ghiasuddin, Kimata, & Patelesio, 2012; Zimmer, Bogenschutz, Meier, & Rolf, 2009) that examine various outcomes. As of September 2012, there were 141 completed HT studies and six studies known to be in progress (Megel et al., 2012).

A proposed model of how HT may promote positive changes in client symptoms follows. A trained HT practitioner sends coherent energy waves from provider hands to the client. This affects the incoherent energy patterns that cause disease or imbalance in the client's energy field and body. Due to a resonant effect, the incoherent energy pattern shifts to a healthier, coherent pattern affecting the client's circulatory, endocrine, and nervous systems, and/or other unidentified mechanisms, promoting positive client responses with the potential to restore optimal health. The HT practitioner moves and repatterns a client's energy field, promoting a more open and symmetric pattern to enhance the client's perceived sense of well-being. This movement of energy may stimulate physiological, neurochemical, and psychological changes that promote positive effects on pain, anxiety, wound healing, immune system function, depression, and sense of well-being.

actual change in frequency

INTERVENTION

Techniques

Nearly 30 HT techniques are taught in the HT curriculum, from the simple to the complex. The HT practitioner determines which to use after an assessment of the client's expressed needs, symptoms presented, and results of an energy field hand scan. These strategies range from localized to full-body techniques. Exhibit 24.1 lists several basic techniques, along with indications and brief descriptions of the procedures. These techniques, which treat a wide range of client symptoms, should be practiced in a supervised setting with an instructor before working with a client. Most of the HT techniques involve two basic types of hand gestures (called magnetic passes) that are described in terms of "hands in motion" (used to clear congestion or density from the energy field) or "hands still" (used to reestablish energy flow and balance) (Schommer & Larrimore, 2010). In the hands-in-motion gestures, the hands make gentle brushing or combing motions, usually downward and outward, to remove congested energy from the field. The hands remain relaxed, palms facing downward toward the patient, between 1 inch and 6 inches above the skin or clothing. The hand strokes may be slow and sweeping or short and rapid. In the hands-still position, the practitioner holds hands over an area of the client's body for 1 to several minutes, either lightly touching the skin or just above it. The practitioner uses "intent" to facilitate a transfer of energy to the specific body part of the client from a "universal source" of energy, with the practitioner as the conduit of this energy.

Although several of the HT techniques can be done with the client in a seated position, most are done while the client is lying down fully dressed in the most relaxed state possible, to promote a more profound effect. The practitioner briefly describes HT and the procedure plan, invites the client to ask any questions at any time, and receives permission to do the treatment and to touch the client. HT therapists practice holistic principles that encourage openness in communication during the healing process, enhancing the depth of the healing experience (McKivergin, 2009).

Measurement of Outcomes

HT outcomes that have been measured include:

- Patient satisfaction
- Anxiety and stress reduction
- Improved mood and reduced fatigue and nausea in cancer patients
- Pain reduction
- Improved sense of well-being

Exhibit 24.1. *Basic Healing Touch Techniques*

Techniques	Indications	Brief Description of Procedure
Full-body techniques		
Basic HT sequence	Promote relaxation Reduce pain Lower anxiety, tension, and stress Facilitate wound healing Promote restoration of the body Promote a sense of well-being	1. Assess client's energy field with a hand scan over the body. 2. Use magnetic passes in client's energy field (hands in motion and/or hands still) to move congestion and density from the field. 3. Reassess client's energy field with hand scan to determine effects of intervention. 4. Ground the client to the present moment and to feel connection to the earth.
Magnetic clearing	Clear the body's energy field of congestion and emotional debris Used for: history of drug use, postanesthesia, chronic pain, trauma, systemic disease, after breathing polluted air, history of smoking, environmental sensitivities, emotional clearing and release of unresolved feelings (e.g., anger, fear, worry, tension), chemotherapy or radiation, and kidney dialysis	1. Assess client's energy field with a hand scan over the body. 2. Place hands 12 inches to 18 inches above the top of client's head with fingers spread, relaxed and curled, thumbs touching or close together. 3. Move hands very slowly in long continuous raking motions over the body from above the head to off the toes, 1 inch to 6 inches above the body, each sweep taking about 30 sec (work the middle of the body first, followed by each side). 4. Procedure is repeated 30 times and takes about 15 minutes. 5. Reassess client's energy field with hand scan to determine effects of intervention. 6. Ground the client to the present moment and to feel connection to the earth.
Full-body techniques		
Chakra connection (Joy, 1979)	Connects, opens, and balances the energy centers (chakras), enhancing the flow of energy throughout the body.	1. Assess client's energy field with a hand scan over the body. 2. Place hands on or over the minor energy centers (chakras) on the extremities and the major energy centers (chakras) on the trunk in a defined sequential manner, holding each area for at least 1 minute. 3. Reassess client's energy field with hand scan to determine effects of intervention. 4. Ground the client to the present moment and to feel connection to the earth.

(continued)

Exhibit 24.1. *Basic Healing Touch Techniques (continued)*

Techniques	Indications	Brief Description of Procedures
Chakra spread	Open the energy centers (chakras) producing a deep clearing of energy blocks Used for: physical or emotional pain, pre- and postmedical procedures/surgery, severe stress reactions, the terminally ill, stress, and assisting in coping with various life transitions	1. Assess client's energy field with a hand scan over the body. 2. Hold the client's feet, then hands, one by one in a gentle embrace for at least 1 minute. 3. Place hands (palms up) above each energy center (chakra), moving the hands slowly downward toward the chakra, then spreading the hands outward as far as possible; motion is repeated three times for each energy center, moving from the upper to the lower chakras. 4. Repeat entire sequence two more times. 5. Reassess client's energy field with hand scan to determine effects of intervention. 6. End treatment with holding the client's hand and heart center (procedure is done in silence and takes 10 min–15 min; is used very carefully by experienced practitioners for special needs and sacred moments in healing).
Localized techniques		
Energetic ultrasound	Breaks up congestion, energy patterns, and blockages Relieves pain Assists in stopping internal bleeding, sealing lacerations, healing fractures, and joint injuries Assists in breaking up bronchitis and sinus congestion	1. Hand scan client's localized area to assess energy field. 2. Hold the thumb and first and second fingers together, directing energy from the palm down the fingers. 3. Imagine a beam of light coming from the fingers of one hand into the client's body. 4. Place opposite hand behind the body part being worked on.
	Assists in stimulating return of bowel motility after surgery	5. Move the hand in any direction over the affected part, continuously moving for 3 minutes to 5 minutes. 6. Repeat hand scan to determine effect of intervention.
Energetic laser	Cuts, seals, and breaks up congestion in the energy field Relieves pain Helps stop bleeding Assists in wound repair	1. Hand scan client's localized area to assess energy field. 2. Hold one or more fingers still and pointed toward the problem area. 3. Use for a few seconds to a minute. 4. Repeat hand scan to determine effect of intervention.

(continued)

Exhibit 24.1. *Basic Healing Touch Techniques (continued)*

Techniques	Indications	Brief Description of Procedures
Mind clearing	Promotes relaxation and focuses or quiets the mind	1. Hold fingertips or palms on designated parts of the neck and head, holding each part 1 minute to 3 minutes. 2. Gently massage mandibular joint. 3. End with light sweeping touches across the forehead and cheeks three times and a gentle hold around the jaw.
Localized techniques		
Pain drain	Eases pain or energy congestion	1. Place left hand on area of pain or energy congestion and right hand downward away from body. 2. Siphon off congested energy from painful area through left hand and out right hand. 3. Place right hand on painful or congested area and place left hand upward in the air to bring in healing energy from the universal energy field (each position is generally held for 3 min–5 min).
Wound sealing	Repairs energy field leaks that occur from the physical body experiencing trauma, incisions, or childbirth	1. Hand scan body above a scar or injury to determine whether any leaks of energy are felt coming from the site (may feel like a column of cool air).
		2. Move hands over the area, gathering energy. 3. Bring gathered energy down to the client's skin over the injury and hold for 1 minute with hands. 4. Rescan the area to determine that the energy field feels evenly symmetrical over the entire body.

Note: Each technique begins with determining the client's specific need for HT and obtaining client permission. Mutual goals are set. This is followed by the practitioner centering, physically and psychologically, and setting the intention for the client's highest good. Assessment of energy-field disturbances are determined. Each technique ends with evaluating the energy field and the client's experience and asking for feedback.

Adapted from Hover-Kramer (2002) and Schommer and Larrimore (2010).

- Reduction in PTSD, and hostility and cynicism in postdeployed active military
- Decrease in depression
- Positive changes in blood pressure, blood glucose, and salivary immunoglobulin A
- Decreased length of hospitalization and adverse periprocedural outcomes after cardiac procedures

- Diminished agitation levels in dementia patients
- Improved behaviors of patients with Alzheimer's disease
- Improved functional status for patients with mobility issues
- Stress recovery in a neonatal intensive care unit

A current study is examining measuring magnetic field activity during an HT session (Moga, 2012). Until a reliable and easily available tool is developed to measure changes in the energy system, objective measurement of changes in the flow of an energy field is not possible. Practitioners do report a change in clients' energy fields that they perceive through the use of their senses, most commonly through touch.

Outcomes measured must reflect the specific client need and presenting symptoms, and the particular HT technique used to treat. Client outcomes have included such things as:

- Measuring patient satisfaction and well-being using Likert-type scale responses
- Visual analog scales (particularly for pain)
- Pain scales
- Measures of posttraumatic stress effects
- Chronic pain scales
- Hostility
- Depression
- Cardiovascular variables (heart rate, systolic/diastolic blood pressure, and mean arterial blood pressure)
- Oxygenation variables (pH, CO_2, PO_2, and HCO_3)
- Recovery measures
- Physical functional measures
- Degree of learning
- Health-related quality of life
- Immunoglobulin concentrations pre- and post-treatments

It is difficult to determine whether the outcome of the HT intervention is due solely to the treatment or to other factors as well. The effect of the practitioner's presence has always been considered a confounding variable affecting client outcome, but this is also true in many nursing interventions.

Precautions

Precautions to be aware of when using HT techniques include the following:

- The energy fields of infants, children, older people, the extremely ill, and the dying are sensitive to energy work, so treatments should be gentle and time limited.

■ Gentle energy treatments are also required for pregnant women because the energy field also includes the fetus.

■ Energy work with a cancer patient should be focused on balancing the whole field rather than concentrating on a particular area.

■ The effect of medications and chemicals in the body may be enhanced with energy work so one must be alert to the possibility of side effects and sensitivity reactions to these substances.

It is recommended that experienced practitioners work with clients in the above situations. However, to help develop a knowledgeable practice, a student or an apprentice in HT can provide treatments in these situations if supervised by a mentor (Umbreit, 2000). HT is not considered a curative treatment and must always be used in conjunction with conventional medical care. However, practitioners and clients have reported that clients have experienced a sense of healing at a more holistic level of mind, body, and spirit, even if a cure is not possible. Umbreit (2000) reports anecdotal comments from clients that include feeling "wonderful," "relaxed," "peaceful," "in a meditative state," "warm," "soothed," "safe," "reassured," "more balanced," "mellow," "happier with life," "as if all my tension was melting," and a "sense of inner peace." Slater (2009) states, "after a session, most people experience a sense of relaxation, lessened stress, increased energy, and other signs of increased vitality" (p. 664). Because HT is a noninvasive intervention, these clients' responses have enormous implications for improving quality of life in their striving toward wellness.

USES

HT interventions have been used on all age groups, from the neonate to the older adult. Besides the general curriculum for learning HT, there are also classes available for specifically working with pregnant women, infants, and children (Kluny, 2012). Healing Touch is being used within diverse health care facilities: hospitals, long-term-care facilities, private practices, hospices, clinics, schools of nursing, communities, and spas (Healing Touch International, 2012d). Models of delivering services range from volunteer to staff-provided programs. There are also well-established community service models that provide support for individuals with cancer while they are receiving conventional medical treatment (L. Anselme, personal communication, 2005).

HT interventions have been supported by a limited number of rigorous research studies; the majority of reports are from anecdotal stories in a variety of clinical situations in all age groups and states of illness or wellness (Bulbrook, 2000; Hover-Kramer, 2002; Scandrett-Hibdon et al., 1999; Umbreit, 2000) and from studies that unfortunately were missing some vital information, which led to problems with both internal and external validity (Wardell & Weymouth, 2004). HT studies have shown positive results in the following clinical situations:

■ Reduction of anxiety and stress
■ Promotion of relaxation
■ Reduction in acute and chronic pain
■ Acceleration of postoperative recovery
■ Aid in preparation for medical treatments and procedures
■ Improvement of cancer treatment side effects
■ Reduction in symptoms of depression
■ Promotion of a sense of well-being
■ Reduction in agitation levels
■ Improvement of PTSD symptoms
■ Improvement in quality of life physically, emotionally, relationally, and spiritually

Exhibit 24.2 lists several research studies that have supported the use of HT interventions in some of these clinical situations over the past 16 years. Many studies are not published in medical, nursing, or psychology journals, but information can be accessed through Healing Touch International's research department (www.healingtouchinternational .org). The research continues to be controversial because the exact mechanism of action cannot be seen or easily explained in our Western view of what constitutes sound scientific research, and few double-blind studies have been done in this area.

Exhibit 24.2. *Selected Research Studies Using Healing Touch Interventions (1996–2012)*

Uses	Selected Sources
Anxiety/stress reduction	Dubrey (2012a); Gehlhaart and Dail (2000); Guevara, Silva, and Menidas (2012); Taylor (2001); Wilkinson et al. (2002)
Pediatrics: Promotion of relaxation/relief of anxiety, stress, pain, depression, fatigue, spasticity	Kemper et al. (2012); McDonough-Means et al. (2009); Speel (2012); Verret (2000); Wong et al. (2012); Zimmer et al. (2009)
Acute and chronic pain reduction	Cordes, Proffitt, and Roth (2012); Darbonne (2012); Diener (2001); Hardwick (2012); Hjersted-Smith and Jones (2012); Kiley (2012); Merritt and Randall (2012);

(continued)

Exhibit 24.2. *Selected Research Studies Using Healing Touch Interventions (1996–2012) (continued)*

	Peck (2007); Protzman (2012); Slater (2012); Wardell (2000); Wardell et al. (2006); Wardell, Rintala, and Tan (2008); Welcher and Kish (2001); Weymouth and Sandberg-Lewis (2000)
Acceleration of postoperative recovery	Laffey and Neizgoda (2012); MacIntyre et al. (2008); Silva (1996)
Aid in medical procedures/ treatments	Seskevich et al. (2004)
Improvement of cancer treatment side effects and general well-being in cancer patients	Cook et al. (2004); Danhauer et al. (2008); Post-White et al. (2003); Rexilius, Mundt, Megel, and Agrawal (2002); Turner (2012)
Mental health	Bradway (1998); Dubrey (2012b); Van Aken (2012)
Older adults	Decker, Wardell, and Cron (2012); Gehlhaart and Dail (2000); Ostuni and Pietro (2012); Peck (2007); Wang and Hermann (2006)
PTSD	Guevara et al. (2012); Jain et al. (2012)
Personal growth and transformation; spiritual meaning and awareness	Geddes (1999); Wardell (2001); Ziembroski, Gilbert, Bossarte, and Guldbery (2003)

CULTURAL APPLICATIONS

HT is being taught and practiced in 37 countries around the world, including impoverished communities with few economic resources, with more countries continuing to request HT education each year. As of 2012, HT has been taught in Argentina, Australia, Belize, Bermuda, Bolivia, Cambodia, Canada, Colombia, Denmark, Ecuador, El Salvador, England, Finland, France, Germany, Guatemala, Hungary, India, Ireland, Italy, Japan, Korea, Mexico, Nepal, Netherlands, New Zealand, Nicaragua, Perú, Romania, South Africa, Sweden, Tanzania, Thailand, Tibet, Trinidad/ Tobago, Uganda, and the United States (*Energy* magazine, July 2011; *Energy* magazine, October/December, 2011). The skills of HT can be communicated across cultures by appropriately adapting teaching styles to the culture and available resources. The HT students are then able to use their skills in their communities: in a hospital setting, clinic, homes, rural areas, villages, and places where health care may be limited and living conditions very difficult. Even in impoverished places of the world, where strife, abject poverty, and hidden hopelessness pervade daily life, learning and practicing HT has helped empower the people to address their serious social and public health issues by decreasing their suffering, especially where women and children are marginalized (Starke, 2008). HT has offered tools to address difficult situations and ways to work in the absence of medications (Goff, 2007). Sidebar 24.1 describes the use of HT in Perú.

M. J. Frost (personal communication, November 30, 2012), certified holistic nurse, certified HT practitioner/instructor, has found her work internationally as an HT instructor unparalleled in her life, filled with rewarding moments with beautiful people from diverse cultures. In Romania, she taught classes to volunteers who would take HT to individuals, families, and orphans healing from the trauma of the newly fallen Communist dictator and years of oppression. In South Africa, she taught caregivers of orphans whose parents had died of HIV/AIDS, and some of whom had been infected through the birth process. Another venue was a care agency outside of Johannesburg, from which home caregivers walked out into refugee camps to use their new HT skills, along with personal care, to ease many suffering and dying of AIDS and TB. She traveled up into the Himalayan range to work with Tibetan refugees and offer HT to those who had been imprisoned by the Chinese. She taught classes to women, men, and Tibetan medical students; and she has stated that HT is a universal language, understood by all.

Sidebar 24.1. *Healing Touch in Perú*

Margaret Kehoe, Lima, Perú

HT classes were first brought to Perú in 2000 at the request of religious sisters who worked with the isolated and very poor. In 2005, they created the Promoting Holistic Health organization to partner with Healing Touch International and Energy Medicine partnerships, extending HT to more regions in Perú, Chile, Argentina, and Ecuador. Their purpose was to provide HT education and scientific investigation about the effectiveness of these therapies, focusing on service toward those parts of Latin America that are most marginalized. In Lima, there are three HT centers in shantytowns; clients who are unable to pay get the services for free. A bridge has been formed between those who have and those who have not, financially. Many clients who are able to pay for services have never really known about poverty; once they face their fears, these same people become actively engaged in helping bring about justice and change in the shantytowns. This has brought together cultures within a culture, allowing healing to take place not only at a personal level but also at an indigenous level.

(continued)

> ### Sidebar 24.1. *Healing Touch in Perú (continued)*
>
> One of these centers also works with children and youth who have very basic living conditions and little access to health care. These children are growing up with a totally different attitude toward health care; they have a very new idea of themselves, who they are, and also their capacity to heal. The ripple is having tremendously important effects in the homes and in the neighborhoods where the children live. The largest influence of HT for all who receive it would be the change in how these people see themselves. Before they seemed caught up in their scarcity; however, once they awaken to their abundance, their lives turn around. This is a huge step culturally because in two thirds of these countries, those who have been made poor are kept poor by those in power. HT is helping to change that at a grassroots level.
>
> It is the heart-centered approach to healing that attracts the Latin American people to HT. HT practitioners work in more affluent areas of Latin America as well. The practitioners speak about the hope, the richness, and the transformation that their clients have received though HT treatments. What is happening through HT in Latin America is just beginning and to be part of this shift in consciousness is a wonderful privilege.

FUTURE RESEARCH

Research studies and anecdotal cases in HT offer promising yet certainly not conclusive data on the positive outcomes from this complementary therapy. Qualitative responses from clients have been especially important in helping guide the direction of the research and may provide insight into the phenomenon of energy exchange in the future. Some of the problems encountered in nursing research include insufficient funding to support the work, multiple variables that are hard to control in a clinical setting versus a laboratory setting, and the use of small sample sizes that can be easily affected by highly variable data and sampling error.

There is the additional difficulty of testing the efficacy of an energy-based therapy in which the energy exchange between practitioner and client cannot be seen by most people, but is only observed as subjective responses from clients. The whole conceptual framework of energy fields and energy exchange does not fit the cause–effect model that Western science is focused on. Rogers's theory (1990) speaks about energy changing, exchanging, and patterning, one moment in time never replicating itself. The focus is on nature's restoring universal order and balance, and restoring energy balance is the goal of HT. This is a huge area of research that obviously will require a multidisciplinary effort by Western and Eastern medicine, quantum physics, biology, psychology, philosophy, spirituality, and nursing. Outcome studies, as well as studies of mechanism, will help support the development and understanding of the phenomenon of energy exchange. There are mediating factors that may contribute to decrease in pain intensity, anxiety reduction, acceleration of healing, immune system enhancement, diminished depression, and increased sense of well-being. More studies that measure some of these mediating mechanisms are recommended.

The choice of valid instruments for measuring outcomes is critical in HT studies. Results can be skewed in either direction if the instruments are not reliable. However, to obtain subject cooperation when working with persons who are ill, measuring instruments must be easy to use and not burdensome to patients who are already facing difficulties.

Other challenges to be controlled in conducting HT research studies include the experience of the HT practitioner, the phenomenon of the caregiver's "presence," the type of HT treatment modality chosen, the length and number of treatments, when the treatment is done, and when measurements are done, and longer term effects of HT. There is a wide range of skill levels of HT practitioners from novice to certified practitioner and comparable skill level is important in planning a research study. It is important to note that "the deepest and longest lasting healing will be at the hands of a healer who has the greatest breadth and depth of training, practice, and personal healing" (Slater, 2009, p. 649). The phenomenon of presence of the HT practitioner may also affect the outcome of the research and needs to be controlled in the study design. Because there are many HT interventions that can be used, a research study may need to be consistent in the type of therapy chosen. The challenge with length and number of treatments is that, under normal circumstances, an HT intervention is not used for a prescribed length of time or number of treatments. The work is done until the practitioner intuitively determines that it is time to stop or that no more treatments are needed. Research could restrict this professional decision-making process. Choosing when to give an HT treatment and when to measure outcomes and ascertaining how long the outcome may last continue to be challenging. Experienced HT practitioners must have input into determining these timelines by observing patterns they may typically see in their own professional practice.

The next steps for research must build on the studies already completed. Replication of studies would help strengthen the validity of HT. The following are questions related to specific areas to build on:

- Is HT equally effective in acute versus chronic pain? How long and how frequent do treatments need to be for the client to report a decrease in pain? How long does this improvement last?
- How is postoperative recovery affected by administering HT (pain relief, wound healing, restoring of bowel function, ease of physical activity, length of stay in the hospital)?
- Does HT have a positive effect on degenerative diseases such as arthritis, multiple sclerosis, fibromyalgia, stroke, immune deficiency disorders, chronic lung conditions, and living with a cancer diagnosis?
- Does HT assist in managing the side effects of treatments in cancer patients?
- What are the psychological and spiritual benefits reported by HT recipients?
- What is the impact of HT as a complement to help eliminate PTSD and depression in our military and others who have experienced trauma?
- What tools are effective in measuring a change in energy in the recipient before and after HT or an exchange of energy between practitioner and recipient?
- Does HT reduce medical costs for pharmaceuticals, hospital stays, and clinic time?

In the quest to examine the impact of HT scientifically, care must be taken so as not to be too quick to dismiss the overwhelming positive client feedback from its clinical application. Creativity is necessary in conducting research of this phenomenon that cannot be seen by the naked eye, but is so often felt by the human spirit.

WEBSITES

For more information on HT:

American Holistic Nurses Association (AHNA)
(www.ahna.org)

Healing Touch International
(www.healingtouchinternational.org)

Healing Touch Program
(www.healingtouchprogram.com)

For more information on Therapeutic Touch
(www.therapeutictouch.org)

REFERENCES

Bailey, A. (1984). *Esoteric healing.* Albany, NY: Lucis Trust.

Bradway, C. (1998). The effects of healing touch on depression. *Healing Touch Newsletter: Research Edition, 8*(3), 2.

Brennan, B. (1986). *Hands of light.* New York, NY: Bantam.

Bruyere, R. L. (1989). *Wheels of light.* New York, NY: Simon & Schuster.

Bulbrook, M. J. (2000). *Healing stories to inspire, teach and heal.* Carrboro, NC: North Carolina Center for Healing Touch.

Carpenito, L. J. (2013). *Nursing diagnosis: Application to clinical practice* (14th ed., pp. 252–255). Philadelphia, PA: Lippincott, Williams, and Wilkins.

Cook, C., Guerrerio, J., & Slater, V. (2004). Healing touch and quality of life in women receiving radiation treatment for cancer: A randomized controlled trial. *Alternative Therapies, 10*(3), 34–41.

Cordes, P., Proffitt, C., & Roth, J. (2012). The effect of healing touch therapy on the pain and joint mobility experienced by patients with total knee replacements. In M. Megel, J. G. Anderson, D. Lu, & N. Strybol (Eds.), *Healing touch research survey* (14th ed., pp. 67–68). Lakewood, CO: Healing Touch International.

Danhauer, S. C., Tooze, J. A., Holder, P., Miller, C., Jesse, M. T., Carroll, S., . . . Kemper, K. J. (2008). Healing touch as a supportive intervention for adult acute leukemia patients: A pilot investigation of effects on distress and treatment-related symptoms. *Journal of the Society for Integrative Oncology, 6*(3), 89–97.

Darbonne, M. (2012). The effects of healing touch modalities on patients with chronic pain. In M. Megel, J. G. Anderson, D. Lu, & N. Strybol (Eds.), *Healing touch research survey* (14th ed., pp. 76–77). Lakewood, CO: Healing Touch International.

Decker, S., Wardell, D. W., & Cron, S. G. (2012). Using a healing touch intervention in older adults with persistent pain: A feasibility study. *Journal of Holistic Nursing, 30*(3), 205–213.

Diener, D. (2001). A pilot study of the effect of chakra connection and magnetic unruffle on perception of pain in people with fibromyalgia. *Healing Touch Newsletter: Research Edition, 1*(3), 7–8.

Dowd, T., Kolcaba, K., Steiner, R., & Fashinpaur, D. (2007). Comparison of a healing touch, coaching, and a combined intervention on comfort and stress in younger college students. *Holistic Nursing Practice, 21*(4), 194–202.

Dubrey, R. (2012a). A quality assurance project on the effectiveness of healing touch treatments as perceived by patients at the wellness institute. In M. Megel, J. G. Anderson, D. Lu, & N. Strybol (Eds.), *Healing touch research survey* (14th ed., p. 89). Lakewood, CO: Healing Touch International.

Dubrey, R. (2012b). The effect of healing touch on in-patients going through stage 1 recovery from alcoholism. In M. Megel, J. G. Anderson, D. Lu, & N. Strybol (Eds.), *Healing touch research survey* (14th ed., pp. 105–106). Lakewood, CO: Healing Touch International.

Duerden, T. (2004). An aura of confusion. Part 2: The aided eye—"Imaging the aura?" *Complementary Therapies in Nurse Midwifery, 10,* 116–123.

Energy Magazine. (2011, July). Healing touch around the world (pp. 8–9). San Antonio, TX: Healing Touch Program.

Energy Magazine. (2011, October/December). My reflections of healing touch in Uganda (pp. 28–29). San Antonio, TX: Healing Touch Program.

Engebretson, J., & Wardell, D. W. (2002). Experience of a reiki session. *Alternative Therapies, 8*(2), 48–53.

Eschiti, V. (2007). Healing touch: A low-tech intervention in high-tech settings. *Dimensions of Critical Care Nursing, 26*(1), 9–14.

Feinstein, D., & Eden, D. (2008). Six pillars of energy medicine: Clinical strengths of a complementary paradigm. *Alternative Therapies, 14*(1), 44–54.

Forbes, M. A., Rust, R., & Becker, G. J. (2004). Surface electromyography (EMG) as a measurement for biofield research: Results from a single case study. *Journal of Alternative & Complementary Medicine, 10*(4), 617–626.

Geddes, N. (1999). The experience of personal transformation in healing touch practitioners: A heuristic inquiry. *Healing Touch Newsletter, 9*(3), 5.

Geddes, N. (2002). Research related to healing touch. In D. Hover-Kramer (Ed.), *Healing touch: A guidebook for practitioners* (2nd ed., pp. 24–40). Albany, NY: Delmar.

Gehlhaart, C., & Dial, P. (2000). Effectiveness of healing touch and therapeutic touch on elderly residents of long term care facilities on reducing pain and anxiety level. *Healing Touch Newsletter, 0*(3), 8.

Goff, R. (2007). Carrying light into South Africa. *Healing Touch International, Inc. Quarterly Newsletter, 1*, 6–7.

Guevara, E., Silva, C., & Menidas, N., (2012). The effect of healing touch therapy on post-traumatic stress disorder (PTSD) symptoms on domestic violence abused Mexican women. In M. Megel, J. G. Anderson, D. Lu, & N. Strybol (Eds.), *Healing touch research survey* (14th ed., pp. 106–107). Lakewood, CO: Healing Touch International.

Hardwick, M. E. (2012). Nursing intervention using healing touch in bilateral total knee arthroplasty. In M. Megel, J. G. Anderson, D. Lu, & N. Strybol (Eds.), *Healing touch research survey* (14th ed., p. 68). Lakewood, CO: Healing Touch International.

Healing Touch International. (2012a). *The history of healing touch.* Retrieved December 11, 2012, from www.healingtouchinternational.org

Healing Touch International. (2012b). *What is healing touch?* Retrieved December 11, 2012, from www.healingtouchinternational.org

Healing Touch International. (2012c). *Healing touch scope of practice.* Retrieved December 12, 2012, from www.healingtouchinternational.org

Healing Touch International. (2012d). *Where is healing touch used?* Retrieved December 12, 2012, from www.healingtouchinternational.org

Healing Touch Program. (2012a). *What is healing touch?* Retrieved December 12, 2012, from www.healingtouchprogram.com

Healing Touch Program. (2012b). *Who can practice healing touch?* Retrieved November 23, 2012, from www.healingtouchprogram.com

Hjersted-Smith, C., & Jones, S. (2012). The effects of healing touch on pain and anxiety with end stage liver disease. In M. Megel, J. G. Anderson, D. Lu, & N. Strybol (Eds.), *Healing touch research survey* (14th ed., pp. 83–84). Lakewood, CO: Healing Touch International.

Hover-Kramer, D. (2002). *Healing touch: A guidebook for practitioners* (2nd ed.). Albany, NY: Delmar.

Hover-Kramer, D., Mentgen, J., & Scandrett-Hibdon, S. (1996). *Healing touch: A resource for health care professionals.* Albany, NY: Delmar.

Hutchison, C. (1999). Healing touch: An energetic approach. *American Journal of Nursing, 99*(4), 43–48.

Jackson, C., & Keegan, L. (2009). Touch. In B. Dossey & L. Keegan (Eds.), *Holistic nursing: A handbook for practice* (5th ed., pp. 347–366). Sudbury MA: Jones & Bartlett.

Jain, S., McMahon, G. F., Hasen, P., Kozub, M. P., Porter, V., King, R., & Guarneri, E. M. (2012). Healing touch with guided imagery for PTSD in returning active duty military: A randomized controlled trial. *Military Medicine, 177* (9), 1015–1021.

Joy, B. (1979). *Joy's way.* New York, NY: G. P. Putnam's Sons.

Kemper, K., Fletcher, N., Hamilton, C., & McLean, T. (2012). Impact of healing touch on pediatric oncology outpatients: A pilot study. In M. Megel, J. G. Anderson, D. Lu, & N. Strybol (Eds.) *Healing touch research survey* (14th ed., pp. 19–20). Lakewood, CO: Healing Touch International.

Kiley, S. (2012). The evaluation of healing touch for headache pain. In M. Megel, J. G. Anderson, D. Lu, & N. Strybol (Eds.), *Healing touch research survey* (14th ed., p. 78). Lakewood, CO: Healing Touch International.

Kluny, R. (2012). *Healing touch for babies.* Retrieved December 12, 2012, from www .healingtouchforbabies.com

Krieger, D. (1979). *The therapeutic touch: How to use your hands to help or to heal.* New York, NY: Simon & Schuster.

Krieger, D. (1993). *Accepting your power to heal.* Santa Fe, NM: Bear & Co.

Krucoff, M., Crater, S., Gallup, D., Blankenship, J., Cuffe, M., Guarneri, M., . . . Lee, K. (2005). Music, imagery, touch, and prayer as adjuncts to interventional cardiac care: The monitoring and actualization of noetic trainings (MANTRA) II randomized study. *Lancet, 366*(9481), 211–217.

Krucoff, M., Crater, S., Green, C., Massa, A., Seskevich, J., Lane, J., . . . Koenig, H. (2001). Integrative noetic therapies as adjuncts to percutaneous intervention during unstable coronary syndromes: Monitoring and actualization of noetic training (MANTRA) feasibility pilot. *American Heart Journal, 142*(5), 760–769.

Laffey, E., & Neizgoda, J. (2012). Wound care and complementary medicine: The impact of healing touch. A case study. In M. Megel, J. G. Anderson, D. Lu, & N. Strybol (Eds.), *Healing touch research survey* (14th ed., pp. 101–102). Lakewood, CO: Healing Touch International.

MacIntyre, B., Hamilton, J., Fricke, T., Ma, W., Mehle, S., & Michel, M. (2008). The efficacy of healing touch in coronary artery bypass surgery recovery: A randomized clinical trial. *Alternative Therapies in Healing and Medicine, 14*(4), 24–32.

Maville, J., Bowen, J., & Benham, G. (2008). Effect of healing touch on stress perception and biological correlates. *Holistic Nursing Practice, 22*(2), 103–110.

McDonough-Means, S. I., Edde, E. L., & Bell, I. R. (2009). Healing touch shows potential stress mitigation in ill neonates [Abstract]. *Journal of Developmental and Behavioral Pediatrics, 30*(6). doi:10.1097/DBP,0b013e3181c77898

McKivergin, M. (2009). The nurse as an instrument of healing. In B. Dossey & L. Keegan (Eds.), *Holistic nursing: A handbook for practice* (5th ed., pp. 721–738). Sudbury, MA: Jones & Bartlett.

Megel, M. E., Anderson, J. G., Lu, D., & Strybol, N. (2012). *Healing touch research survey* (14th ed.). Lakewood, CO: Healing Touch International.

Merritt, P., & Randall, D. (2012). The effect of healing touch and other forms of energy work on cancer pain. In M. Megel, J. G. Anderson, D. Lu, & N. Strybol (Eds.), *Healing touch research survey* (14th ed., p. 24). Lakewood, CO: Healing Touch International.

Moga, M. (2012). Environmental DC magnetic field activity and healer-client feedback as measures of bioenergy during healing touch therapy. In M. Megel, J. G. Anderson, D. Lu, & N. Strybol (Eds.), *Healing touch research survey* (14th ed., p. 121). Lakewood, CO: Healing Touch International.

NCCAM: National Center for Complementary and Alternative Medicine. (2012, May). *Energy medicine: An overview.* Retrieved December 9, 2012, from www.nccam.nih.gov

Oschman, J. (2008, September). *Validating the heart's work.* Paper presented at the Healing Touch International Conference, Milwaukee, WI.

Oschman, J. L. (2000). *Energy medicine: The scientific basis.* Dover, NH: Churchill Livingston.

Oschman, J. L. (2009). Toward a scientific understanding of energy healing. In D. Hover-Kramer (Ed.), *Healing touch guidebook* (pp. 59–72). San Antonio, TX: Healing Touch Program.

Ostuni, E., & Pietro, M. J. (2012). Effects of healing touch on nursing home residents in later stages of Alzheimer's. In M. Megel, J. G. Anderson, D. Lu, & N. Strybol (Eds.), *Healing touch research survey* (14th ed., pp. 48–49). Lakewood, CO: Healing Touch International.

Peck, S. (2007). Aftermath of an unexpected, unexplained and abrupt termination of healing touch and extrapolation of related costs. *Complementary Health Review, 12*(144), 144–160.

Post-White, J., Kinney, M. E., Savik, K., Gau, J. B., Wilcox, C., & Lerner, I. (2003). Therapeutic massage and healing touch improve symptoms in cancer. *Integrative Cancer Therapies, 2*(4), 332–344.

Protzman, L. (2012). The effect of healing touch on pain and relaxation. In M. Megel, J. G. Anderson, D. Lu, & N. Strybol (Eds.), *Healing touch research survey* (14th ed., pp. 48–49). Lakewood, CO: Healing Touch International.

Rexilius, S., Mundt, C., Megel, M., & Agrawal, S. (2002). Therapeutic effects of healing touch and massage therapy on caregivers of autologous hematopoietic stem cell transplant patients. *Oncology Nursing Forum, 29*(3), 1–14.

Rogers, M. (1990). Nursing: Science of unitary, irreducible, human beings: Update 1990. In E. A. M. Barrett (Ed.), *Vision of Rogers' science-based nursing* (pp. 5–11). New York, NY: National League for Nursing.

Scandrett-Hibdon, S. (1996). Research foundations. In D. Hover-Kramer, J. Mentgen, & S. Scandrett-Hibdon (Eds.), *Healing touch: A resource for health care professionals* (pp. 27–42). Albany, NY: Delmar.

Scandrett-Hibdon, S., Hardy, C., & Mentgen, J. (1999). *Energetic patterns: Healing touch case studies* (Vol. 1). Lakewood, CO: Colorado Center for Healing Touch.

Schommer, B., & Larrimore, D. (2010). *HTI healing touch certificate program level 1 student workbook.* Lakewood, CO: Healing Touch International.

Schwartz, G. E. (2007). *The energy healing experiments.* New York, NY: Atria Books.

Seskevitz, J., Crater, S., Lane, J., & Krucoff, M. (2004). Beneficial effects of noetic therapies on mood before percutaneous intervention for unstable coronary symptoms. *Nursing Research, 53*(2), 116–121.

Silva, C. (1996). The effects of relaxation touch on the recovery level of postanesthesia abdominal hysterectomy patients. *Alternative Therapies, 2*(4), 94.

Slater, V. (2009). Energy healing. In B. Dossey & L. Keegan (Eds.), *Holistic nursing: A handbook for practice* (5th ed., pp. 647–673). Sudbury, MA: Jones & Bartlett.

Slater, V. (2012). Safety, elements, and effects of healing touch on chronic non-malignant abdominal pain. In M. Megel, J. G. Anderson, D. Lu, & N. Strybol (Eds.), *Healing touch research survey* (14th ed., pp. 84–85). Lakewood, CO: Healing Touch International.

Speel, L. (2012). A pilot study on the effect of healing touch–mind cleaning and magnetic unruffling on high school students with mental and physical disabilities. In M. Megel, J. G. Anderson, D. Lu, & N. Strybol (Eds.), *Healing touch research survey* (14th ed., pp. 96–98). Lakewood, CO: Healing Touch International.

Starke, B.A. (2008, July). Presence in Nepal. *Energy Magazine, 25*, 11–14.

Taylor, B. (2001). The effect of healing touch on the coping ability, self esteem, and general health of undergraduate nursing students. *Complementary Therapies in Nursing and Midwifery, 7*(1), 34–42.

Therapeutic Touch. (2004). *What is therapeutic touch?* Retrieved December 9, 2012, from www.therapeutictouch.org

Turner, K. (2012). Preliminary data analysis of the healing touch partners program. In M. Megel, J. G. Anderson, D. Lu, & N. Strybol (Eds.), *Healing touch research survey* (14th ed., pp. 27–29). Lakewood, CO: Healing Touch International.

Umbreit, A. (2000). Healing touch: Applications in the acute care setting. *AACN Clinical Issues, 11*(1), 105–119.

Van Aken, R. (2012). The experiential process of healing touch for people with moderate depression. In M. Megel, J. G. Anderson, D. Lu, & N. Strybol (Eds.), *Healing touch research survey* (14th ed., pp. 108–109). Lakewood, CO: Healing Touch International.

Verret, P. (2000). Healing touch as a relaxation intervention in children with spasticity. *Healing Touch Newsletter: Research Edition, 0*(3), 6–7.

Wang, K., & Hermann, C. (2006). Pilot study to test the effectiveness of healing touch on agitation levels in people with dementia. *Geriatric Nursing, 27*(1), 42–40.

Wardell, D. (2000). The trauma release technique: How it is taught and experienced in healing touch. *Alternative and Complementary Therapies, 6*(1), 20–27.

Wardell, D. (2001). Spirituality of healing touch participants. *Journal of Holistic Nursing, 19*(1), 71–86.

Wardell, D., Rintala, D., Tan, G., & Duan, A. (2006). Pilot study of healing touch and progressive relaxation for chronic neuropathic pain in persons with spinal cord injury. *Journal of Holistic Nursing, 24*(4), 231–240.

Wardell, D., Rintala, D., & Tan, G. (2008). Study descriptions of healing touch with veterans experiencing chronic neuropathic pain from spinal cord injury. *Explore, 4*(3), 187–195.

Wardell, D. W., & Weymouth, K. F. (2004). Review of studies of healing touch. *Journal of Nursing Scholarship, 36*(2), 147–154.

Watson, J. (1985). *Nursing: The philosophy and science of caring.* Boulder, CO: Associated University Press.

Welcher, B., & Kish, J. (2001). Reducing pain and anxiety through healing touch. *Healing Touch Newsletter, 1*(3), 19.

Weymouth, K., & Sandberg-Lewis, S. (2000). Comparing the efficacy of healing touch and chiropractic adjustment in treating chronic low back pain: A pilot study. *Healing Touch Newsletter, 00*(3), 7–8.

Wilkinson, D., Knox, P., Chatman, J., Johnson, T., Barbour, N., Myles, Y., & Reel, A. (2002). The clinical effectiveness of healing touch. *Journal of Alternative and Complementary Medicine, 8*(1), 33–47.

Wong, J., Ghiasuddin, A., Kimata, C., & Patelesio, B. (2012). The psychosocial and hematological impact of healing touch on pediatric oncology patients: A randomized, prospective intervention study. In M. Megel, J. G. Anderson, D. Lu, & N. Strybol (Eds.), *Healing touch research survey* (14th ed., pp. 30–37). Lakewood, CO: Healing Touch International.

Ziembroski, J., Gilbert, N., Bossarte, R., & Guldbery, G. (2003). Healing touch and hospice care: Examining outcomes at the end of life. *Alternative and Complementary Therapies, 9*(3), 146–151.

Zimmer, M. H., Bogenschutz, L., Meier, M. E., & Rolf, W. G. (2009). Effect of healing touch on children's pain and comfort in the postoperative period [Abstract]. *Alternative Therapies in Health and Medicine, 15*(3), S186.

We all have access to universal energy.

Chapter 25: Reiki

DEBBIE RINGDAHL

Emphasis is on healing not cure healing on other levels besides physical

Reiki is an energy-healing method that can be used as an integrative therapy for a broad range of acute and chronic health problems. Increasingly, it is gaining acceptance as an adjunct to management of chronic conditions: pain management, hospice and palliative care, and stress reduction. In 2003, Miles and True described 24 hospitals and community-based programs in the United States that use Reiki in the areas of general medicine, surgery, treatment of HIV/AIDS and cancer, and older adult and hospice care, as well as for staff and family members. In 2013, the Center for Reiki Research identified 75 hospitals, medical clinics, and hospice programs where Reiki was offered as part of standard practice. This author notes that only one of five area health care facilities using Reiki is listed, suggesting a greater usage of Reiki than these numbers indicate.

The 2010 Complementary and Alternative Medicine Survey of Hospitals (Ananth, 2011) reported that Reiki and Therapeutic Touch were offered in 21% of inpatient settings surveyed. A 2007 national survey found that 1.2 million adults and 161,000 children received one or more energy-healing sessions such as Reiki in the previous year (Barnes, Bloom, & Nahin, 2008). The National Institutes for Health (NIH) recently completed clinical trials investigating Reiki use for fibromyalgia, AIDS, painful neuropathy, stress, and prostate cancer (NCCAM, 2013).

According to the National Center for Complementary and Alternative Medicine (NCCAM), Reiki is a biofield therapy. Therapies in this category affect energy fields that both surround and interpenetrate the human body. Bioenergy therapies involve touch or placement of the hands into a biofield, the existence of which has not been scientifically proven (NCCAM, 2011). Several biofield therapies have been introduced into clinical care over the

419

past few decades, representing a renewed interest in the therapeutic use of intentional touch in clinical practice. Reiki, Therapeutic Touch (TT), and Healing Touch (HT) are all biofield therapies that are used to support the healing process. Although each has its own history, techniques, and practice standards, they share many similarities. All three traditions include the fundamental assumption that a universal life force sustains all living organisms (Hover-Kramer, 1996; Macrae, 1987; Ringdahl, 2010) and that human beings have an energetic and spiritual dimension that is a part of the healing process (Anderson & Taylor, 2011b). The focus is on balancing the energies of the total person and stimulating the body's own natural healing ability, rather than on the treatment of specific physical diseases (Anderson & Taylor, 2011b; Macrae, 1987; Ringdahl, 2010). The common thread that exists among these modalities lies in their capacity to reduce stress, promote relaxation, and mitigate pain.

A Reiki practitioner does not need to be prepared as a health care practitioner; however, nurses, physical therapists, massage therapists, and physicians who practice Reiki may have greater access and acceptability within the health care system in performing hands-on treatments. Additionally, Reiki practice by nurses supports a high-touch practice model in a high-tech practice environment. The Institute of Medicine (IOM) 2009 Summit on Integrative Medicine and the Health of the Public identified that empathy and compassion enhanced care and improved outcomes with grade A evidence (IOM, 2010). Although this evidence is not specific to physical touch, research suggests that recipients of touch therapies frequently experience an integration of mind, body, and spirit that promotes feelings of well-being (Engebretson & Wardell, 2002). Jean Watson's conceptualization of the reciprocal nature of caring also supports the value of Reiki touch in providing nursing care (Brathovde, 2006).

The origins of Reiki are unclear, but Reiki historians generally agree that this therapy may have its roots in hands-on healing techniques that were used in Tibet or India more than 2,000 years ago. Reiki emerged in modern times around 1900 through the work of a Japanese businessman and practitioner of Tendai Buddhism, Mikao Usui (Miles, 2006). According to William Lee Rand (2000), founder of The International Center for Reiki Training, Usui searched many years for knowledge of healing methods until he had a profound, transformative experience and received direct revelation of what became known as Reiki. Following this experience, Usui worked with the poor in Kyoto and Tokyo, teaching classes and giving treatments in what he called "The Usui System of Reiki Healing." One of Dr. Usui's students, Chujiro Hayashi, wrote down the hand positions and suggested ways of using them for various ailments.

Mrs. Hawayo Takata is credited with the spread of Reiki in the Americas and Europe. In 1973, Mrs. Takata began to train Reiki teachers (Miles, 2006). The Reiki Alliance, a professional organization of Reiki masters, grew from 20 to nearly 1,000 members between 1981 and 1999 (Horrigan, 2003).

3 levels. Can self heal

DEFINITION

The word *Reiki* is composed of two Japanese words—*rei* and *ki*. *Rei* is usually translated as universal, although some authors suggest that it also has a deeper connotation of all-knowing spiritual consciousness. *Ki* refers to life force energy that flows throughout all living things, known in certain other parts of the world as *Chi*, *prana*, or *mana*. When *Ki* energy is unrestricted, there is thought to be less susceptibility to illness or imbalances of mind, body, or spirit (Rand, 2000). In its combined form, the word *Reiki* is taken to mean spiritually guided life force energy or universal life force energy.

The mind–body component to Reiki healing is evidenced in the underlying belief that the deepest level of healing occurs through the spirit. The emphasis is on healing, not cure, which is believed to occur by Reiki energy connecting individuals to their own innate spiritual wisdom and "highest good." Reiki is considered a nondirective healing tradition: Reiki energy flows through, but is not directed by, the practitioner, leaving the healing component to the individual receiving the treatment.

Reiki is not only a healing technique, but a philosophy of living that acknowledges mind–body–spirit unity and human connectedness to all things. This philosophy is reflected in the Reiki principles for living: "Just for today do not worry. Just for today do not anger. Honor your teachers, parents, and elders. Earn your living honestly. Show gratitude to all living things" (Mills, 2001). These principles further support the value of living with intention, self-awareness, and in the present moment.

The ability to practice Reiki is transmitted in stages directly from teacher to student via initiations called attunements. This attunement process differentiates Reiki from other hands-on healing methods. During attunements, teachers open up the students' energy channels by using specific visual symbols that were revealed to Dr. Usui. There are three degrees of attunement preparatory to achieving the status of Master Teacher, at which stage the practitioner is considered fully open to the flow of universal life force energy. By tradition, the Usui Reiki symbols and their Japanese names are confidential. This arises from the sacred nature of the techniques rather than from proprietary motives; the symbols are believed not to convey Reiki energy if used by noninitiates.

Level I Reiki is taught as a hands-on technique that includes basic information about Reiki history, application, principles, and hand positions. In Level II, students are taught symbols that allow transfer of energy through space and time, also known as absentee or distance healing. The higher vibration of energy available at Level II is considered to work at a deeper level of healing and with greater intuitive awareness. Level III, or the mastery level, is typically achieved through an apprenticeship with a Reiki Master, and includes more in-depth study of Reiki practice and teaching. At all levels, Reiki skill develops through years of committed practice.

In recent years, additional branches of Reiki with further degrees of attunement have developed; two of these are Karuna Reiki and Reiki Seichim. There are currently no uniform standards in Reiki education, either at the national or international level. Because of the noninvasive nature of the treatments, this does not present problems in Reiki hands-on practice, but may contribute to variable levels of professionalism among practitioners. This lack of standardization may also pose problems when working to develop practice standards for integration of Reiki into the conventional health care system.

SCIENTIFIC BASIS

Researchers have attempted to study the biological effects of biofields on biomolecules, in vitro cells, bacteria, plants, and animals, as well as clinical effects on hemoglobin, immune functioning, and wound healing (Movaffaghi & Farsi, 2009). There is increasing evidence that living systems are sensitive to bioinformation and that biofield therapies can influence diverse cellular and biological systems (Abbot, 2000; Bowden, Goddard, & Gruzelier, 2010). The notion that cellular and molecular changes occur within the energy spectrum of biofields is congruent with the view that subtle energy shifts may manifest as a physiological cause or effect and also play a role in inter- and intracellular communication (Movaffaghi & Farsi, 2009). Morse and Beem (2011) reported a case with an increase in absolute neutrophil count following Reiki, resulting in toleration of interferon and subsequent clearance of hepatitis C virus.

There have also been studies focused on identifying the physical properties of biofields in order to determine potential mechanisms of action (Movaffaghi & Farsi, 2009). An emerging body of evidence confirms the existence of energy fields and suggests new ways of measuring energy, although these are not specific to Reiki. Traditional electrical measurements such as electrocardiograms and electroencephalograms can now be supplemented by biomagnetic field mapping to obtain more accurate information about the human condition. Electromagnetic information has been used to both diagnose and treat disease (Oschman, 2002).

Superconducting quantum interference devices have been used to show the effect of disease on the magnetic field of the body, and pulsating magnetic fields have been used to improve healing (Oschman, 2002). In a small experimental study of the effects of one type of energy therapy, researchers found consistent, marked decreases in gamma rays measured at several sites within intervention subjects' electromagnetic fields during treatment (Benford, Talnagi, Doss, Boosey, & Arnold, 1999). Charman's research (2000) suggests that intention to heal transmits measurable wave patterns to recipients. These studies suggest that in the future it may be possible to directly measure subtle elements of the human energy field and to elucidate mechanisms by which Reiki and other energy-healing techniques lead to changes in health outcomes.

A Reiki treatment commonly puts the recipient's body into a state of relaxation, presumably by downregulating autonomic nervous system tone, which lowers blood pressure and relieves tension and anxiety (Meland, 2009). Mackay, Hansen, and McFarlane (2004) concluded that Reiki has some effect on the autonomic nervous system by comparing heart rate, cardiac vagal tone, blood pressure, cardiac sensitivity to bar reflex and breathing activity among three groups of subjects: those resting, receiving Reiki, or receiving placebo Reiki. Friedman, Burg, Miles, Lee, and Lampert (2010) found an increase in high-frequency heart rate variability in patients recovering from acute coronary syndrome who received Reiki compared with those listening to music or resting. Kerr, Wasserman, and Moore (2007) theorize that sensory reorganization is the mechanism for pain and stress reduction that occurs with touch healing therapies. To date, the strongest support for the measurable physiological effect of Reiki was demonstrated in an animal model (Baldwin & Schwartz, 2006; Baldwin, Wagers, & Schwartz, 2008).

Methodological problems, which hinder the interpretation of results, have been identified in a number of studies. Although case studies and anecdotal examples have been relatively consistent in reporting positive responses to Reiki treatments, this does not represent the scientific rigor that is demanded within an evidence-based health care system. Efforts to strengthen research design and mitigate the confounding effects of human touch have led to the development of sham or placebo Reiki (Mansour, Beuche, Laing, Leis, & Nurse, 1999), now frequently incorporated into randomized controlled trials.

It has also been speculated that energy healing impacts outcome in a way that is difficult to measure. "The phenomenon of energy has a qualitative nature and can never be completely knowable, measurable, or ultimately predictable" (Todaro-Franceschi, 2009, p. 135). Engebretson and Wardell (2002) concluded that many research models are not complex enough to capture the experience of a Reiki session. In their qualitative study they found that participants had a diverse and descriptive language that accompanied their experience, creating a more complete picture of the subjective experience of a Reiki session.

Rogers's Science of Unitary Human Beings has been used as a theoretical framework for understanding the experience of Reiki. This theory connects scientific principles of energy as matter to the human energy field and energetic interconnections that occur in the environment (Ring, 2009; Vitale, 2007).

INTERVENTIONS

Technique

The Reiki practitioner acts as a conduit for this healing-intended energy to self or others. A Level I Reiki practitioner employs a series of 12 to 15 hand positions for a full session and six to seven hand positions for a seated session (Exhibit 25.1). A Level II Reiki practitioner also uses hand positions, but may use various Reiki symbols to focus the *Ki* energy or perform distance healings. If touch is contraindicated for any reason, the hands can be held 1 inch to 4 inches above the body. A full Reiki session usually lasts 45 minutes to 90 minutes and a seated session usually lasts 15 minutes to 20 minutes. Reiki practitioners, especially if they are nurses working in a clinical setting, often do not have the luxury of providing a full session. At such times, shorter and more targeted treatments may be offered for specific purposes. In *The Original Reiki Handbook of Dr. Mikao Usui* (Petter, 1999), the use of particular hand positions is recommended for addressing specific health problems.

Reiki energy flows through the hands without employing cognitive, emotional, or spiritual skills. The attunement process provides access to the energy without requiring ongoing practice or conscious intention. This makes Reiki particularly easy to learn and simple to use. Potter (2003) compared her experience with therapeutic touch after receiving a Level I attunement. She found that her work became less directive and the effort to stay centered was no longer a concern.

Guidelines for Hands-On Reiki Session

The recipient may sit or lie down, and either method is suitable for Reiki practice. Because Reiki tends to be very relaxing it is often preferable to lie down, but a seated session may be more practical if a table or bed is not available.

Exhibit 25.1. *Reiki Seated Session*

(Each hand position is held for approximately 2–3 min)

1. General approach: Use touch therapy competencies: *apply hands for approximately 2 to 3 minutes of light touch in each hand position*; vary positions and duration based on individual needs
2. Hands on shoulders (introduction to light touch)
3. One hand on forehead, one hand on upper nape of neck
4. One hand on chest, other hand on upper back
5. One hand around each on ankle
6. Hands on shoulders (conclusion to light touch)

Patients typically remain clothed during a Reiki treatment. A massage table or hospital bed for a full session is ideal, providing comfort for both client and practitioner. After practitioners center themselves and establish intent to heal with Reiki, the energy flows automatically from their hands without cognitive effort. The hands rest gently on the person's body with the fingers touching so that each hand functions as a unit. Reiki can also be provided with the hands 2 inches to 3 inches off the body. The sequence of hand positions may vary, but will generally include all seven major *chakras* and the endocrine glands. The success of a Reiki treatment does not depend on the use of certain hand positions, for the *Ki* energy goes where it is needed.

In clinical practice, four basic principles of physical touch should be considered: (1) ask permission to touch, (2) provide basic information about what you will be doing, (3) describe anticipated benefits and range of outcomes, (4) assure the right to decline or discontinue receiving physical touch. Standards of practice have been developed by several professional Reiki organizations and include ethics related to intention, healing environment, healing principles, and the nondiagnostic nature of the work (International Association of Reiki Professionals [IARP], 2010; International Center for Reiki Training [ICRT], 2012). The American Holistic Nursing Association (2007) developed scope and standards of practice for holistic nursing, but these are not specific to any one integrative therapy. In the book *Creating Healing Relationships: Professional Standards for Energy Therapy Practitioners,* Hover-Kramer (2011) describes parameters for level of competence, record keeping, professional responsibility, boundaries, confidentiality, marketing, and informed consent. General competencies for Reiki practice are provided in Exhibit 25.2.

Exhibit 25.2. *Reiki Practice Competencies*

1. Ask permission to touch before any encounter.
2. Provide basic information about what you will be doing, including use of light touch, basic hand positions, length of session.
3. Describe the areas of the body you will be touching and what sensations the client may experience. Ask whether there are areas they would prefer not to be touched.
4. Describe anticipated benefits and range of outcomes.
5. Let them know you will stop at any time. Ask whether they prefer to be wakened if they fall asleep.
6. Create an environment that promotes feelings of safety. If possible, assure privacy. In a hospital setting, consider putting a sign on the door asking to not be disturbed.
7. Clearly communicate that Reiki practice is not diagnostic or used to treat specific disease conditions.

In an effort to provide guidelines to assure safety and protection of the public using integrative therapies, a diverse group of complementary and alternative providers, health care providers, ethicists, legal consultants, health policy specialists, and consumers recently developed ethical guidelines for boundaries of touch in the practice of complementary medicine (Schiff et al., 2010). They provided guiding principles and ethical rules addressing behavior and language regarding inappropriate touch and exposure, as well as right of the client to discontinue treatment.

As more health care institutions offer complementary therapies, policies and guidelines must be developed that provide standards for implementation. Brill and Kashurba (2001) provide an outline for starting a Reiki program in a health care facility, including development of program objectives, training health care providers, and tracking and reporting outcomes. Reiki practice at a Magnet-designated facility in Pennsylvania requires evidence of competency in Reiki practice and adherence to written hospital policy when administering Reiki (Kryak & Vitale, 2011). A protocol for Reiki use in the operating room was developed at a hospital in New Hampshire following a request to have a Reiki practitioner present during surgery (Sawyer, 1998). This author developed a Reiki protocol for use by nurses providing care to chemotherapy patients (Ringdahl, 2008).

Measurement of Outcomes

Recipients' subjective feelings during a Reiki session are not considered indications of effectiveness. Patients may feel sensations similar to those of the practitioner, but they may also feel nothing. Sensations may include heat, cold, numbness, involuntary muscle twitching, heaviness, buoyancy, trembling, throbbing, static electricity, tingling, color, and heightened or decreased awareness of sound (Engebretson & Wardell, 2002). It is not uncommon for clients to fall asleep during a treatment with reports of increased relaxation, peacefulness, and reconnecting to their center. These subjective feelings are supported in research studies that demonstrate physiological and psychological evidence of stress reduction following a Reiki session (Bowden et al., 2010; Caitlin & Taylor-Ford, 2011; Engebretson & Wardell, 2002; Friedman et al., 2010; Potter, 2003; Richeson, Spross, Lutz, & Peng, 2010; Ring, 2009; Shore, 2004; Vitale & O'Connor, 2006; Wardell & Engebretson, 2001; Witt & Dundes, 2001).

Reiki research outcomes are focused primarily on reducing stress and pain, increasing relaxation and an overall sense of well-being, particularly in the area of chronic disease and pain management. Application of Reiki for pain management among patients with cancer, undergoing rehabilitation, and recovering from surgery has been the focus of several studies (Beard et al., 2010; Birocco et al., 2012; Dressen & Singh, 2000; Olson, Hanson, & Michaud, 2003; Pocotte, & Salvador, 2008; Shiftlett, Nayak, Bid, Miles, & Agostinelli, 2002; Tsang, Carlson, & Olson, 2007; Vitale & O'Connor, 2006).

Achieving institutional approval for Reiki use requires both evidence of safety and effectiveness and the development of policies or clinical guidelines. In a Cochrane Database Systematic Review of touch therapies for pain relief in adults (So, Jiang, & Qin, 2008), the authors concluded that, although the studies were inconclusive, the evidence supports the use of touch therapies for pain relief and there were no adverse effects identified. Five systematic reviews on Reiki research representing 24 studies and nine randomized controlled trials (RCTs) resulted in the following: four studies demonstrated pain reduction, two studies showed decreased depression and anxiety, and one study showed decreased fatigue and quality of life among cancer patients (Herron-Marx, Price-Knol, Burden, & Hicks, 2008; Jain & Mills, 2010; Lee, Pittler, & Ernst, 2008; vanderVaart, Gijsen, de Wildt, & Koren, 2009; Vitale, 2007). The variation in populations and outcomes measured serves to reinforce the notion that Reiki may have application among populations with diverse health needs. This author served as coinvestigator in a study testing feasibility, acceptability, and safety of Reiki touch for premature infants (Duckett, 2008), a new area of Reiki application.

Physiological outcome measures examined in other studies involving touch, such as hematologic tests, blood pressure and heart rate, bioelectric measures, wound healing rate, inhibition of harmful microorganisms, and body temperature changes, are also appropriate for Reiki. Psychological measures, including perceived pain, cognitive function, memory, and levels of anxiety, depression, or hostility are equally important.

Although both hands-on and distance healing are forms of energy healing, the presence of touch has the capacity to confound the research results, as all touch may have some healing properties. A review of studies of the efficacy of distance healing (Astin, Harkness, & Ernest, 2000) identified both methodological limitations and positive outcomes meriting further study. Shore (2004) compared outcomes between hands-on and distant Reiki healing, and found a greater reduction in depression symptoms with distance healing.

Precautions

No serious adverse effects of Reiki treatments have been published. Some patients, however, may experience emotional release that may be uncomfortable or disturbing. Therefore, practitioners must be prepared to provide assistance and appropriate referrals if emotional distress persists. Moreover, some individuals may dislike being touched. Practitioners can avoid this discomfort by assessing the person's level of comfort with touch and taking into account gender and cultural considerations. Few patients who are fully informed object to the therapy; this is true even among vulnerable populations such as victims of torture (Kennedy, 2001) or those with long-term mental health problems (Collinge, Wentworth, & Sabo, 2005), in whom responses to Reiki have been favorable.

USES

An enlarging body of literature supports the use of Reiki as a stress-reduction and relaxation technique. Therapies that contribute to a relaxation response have the potential for enhancing overall well-being as well as reducing the physiological effects of stress. The range of potential practical applications with patients is broad and depends on the setting. Reiki has been used in hospice and palliative care, among cancer patients, in HIV/AIDS programs, for pre- and postoperative patients, and in stroke rehabilitation. The common theme described in many of these programs is the benefit of Reiki for pain relief, stress and anxiety reduction, and promoting relaxation. Reiki may have particular application for people suffering from chronic physical and mental health conditions, such as fibromyalgia and depression and within mental health settings and long-term-care facilities. A study by Shore (2004) provides evidence that Reiki may reduce symptoms of depression that last as long as 1 year following treatment. Collinge et al. (2005) piloted the use of Reiki and three other modalities for long-term mental health patients undergoing psychotherapy, demonstrating high levels of satisfaction and significant changes in four dimensions of trauma recovery.

Energy touch therapies are considered to be within the scope of nursing practice and touch is recognized in the Nursing Interventions Classification Code as a nursing function (Wardell & Engebretson, 2001). In the past 10 years, many professional organizations and state boards of nursing have developed statements that provide parameters for integrative therapy use by nurses, reinforcing the notion that integrative nursing care is often accompanied by the use of specific complementary modalities. Several authors have documented effective use of Reiki in the direct provision of nursing care (Brill & Kashurba, 2001; Engebretson, 2002; Gallob, 2003; Lipinski, 2006; Pierce, 2007; Vitale, 2006). Increased evidence of efficacy and support for integrative nursing practice supports a shift to greater nursing engagement in Reiki practice, including informal application in all clinical encounters.

Within hospitals, the introduction of Reiki into patient care has primarily been initiated through volunteers; however, increasingly there is support for embedding these modalities into direct care through educational programs for health care providers (Ernst & Ferrer, 2012; Kryak & Vitale, 2011). Access to Reiki within a hospital setting may also exist through an integrative health team that provides a variety of services through a nurse and physician referral system that includes Reiki (Knutson & Weiss, 2009) Ambulatory care models for integrative therapies exist primarily through contracting with complementary and alternative medicine (CAM) practitioners to provide specific services. These services may exist within an integrative care clinic that has a specialty focus, such as oncology or women's health. Exhibit 25.3 provides a list of

Exhibit 25.3. *Applications for Reiki in Clinical Settings*

Application	Reference
Promoting relaxation in labor and delivery	Mills (2003); Rakestraw (2009)
HIV/AIDs	Schmehr (2003)
Supporting pre- and postoperative surgical patients	Hulse, Stuart-Shor, and Russo (2010); Potter (2007); Sawyer (1998); Vitale and O'Connor (2006); VanderVaart et al. (2011); Wirth, Brenlan, Levine, and Rodriguez (1993)
Hospice and palliative care	Burden, Herron-Marx, and Clifford (2005); Hemming and Maher (2005); Mramor (2004)
Supporting oncology patients	Anderson and Taylor (2012); Beard et al. (2010); Birocco et al (2012); Bossi, Ott, and DeCristofaro (2008); Caitlin and Taylor-Ford (2011); Coakley and Barron (2012); Pierce (2007); Tsang et al. (2007)
Pain management	Dressen and Singh (2000); Gillipsie, Gillipsie, and Stevens (2007); Lee (2008); Olson et al. (2003); Park, McCaffrey, Dunn, and Goodman (2011); So et al. (2008)
Decreasing depression and/or anxiety and stress levels	Shore (2004); Witt and Dundes (2001)
Trauma, posttraumatic stress disorder	Collinge et al. (2005); Dey and Emanuel (2008); Kennedy (2001)
Enhancing immune function	Bowden et al. (2010); Wardell and Engebretson (2001)
Promoting wound healing	Papantonio (1998)
Rehabilitation	DiNucci (2005); Hall (2004); Pocotte and Salvador (2008); Schiflett et al. (2002)
Support for nursing home residents	Richeson et al. (2010); Thomas (2005)
Improving hematologic measures	Morse and Beem (2011); Wirth, Chang, Eidleman, and Paxton (1996)
Cardiovascular disease management	Anderson and Taylor (2011a); Friedman et al. (2010); Sharma, Sanghvi, Mehta, and Trehan (2000)
Cognitive impairment	Crawford, Leaver, and Mahoney (2006); Meland (2009); Silva (2002)
Critical care	Toms (2011)
Fibromyalgia	Assefi, Bogart, Goldberg, and Buchwald (2008)
Self-care and stress reduction for health care providers	Brathovde (2006); Cuneo et al. (2011); Diaz-Rodriquez et al. (2011); Fortune and Price (2003); Natale (2010); Raingruber and Robinson (2007); Vitale (2009); Whelan and Wishnia (2003)

populations/settings in which Reiki has been used. In a biomedical treatment setting, Reiki is best seen as a complementary healing modality, whereas in other circumstances it can either be used alone or along with other approaches.

Self-Treatment and Practitioner Benefits

One of the more unique features of Reiki therapy is its capacity to self-treat. A Reiki practitioner can self-treat by using hand positions on the head, abdomen, chest, or other areas of the body, reducing pain and/or increasing a sense of relaxation. The concepts of empowerment and self-treatment have particular value when considering chronic health problems. For some Reiki practitioners, teaching their clients Level I Reiki provides the clients with a greater sense of control over some of their health problems, including pain management and stress reduction (Miles & True, 2003; Mills, 2001). This author teaches Levels I and II to clients with a variety of health problems, including fibromyalgia, mood disorders, cancer, and neurological problems such as advanced amyotrophic lateral sclerosis (ALS). Clients with physical limitations may gain particular benefits from learning Level II, or distance healing.

Additionally, those using Reiki receive the benefits of the therapies while performing them on patients. Reiki practitioners report feeling energized, relaxed, and/or more centered after performing a Reiki treatment. Research on Reiki use by nurses has demonstrated positive effects on the practitioner, including greater job satisfaction and increase in caring behaviors (Brathovde, 2006; Fortune & Price, 2003; Whelan & Wishnia, 2003). The increased sense of well-being that occurs when giving and receiving Reiki may influence the patient/nurse relationship and create a less stressful work environment.

Reiki may also be used for health care provider self-care, with the potential for reducing stress (Fortune & Price, 2003; Whelan & Wishnia, 2003). Several research studies have shown beneficial effects of Reiki for nurses in positively influencing well-being, quality of care, stress reduction (Cuneo et al., 2011; Raingruber & Robinson, 2007), and burnout (Diaz-Rodriquez et al., 2011).

CULTURAL ASPECTS

Energy and touch therapies are found in the health traditions of most cultures. Like Reiki, *Johre* originated in Japan. It is a spirituality-based energy modality that aims to release negativity from the individual's spiritual self (Brooks, Schwartz, Reece, & Nangle, 2006). *Anagami* healing practices include massage, bone-setting, and curing sprains (Joshi, 2004).

The healing practices of Siberian shamans include touching the sore place of a person with a bundle of twigs or blowing the disease out of the dwelling, shaking off the illness, or banishing the illness by ringing a bell (Sem, 2009). Shamanic healing practices can also include the shaman sucking directly on the skin over the area where the harmful spiritual intrusion is thought to reside or seeking to remove this harmful spirit by cupping the hands over the area (Shamanic Healing, 2009).

Although health care workers may find that some of the energy and healing practices used in non-Western cultures differ greatly from Western health practices and even from the more frequently used complementary therapies, respecting the person's belief in these practices is important in the healing process. The patient's strong belief in the unity of body and spirit warrants the nursing staff to find ways to include these therapies in the care regimen unless these interfere with needed medical therapies.

Sidebar 25.1 details the current use of Reiki in Japan, the country in which the therapy originated.

Sidebar 25.1. *Reiki Practice in Japan*

Ikuko Ebihara, Japan

Reiki was started in Japan by Dr. Mikao Usui. The practice was forgotten after World War II until it was imported back from abroad in the 1990s. The traditional Usui Reiki has been regaining popularity in Japan since then, but the acceptance has been slow.

People in Japan find Reiki practitioners and masters by word of mouth and Internet search. The common reason for seeking Reiki practice is to restore mind and body balance; it is not for seeking remedies for physical discomfort. Reiki does not have any national standards; it is not recognized as a medical or physiotherapeutic practice.

There are numerous traditional medicines in Japan but only a limited number of therapies are nationally recognized. Judo therapies, acupuncture, and moxibustion are examples of nationally recognized practices; they have national certification systems. Insurance and reimbursement are available for such therapies; however, even though they are reimbursable, they are not usually provided at hospitals. Western medicine and Japanese traditional medicines are governed by different regulations. Patients may visit both care providers.

In Japan, as in most Western countries, Western and alternative practices are rarely provided by the same health care organizations.

FUTURE RESEARCH

The trajectory of Reiki research has enjoyed a significant acceleration within the past decade and researchers are developing more improved methodology and research designs. The Center for Reiki Research website and The Touchstone Project provide a clearinghouse for disseminating current Reiki research information for practitioners and researchers. The Touchstone Project has a process to systematically analyze published, peer-reviewed studies of Reiki, and currently has results from 38 studies accessible online (Baldwin et al., 2010). Analysis of these studies has generated data supporting Reiki as a noninvasive tool for healing at the physical and nonphysical levels, particularly in alleviating of pain, depression, and anxiety.

However, most published research on Reiki has been conducted with small, nonrandom, convenience samples, raising questions about the validity and generalizability of findings. Outcomes for touch therapies such as Reiki are typically not disease specific and establishing an appropriate time frame to detect effect is variable (Engebretson & Wardell, 2007). Further experiments are required with greater numbers of subjects to provide the statistical power necessary for meaningful interpretation (Baldwin et al., 2010).

New models of research that enlarge our definition of outcomes need to be explored (Schiller, 2003). Clinical evaluation of Reiki represents a challenge using our current standards of assessment. Combining subjective and physiological measures in such research studies will allow broader assessment of the effects of Reiki (Liverani, Minelli, & Ricciuti, 2000). Because the goals of Reiki may be broader than symptom relief and include concepts of physiological and psychological balance, qualitative studies that can address values and meaning are also important, as evidenced in the research by Wardell and Engebretson (2001).

Forgues (2009) reviewed key methodological issues that exist in energy-based therapy (EBT) research studies, including the challenges in verification of effectiveness and use of appropriate research methodology. There remains ongoing debate among researchers about whether the current scientific research model works with EBT research and whether all therapies should be held to the same standard. Randomized controlled trials are considered the current gold standard of research, and EBT integration into clinical practice requires this level of rigorous research (Ernst, 2003). An analysis grid was developed by Forgues (2009) to assess methodological quality, EBT specificity, and treatment effectiveness.

Vitale (2007) identified limitations in research design and the use of linear research methods as problematic in conducting Reiki research.

Current outcome measures may not accurately reflect or measure all aspects of a Reiki treatment. Lack of standardization in Reiki practice also impacts reliability and validity. Some research studies do not identify all components of the Reiki intervention used, including length of treatment, type of treatment, or level/training of the Reiki practitioner. There is a need to develop research designs that consider more subtle and longer-lasting outcomes than those that have typically been used. If energy treatment works on a different level from the conventional medical model, the results may not be as dramatic and may require larger groups and a longer treatment period to show a positive outcome (Nield-Anderson & Ameling, 2000).

Additional information about Reiki can be obtained on the websites found in Exhibit 25.4. Suggested questions for future research include:

■ What are the physiological and/or psychological effects of Reiki treatments for specific conditions when used alone or in conjunction with other therapies?
■ What is the relative effectiveness of noncontact Reiki (distance healing) and hands-on Reiki?
■ What is the best way to use Reiki in providing stress reduction for health care providers?
■ Is the traditional gold standard of randomized controlled trials appropriate for evaluating Reiki?

Exhibit 25.4. *Websites*

Center for Reiki Research
(www.centerforreikiresearch.org)

The International Association of Reiki Professionals (IARP)
(www.iarp.org)

The International Center for Reiki Training (ICRT)
(www.reiki.org)

Reiki in Medicine
(www.reikiinmedicine.org)

Reiki online module, Taking Charge of Your Health, University of Minnesota Center for Spirituality and Healing
(www.takingcharge.csh.umn.edu/explore-healing-practices/reiki)

The Touchstone Process
(www.centerforreikiresearch.org/RRTouchstone.aspx)

REFERENCES

Abbot, N. C. (2000). Healing as a therapy for human disease: A systematic review. *Journal of Alternative and Complementary Medicine, 6*(2), 159–169.

American Holistic Nurses Association and American Nurses Association. (2007). *Holistic nursing: Scope and standards of practice.* Silver Springs, MD: Nursebooks.org

Ananth, S. (2011). *2010 complementary and alternative medicine survey of hospitals.* Alexandria, VA: Samueli Institute.

Anderson, J. G., & Taylor, A. G. (2011a). Biofield therapies in cardiovascular disease management: A brief review. *Holistic Nursing Practice, 25*(4), 199–204.

Anderson, J. G., & Taylor, A. G. (2011b). Effects of healing touch in clinical practice: A systematic review of randomized clinical trials. *Journal of Holistic Nursing, 29*(3), 221–228.

Anderson, J.G., & Taylor, A.G. (2012). Biofield therapies and cancer pain. *Clinical Journal of Oncology Nursing, 16*(1), 43–48.

Assefi, N., Bogart, A., Goldberg, J., & Buchwald, D. (2008). Reiki for the treatment of fibromyalgia: A randomized controlled trial. *Journal of Alternative and Complementary Medicine, 14*(9), 1115–1122.

Astin, J., Harkness, E., & Ernst, E. (2000). The efficacy of "distant healing": A systematic review of randomized trials. *Annals of Internal Medicine, 132*(11), 903–910.

Baldwin, A. L., & Schwartz, G. E. (2006). Personal interaction with a Reiki practitioner decreases noise-induced microvascular damage in an animal model. *Journal of Complementary and Alternative Medicine, 12*(1), 15–22.

Baldwin, A. L., Vitale, A., Brownell, D., Scicisnski, J., Kearns, M., & Rand, W. (2010). The touchstone process: An ongoing critical evaluation of reiki in the scientific literature. *Holistic Nursing Practice, 24*(5), 260–276.

Baldwin, A. L., Wagers, C., & Schwartz, G. E. (2008). Reiki improves heart rate homeostasis in laboratory rats. *Journal of Alternative and Complementary Medicine, 14*(4), 417–422.

Barnes, P. M., Bloom, B., & Nahin, R. (2008). Complementary and alternative medicine use among adults and children, United States, 2007. *CDC National Health Statistics Report #12.*

Beard, C., Stason, W. B., Wang, Q., Manola, J., Dean-Clower, E., Dusek, J. A., . . . Benson, H. (2010). Effects of complementary therapies on clinical outcomes in patients being treated with radiation therapy for prostate cancer. *Cancer, 117*(1), 96–102.

Benford, M. S., Talnagi, J., Doss, D. B., Boosey, S., & Arnold, L. E. (1999). Gamma radiation fluctuations during alternative healing therapy. *Alternative Therapies, 5*(4), 51–56.

Birocco, N., Guillame, C., Storto, S., Ritorto, G., Catino, C., Gir, N., . . . Ciuffreda, L. (2012). The effects of Reiki therapy on pain and anxiety in patients attending a day oncology and infusion services unit. *American Journal of Hospice and Palliative Care, 29*(4), 290–294.

Bossi, L. M., Ott, M. J., & DeCristofaro, S. (2008). Reiki as a clinical intervention in oncology nursing practice. *Clinical Journal of Oncology Nursing, 12*(3), 489–494.

Bowden, D., Goddard, L., & Gruzelier, J. (2010). A randomised controlled single-blind trial of the effects of Reiki and positive imagery on well-being and salivary cortisol. *Brain Research Bulletin, 81,* 66–72.

Brathovde, A. (2006). A pilot study: Reiki for self-care and healthcare providers. *Holistic Nursing Practice, 20*(2), 95–101.

Brill, C., & Kashurba, M. (2001). Each moment of touch. *Nursing Administration Quarterly, 25*(3), 8–14.

Brooks, A. J., Schwartz, G., Reece, K., & Nangle, G. (2006). The effect of *johrei* healing on substance abuse recovery: A pilot study. *Journal of Alternative and Complementary Medicine, 12,* 625–631.

Burden, B., Herron-Marx, S., & Clifford, C. (2005). The increasing use of Reiki as a complementary therapy in specialist palliative care. *International Journal of Palliative Care Nursing, 11*(5), 248–253.

Caitlin, A., & Taylor-Ford, R.L. (2011). Investigation of standard care versus sham Reiki placebo versus actual Reiki therapy to enhance comfort and well-being in a chemotherapy infusion center. *Oncology Nursing Forum, 38*(3), E212–E220.

Center for Reiki Research. (2013). Reiki in hospitals. Retrieved February 19, 2013, from http://www.centerforreikiresearch.org/HospitalList.aspx

Charman, R. A. (2000). Placing healers, healees, and healing into a wider research context. *Journal of Alternative and Complementary Medicine, 6*(2), 177–180.

Coakley, A. B., & Barron, A. M. (2012). Energy therapies in oncology nursing. *Seminars in Oncology Nursing, 28*(1), 55–63.

Collinge, W., Wentworth, R., & Sabo, S. (2005). Integrating complementary therapies into community mental health practice: An exploration. *Journal of Alternative and Complementary Medicine, 11,* 569–574.

Crawford, S. E., Leaver, V. W., & Mahoney, S. D. (2006). Using Reiki to decrease memory and behavior problems in cognitive impairment and mild Alzheimer's disease. *Journal of Alternative and Complementary Medicine, 12*(9), 911–913.

Cuneo, C., Cooper, M., Drew, C., Naoum-Heffernan, C., Sherman, T., & Walz, K. (2011). The effect of Reiki on work-related stress of the registered nurse. *Journal of Holistic Nursing, 29*(1), 33–43.

Dey, M., & Emanuel, M. (2008). Reiki for veterans. *Reiki News Magazine, 7*(4), 41–43.

Diaz-Rodriquez, L., Arroyo-Morales, M., Cantarero-Villanueva, I., Fernandez-Lao, C., Polley, M., & Fernandez-de-las-Penas, C. (2011). The application of Reiki in nurses diagnosed with burnout syndrome has beneficial effects on concentration of salivary IgA and blood pressure. *Latin American Journal of Nursing, 19*(5), 1132–1138.

DiNucci, E. (2005). Energy healing: A complementary treatment for orthopaedic and other conditions. *Orthopaedic Nursing, 24*(4), 259–269.

Dressen, L. J., & Singh, S. (2000). Effects of Reiki on pain and selected affective and personality variables of chronically ill patients. *Subtle Energies and Energy Medicine, 9*(1), 53–82.

Duckett, L. (2008). Testing feasibility, acceptability, and safety of Reiki touch for premature infants. Minneapolis, MN: University of Minnesota IRB application.

Engebretson, J. (2002). Hands on: The persistent metaphor in nursing. *Holistic Nursing Practice, 16*(4), 20–35.

Engebretson, J., & Wardell, D. (2002). Experience of a Reiki session. *Alternative Therapies, 8*(2), 48–53.

Engebretson, J., & Wardell, D. (2007). Energy-based modalities. *Nursing Clinics of North America, 42,* 243–259.

Ernst, E. (2003). Obstacles to research in complementary and alternative medicine. *Medical Journal of Australia, 179*(6), 279–280.

Ernst, L. S., & Ferrer, L. (2012). Reflection of a 7-year patient care program: Implementing and sustaining an integrative hospital program. *Journal of Holistic Nursing, 27*(4), 276–281.

Forgues, E. (2009). Methodological issues pertaining to the evaluation of energy-based therapies, avenues for a methodological guide. *Journal of Complementary and Integrative Medicine, 6*(1), 1–17.

Fortune, M., & Price, M. (2003, Spring/Summer). The spirit of healing: How to develop a spiritually based personal and professional practice. *Journal of New York State Nurses Association, 34*(1), pp. 32–38.

Friedman, R. S. C., Burg, N. M., Miles, P., Lee, F., & Lampert, R. (2010). Effects of Reiki on autonomic activity after acute coronary syndrome. *Journal of the American College of Cardiology, 56,* 995–996.

Gallob, R. (2003). Reiki: A supportive in nursing practice and self-care for nurses. *Journal of the New York State Nurses Association, 34*(1), 9–13.

Gillipsie, E., Gillipsie, B., & Stevens, M. (2007). Painful diabetic neuropathy: Impact of an alternative approach. *Diabetes Care, 30,* 999–1001.

Hall, M. (2004) Treating stroke and other neurological disorders. *Reiki News Magazine, 3*(2), 38–42.

Hemming, L., & Maher, D. (2005). Complementary therapies in palliative care: A summary of current evidence. *British Journal of Community Nursing, 10*(10), 448–452.

Herron-Marx, S., Price-Knol, F., Burden, B., & Hicks, C. (2008). A systematic review of the use of Reiki in health care. *Alternative and Complementary Therapies, 14*(1), 37–42.

Horrigan, B. (2003). Pamela Miles: Reiki vibrational healing. *Alternative Therapies, 9*(4), 75–83.

Hover-Kramer, D. (1996). *Healing touch: A resource for health care professionals.* New York, NY: Delmar.

Hover-Kramer, D. (2011). *Creating healing relationships: Professional standards for energy therapy practitioners.* Santa Rosa, CA: Energy Psychology Press.

Hulse, R. S., Stuart-Shor, E. M., & Russo, J. (2010). Endoscopic procedure with a modified Reiki intervention. *Journal of Gasteroenterology Nursing, 33*(1), 20–26.

Institute of Medicine of the National Academies. (2010). *Integrative medicine and the health of the public: A summary of the February 2009 summit.* Washington, DC: National Academies Press.

International Association of Reiki Professionals (IARP). (2010). *Code of ethics for Reiki practitioners and Reiki master teachers.* Retrieved from www.iarp.org/IARPReikiCodeofEthics.html

International Center for Reiki Training (ICRT). (2012). *ICRT reiki membership code of ethics.* Retrieved August 20, 2012, from www.reikimembership.com/Code_of_Ethics.aspx

Jain, S., & Mills, P. J. (2010). Biofield therapies: Helpful or full of hype? A best evidence systhesis. *International Journal of Behavioral Medicine, 17,* 1–16.

Joshi, V. (2004). Human spiritual agency in angami healing. Part 1. Divinational healers. *Anthropology and Medicine, 11,* 269–291.

Kennedy, P. (2001). Working with survivors of torture in Sarajevo with Reiki. *Complementary Therapies in Nursing and Midwifery, 7*(1), 4–7.

Kerr, C. E., Wasserman, R. H., & Moore, C. I. (2007). Cortical dynamics as a therapeutic mechanism for touch healing. *Journal of Alternative Complementary Medicine, 13*(1), 59–66.

Knutson, L., & Weiss, P. (2009). Exploring integrative medicine: The story of a large, urban, tertiary care hospital. In B. Dossey & L. Keegan (Eds.), *Holistic nursing: A handbook for practice* (6th ed., pp. 523–529). Sudbury, MA: Jones & Bartlett.

Kryak, E., & Vitale, A. (2011). Reiki and its journey into a hospital setting. *Holistic Nursing Practice, 25*(5), 238–245.

Lee, M. S. (2008). Is reiki beneficial for pain management? *Focus on Alternative and Complementary Therapies, 12*(2), 78–81.

Lee, M. S., Pittler, M. H., & Ernst, E. (2008). Effects of Reiki in clinical practice: A systematic review of randomized control trials. *International Journal of Clinical Practice, 62*(6), 947–954.

Lipinski, K. (2006). Finding Reiki: Applications for your nursing practice. *Beginnings, 26*(1), 6–7.

Liverani, A., Minelli, E., & Ricciuti, A. (2000). Subjective scales for the evaluation of therapeutic effects and their use in complementary medicine. *Journal of Alternative and Complementary Medicine, 6*(3), 257–264.

Mackay, N., Hansen, S., & McFarlane, X. O. (2004). Autonomic nervous system changes during Reiki treatment: A preliminary study. *Journal of Alternative and Complementary Medicine, 10*(6), 1077–1081.

Macrae, J. (1987). *Therapeutic touch: A practical guide.* New York, NY: Alfred A. Knopf.

Mansour, A. A., Beuche, M., Laing, G., Leis, A., & Nurse, J. (1999). A study to test the effectiveness of placebo Reiki standardization procedures developed for a planned Reiki efficacy study. *Journal of Alternative and Complementary Medicine, 5*(2), 153–164.

Meland, B. (2009). Effects of Reiki on pain and anxiety in the elderly diagnosed with dementia: A series of case reports. *Alternative Therapies, 15* (4), 56–57.

Miles, P. (2006). *Reiki: A comprehensive guide.* New York, NY: Jeremy P. Tarcher/Penguin.

Miles, P., & True, G. (2003). Reiki—Review of a biofield therapy: History, theory, practice, and research. *Alternative Therapies, 9*(2), 62–72.

Mills, J. (2001). *Tapestry of healing: Where Reiki and medicine intertwine.* Green Valley, AZ: White Sage Press. Retrieved from www.TapestryofHealing.Com

Mills, J. (2003). How I introduced Reiki treatments into my obstetrics and gynecologic practice. *Reiki News, 2*(2), 16–21.

Morse, M. L., & Beem, L. A. W. (2011). Benefits of Reiki therapy for a severely neutropenic patient with associated influences on a true random number generator. *Journal of Alternative and Complementary Medicine, 17*(12), 1180–1190.

Movaffaghi, Z., & Farsi, M. (2009). Biofield therapies: Biophysical basis and biological regulations? *Complementary Therapies in Clinical Practice, 15*, 35–37.

Mramor, J. (2004, February/March). Reiki in hospice care: Miranda's story. *Massage and Bodywork*, 51–59.

Natale, G. W. (2010). Reconnecting to nursing through reiki. *Creative Nursing, 16*(4), 171–176.

National Center for Complementary and Alternative Medicine (NCCAM). (2011). *What is complementary and alternative medicine?* Retrieved August 18, 2012, from http://nccam.nih.gov/heatlh/whatiscam

National Center for Complementary and Alternative Medicine (NCCAM). (2013). *NCCAM clinical trials on Reiki.* Retrieved February 12, 2013, from http://clinicaltrials.gov/search/term=%28NCCAM%29+%5BSPONSOR-COLLABORATORS%5D+%28reiki%29+%5BTREATMENT%5D?recruiting=false

Nield-Anderson, L., & Ameling, A. (2000). The empowering nature of Reiki as a complementary therapy. *Holistic Nursing Practice, 14*(3), 21–29.

Olson, K., Hanson, J., & Michaud, M. (2003). A phase II trial of Reiki for the management of pain in advanced cancer patients. *Journal of Pain and Symptom Management, 26*(5), 990–997.

Oschman, J. (2002). Clinical aspects of biological fields: An introduction for health care professionals. *Journal of Bodywork and Movement Therapies, 6*(2), 117–125.

Papantonio, C. (1998). Alternative medicine and wound healing. *Ostomy/Wound Management, 44*(4), 44–55.

Park, J., McCaffrey, R., Dunn, D., & Goodman, R. (2011). Managing osteoarthritis: Comparisons of chair yoga, Reiki, and education (pilot study). *Holistic Nursing Practice, 25*(6), 316–326.

Petter, F. (1999). *The original reiki handbook of Dr. Mikao Usui.* Twin Lakes, WI: Lotus Press.

Pierce, B. (2007). The use of biofield therapies in cancer care. *Clinical Journal of Oncology Nursing, 11*(2), 253–258, 269–273.

Pocotte, S., & Salvador, D. (2008). Reiki as a rehabilitative nursing intervention for pain management: A case study. *Rehabilitation Nursing, 33*(6), 231–232.

Potter, P. (2003). What are the distinctions between Reiki and therapeutic touch? *Clinical Journal of Oncology Nursing, 7*(1), 89–91.

Potter, P. (2007). Breast biopsy and distress: Feasibility of testing a Reiki intervention. *Journal of Holistic Nursing, 25,* 238–248.

Raingruber, B., & Robinson, C. (2007). The effectiveness of tai chi, yoga, meditation, and Reiki healing sessions in promoting problem solving abilities of registered nurses. *Issues in Mental Health Nursing, 28,* 1141–1155.

Rakestraw, T. (2009). Reiki: The energy doula. *Midwifery Today International Midwife, 92,* 16–17.

Rand, W. (2000). *Reiki, the healing touch: First and second degree manual.* Southfield, MI: Vision.

Richeson, N., Spross, J., Lutz, K., & Peng, C. (2010). Effects of Reiki on anxiety, depression, pain, and physiological factors in community-dwelling older adults. *Research in Gerontological Nursing, 3*(3), 187–199.

Ring, M. E. (2009). Reiki and changes in pattern manifestations. *Nursing Science Quarterly, 22*(3), 250–258.

Ringdahl, D. (2008). *Implementation of a hospital-based Reiki program* (Unpublished University of Minnesota DNP project). Minneapolis, MN: University of Minnesota.

Ringdahl, D. (2010). Reiki. In M. Snyder & R. Lindquist (Eds.), *Complementary and alternative therapies in nursing* (6th ed., pp. 271–286). New York, NY: Springer Publishing Company.

Sawyer, J. (1998). The first Reiki practitioner in our OR. *AORN Journal, 67*(3), 674–676.

Schiff, E., Ben-Arye, E., Shilo, M., Levy, M., Schachter, L., Weitchner, N., . . . Stone, J. (2010). Development of ethical rules for boundaries of touch in complementary medicine–Outcomes of a delphi process. *Complementary Therapies in Clinical Practice, 16,* 194–197.

Schiller, R. (2003). Reiki: A starting point for integrative medicine. *Alternative Therapies in Health and Medicine, 9*(2), 20–21.

Schmehr, R. (2003). Enhancing the treatment of HIV/AIDS with Reiki training and treatment. *Alternative Therapies, 9*(2), 120–121.

Sem, T. (2009). Shamanic healing rituals. *Messages from the Museum Directors, Illinois State Museum.* Retrieved March 12, 2009, from http://www.museum.state.il.us/exhibits/changing/journey/healing.html

Shamanic Healing. (2009). *Earth shamans.* Retrieved March 12, 2009, from http://www.geocities.com/athens/troy/7922?SHAMANHEALER.html?200911

Sharma, V. G., Sanghvi, C., Mehta, Y., & Trehan, N. (2000). Efficacy of Reiki on patients undergoing coronary artery bypass graft surgery. *Annals of Cardiac Anaesthesia, 3*(2), 12–18.

Shiflett, S., Nayak, S., Bid, S., Miles, P., & Agostinelli, M. (2002). Effect of Reiki treatment as functional recovery in patients in post stroke rehabilitation: A pilot study. *Journal of Alternative and Complementary Medicine, 8*(6), 755–763.

Shore, A. G. (2004). Long-term effects of energetic healing on symptoms of psychological depression and self-perceived stress. *Alternative Therapies, 10*(3), 42–48.

Silva, T. (2002). Treating Alzheimer's disease with Reiki. *Reiki News Magazine, 1*(2), 37–39.

So, P., Jiang, Y., & Qin, Y. (2008). Touch therapies for pain relief in adults. *Cochrane
Database of Systematic Reviews, 4*: CD006535. doi:10.1002/1465158

Thomas, T. (2005). Reiki adds a new dimension to the term "quality of life" in the nursing home community. *American Journal of Recreation Therapy,* Fall, 43–48.

Todaro-Franceschi, V. (2009). Energy: A bridging concept for nursing science. *Nursing
Science Quarterly, 14*(2), 132–140.

Toms, R. (2011). Reiki therapy: A nursing intervention for critical care. *Critical Care
Nursing Quarterly, 34*(3), 213–217.

Tsang, K. L., Carlson, L. E., & Olson, K. (2007). Pilot crossover of Reiki versus rest for
treating cancer-related fatigue. *Integrative Cancer Therapies, 6*(1), 25–35.

vanderVaart, S., Berger, H., Tam, C., Goh, Y. H., Gijsen, V., de Wildt, S. N., . . . Koren, G.
(2011). The effect of distant Reiki on pain in women after elective Caesarean section: A double-blinded randomized controlled trial. *BMJ Open*: 1:e000021. doi.
1136/bmjopen-2010-000021

vanderVaart, S., Gijsen, V. M., de Wildt S. N., & Koren, G. (2009). A systematic review
of the therapeutic effects of Reiki. *Journal of Alternative and Complementary Medicine,
15*(11), 1157–1169.

Vitale, A. (2006). The use of selected energy touch modalities as supportive nursing
interventions: Are we there yet? *Holistic Nursing Practice, 20*(4), 191–196.

Vitale, A. (2009). Nurses' lived experiences of Reiki for self-care. *Holistic Nursing
Practice, 23,* 129–145.

Vitale, A. T. (2007). An integrative review of Reiki touch therapy research. *Holistic
Nursing Practice, 21*(4), 167–179.

Vitale, A. T., & O'Connor, P. C. (2006). The effect of Reiki on pain and anxiety in women
with abdominal hysterectomies: A quasi-experimental pilot study. *Holistic Nursing
Practice, 20*(6), 263–274.

Wardell, D., & Engebretson, J. (2001). Biological correlates of Reiki touch healing.
Journal of Advanced Nursing, 33(4), 439–445.

Whelan, K. M., & Wishnia, G. S. (2003). Reiki therapy: The benefits to a nurse-Reiki
practitioner. *Nursing Practice, 17*(4), 209–217.

Wirth, D., Brenlan, D., Levine, R., & Rodriguez, C. (1993). The effect of complementary
healing therapy on postoperative pain after surgical removal of impacted third
molar teeth. *Complementary Therapies in Medicine, 1,* 133–138.

Wirth, D. P., Chang, R. J., Eidelman, W. S., & Paxton, J. B. (1996). Haematological indicators of complementary healing intervention. *Complementary Therapies in Medicine,
4*(1), 14–20.

Witt, D., & Dundes, L. (2001). Harnessing life energy or wishful thinking? *Alternative
and Complementary Therapies, 10,* 304–309.

Chapter 26: Acupressure

PAMELA WEISS-FARNAN

*T*ouch has been central to the practice of nursing since its inception. This chapter describes a form of touch—and its application in nursing care—known in traditional Chinese medicine (TCM) as acupressure. This method of treatment is common in many cultures. As Dossey, Keegan, and Guzzetta (2000) note, "all cultures have demonstrated that some form of rubbing, pressing, massaging or holding are [sic] natural manifestations of the desire to heal and care for one another" (p. 615). Acupressure is also integral to the practice of *shiatsu, tui na, tsubo,* and *jin si ju jitsyu.*

DEFINITIONS

Acupressure is defined by Gach (1990) as "an ancient healing art that uses the fingers to press certain points on the body to stimulate the body's self-curative abilities" (p. 3). To assist the reader, the following definitions are also provided:

- *Acupuncture*—"[a] procedure used in or adapted from Chinese medical practice in which specific body areas are pierced with fine needles for therapeutic purposes or to relieve pain or produce regional anesthesia" (FreeDictionary, 2009).
- *Auricular Acupuncture*—"also called ear acupuncture, applies the principles of acupuncture to specific points on the ear" (FirstHealth of Andover, 2009).
- *Jin Shin Jyutsu*—"a nonmassage form of shiatsu—using pressure points to harmonize the flow of energy through the body" (Health Education Alliance for Life and Longevity [HEALL], 2006).

- *Meridians*—"Any of the longitudinal lines or pathways on the body along which the acupuncture points are distributed." (Answers.com, 2013).
- *Moxibustion*—"[t]he burning of moxa or other substances on the skin, to treat diseases or to produce analgesia" (FreeDictionary, 2009).
- *Qi* (pronounced *chee*)—"[t]he vital force believed in Taoism and other Chinese thought to be inherent in all things. The unimpeded circulation of Chi (Qi) and a balance of its negative and positive forms in the body are held to be essential to good health in traditional Chinese medicine" (FreeDictionary, 2009).
- *Shiatsu*—"A form of therapeutic massage in which pressure is applied with the thumb and palms to those areas of the body used in acupuncture. Also called acupressure" (FreeDictionary, 2009).

TRADITIONAL CHINESE MEDICINE

TCM is an ancient system of health developed more than 3,000 years ago in Asia. This system is based on the concept that *Qi* flows throughout the body and that balance of *yin* and *yang* forces represents health and well-being. As Kaptchuk (1983) describes it:

> This system of care is based on ancient texts and is the result of a continuous process of critical thinking, as well as extensive clinical observation and testing. It represents a thorough formulation and reformulation of material by respected clinicians and theoreticians. It is also, however, rooted in the philosophy, logic and sensibility, and habits of a civilization entirely foreign to our own. It has therefore developed its own perception of the body and health and disease. (p. 2)

The focus of care within this system is to restore balance in the body. To do so, *yin* and *yang* must be balanced. *Yin* aspects are associated with cold, passivity, interiority, and decreases. *Yang* aspects are associated with warmth, activity, external forces, and increases. *Yin* and *yang* are always in relation to each other (Kaptchuk, 1983). According to this conceptualization, they are in continuous flux and there is always *yin* within *yang* and *yang* within *yin*.

Unschuld (1999) reflects that TCM theory is a mixture of beliefs that pathogenic influences from the outside combine with the lack of balance or harmony within the person and result in illness. TCM is also concerned with the concept of *Qi*. *Qi* flows in the body through specific pathways identified as meridians or channels. If the *Qi* is blocked or diminished, a person experiences pain or illness.

There are 12 bilateral meridians and eight extra meridians. All meridians have an exterior and an interior pathway and are named according to the organ system. Located on the meridians are specific points. In the 12 major meridians, the points are bilateral and in the West are called acupuncture points. This nomenclature implies that the points are designated for needle insertion and does not fully reflect the TCM concept of the point.

Acupuncture points are also used for acupressure. The points do not have a corresponding anatomic structure but are described by their location relative to other anatomical landmarks. This contributes to the skepticism of many Western-trained scientists about their existence. In Chinese, the name of the point usually is descriptive of its function or location. Mistranslation over the years has often limited the substantial amount of the anatomical basis for the nomenclature of points and the apparent knowledge of anatomy of Chinese scholars (Schnorrenberger, 2006).

There are 365 (Kaptchuk, 1983) to 700 (Yang, 2006) major points on the meridians. Dr. Yang, Jwing-Ming stated that 108 points could be stimulated using the fingers. In a traditionally formulated TCM treatment plan, whether the modality is needles or pressure, the points are combined to achieve maximum benefit for the patient. Rarely is only one point used. There are also points that should not be stimulated, especially during pregnancy, which are referred to as "forbidden points."

SCIENTIFIC BASIS

Western medicine is the dominant system of health care in the United States. It is characterized by hospitals; clinics; pharmaceutical resources; and a workforce of physicians, nurses, specialized therapists, and various support service personnel. There are many differences between Western medicine and TCM that become more evident as nurses seek to add TCM modalities to their practice. Western medicine emphasizes disease, causal agents, and treatments that are designed to control or destroy the cause of disease (Kaptchuk, 1983). Once a causal agent or mechanism is identified, treatment plans are developed that focus on the agent or mechanism as a consistent factor in all human manifestations of the disease. In Western journals, almost all studies using the modality of acupuncture and acupressure emphasize the specific effects of needling one point known to address a specific symptom. Medical researchers are eager to find the mechanism by which acupuncture alleviates the symptoms. Some of the mechanisms have been suggested in Western medical research (National Center for Complementary and Alternative Medicines [NCCAM], 2000; National Institutes of Health [NIH], 1997). The therapeutic effect that seems to be produced by stimulation of the points with needles or with pressure may be due to the following:

■ Conduction of electromagnetic signals that may start the flow of pain-killing biochemicals, such as endorphins, and of immune system cells to specific sites in the body that are injured or vulnerable to disease (Dale, 1997; Takeshige, 1989; Wu, Zhou, & Zhou, 1994).

- Activation of opioid systems, which also reduces pain (Han, 1997).
- Changes in brain chemistry, sensation, and involuntary responses by changing the release of neurotransmitters and neurohormones in a health-promoting way (Han, 2003; Wu, 1995).

More sophisticated tools have been used recently to further explore the mechanism of acupressure/acupuncture. Recent meta-analyses indicate that changes in brain chemistry and brain imaging occur during stimulation of the points (Huang et al., 2012; Liang, Chen, & Cooper, 2012).

The scientific research into an underlying mechanism demonstrates one of the differences between Western medicine and the TCM system. The focus in TCM is the imbalance in the patient, and the causality is always multifactorial. The function of the points is described in terms of TCM diagnosis. For example, Western medicine research has focused on pericardium 6, or *nei guan*, for the treatment of nausea. In English its name means "inner border gate." Lade (1986) describes the point:

> The name refers to the point's role as the gateway or connecting point of the triple burner channel and the yin-linking vessel. Inner refers to the palmar aspect of the forearm and to the point's location on the yin channel. The actions of this point are: to regulate and tonify the heart, transform heart phlegm, facilitate qi flow, regulate the yin-linking vessel and clear heart fire, redirect rebellious qi downward, expand and relax the chest and benefit the diaphragm. The indications for use of the point are: asthma, bronchitis, pertussis, hiccups, vomiting, diaphragmatic spasms, intercostal neuralgia, chest fullness, and pain and dyspnea. (pp. 196, 197)

Whereas Western medicine focuses on the treatment of nausea for this point, the TCM paradigm suggests multiple uses. In TCM theory, nausea is considered rebellious *Qi* (*Qi* that flows in the wrong direction). Nausea and vomiting are examples of this. *Nei guan* (pericardium 6) is used as one of the points in the treatment of a patient who presents with nausea. In TCM theory, nausea is considered one of the external manifestations of the imbalance; however, in an authentic TCM treatment, a practitioner would evaluate the imbalances that set up the manifestation and treat the underlying condition. Therefore, a combination of points to treat nausea would be used, possibly including other primary points for antiemesis (Hoo, 1997): Stomach 36 on the stomach meridian located on the knee, Ren 12 on the ren/conception meridian located on the upper abdomen, or the Spleen 4 on the spleen meridian located on the foot. Application of multiple acupoints may be more effective for the treatment of nausea; however, in Western medicine, the focus on finding the single active point or the mechanism creates an almost insurmountable challenge to the fullest application of the therapy.

In 1997, the National Institutes of Health held the first consensus conference on acupuncture. The conference concluded that:

> Acupuncture is effective in the treatment of adult nausea and vomiting in chemotherapy and probably pregnancy and in postoperative dental pain. The conference members stated there is an indication that acupuncture may be helpful in the treatment of addiction, stroke rehabilitation, headache, menstrual cramps, tennis elbow, fibromyalgia, myofascial pain, osteoarthritis, low back pain, carpal tunnel syndrome, and asthma, in which acupuncture may be useful as an adjunct treatment or an acceptable alternative or be included in a comprehensive management program. (NIH, 1997)

Research evidence underlying the use of the point called *nei guan* (pericardium 6) for nausea is reviewed in the text that follows. This NIH statement was the springboard for increasing the number of studies completed for the treatment of nausea and vomiting that include the use of devices to apply pressure or stimulation to pericardium 6. These devices included an elastic bracelet with a pressure button called Sea-Bands® or an electrical stimulation device called a ReliefBand®.

In recent years, the research focusing on the effectiveness of pericardium 6 for the treatment of nausea and vomiting have increased. Exhibit 26.1 demonstrates that current studies continue to find conflicting results about the effectiveness of using pericardium 6 for the treatment of nausea and vomiting from any condition. Meta-analyses published by the Cochrane Collaborative conclude that inclusion of acupressure for multiple symptoms may be useful but more rigorous trials are required. (Griffiths et al., 2012; Lee & Frazier, 2011; Robinson, Lorenc, & Liao, 2011).

Exhibit 26.1. *Sample of Studies Using P6 for Nausea*

Condition	Modality	Author/Date	Conclusion
Radiation-related nausea	Acupuncture pressure bands	Roscoe et al. (2009)	Acupressure bands and information about their use were effective in reducing nausea in radiation-induced nausea.
Chemotherapy-induced nausea and vomiting in patients with breast cancer	Three treatment groups: control, acupressure on P6 only, or nurse-led counseling and acupressure P6	Suh (2012)	The synergistic effects of nurse counseling and use of acupressure on P6 was effective in reducing chemotherapy-induced nausea.

(continued)

Exhibit 26.1. *Sample of Studies Using P6 for Nausea (continued)*

Condition	Modality	Author/Date	Conclusion
Vertigo	Comparison of two groups with acupressure on P6 and on group with incorrect acupressure point	Alessandrini, Napolitano, Micarelli, de Padova, and Bruno (2012)	P6 acupressure device (Sea-Band) improved neurovegetative symptoms in patients with spontaneous and provoked vertigo.
Migraine-associated nausea	Application of Sea-Band	Allais et al. (2012)	The application of the Sea-Bands was effective in controlling the nausea when applied with a migraine attack.
Postoperative nausea and vomiting after strabismus surgery	Acupressure on P6 using acupressure pressure band compared to ondansetron and metoclopramide	Ebrahim Soltani et al. (2010)	Acupressure on P6 caused a significant reduction in the postoperative nausea and vomiting after strabismus surgery, as well as the medications metoclopramide and ondansetron for patients 10 years of age or older.
Preoperative treatment to limit postoperative nausea and vomiting	Literature review	Pettersson and Wengstrom (2012)	Systematic review concluded that preoperative acupressure and acupuncture seemed to prevent postoperative nausea and could be used to do further research and improve practice.
Nausea and vomiting in women undergoing regional anesthesia for Caesarean section	Acupressure	Griffiths et al. (2012)	Meta-analysis indicated that acupressure is effective in reducing nausea but not vomiting in women receiving regional anesthesia for C-section.
Nausea and vomiting of pregnancy	Direct pressure or the use of Sea-Bands	Ebrahimi, N., Maltepe, C., and Einarson, A. (2010)	Although there was weak evidence that pressure at P6 was effective, it was supported because it was noninvasive and inexpensive.

Exhibit 26.2 presents a brief overview of recent studies examining the use of acupressure in a variety of patients. The conditions treated include: insomnia, as part of weight loss program, postoperative pain control and range of motion improvement in total knee replacements, reduction in heart rate in poststroke rehabilitation care, student anxiety,

Exhibit 26.2. *Sample of Studies of Effective Uses of Acupuncture/Acupressure*

Condition	Modality	Author/Date	Conclusion
Insomnia	Stimulation of Heart 7 on the inner wrist with either acupuncture or acupressure	Litscher et al. (2012)	Stimulation of Heart 7 acupuncture point reduced heart rate variability and improved ability of the subjects to sleep.
Making healthful life choices	Shiatsu	Long (2009)	When Shiatsu was added to a health-promotion program, more individuals changed to a more healthful lifestyle.
Total knee replacement postoperative and range of motion	Acupressure with use of magnetic beads to ear Shen Men and Subcortex points.	Chang et al. (2012)	The applied acupressure to the ear points decreased the demand for opioid pain relief and improved passive range of motion.
Abdominal obesity in adolescent subjects	Auricular acupressure with vaccaria seed or magnetic pearl	Hsieh, Su, Fang, and Chou (2012)	The study group demonstrated a greater abdominal circumference decrease than the nontreatment group.
Cardiovascular benefits of reduced heart rate in stroke patients	Use of practitioner-selected acupressure points	McFadden and Hernández (2010)	Patients receiving active acupressure treatments demonstrated a reduction of heart rate when compared to the placebo treatments. There was no treatment effect on blood pressure, which the authors hypothesized was due to the patients already receiving hypotensive medications.
Pain conditions and autonomic functions of women with chronic neck pain	Acupressure on local gall bladder (GB 21), small intestine (SI 14 and SI 15), and distal points large intestine (LI 4, LI 10, and LI 11)	Matsubara et al. (2011)	Acupressure can reduce pain and influence autonomic nervous systems as measured by heart rate.
Preoperative anxiety	Acupressure massage on the points Yin tang, placing a plastic bead on ear Shen Men, followed by pressure on point Yin tang	Valiee et al. (2012)	The acupressure group resulted in a clinical reduction of anxiety when compared to the control group. Further study is warranted.

(continued)

Exhibit 26.2. *Sample of Studies of Effective Uses
of Acupuncture/Acupressure (continued)*

Condition	Modality	Author/Date	Conclusion
Recovery of motor function for stroke patients	Routine poststroke care and two-phase acupressure intervention with daily acupressure protocol for the first month in hospital, and weekly treatments after discharge	Yue, Jiang, and Wong (2012)	Nurse-led acupressure demonstrated improvement in activities of daily living and motor scores, when compared to the control group by the third month.
Primary dysmenorrhea	Self-administered acupressure on Spleen (Sp) 6 and Sp 8	Gharloghi, Torkzahrani, Akbarzadeh, and Heshmat (2012)	Pain relief lasted for 2 hours after the self-administered treatment and systemic symptoms also were reduced.
Stress reduction in college students	Subjects were placed in three treatment groups. One group received acupressure from a trained practitioner, one group received sham acupressure, and one group was given relaxation music and rest.	McFadden, Healy, Hoversten, Ito, and Hernández (2012)	No significant differences were found among the groups, with all groups demonstrating a reduction in stress measurements. Further study is needed to determine what dose of acupressure treatment produces the best effect.
Children undergoing hematopoietic cell transplant (pain, nausea, relaxation, and greater ease of falling asleep)	Patients received semi-standardized Swedish massage and acupressure on nine points: Pericardium (PC) 6, Stomach (ST) 36, Large Intestine (LI) 4, Spleen (SP) 6, Bladder (BL) 62, Kidney (KI) 6, Heart (HE) 7, Conception Vessel (CV) 17 and Liver (LV) 3	Ackerman et al. (2012)	The massage and acupressure helped relieve the patients' symptoms, and the parents felt an increased competence in helping their children. Parent stress was relieved, and there was improved connection between child and parent.
Weight-loss maintenance	Acupressure using the Tapas Acupressure Technique (light acupressure to a series of specific points)	Elder et al. (2012)	Participants who participated in the treatment had greater initial weight loss, but had no difference in weight regain after 6 months.

neck pain in women, and anxiety in pediatric patients' parents. Many of the studies were done outside of the United States, where the cultural barriers about the use of this ancient type of medicine are lower because the use of acupressure is an accepted part of the cultural health practices.

Pediatric patients have not been studied extensively using acupuncture as an intervention; however, in the framework of TCM, children are considered sensitive to any type of energy and may enjoy the same benefits that are found in adult populations. Acupressure is less invasive than other treatments and may be more acceptable to pediatric patients.

The number of studies continues to increase, and yet scarce funding has yielded studies with small sample sizes, thus limiting their power and generalizability. However, these limited studies do provide the incentive for nurses to consider incorporating acupressure techniques into their practices because it is a noninvasive treatment that may have a salutary impact on patient outcomes.

INTERVENTION

A diagnostic process is used to choose the correct points to stimulate. In TCM, the process includes an extensive history, observing the patient's appearance and demeanor, noticing the patient's odor, checking the tongue, palpating the abdomen and points on the body, and palpating the pulses at the radial location on the wrists. A diagnosis is formulated and a treatment plan, which may use a variety of techniques, is implemented. Nurses will not follow this process and will therefore be using a Western, symptom-based system of determining the correct treatment plan.

Guidelines for Use

Nurses can incorporate acupressure into the care of patients by using some common points that have specific actions to relieve common symptoms. The nurse can treat the patient with acupressure or teach the patient or family members how to use acupressure as part of a care plan.

Prior to touching any patient, the nurse must assess the readiness of the client. Shames and Keegan (2000) recommend the following assessment of clients:

- Perception of mind–body situation
- Pathophysiological problems that may require referral
- History of psychological disorders
- Cultural beliefs about touch
- Previous experience with body therapies (p. 264)

Each point is located using an anatomical marker. There are many books describing point location. The standard measure is the *cun*, which is different for each individual. One *cun* for a particular patient is defined as the "width of the interphalangeal joint of the patient's thumb" or as the " distance between the two radial ends of the flexor creases of a flexed middle finger of the patient. Two cun is the width of the index finger, the middle finger, and the ring finger" (Hoo, 1997).

Stimulating the Point

There are several different types of techniques to stimulate the points, according to Gach:

- *Firm stationary pressure*—using the thumbs, fingers, palms, the sides of hands, or knuckles
- *Slow motion kneading*—using the thumbs and fingers along with the heels of the hands to squeeze large muscle groups
- *Brisk rubbing*—using friction to stimulate the blood and lymph
- *Quick tapping*—using the fingertips to stimulate muscles on unprotected areas of the body such as the face (1990, p. 9)

Evaluating Acupressure's Effect

Gach has developed guidelines for assessing results. The elements of the assessment include:

- Identifying the problems being addressed with acupressure
- Identifying the points being used for the treatment
- The length of time for the acupressure
- Identifying what makes the condition worse (e.g., standing, cold weather, menstruation, constipation, lack of exercise, stress, traveling, and other variables)
- Describing the changes experienced by the patient after 3 days and after 1 week of treatment
- Describing the changes in the condition and overall feeling of well-being (1990, p. 13)

USES

There are many uses for acupressure. Some conditions for which it has been used are shown in Exhibit 26.2. The use of acupuncture for nausea, pain, and gastrointestinal disorders is described below.

Nausea

Point: Pericardium 6 *(Nei Guan, "Inner Gate")*

Location: Pericardium 6 is located on the inner aspect of the wrist 2 *cun* (units) proximal to the transverse crease of the wrist between the tendons of the palmaris longus and flexor carpi radialis muscles (Lade, 1986). Have

Exhibit 26.3. *Pressure Point Pericardium 6. This Point Has Multiple Functions and Is One of the Most Important Points.*

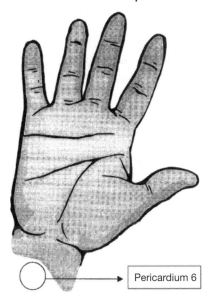

Pericardium 6

the patient place the middle three fingers (index, middle, and ring fingers) on the opposite hand that is palm upward. The point under the ring finger between the two tendons is pericardium 6 (see Exhibit 26.3).

Functions: Its functions were outlined previously in the discussion on the research on this point.

Method of Stimulation: The point can be stimulated using firm pressure either with a rotating pattern with the thumb or the static pressure of a Sea-Band.

Indications in Nursing: This point can be used for the treatment of nausea in many situations, but research, as cited previously, has focused on postoperative nausea, the nausea of pregnancy, and the nausea accompanying chemotherapy.

Pain and Gastrointestinal Disorders

Point: Large Intestine 4 (LI 4) *(Hoku, "Joining the Valley")*

Location: This point is on the back of the hand halfway between the junction of the first and second metacarpal bones, which form a depression or valley when the thumb is abducted (Lade, 1986). There are two ways to locate this point easily. Have the patient hold the hand with the thumb touching the index finger; hold the hand at eye level and the highest mound at the base of the thumb and index finger is the location of LI 4. Or, instruct the patient to place the thumb of one hand in the web between the thumb and index finger of the opposite hand. The patient should match the first crease on the thumb of one hand to the web of the other and then rotate the thumb to touch the fleshy area between the index finger and the thumb. The point is where the tip of the thumb touches the area between the thumb and the index finger.

Functions: This point has multiple functions and is one of the most important points of the body. It alleviates pain, tones *Qi*, and generates protective *Qi* (in Western medicine this would be considered an immune system-building function); moistens the large intestine and in so doing relieves diarrhea or constipation; clears the nose; regulates the lungs in asthma, bronchitis, or the common cold; and expedites labor. This point is contraindicated in pregnancy because of the latter function (Lade, 1986, pp. 40–41).

Method of Stimulation: Firm pressure can be applied on this point with a rotating thumb massage technique. This point is often sensitive and the patient will report a feeling of discomfort. This is normal and not indicative of a problem.

Indications in Nursing: This point will relieve any pain in the body. In addition, persons with diarrhea or constipation may feel relief because stimulating the point balances the gastrointestinal functions. This point can be used to induce labor and, coupled with its pain-relieving effect, may be helpful.

Precautions

There are overall guidelines and precautions carefully outlined by Michael Reed Gach (1990) in his book *Acupressure Potent Points*:

- Never press any area in an abrupt, forceful, or jarring way. Apply finger pressure in a slow, rhythmic manner to enable layers of tissues and the internal organs to respond (p. 11).
- Use abdominal points cautiously, especially if the patient is ill. Avoid the abdominal area altogether if the patient has a life-threatening disease, especially intestinal cancer, tuberculosis, or leukemia. Avoid the abdominal area during pregnancy (pp. 11–12).
- During pregnancy, strong stimulation of certain points should be avoided: LI 4 (fourth point on the large intestine meridian), K 3 (third point on the kidney meridian), and SP 6 (sixth point on the spleen meridian). Each of these points may have an effect on the pregnancy (p. 192).
- Lymph areas such as the groin, the area of the throat just below the ears, and the outer breast near the armpits are very sensitive. Touch these areas lightly (p. 12).
- Do not work directly on a serious burn, ulcer, or area of infection.
- Do not work directly on a newly formed scar. New surgical or other wounds should not be touched directly. Continuous holding on the periphery of the injury will stimulate the injury to heal (p. 12).

■ After an acupressure treatment, tolerance to cold is lowered and the energy of the body is focused on healing, so advise the patient to wear warm clothes and keep out of drafts (p. 12).

■ Use acupressure cautiously in persons with a new acute or serious illness (p. 12).

■ Acupressure is not a sole treatment for cancer, contagious skin disease, or sexually transmitted disease (pp. 11–12).

■ Brisk rubbing, deep pressure, or kneading should not be used for persons with heart disease, cancer, or high blood pressure (Gach, 1990, p. 9).

CULTURAL CONSIDERATIONS

Nurses work with patients from differing cultural backgrounds. Multiple cultures throughout the world use manual therapies to either promote or maintain health or to treat illness. Although the therapies are part of the indigenous healing methods used by different groups of people, currently they are classified as complementary and alternative medicine (CAM) in the United States. However, within many cultures, individuals and families treat manual therapies as mainstream and integral to their health practices. Such remains the case in mainland China. The contemporary use of acupressure in northern China is described in Sidebar 26.1.

Folk and indigenous healing practices are common not only for the people of Asian origin (Chinese, Thai, Cambodian, Vietnamese, and Japanese), but also for almost every other culture. The practices include massage: pressure, rubbing, stretching and pulling the skin, with and without herbal preparations, oils, or poultices. For example, many indigenous practices are focused on preparing for childbirth. To illustrate, in Oaxaca (a Mexican state), a practice called *sobada* massage is used as a diagnostic tool for gestational age, and to relieve the aches and pain of pregnancy and delivery, and then stimulating the baby immediately after birth. In India, infant massage with various oils is a regular practice and recent research has confirmed that massage with coconut oil enhances the baby's weight gain (Sankaranarayanan, 2005).

Although Western-trained nurses may not understand how different cultural groups incorporate skin massage and rubbing and may misinterpret what they may observe, it is important for the nurse to allow the family to express the types of practices they use as part of their routine caring for each other and their children (Davis, 2000). Struthers (2008) emphasized that there is a "need for nurses and other health care providers to become knowledgeable regarding traditional indigenous health care that their clients may be receiving—to foster open communication" (p. 74). What the practices are called will vary from one cultural group to another, but each uses skin stimulation as part of health routines and family bonding.

Sidebar 26.1. *Use of Acupressure in China*

Fang Yu, Siping, Jilin Province, China

TCM has been practiced for more than 3,000 years, and is still very popular in China and many Asian countries. To achieve better therapeutic effects, TCM practitioners often combine two or more treatment methods. In China, as elsewhere, the wide use of acupressure is founded in its unique feature of not requiring any medical facilities, equipment, or devices; hence, acupressure can take place at any place and time. The acupunctural points used in the treatment may or may not be in the same area of the body as the targeted symptom. Early healers had found that certain techniques of rubbing and pressing could relieve symptoms such as hemorrhage, pain, and swelling. The selection and effectiveness of such points are grounded in how they stimulate the channels and collaterals to bring about relief by rebalancing *yin* and *yang* as well as *Qi* (life energy in TCM) and blood. Fingers used for rubbing and pressing can be a single finger (often thumb or middle finger), double fingers (two thumbs, two middle fingers, one thumb and one middle finger, or one thumb and one index finger), or multiple fingers.

The role and popularity of acupressure has shifted over the past 30 years in China. Prior to the economic reform in 1978, acupressure was used widely for the treatments of common ailments and diseases, especially in rural regions where there was a significant shortage of doctors and limited access to health care. Many practitioners learned from their parents and local elders to use acupressure to treat back pain, headache, stomach pain, and *Bi Zheng* (painful obstruction syndrome). My cousin, who is 4 years older than me, injured his lower back at work in his late teens, and was treated by local acupressure practitioners for years to relieve his pain. I had even learned to press some pressure points occasionally, when he was in minor pain or discomfort and did not feel it warranted a visit to a practitioner. Although my cousin has continued to experience episodes of back pain up to this day, he has never resorted to surgeries, especially after the effects of the 1978 economic reform rippled through the whole country and made complementary medicine even more accessible than ever.

With heightened awareness of health and increasing financial means, the Chinese have made acupressure a national sensation and part of everyone's daily life. Spas and foot parlors that boast acupressure-based techniques for promoting wellness, correcting suboptimal health states, preventing diseases, and treating ailments have sprung up like the bamboo shoots after a spring rain. They are popular and affordable places for even the ordinary Chinese to relax and socialize. Spas and

(continued)

> **Sidebar 26.1.** *Use of Acupressure in China (continued)*
>
> foot parlors employ cheap labor: often migrant farmers and laid-off city dwellers with limited education. These workers have typically received targeted on-the-job acupressure training from their employers in order to perform their duties. Foot acupressure (reflexology) parlors are now in almost every town and city in China; the latest statistics suggest that foot acupressure parlors dot the streets of Shanghai every 1,500 feet. Some foot acupressure establishments are so successful, they have become publicly traded companies on the New York Stock Exchange in the United States. My recent trips to China would have been incomplete if I had not visited a beauty spa and a foot parlor to get an acupressure-based back massage and a foot massage.

FUTURE RESEARCH

There are many areas of research in which the methods of traditional Chinese medicine and the underlying theory can be tested using Western medical research techniques. Research questions about the usefulness of acupressure strategies can be posed in many areas of nursing, including their use for palliative care, rehabilitation nursing, support of women in labor, and health promotion and disease prevention programs. Gach (2004) has expanded his self-care manuals to include trauma, stress, and common emotional imbalances.

Acupressure is used by millions of persons around the world. Incorporating this technique into nursing care plans will unite us in the commonality we share—the desire to relieve human suffering.

Author's Notes

ReliefBand used in some of the studies has been discontinued, and replaced by a product named Reletex. Product information at www.aeromedix.com can be accessed.

Sea-Bands continue to be available under that brand name. Information at www.sea-band.com can be accessed.

WEBSITES

Acupressure.com

Gives an overview of acupressure, with excellent basic information. Also, the site of a newsletter from Michael Reed Gach.
(www.acupressure.com)

PointFinder: The Online Acupressure Guide

Excellent drop-down symptoms charts with illustrated acupressure points treatments. (onlineartdirector.com/pointfinder)

The Essential Guide to Acupuncture in Pregnancy and Childbirth

Shares personal stories of women who used acupressure/acupuncture. Discusses research studies that support the use or acupressure. (acupuncture.rhizome.net.nz)

REFERENCES

Ackerman, S. L., Lown, E. A., Dvorak, C. C., Dunn, E. A., Abrams, D. I., Horn, B. N., . . . Mehling, W. E. (2012). Massage for children undergoing hematopoietic cell transplanation: A qualitative report. *Evidence Based Complementary and Alternative Medicine* (pp. 1–9) doi:10.1155/2012/792042

Alessandrini, M., Napolitano, B., Micarelli, A., de Padova, A., & Bruno, E. (2012). P6 acupressure effectiveness on acute vertginous patients: A double blind randomized study. *Journal of Alternative and Complementary Medicine, 18*(12), 1121–1126.

Allais, G. R., Rolando, S., Gabellari, I. C., Burzio, C., Airola, G., Borgogno, P., . . . Benedetto, C. (2012). Acupressure in the control of migraine-associated nausea. *Neurolological Sciences, 33*(Suppl. 1), S207–S210.

Answers.com. (2013). Retrieved August 17, 2013, *Meridian* from http://www.answers/topic/meridian.com

Chang, L.-H., Hsu, C.-H., Jong, G.-P., Ho, S., Tsay, S.-I., & Lin, K.-C. (2012). Auricular acupressure for managing postoperative pain and knee motion in patients with total knee replacement: A randomized sham control study. *Evidence-Based Complementary and Alternative Medicine* (pp. 1–7) doi:10.1155/2012/528452

Dale, R. (1997). Demythologizing acupuncture. Part 1: The scientific mechanisms and the clinical uses. *Alternative and Complementary Therapies Journal, 3*(2), 125–131.

Davis, R. (2000). Cultural health care or child abuse? The Southeast Asian practice of cao gio. *Journal of the Academy of Nurse Practitioners, 3*(2), 125–131.

Dossey, B. M., Keegan, L., & Guzzetta, C. E. (2000). *Holistic nursing: A handbook for practice.* Gaithersburg, MD: Aspen.

Ebrahim Soltani, A., Mohammadinasab, H., Goudarzi, M., Arbabi, S., Mohtaram, R., Afkham, K., & Darbi, M. E. (2010). Acupressure using ondansetron versus metocolpramide on reduction of postoperative nausea and vomiting after strabismus surgery. *Archives of Iranian Medicine, 13*(4), 288–293.

Ebrahimi, N., Maltepe, C., & Einarson, A. (2010). Optimal mangement of nausea and vomiting in pregnancy. *International Journal of Women's Health, 2*, 241–248.

Elder, C. R., Gullion, C. M., DeBar, L. L., Funk, K., Lindberg, N. M., Rittenbaugh, C., . . . Stevens, V. J. (2012). Randomized trial of tapas acupressure for weight loss maintenance. *BMC Complementary and Alternative Medicine, 12*(19), 1–12.

FirstHealth. (2009). *First health of Andover.* Retrieved August 17, 2013, from http://firsthealthandover.com

FreeDictionary. (2009, October 26). *Freedictionary*. Retrieved October 26, 2009, from http://www.thefreedictionary.com: http://www.thefreedictionary.com

Gach, M. (1990). *Acupressure potent points*. New York, NY: Bantam Books.

Gach, M. (2004). *Acupressure: A self care guide for trauma, stress and common emotional imbalances*. New York, NY: Bantam Books.

Gharloghi, S., Torkzahrani, S., Akbarzadeh, A. R., & Heshmat, R. (2012). The effects of acupressure on severity of primary dysmenorrhea. *Patient Preference and Adherence, 6*, 137–142.

Griffiths, J. D., Gyte, G. M. L., Paranjothy, S., Brown, H. C., Broughton, H. K., & Thomas, J. (2012). Interventions for preventing nausea and vomiting in women undergoing regional anaesthesia for caesaren section. Cochrane Database of Systematic Reviews 2012, Issue 9. Art. No.: CD007579. doi: 10.1002/14651858.CD007579.pub2

Han, J.-S. (1997). *Acupuncture activates endogenous systems of analgesia*. National Institutes of Health Consensus Conference on Acupuncture: Program and abstracts. Bethesda, MD: National Institutes of Health, 55–60.

Han, J-S. (2003). Acupuncture: Neuropeptide release produced by electrical stimulation of different frequencies. *Trends in Neurosciences, 26*(1), 17–22.

Health Education Alliance for Life and Longevity. (2006, October 26). *Health Education Alliance for Life and Longevity*. Retrieved October 26 2006, from HEALL: http://www.heall.com

Hoo, J. J. (1997). Acupressure for hyperemesis gravidarum. *American Journal of Obstetrics and Gynecology, 176*(6), 1395–1396.

Hsieh, C. H., Su, J., Fang, Y. W., & Chou, P. H. (2012). Efficacy of two different materials used for auricular acupressure on weight reduction and abdominal obesity. *American Journal of Chinese Medicine, 40*(4), 713–720.

Huang, W., Pach, D., Napadow, V., Park, K., Long, X., Neumann, J., . . . Witt, C. M. (2012, April 9). Characterizing acupuncture stimuli using brain imaging with fMRI-a systematic review and meta-analysis of the literature. *PloS One, 7*(4), e32960. Retrieved from 10.1371/journal.pone.0032960

Kaptchuk, T. J. (1983). *The web that has no weaver*. Boston, MA: Congdon & Weed.

Lade, A. (1986). *Images and functions*. Seattle, WA: Eastland.

Lee, E. J., & Frazier, S. (2011). The efficacy of acupressure for symptom management. *Journal Pain and Symptom Management, 42*(4), 589–603.

Liang, F., Chen, R., & Cooper, E. L. (2012). Neuroendocrine mechanisms of acupuncture. *Evidence-Based Complementary and Alternative Medicine*, 2012: 792793, doi:10.1155/2012/792793

Litscher, G., Cheng, G., Cheng, W., Wang, L., Niu, Q., Feng, X., . . . Kuang, H. (2012). Sino-European transcontinental basic and clinical high-tech acupuncture studies-part 2: Acute stimulation effects on heart rate and its variability in patients with insomnia. *Evidence-Based Complementary and Alternative Medicine, 2012*: 2012(4):916085-916085

Long, A. F. (2009). The potential of complementary and alternative medicine in promoting well-being and critical health literacy: An observational study of shiatsu. *BMC Complementary and Alternative Medicine*. Retrieved October 26, 2012, from http:www.biomedcentral.com/1472-6882/9/19

Matsubara, T., Arai, Y.-C. P., Shiro, Y., Shimo, K., Nishihara, M., Satao, J., & Ushida, T. (2011). Comparative effects of acupressure at local and distal acupuncture points on pain conditions and autonomic function in females with chronic neck pain. *Evidence-Based Complementary and Alternative Medicine*, 2011: 543291. Published online 2010 September 23. doi: 10.1155/2011/543291

McFadden, K. L., Healy, K. M., Hoversten, K. P., Ito, T. A., & Hernández, T. (2012). Efficacy of acupressure for non-pharmacological stress reduction in college students. *Complementary Therapies in Medicine, 20*(4), 175–182.

McFadden, K. L., & Hernández, T. D. (2010). Cariovascular benefits of acupressure (Jin Shin) following stroke. *Complementary Therapies in Medicine, 18*(2), 42–48.

National Center for Complementary and Alternative Medicine. (2000). *Acupuncture information and resources.* Retrieved July 31, 2009, from http://nccam.nih.gov/health/ acupuncture/

National Institutes of Health. (1997). *NIH Consensus Development Conference Statement. Acupuncture.* Retrieved April 30, 2004, from http://consensus.nih.gov/1997/1997Acupuncture107html.htm

Pettersson, P. H., & Wengström, Y. (2012). Acupuncture prior to surgery to minimize postoperative nausea and vomiting: A systematic review. *Journal of Clinical Nursing, 21*(13–14), 1799–1805.

Robinson, N., Lorenc, A., & Liao, X. (2011). The evidence for shiatsu: A systematic review of shiatsu and acupressure. *BMC Complementary and Alternative Medicine, 11*(88), 1–14.

Roscoe, J. A., Bushnow, P., Jena-Pierre, P., Heckler, C. E., Purnell, J. Q., Chen, Y., . . . Morrow, G. R. (2009). Acupressure bands are effecting in reducing radiation therapy-related nausea. *Journal of Pain Symptom Management, 38*(3), 381–389.

Sankaranarayanan, K. M. (2005). Oil massage in neonates: An open randomized controlled study of coconut versus mineral oil. *Indian Pediatric, 42*(9), 877–884.

Schnorrenberger, C. C. (1996). Morphological foundations for acupuncture: An anatomical nomenclature of acupuncture structures. *Acupuncture in Medicine, 14*(2), 89–103.

Shames, K., & Keegan, L. (2000). Touch: Connecting with the healing power in 2000. In B. Dossey, L. Keegan, & C. E. Guzzetta (Eds.), *Holistic nursing* (3rd ed., pp. 613–635). Gaithersburg, MD: Aspen.

Struthers, R. (2008). The experience of being an Anishinabe man healer: Ancient healing in the modern world. *Journal of Cultural Diversity, 15*(2), 70–75.

Suh, E. E. (2012). The effects of P6 acupressure and nurse provided counseling on chemotherapy-induced nausea and vominting in patients with breast cancer. *Oncology Nursing Forum, 39*(1), E1.

Takeshige, C. (1989). Mechanism of acupuncture analgesia based on animal experiments: Scientific bases of acupuncture. Berlin, Germany: Springer-Verlag.

Unschuld, P. U. (1999). The past 1,000 years of Chinese medicine. *Lancet, 354*(Suppl. SIV9).

Valiee, S., Bassampour, S. S., Nasrabadi, A. N., Pouresmaeil, Z., & Mehran, A. (2012). Effect of acupressure on preoperative anxiety: A clinical trial. *Journal of PeriAnesthesia Nursing, 27*(4), 259–266.

Wu, B. (1995). Effect of acupuncture on the regulation of cell-mediated immunity in patients with malignant tumors [in Chinese]. *Zhen Ci Yan Jiu, 20*(3), 67–71.

Wu, B., Zhou, R. X., & Zhou, M. S. (1994). Effect of acupuncture on interleukin-2 level and NK cell immunoactivity of perhieral blood of malignant tumor patients. *Zhongguo Zhong Xi Yi Jie He Za Zhi, 14*(9), 537–539.

Yang, J-M. (2006). *Chinese qigong massage* (2nd ed.). Boston, MA: Yang's Martial Arts Academy (YMAA) Publication Center, Inc.

Yue, S., Jiang, X., & Wong, T. (2012). Effects of nurse-led acupressure programme for stroke patients in China. *Journal of Clinical Nursing, 22*(7–8), 1182–1188.

Chapter 27: Reflexology

Thora Jenny Gunnarsdottir

Reflexology is a complex complementary alternative therapy used globally for symptom management and for increasing well-being. In reflexology, the whole body has been mapped out in the hands and in the feet and can be manipulated directly using specific massage techniques. The corresponding areas on the feet are easier to locate because they cover a larger area and are more specific, rendering them easier to work on than the hands. In this chapter the main focus is on reflexology of the feet. Reflexology shares the philosophical base of holism congruent with nursing. As such, it provides nurses with an important tool to increase the healing mechanisms in their patients. Reflexology can be a prime tool in supplying caring, presence, and showing compassion in combination with a feeling of doing something that may help a patient to become more whole and feel better. This gentle intervention has been shown to affect some symptoms, but the scientific basis behind reflexology needs to be further established.

DEFINITION

Reflexology is defined as a holistic healing technique aimed at treating the individual as an entity, incorporating the body, mind, and spirit. It is a specific pressure therapy that works on precise reflex points of the feet that correspond to other body parts as depicted in Exhibit 27.1. Because the feet represent a microcosm of the body, all organs, glands, and other body parts are laid out in a similar arrangement on the feet (Dougans, 2005). Different definitions have been put forth, but they all

Exhibit 27.1. *Relationship of Body Parts With Reflexology Points on the Feet*

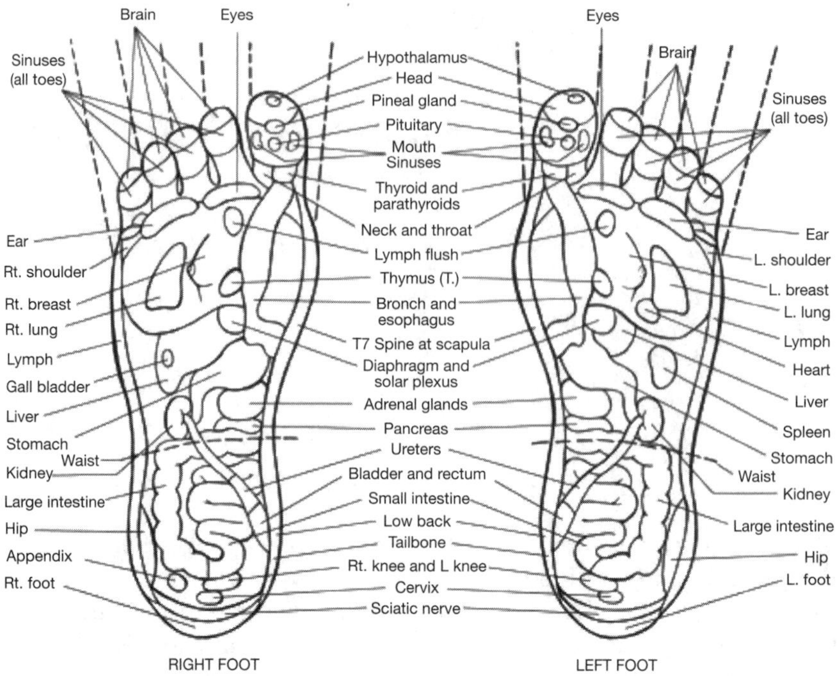

Brain   Eyes   Eyes

Sinuses
(all toes)

Hypothalamus
Head
Pineal gland
Pituitary
Mouth
Sinuses

Brain

Sinuses
(all toes)

Thyroid and
parathyroids
Neck and throat
Ear
Lymph flush
Rt. shoulder
Thymus (T.)
Rt. breast
Bronch and
esophagus
Rt. lung
T7 Spine at scapula
Lymph
Diaphragm and
solar plexus
Gall bladder
Adrenal glands
Liver
Pancreas
Stomach
Ureters
Waist
Kidney
Bladder and rectum
Large intestine
Small intestine
Hip
Low back
Appendix
Tailbone
Rt. foot
Rt. knee and L knee
Cervix
Sciatic nerve

Ear
L. shoulder
L. breast
L. lung
Lymph
Heart
Liver
Spleen
Stomach
Waist
Kidney
Large intestine
Hip
L. foot

RIGHT FOOT   LEFT FOOT

Source: Retrieved April 27, 2013, from www.dummies.com/how-to/content/foot-reflexology-map.html

express the basic principle behind reflexology—the soles of the feet and the palms of the hands are connected to all parts of the human body, including its internal organs; by applying specific pressure strategies to the soles of the feet, healing effects can be induced throughout the entire body.

The International Institute of Reflexology defines reflexology as a science that deals with the principle that there are reflex areas in the feet, and stimulating them properly can help many health problems in a natural way—a type of preventative maintenance (International Institute of Reflexology, 2012). Furthermore, the institute emphasizes that its purpose is not to treat or diagnose for any specific medical disorder but to promote better health and well-being. Kunz and Kunz (2003) state that the pressure techniques stimulate specific reflex areas on the feet and hands with the intention of invoking a beneficial response in other parts of the body. The literature also suggests that reflexology is useful for achieving and maintaining health, enhancing well-being, and relieving the symptoms of illness and disease (Tiran, 2002).

Definitions of reflexology convey that the basic principle behind reflexology is that the extremities are connected to all other parts and internal organs of the human body, and that there is a relationship among organs, systems, and processes. By using specific pressure strategies on the foot or hand, healing the whole body is possible. The left foot/hand represents the left side of the body and the right foot/hand represents the right side of the body. Numerous schools of reflexology have been established throughout the world.

SCIENTIFIC BASIS

The foundations of reflexology can be traced to two different theories or schools of thought documented in the reflexology literature. The first theory originated in traditional Chinese medicine (TCM) and the second one in a Western technique known as *zone therapy*.

Traditional Chinese Medicine

Reflexology is thought to be Eastern in origin (Dougans, 2005), and it is congruent with the principle of organ representation from TCM: "the whole represents itself in the parts" (Kaptchuk, 2000). This statement means that the feet are seen as a microcosm of the body, as a kind of holographic image in which all organs, glands, and other body parts are mirrored on the soles of the feet. The idea that the whole body can be represented in its parts is not new. For example, tongue diagnosis has been documented in China for at least 2,000 years. It is also evident in the iris of the eye, the face, and the ear (Maciocia, 2005).

TCM posits that there are a number of invisible energy pathways, or meridians, within the body that carry an energy called *Qi*, which is the vital energy behind all processes. All organs are interconnected with each other by a meridian network system and, to maintain health, energy needs to be flowing in balance. Factors impeding the free circulation of *Qi* are divided into categories of excess and deficiency. *Excess* refers to the presence of something that is too much for the individual to handle—too much food to digest, too much waste to eliminate, and so forth. *Deficiency* refers to the absence or relative insufficiency of one or more aspects of the life energies necessary for sustaining health and well-being. A deficiency or excess of life energy can allow outside factors to overwhelm the individual, thus inducing pathology and leading to pain and illness (Maciocia, 2005).

In a healthy person with energy in balance, the feet feel soft when palpated and should have the same texture in every area. When an area is felt to be empty or is lacking in texture when palpated, it is an indication of deficiency in the energy of that particular organ or area in the body. If an area feels stiff and hard in texture when palpated, it indicates an excess of energy. If a lack of energy is found in one area, this means that some other area has too much energy because the energy must be in balance. On empty areas, it is necessary to slowly build aggressive pressure to increase the energy flow, and more vigorous, light but firm pressure is applied on the area that has too much energy to direct the flow out and away from this area. In that way, reflexology redirects excess energy from one area into another where there is an apparent deficiency, so as to supplement a deficiency or to subdue an excess pattern.

Zone Therapy

The second theory, often referred to as zone therapy, originated in the West. At the beginning of the 20th century, Dr. William Fitzgerald found that pressure applied to some parts of the feet induced anesthesia in specific parts of one's body. He then determined that the entire body and all its organs were laid out in a certain configuration on the soles of the feet. He divided the body into 10 longitudinal zones, running from the top of the head to the toes, and proposed that parts of the body within a certain zone were linked with one another—hence the name *zone therapy*.

An American therapist, Eunice Ingham, is credited with establishing reflexology in its present form (Ingham, 1984). She used the zones as a guiding map, but began to chart the feet according to where pressure would produce distinct effects in the body. She developed a map of the entire body on the feet and called the areas *reflexes*. Her proposition was that when the bloodstream becomes blocked with waste materials or excess acid, calcium deposits start to form in the nerve endings, impeding the normal circulation of the blood and creating an imbalance in the various parts of the body, depending on the location of the blockage. She believed that by using the specific pressure of reflexology, the calcium deposits on the feet could be detected as "gritty areas" that may feel painful when touched. Ingham describes these as "particles of frost" or "crystal blocks" when examined under a microscope. The pressure and massage techniques taught in reflexology are designed to dissipate these formations and break down their crystalline structures. By doing so, the corresponding area connected with this particular nerve ending will receive an added supply of blood. In this way, the circulatory and lymphatic systems are stimulated, thus encouraging the release and removal of toxins, and the body starts to heal itself. Other theories have been considered in the literature but are not detailed in this chapter.

No theoretical framework for reflexology has been directly proven, which may partially explain why there is not universal agreement on how to classify reflexology. The National Center for Complementary and

Alternative Medicine classifies reflexology as a manipulative and body-based method (NCCAM, 2012).

INTERVENTION

The patient will be lying comfortably, covered by a blanket, somewhat higher than the chair in which the reflexologist sits, and will have pillows under the knees and the head to induce relaxation. In addition, the patient will be barefoot and in a comfortable position, with any tight clothes loosened so as not to hinder circulation. Then the patient will be assessed continuously for tolerance to the amount of pressure applied. The pressure needs to be firm enough to activate the body's healing potentials but must also be tolerable to the patient. Sensitivity varies in each individual, and the feet usually become more sensitive with subsequent treatments. Each area is worked, finishing the toe area on the one foot and then treating the toe area on the other foot, and so on, going from one foot to the other.

Although it is emphasized that reflexology is to be applied to the feet as a whole, it is important to work specifically on several systems of the body. These specific systems are, for example: the digestive system to increase proper elimination; the lymphatic system, to increase the clearance of waste materials; the bladder and kidneys, to increase urine and energy flow (the kidneys are one source of Qi); the solar plexus (where feelings and emotions are stored), to increase relaxation; all internal glands, to stimulate their respective functions; and the lungs, to increase oxygen consumption. A foot map with physical locations and corresponding body systems is illustrated in the interactive website (www.dk.co.uk/static/cs/uk/11/features/reflexology/footchart.html). By using reflexology on these body systems, the reflexologist is both increasing circulation and elimination and affecting the flow of Qi because all organs are interconnected with each other by meridians.

Techniques

There are several techniques used, depending on the area of the foot. One hand supports the foot while the fingers and the thumb of the other hand massage the skin. A period of 45 minutes to 1 hour is estimated to be enough time to perform the reflexology on both feet and will allow for extra time to work on specific areas that need further care. At the end of each session the receiver is encouraged to relax for several minutes. There are some standard pressure procedures for working on the reflexes of the feet. The two techniques described here are thumb-walking and hook and back-up (Kunz & Kunz, 2003). Other grips can be used, depending on the area of the foot in question. It is important not to forget any area and to finish one area before starting the next one (see Exhibit 27.2).

Exhibit 27.2. *Techniques*

Thumb-Walking

The goal of the thumb-walking technique is to apply a constant, steady pressure to the surface of the foot or the hand:

1. With the other hand (holding hand) stretch the sole of the foot. Rest the working thumb on the sole and your fingers on the top of the foot. Drop your wrist to create leverage, which exerts pressure with the thumb.
2. Bend and unbend the thumb's first joint, moving it forward a little bit at a time. When your working hand feels stretched, reposition it and continue walking it forward. Take a little step forward with each unbend. The goal is to work with a small area in each step to create a feeling of constant, steady pressure. Always walk in a forward direction, not backward. Keep your thumb slightly cocked as you work to prevent overextending it.

Hook and Back-Up

The hook and back-up technique is used to work a specific point rather than to cover a larger area. It is a relatively stationary technique, with only small movements of the working thumb involved. To avoid digging your fingernail into the flesh, apply pressure using more of the flat of the thumb:

1. Support and protect the area to be worked with the holding hand. The hand wraps around the area while the thumb and fingers hold it in place. Place the fingers of the working hand over those of the holding hand.
2. Place the working thumb in the center of the area to be worked. Hook and back-up, using the edge of the thumb.

Adapted from Kunz and Kunz (2003).

Measurement of Outcomes

The philosophy behind reflexology states that it affects the body as whole; however, based on the literature, more studies have measured physiological or psychological outcomes of reflexology than its overall effects. It is important to measure the effect of reflexology over a number of sessions to gain insight into its overall benefits.

Precautions

Reports from people have indicated reflexology to be a largely pleasant experience, leaving them both calm and relaxed. However, it must be emphasized that many do not like to have their feet touched and approval from the patient is needed before starting. Before beginning reflexology, the condition of the feet must be examined for swelling, color, ulcerations, toe deformities, and odor. The physical condition of the person is also very important; hence, the health history is reviewed. The therapist must be careful about the pressure of the massage, if there is a problem regarding the blood flow to the limbs because of diabetes, neurological diseases, or arteriosclerosis. Older adults may require special precautions, due to such concerns as restricted movement, incontinence, arthritis, and aching joints. When dealing with such conditions, it may be better to consider the person's comfort and feel of the touch as the primary goals. Children have also been participants in research, where the effects of reflexology on constipation were reported on 3- to 14-year-olds without any adverse effects.

Some symptoms of adverse effects after undergoing complementary therapy are often referred to as "healing crisis." This is said to present frequently during and immediately following treatment as localized or distal pain, perspiration or shivering, and changes in the heart rate, respiration, or temperature. This phenomenon is also described as a cleansing process. The treatment is believed to activate the body's healing power; accumulated waste products and toxins, which have often lain dormant in the body, are released into the bloodstream. In one study where the effects of reflexology on fibromyalgia syndrome were studied, the participants were specifically observed and asked about healing crisis as part of the reflexology treatment (Gunnarsdottir & Jonsdottir, 2010). The participants, six women who were given 10 reflexology treatments, described several symptoms as healing crisis: headaches, increased thirst, increased pain, increased urination, more frequent bowel movements, aggravated skin conditions, increased perspiration, fatigue, feverishness, dizziness, and exhaustion, and also increased energy. These symptoms appeared during the early stages and lasted for 1 or 2 days each time. Due to reports of such reactions, it must be emphasised that reflexologists may need to be extra careful when applying reflexology on people who are seriously ill, such as cancer patients, because they may not tolerate a healing crisis well. It is also important to explain to people what can be expected after a treatment.

USES

Research testing the effects of reflexology is limited and includes studies of many approaches to practices of reflexology. Some conditions for which it has been used are listed in Exhibit 27.3.

Exhibit 27.3. *Uses of Reflexology*

Decrease pain (Hodgson & Andersen, 2008; Stephenson, Dalton, & Carlson, 2003; Stephenson, Swanson, Dalton, Keefe, & Engle, 2007)

Decrease symptoms of fibromyalgia (Gunnarsdottir & Peden-McAlpine, 2010)

Decrease anxiety (Gambles, Crooke, & Wilkinson, 2002; Quattrin et al., 2006; Stephenson et al., 2007)

Reduce physiologic distress in elderly (Hodgson & Andersen, 2008)

Improve well-being in people with Parkinson disease (Johns, Blake, & Sinclair, 2010)

Improve the quality of life (Gambles et al., 2002; Milligan, Fanning, Hunter, Tadjali, & Stevens, 2002)

Alleviate effects of stress (Milligan et al., 2002)

Reduce the symptoms of multiple sclerosis (Mackereth, Booth, Hillier, & Caress, 2008; Siev-Ner, Gamus, Lerner-Geva, & Achiron, 2003)

Promote relaxation (Gambles et al., 2002; Milligan et al., 2002; Ross et al., 2002)

Improve constipation (Bishop, McKinnon, Weir, & Brown, 2003; Woodward, Norton, & Barriball, 2010)

Improve sleep (Gambles et al., 2002; Milligan et al., 2002)

Effect on hemodynamic variables (Jones, Thomson, Irvine, & Leslie, 2012)

The duration of the effects of reflexology on pain was tested on patients with various types of cancer. The immediate effects on pain were supported, but the pain-relieving effects were not significant at 3 hours and 24 hours after the reflexology session (Stephenson, Dalton, & Carlson, 2003). In a study by Ross and colleagues (2002), the effects of reflexology on anxiety and depression were compared with those of simple foot massage on two groups of cancer patients. These cancer patients received six sessions of intervention, and depression and anxiety were measured at baseline and within 24 hours after each session. No significant differences were found between the groups with respect to anxiety and depression, but both groups indicated experiencing relaxing effects from the treatment.

A case study design was used to test the effects of reflexology on six cases of women with fibromyalgia (Gunnarsdottir & Peden-McAlpine, 2010). Each case had 10 sessions of reflexology over a period of 10 weeks.

Data were collected by observation, interviews, and diaries and then analyzed within each case and across cases. The findings showed that symptoms of pain in multiple areas started to localize and decrease in severity. The areas that responded best were the head, shoulders, neck, and arms.

In a study by Hodgson and Andersen (2008), 21 nursing home residents with dementia were given four reflexology treatments over 4 weeks. The primary efficacy endpoint that was obtained was a significant reduction of physiological distress as measured by salivary alpha-amylase. Furthermore, the residents demonstrated significant reduction in observed pain during the study period.

Quality of life (QOL) has been found to be enhanced in cancer patients after reflexology. To investigate patient satisfaction with reflexology therapy and its impact on QOL, an audit was undertaken in a Scottish hospice (Milligan et al., 2002). Twenty cancer patients completed self-report questionnaires after receiving from three to more than five reflexology sessions from a nurse trained in the therapy. The patients reported that reflexology reduced pain, improved sleep, enhanced relaxation, and reduced stress. In England, a similar study took place in which 34 cancer patients under palliative care were asked to comment about the reflexology therapy they had received (Gambles et al., 2002). The patients received from four to six individually tailored reflexology interventions. They commented on reflexology as being emotionally beneficial in reducing anxiety and tension, improving sleep, and coping with the side effects of medications.

Patients with multiple sclerosis (MS) tend to suffer from a variety of chronic muscular symptoms, and two studies have reported improvements in symptoms after sessions of reflexology. Siev-Ner et al. (2003) conducted a randomized controlled clinical trial to determine the effects of reflexology on the symptoms of MS. Statistically significant positive differences in the scores for paresthesia, urinary symptoms, and spasticity were found in the group receiving reflexology compared with the control group. Another study compared the effects of reflexology and progressive muscle relaxation training for 50 people with MS with a crossover design (Johns et al., 2010). Positive effects were found from both treatments on physiological and psychological outcomes.

Domestic partners can be taught by qualified professionals to perform foot reflexology on patients with metastases from cancer. Stephenson et al. (2007) showed that partner-delivered foot reflexology had significant effects, resulting in a decrease of pain and anxiety as compared with a control group that received reading sessions from their partners. Social benefits of such use of reflexology were reported by some participants.

Subjective reports in studies of reflexology are few but suggest that the experience is mostly positive, indicating relaxing, calming, and comforting effects. Patients receiving reflexology frequently experience relaxation as a benefit (Gambles et al., 2002; Milligan et al., 2002), and feel more energy and a sense of well-being (Woodward et al., 2010). Patients have also commented on how reflexology can create space for them to talk about their worries and concerns, which is an important part of the therapy as a whole (Mackereth, Booth, Hillier, & Caress, 2009).

A systematic review of randomized controlled trials was done to explore if reflexology can have specific hemodynamic effects (Jones et al., 2012). The findings indicated that reflexology can have some effect on hemodynamic variables.

CULTURAL APPLICATIONS

The roots of reflexology are embedded in ancient history, when pressure therapies were recognized as preventive and therapeutic. Evidence indicates that therapeutic foot massage has been practiced throughout history by a variety of cultures. The oldest documentation depicting the practice of reflexology was unearthed in Egypt, dating around 2500–2330 BCE. The use of reflex pressure applied to the feet as a healing therapy has been practiced by the North American native peoples for generations.

As discussed earlier in the chapter, there are different perspectives on the effects of reflexology in Eastern and Western cultures. The TCM energy channels are one of the main concepts in both reflexology and acupuncture because in both therapies energy is channeled throughout the body. Energy is channeled through the meridians and through the zones in reflexology. Both practices assert that diseases are caused by blockages in energy channels. In acupuncture/acupressure, energy is stimulated or sedated with needle/finger pressure. Six meridians are present in the feet, where they either end or begin. The other ends of the meridians going from or to the feet start or end in the fingers. Therefore, the meridians in the upper and lower parts of the body are connected.

Reflexology on the whole foot is also done on the acupuncture points there, and thus can help clear congestions in the meridians. It can also be used purposively, as it may be very helpful to push, press, or massage these points to increase energy in the meridians. Such stimulation aids in increasing energy movement along the meridians and in the organs to which they are connected. In this way the use of reflexology is based more on energy and assessment and movement of energy throughout the body. Zone therapy as developed by Eunice Ingham is mostly practiced in Europe and the United States.

Reflexology, reflex zone therapy, and reflexotherapy are all terms that refer to the current use of the treatment, with distinctions apparently being due to scientific, philosophical, and political differences of opinion among authorities. Reflexology has become one of the most common therapies

---

Sidebar 27.1. *Reflexology in Iceland*

Thora Jenny Gunnarsdottir, University of Iceland, Reykjavik, Iceland

In 2000, eight major societies of alternative therapies in Iceland merged into the Association of Complementary and Alternative Medicine in Iceland (ACAMI). Approximately 600 practitioners are members of this organization, whose major goals include: striving for continued progress in the work environment of healers, establishing recognition for therapists, and providing education on issues related to the activities of health professionals in the community (ACAMI, 2012). The organization includes two groups of reflexologists: the Icelandic Association of Reflexology and the Association of the Icelandic Reflexologists.

In 2005, the Ministry of Health in Iceland commissioned a report on the regulatory status and the future direction of alternative therapies in Iceland (Althingi, 2005). All practitioners in ACAMI were required to have certain qualifications to be members of the organization. This has helped to regulate services offered by all healers, including reflexologists. Those who are fully accredited members of both professional associations of reflexologists are also members of ACAMI.

As part of a larger study on the use of health care services in Iceland, the scope of the use of CAM providers was assessed (Helgadottir, Vilhjalmsson, & Gunnarsdottir, 2010). A sample of 1,532 Icelandic adults between the ages of 18 and 75 responded to a survey yielding a 60% response rate. Almost 32% of the respondents reported visiting a CAM provider during the preceding year, an estimated increase of 5% since 1998. The most common therapy was massage; however, visits to reflexologists were ranked number two, with 43% use. This indicates a growing, widespread interest in reflexology in Iceland.

---

practiced by nurses and midwives in the United Kingdom (Mackereth & O'Hara, 2002). The practice of reflexology is on the rise in the United Kingdom, with an estimated 12,500 registered reflexologists and approximately 4.33 million visits per year (Poole, 2002). Reflexology is also a commonly practiced complementary therapy in Iceland, as described in Sidebar 27.1.

FUTURE RESEARCH

In the pursuit of greater integration of complementary therapies into conventional health care, it is inevitable that reflexology will evolve and will need to be adapted to meet the needs of the system in which it finds itself.

Practitioners need to be critical and acknowledge the value of research and inquiry in this process. The scientific basis for reflexology is growing, and promising results of its use for some symptoms are beginning to emerge; however, more rigorous research is needed if it is to be used effectively by nurses in health care settings.

A recent systematic review of reflexology concluded that there is no evidence for any specific effect of reflexology in any conditions, with the exception of urinary symptoms associated with MS (Wang, Tsai, Lee, Chang, & Yang, 2008). However, another critical review on studies of reflexology (Gunnarsdottir & Peden-McAlpine, 2010) suggests that the reasons for limited scientific evidence of reflexology's effects are several. The methods used in the studies differ and are often not adequately explained. The amount of time and frequency of sessions are different and the principle behind reflexology states that it can affect the body as a whole. It is important to measure the effect of reflexology over a number of sessions to gain insight into its overall benefits. The latter phenomenon has not yet been captured in the studies reviewed. There may also be problems with localizations of reflexology points. One researcher, nurse Jenny Jones, has looked specifically at the localization of the heart point and conducted a survey among members of the Association of Reflexologists in the United Kingdom (Jones, Thomson, Lauder, & Leslie, 2012). The findings showed lack of clarity and consistency regarding the indication of reflexology for cardiac patients, inconsistencies in reflexology teaching literature, and marked inconsistencies in the heart point placement.

Nurses are in a primary position to conduct research on reflexology because their holistic background is in tune with the philosophies behind reflexology. Some questions for future research are:

- What are the specifics of reflexology among other complementary therapies, and how can the specifics of reflexology be captured in research?
- What is the mechanism behind reflexology?

The principle behind reflexology states that it can affect the body as a whole. However, it is not clear how these holistic changes come about. It has been pointed out that it is important for researchers in reflexology to identify the foundation or mechanisms of action in order to build a stronger theoretical framework for future studies (Poole, 2002). The scientific basis behind reflexology is growing, and promising results of its use for certain symptoms are beginning to emerge. However, more rigorous research is needed if it is to be used as a standard practice by nurses or other health care practitioners within health care settings. There is an urgent need to explore the experience of having reflexology in order to try to gain more information about what takes place during sessions and how the framework supports the intervention.

WEBSITES

The International Institute of Reflexology, with branches around the world, is the only school licensed to teach the original Ingham method. The late Eunice Ingham originated, researched, and developed reflexology as it is known today. Reflexology has grown to international proportions under the able direction of her nephew, Dwight Byers, today's leading authority.
(www.reflexology-usa.net)

Kevin and Barbara Kunz have developed and maintain two websites offering the basics on reflexology theory and practice, and facts on developments in reflexology research.
(www.reflexology-research.com)
(www.foot-reflexologist.com)

Other selected websites offer additional data, including lists of worldwide reflexology organizations, as well as interactive information on reflexology products and practice.
(www.reflexology.org)
(www.myreflexologist.com)
(www.aor.org.uk)

The International Council of Reflexologists was established in 1990 in Toronto, Ontario, Canada, and holds an international conference on reflexology every other year.
(www.icr-reflexology.org)

REFERENCES

ACAMI. (2012). Association of Complementary and Alternative Medicine in Iceland. Retrieved March 20, 2012, from http://big.is/page29/page29.html

Althingi. (2005, May). *Lög um græðara* [Act on alternative practitioner. Legislation on the Association of Complementary and Alternative Medicine in Iceland] (nr. 34, 11).

Bishop, E., McKinnon, E., Weir, E., & Brown, D. W. (2003). Reflexology in the management of encopresis and chronic constipation. *Pediatric Nursing, 15*(3), 20–21.

Dougans, I. (2005). *Reflexology: The 5 elements and their 12 meridians. A unique approach.* London, UK: Thorsons.

Gambles, M., Crooke, M., & Wilkinson, S. (2002). Evaluation of a hospice based reflexology service: A qualitative audit of patient perceptions. *European Journal of Oncology Nursing, 6*(1), 37–44.

Gunnarsdottir, T. J., & Jonsdottir, H. (2010). Healing crisis in reflexology: Becoming worse before becoming better. *Complementary Therapies in Clinical Practice, 16,* 239–243.

Gunnarsdottir, T. J., & Peden-McAlpine, C. (2010). Effects of reflexology on fibromyalgia symptoms: A multiple case study. *Complementary Therapies in Clinical Practice, 16*, 167–172.

Helgadottir, B., Vilhjalmsson, R., & Gunnarsdottir, T. J. (2010). Notkun óhefðbundinnar heilbrigðisþjónustu á Íslandi [Use of complementary and alternative therapies in Iceland]. *The Icelandic Medical Journal, 96*, 269–275.

Hodgson, N. A., & Andersen, S. (2008). The clinical efficacy of reflexology in nursing home residents with dementia. *Journal of Alternative and Complementary Medicine, 14*(3), 269–275.

Ingham, E. D. (1984). *Stories the feet can tell thru reflexology/Stories the feet have told thru reflexology.* Saint Petersburg, FL: Ingham.

International Institute of Reflexology. (2012). *Reflexology facts USA.* Retrieved October 18, 2012, from http://www.reflexology-usa.net/facts.htm

Johns, C., Blake, D., & Sinclair, A. (2010). Can reflexology maintain or improve the well-being of people with Parkinson's disease? *Complementary Therapies in Clinical Practice, 16*, 96–100.

Jones, J., Thomson, P., Irvine, K., & Leslie, S. J. (2012). Is there a specific hemodynamic effect in reflexology? A systematic review of randomized controlled trials. *Journal of Alternative and Complementary Medicine* (Epub ahead of print). doi:10.1089/acm.2011.0854

Jones, J., Thomson, P., Lauder, W., & Leslie, S. J. (2012). Reported treatment strategies for reflexology in cardiac patients and inconsistencies in the location of the heart reflex point: An online survey. *Complementary Therapies in Clinical Practice, 18*, 145–150.

Kaptchuk, T. J. (2000). *The web that has no weaver: Understanding Chinese medicine.* Chicago: Contemporary Books.

Kunz, K., & Kunz, B. (2003). *Reflexology: Health at your fingertips.* New York, NY: DK.

Maciocia, G. (2005). *The foundations of Chinese medicine* (2nd ed.). London, UK: Elsevier.

Mackereth, P. A., Booth, K., Hillier, V. F., & Caress, A. (2008). Reflexology and progressive muscle relaxation training for people with multiple sclerosis: A crossover trial. *Complementary Therapies in Clinical Practice, 15*, 14–21.

Mackereth, P. A., Booth, K., Hillier, V. F., & Caress, A. (2009). What do people talk about during reflexology? Analysis of worries and concerns expressed during sessions for patients with multiple sclerosis. *Complementary Therapies in Clinical Practice, 15*, 85–90.

Mackereth, P. A., & O'Hara, C. S. (2002). Appreciating preparatory and continuing education. In P. A. Mackereth & D. Tiran (Eds.), *Clinical reflexology* (pp. 17–32). Edinburgh, Scotland: Churchill Livingstone.

Milligan, M., Fanning, M., Hunter, S., Tadjali, M., & Stevens, E. (2002). Reflexology audit: Patient satisfaction, impact on quality of life and availability in Scottish hospices. *International Journal of Palliative Nursing, 8*, 489–496.

National Center for Complementary and Alternative Medicine (NCCAM).(2012). *About NCCAM.* Retrieved November 10, 2012, from http://nccam.nih.gov/health/whatiscam/

Poole, H. (2002). Appreciating preparatory and continuing education. In P. A. Mackereth & D. Tiran (Eds.), *Clinical reflexology* (pp. 61–71). Edinburgh, Scotland: Churchill Livingstone.

Quattrin, R., Zanini, A., Buchini, S., Turello, D., Annunziata, M. A., Vidotti, C., & Brusaferro, S. (2006). Use of reflexology foot massage to reduce anxiety in hospitalized cancer patients in chemotherapy treatment. *Journal of Nursing Management, 14*, 96–105.

Ross, C. S. K., Hamilton, J., Macramé, G., Docherty, C., Gould, A., & Corbeled, M. A. (2002). A pilot study to evaluate the effect of reflexology on mood and symptom rating of advanced cancer patients. *Palliative Medicine, 16,* 544–545.

Siev-Ner, I., Gamus, D., Lerner-Geva, L., & Achiron, A. (2003). Reflexology treatment relieves symptoms of multiple sclerosis: A randomized controlled study. *Multiple Sclerosis, 9,* 356–361.

Stephenson, L. N., Dalton, J. A., & Carlson, J. (2003). The effect of foot reflexology on pain in patients with metastatic cancer. *Applied Nursing Research, 16*(4), 284–286.

Stephenson, L. N., Swanson, M., Dalton, J., Keefe, F. J., & Engle, M. (2007). Partner-delivered reflexology: Effects on cancer pain and anxiety. *Oncology Nursing Forum, 34*(1), 127–132.

Tiran, D. (2002). Reviewing theories and origins. In P. A. Mackereth & D. Tiran (Eds.), *Clinical reflexology* (pp. 5–15). Edinburgh, Scotland: Churchill Livingstone.

Wang, M., Tsai, P., Lee, P., Chang, W., & Yang, C. (2008). The efficacy of reflexology: A systematic review. *Journal of Advanced Nursing, 62*(5), 512–520.

Woodward, S., Norton, C., & Barriball, K. (2010). A pilot study of the effectiveness of reflexology in treating idiopathic constipation in women. *Complementary Therapies in Clinical Practice, 16,* 41–46.

Chapter 28: Magnet Therapy

CORJENA K. CHEUNG

Magnets have been used for healing purposes for centuries in many countries such as China, Egypt, Greece, and India. They are mentioned in the oldest medical text ever found, the Yellow Emperor's *Classic of Internal Medicine* in 2000 BCE, as well as in the ancient Hindu scriptures, the *Vedas* (Whitaker & Adderly, 1998). In Europe during the 16th century, Paracelsus, a German-Swiss physician, theorized that because magnets attract iron they might attract and "draw out" diseases from the body. German physician Franz Mesmer, who is believed to be the father of alternate medicine, claimed that a mysterious fluid, which he called "animal magnetism," had an influence on the body's health and that the planets influenced how animal magnetism worked (Trueman, 2000).

Magnet therapy was popular in the United States in the 18th century, where it was used for treating many ailments of the body, especially in some rural areas where few doctors were available. The introduction of antibiotics, cortisone, and other medications resulted in magnet therapy losing its allure. Since the 1940s, there has been a resurgence of interest in magnet therapy by health professionals (Whitaker & Adderly, 1998). During the 1970s, both magnets and electromagnetic machines became popular among athletes in many countries for treating sports-related injuries (New York University, 2012). Magnetic products such as magnetic mattress pads, bracelets, and necklaces became a rapidly growing industry during that time for a variety of conditions. Although both public and health care professionals were fascinated by the potential therapeutic effects of magnets, it was not until the late 20th century that reports from adequately designed clinical trials of magnets were published. Results of several preliminary studies suggested that both static magnets and electromagnetic therapy may have therapeutic effects. These findings have accelerated research interest in magnet therapy. A recent PubMed search for *magnet therapy* as the keyword yielded only 2,872 articles, and yet more than 2,540,000 links with mostly commercial advertisements were generated via Google. Currently, magnet therapy is one of the most widely used forms of complementary and alternative therapies for the management of chronic pain associated with musculoskeletal disorders. Magnets are often marketed for many different types of pain, including foot pain and back pain from conditions such as arthritis and fibromyalgia (National Center for Complementary and Alternative Medicine [NCCAM], 2012). The modern magnet therapy industry's total sales are estimated at $500 million per year in the United States and $5 billion globally (Winemiller, Billow, Laskowski, & Harmsen, 2005).

Today, energy healing remains a debatable subject in the scientific community. The scientific literature on magnet therapy continues to yield conflicting findings. Scientists continue to try to understand the healing power of magnets, and whether, how, and why magnets work on certain health problems.

DEFINITION

The National Center of Complementary and Alternative Medicine (NCCAM) classified magnet therapy under the domain of energy therapies. Energy therapies operate on the principle that health can be influenced by the subtle realignment of a person's "vital energy"—energy that is innate to all living beings and that, when disordered or blocked, can create disease (Kaptchuk, 1996). The term *magnet* comes from the legend of Greek shepherd Magnes, who about 2,500 years ago discovered mysterious iron deposits attracted to the nails of his sandals while walking in an area near Mount Ida in Turkey. These deposits, which were known to the ancients as lodestones or live-stones, are now known as magnetite (magnetic oxide, Fe_3O_4; Macklis, 1993). Magnet therapy involves the use of magnets of varying sizes and strengths that are placed on the body to relieve pain and treat disease (New York University, 2012).

SCIENTIFIC BASIS

The Earth's magnetic field and the body's bioenergetic field exist. Magnet therapy is based on the premise that all living things exist in a magnetic field (the Earth), and that the human body exists in and generates a magnetic field that has healing powers. According to Oschman (1998), each of the great systems in the body—the musculoskeletal system, the digestive system, the circulatory system, the nervous system, the skin—is composed of connective tissues that have important roles in communication and regulation. The extracellular, cellular, and nuclear matrices throughout the body form an interconnected solid-state network called a "living matrix." Because the main structural components are helical piezoelectric semiconductors, the living matrix generates energetic vibrations, absorbs them from the environment, and conducts a variety of energetic signals from place to place. There are many energetic systems in the living body and many ways of influencing them. The Western concept of *energy* is similar to the concepts *Qi* in traditional Chinese medicine and *Prana* in the Hindu system of traditional medicine (Ayurveda).

Scientists suggest that magnetic fields can influence important biological processes in the following ways: decrease the firing rate of certain neurons, particularly c-type chronic pain neurons; change the rate of enzyme-mediated reactions, which may play a role in inflammatory cascades and free radical generation; modulate intracellular signaling by affecting the functioning of calcium channels in cell membranes; and cause small changes in blood flow (Wolsko et al., 2004). Yet another theory, the Hall effect, has been suggested. The Hall effect refers to positively and negatively charged ions in the bloodstream that become activated by a magnetic field and generate heat-causing vasoconstriction and an increased blood and oxygen supply to the affected area (Whitaker & Adderly, 1998).

Evidence demonstrated that repetitive transcranial magnetic stimulation (rTMS) and pulsed electromagnetic field therapy (PEMF) can affect nerve tissue and organ functions. However, for centuries, the effects of static magnets and low-frequency electromagnetic fields on biological processes have been investigated and debated. According to Frankel and Liburdy (1996), static magnets could affect charged particles in the blood, nerves, and cell membranes or subtly alter biochemical reactions. The question remains, however, whether the effect is strong enough to make a difference.

INTERVENTION

Technique

Permanent (or static) magnets are typically placed directly on the skin or inside clothing or other materials that come into close contact with the body. There are a number of permanent magnets available commercially, in various shapes and forms, for therapeutic purposes. The three most common forms of permanent magnets are plastiform magnets, neodymium magnetic discs, and ceramic magnets. Plastiform magnets are flexible, rubberized magnetic rolls that can be wrapped around an affected extremity or lie along the full length of the spine. Neodymium magnetic discs are light-weight and can be used on the face and on various acupuncture points. Ceramic magnets can be made in any shape and size (Beattie, 2004).

A permanent magnet is either a natural or artificially made magnet that produces magnetic force by the movements of electrons in the atoms of the material that make up the magnet, such as iron or nickel. These materials can be ordered to all lie in one direction (referred to as "north" or "south"). Therefore one large magnetic field can be created where similar poles repel one another and opposing poles attract. The poles are thought to have different effects on the human body. The northern pole is considered negative magnetic energy and is suggested to calm and normalize the body; the southern pole is made up of positive magnetic energy and is believed to be responsible for disordering and overstimulating the biological system (Arizona Unipole Magnetics, 2008a, 2008b). Permanent magnets can be unipolar (one pole of the magnet faces or touches the skin) or bipolar (both poles face or touch the skin, sometimes in repeating patterns). They have magnetic fields that do not change.

Electromagnets are magnets produced by electric current passing through a cylindrical coil of wire, also known as a time-varying magnetic field. Its use is under the supervision of a health care provider. The magnetic strength is directly proportional to the strength of the electric current. When the electric current is discontinued, the wire loses its magnetism.

Pulsed electromagnetism is the process by which alternating electromagnetic fields are delivered in a time-varying manner. The PEMF is primarily used in hospitals, in clinics, and in clinical trials for pain, inflammation, and wound (tissue and bone) healing. Medicare has approved the coverage of PEMF for chronic wound treatment (Medlearn Matters, 2004).

Two other electromagnets being used in clinical settings are the magnetic molecular energizer (MME) and transcranial magnetic stimulation (TMS). MME is a treatment method that consists of the application of high direct current electromagnetic field ranges between 3,000 gauss to 5,000 gauss (explained in the Guidelines section, which follows). An MME device consists of two very large and strong electromagnets, with the patient lying in a focal point between the two electromagnets. It acts as a catalyst to improve chemical reactions occurring in the human body. This form of magnet therapy is used for neurological and neuromuscular ailments such as spinal cord injury, brain injury, stroke impairment, multiple sclerosis, muscular dystrophy, cerebral palsy, Parkinson's disease, Alzheimer's disease, congestive heart failure, and orthopedic conditions involving bone and joint repair (Advanced Magnetic Research Institute, 2005).

TMS delivers electrical stimulation to neural tissue, including cerebral cortex, spinal roots, and cranial and peripheral nerves. It can be applied as single or repetitive pulses of stimulation at various frequencies. Single stimuli can depolarize neurons and evoke measurable effects. Trains of stimuli (repetitive TMS) can modify excitability of the cerebral cortex at the stimulated site and also at remote areas along functional anatomical connections. TMS is primarily used as a treatment option for depression. Performed by a psychiatrist, the noninvasive procedure involves the use of a large electromagnetic coil placed directly against the brain's motor cortex creating electric currents that stimulate nerve cells in the region of the brain involved in mood control and depression. The treatment typically involves five 40-minute treatments each week for up to 6 weeks (Mayo Clinic, 2012). The Food and Drug Administration (FDA) has recently approved TMS treatment for depression, and it is now being explored for treating migraines. The rTMS is also available for depression treatment in Canada, Australia, New Zealand, Israel, and the European Union.

Guidelines

Generally, it is safe to apply permanent magnets for a long period of time. The time of application largely depends on the type and nature of the disease, the age of the individual, and the strength of the magnet. The strength of a magnet is measured in units referred to as gauss (G), or alternatively, units called tesla (T; 1T = 10,000 G), which represents "the number of lines of magnetic force passing through an area of 1 square centimeter" (Whitaker & Adderly, 1998, p. 15). Currently, the Earth's magnetic field is estimated to be about 0.5 G, whereas a refrigerator magnet ranges from 35 G to 200 G. Magnets used for pain intervention usually measure from 300 G to 5,000 G; and MRI machines used to diagnose medical conditions produce up to 200,000 G. Manufacturers are not required to mark the strength of magnets on their products, so the G of a magnet must be checked against the weight a magnet can lift, with 1 kg equivalent to approximately 600 G (Whitaker & Adderly, 1998).

Although it is important to determine the correct strength of a magnet for a therapeutic effect, some practitioners believe that the right choice of polarity (north pole or south pole) is crucial. However, the issue of polarity remains controversial. It is thought that large magnets of more than 2,000 G should be used for short periods of time, ranging from several seconds to about 60 minutes for one application (Beattie, 2004). Exhibit 28.1 lists various ways in which magnets can be applied to the human body. However, these application recommendations have yet to be fully evaluated by long-term clinical testing. It is strongly recommended that magnets not be used as a replacement for conventional medical treatment or as a reason to postpone seeing one's health care provider about any health problems.

Measurement of Outcomes

The type of measurement used to determine the effectiveness of a magnet therapy depends on the purpose of the intervention. A variety of outcome measures have been used. For example, the progression of bone healing has been objectively measured by using x-rays, bone mineral density, and calcium content in bone. Pain relief or stress reduction has been measured by an individual's subjective report on a pain/stress rating scale. The improvement of a sleep disorder can be detected by using polysomnography, a diagnostic test that records a number of physiological variables during sleep. A number of objective measurements that have been used to indicate the change of magnetic field in the body are:

1. The superconducting quantum interference device (SQUID), a sensitive magnetometer for mapping the magnetic fields around the human body, can be used to detect an increase or decrease in the biomagnetic field of the body (Oschman, 1997).
2. Kirlian photography, which is a tool that provides photographs, video, or computer images of energy flow. It introduces a high-frequency, high-voltage, ultra-low current to the object being photographed. This influx of electrical energy amplifies as it travels through the object and makes visible the biological and energetic exchange (Cope, 1980).
3. Natural light emission (biophotons), a low-level light-detection technology that assesses the ultra-weak emission from organisms, which ranges from a few to hundreds of photons per second per square centimeter of tissue could, in fact, be measured. This range might be correlated to changes in health, disease, healing, and altered states of consciousness (Foundation for Alternative and Integrative Medicine [FAIM], 2012).

It is noteworthy that these tools have primarily been used in basic and clinical research. Because reliability and validation studies are scarce, clinical applications of these measurement tools are limited. No device at this time has been consistently found in well-designed studies to yield the measurements of the energy field that correlate well with diagnoses or therapeutic effects. Exhibit 28.1 displays methods in which magnets may be applied.

USES

Use of electromagnets for diagnostic and intervention purposes requires administration by health professionals. Static magnets, alternatively, can be purchased in stores or online. They are available commercially in the form of wraps, belts, mattresses, and jewelry. Individuals can use static magnets independently without any prescriptions.

Acu-magnet therapy is one of the therapies that is commonly practiced in China and Japan. Recent studies on placing magnets on acupuncture sites revealed positive outcomes. A systematic review on acu-magnet therapy using six electronic databases (PubMed, AMED, ScienceDirect College Edition, China Academic Journals, Acubriefs, and the in-house Journal

Exhibit 28.1. *Methods of Application of Magnets*

Mode	Application
Local	Magnets are placed directly on the skin over affected parts
Acu-Site	Local applications with use of acupuncture points
General	Used for whole body or ailments affecting larger body parts
Internal	Magnetic water (ionized water) is ingested
Remote	Wearing magnetic jewelry to treat an ailment remote from the point of application such as a magnetic bracelet for stimulating the thymus gland to boost the immune system

Article Index maintained by the Oregon College of Oriental Medicine Library) was conducted (Colbert et al., 2008). A total of 42 studies met the inclusion criteria. Studies included 32 different clinical conditions ranging from musculoskeletal problems to insomnia in 6,453 patients from 1986 to 2007. A variety of magnetic devices, dosing regimens, and control devices were used. The review reported that 37 of 42 studies (88%) found therapeutic benefit from using acu-magnet therapy, particularly for the management of diabetes (Chen, 2002) and insomnia (Suen, Wong, Leung, & Ip, 2003).

Common Health Conditions Treated With Magnet Therapy

Pain, including both acute (postsurgical) and chronic (arthritis and peripheral neuropathy); inflammatory disorders; and wound healing are conditions in which magnet therapy has been most frequently used. PEMF is more specifically used for treating nonhealing bone. It has also been studied for other medical conditions such as osteoarthritis (OA) and incontinence. rTMS is primarily used for depression and has been investigated for treating emotional illnesses and other brain-related conditions as well. Additional uses of magnets are noted in Exhibit 28.2.

Permanent Magnets

Although articles and books contain testimonials to support the efficacy of permanent magnets on pain, little support has been established from research studies. Findings from systematic reviews of static magnets for pain relief have been contradictory. One review indicated 11 out of 15 (73.3%)

Exhibit 28.2. *Conditions in Which Magnets Have Been Investigated/Used*

Bone and wound healing (Henry, Concannon, & Yee, 2008)
Immune responses (Bouchlaka et al., 2012)
Inflammatory disorders (Sutbeyaz, Sezer, & Koseoglu, 2006)
Menopause (Brockie, 2008)
Migraine (Curtis et al., 2010)
Stroke (Buetefisch, 2007)
Tinnitus (Meng, Liu, Zheng, & Phillips, 2011)

studies found a positive effect of static magnets in achieving analgesia for a wide variety of pain (neuropathic, inflammatory, musculoskeletal, fibromyalgic, rheumatic, and postsurgical; Eccles, 2005). Based on nine randomized placebo-controlled trials, another recent systematic review and meta-analysis suggested static magnets offer no significant effects on pain reduction (Pittler, Brown, & Ernst, 2007). Positive and negative results from studies were spread across magnet strengths. Ideal magnet strength and treatment duration for pain reduction remain unclear. It is noteworthy that many studies were criticized for being of low quality, including small sample size, short duration, and/or were inadequately controlled. The NCCAM (2012) declares that scientific evidence does not support the use of magnets for pain relief.

PEMF

PEMF therapy has been used to stimulate bone repair in nonunion and other fractures since the 1970s. It was granted the "safe and effective" classification by the FDA in 1979. The effect of PEMF on osteoarthritis (OA) remains controversial. A number of recent randomized controlled trials (RCTs) applied PEMF to the treatment of knee OA, and found significant improvements in pain and function (Nicolakis et al., 2002; Thamsborg et al., 2005). However, a recent systematic review of five RCTs reported that PEMF does not significantly reduce the pain of knee OA and that it has little value in the management of knee OA (McCarthy, Callaghan & Oldham, 2006).

Stress incontinence is a prevalent condition among women. It can be triggered by activities such as laughter, physical exercise, sneezing, and coughing. A placebo-controlled study using high-intensity pulsating magnetic fields for 62 women with stress incontinence was conducted with positive results (Fujishiro et al., 2000). PEMF was used to stimulate the nerves that control the pelvic muscles. The results showed that with only one session of magnetic stimulation, 74% of participants experienced significant reduction in the number of urinary leakages over the following week as compared to subjects in the placebo group.

rTMS

A number of studies have evaluated rTMS for the treatment of depression (including severe depression and the depressive phase of bipolar illness), and most found it effective (Fitzgerald et al., 2003; Kauffmann, Cheema, & Miller, 2004). In a more recent study involving 45 participants, rTMS was found to be more effective than the sham (fake) treatment rTMS as an add-on treatment to medication in people with moderate to severe depression (Ray et al., 2011). A recent meta-analysis using 30 double-blind trials involving 1,164 depressed patients reported that real rTMS is significantly more effective than sham rTMS (Schutter, 2008). Another meta-analysis including the results of six controlled trials, which involved a total of 232 patients with schizophrenia resistant to conventional treatment, found that real low-frequency rTMS was significantly better at reducing auditory hallucinations compared to sham rTMS (Tranulis et al., 2008). A systematic review of 10 randomized trials in Parkinson's patients indicated significant benefit for rTMS with higher frequencies (Elahi, Elahi, & Chen, 2008).

As noted earlier, magnets are being used in many countries. Sidebar 28.1 presents information about the use of magnets in Canada.

Sidebar 28.1. *Use of Magnets in Canada*

Linda Lindeke, Edmonton, Alberta, Canada

In general, integrative therapies are more accepted in Canada than in the United States. Perhaps it is because people there have basic health coverage, and so they are willing to pay out of pocket for other kinds of therapies. Also, there are waiting periods for quite a few diagnostics and surgeries, so perhaps people use integrative therapies while waiting for conventional diagnosis and treatments. Another reason may be that Canadian life expectancy is long and so there are many people with aging ailments/chronic conditions who are willing to try therapies that are readily available, nonintrusive, and that might work—if they do not cost exorbitant amounts of money.

(continued)

Sidebar 28.1. *Use of Magnets in Canada (continued)*

Websites

There are many websites in Canada for magnet therapy, including:

- www.magnapak.ca
- www.bioflexmagnets.com
- www.alive.com/articles/view/22345/magnet_therapy

Magnets are used mostly for pain. An interesting use of a kind of magnet therapy that was recently in the news was the use of magnets in the treatment of depression.

In terms of regulation, in 2009 there was an initiative in Canada to regulate magnet therapy but this was abandoned due to lack of evidence that magnets are a valid therapy. The Medical Devices Bureau of the Therapeutic Product Directorate recently completed a review of static magnets sold for therapeutic purposes. A review of the scientific literature by the bureau has determined that there is insufficient published evidence to indicate that static magnets are beneficial for therapeutic purposes. Although magnets are not regulated, people continue to buy and sell them, and claims continue to be publicized that magnets provide some relief from chronic pain.

Precautions

There are some precautions regarding the placement of magnets. Magnets should not be placed over: (a) the heart, as it may cause arrhythmia; (b) the carotid artery, as it may cause lightheadedness and dizziness; (c) the stomach within 60 minutes after a meal, as it may interfere with the normal contraction of the digestive tract; (d) any open wounds with active bleeding, as it may increase bleeding; or (e) any transdermal drug-delivery system or patch, as they may increase the amount of drug circulating in the body. With the exception of magnetic mattresses and mattress pads, most magnets sold for therapeutic purposes do not interfere with the magnetically activated switches present in most pacemakers or defibrillating regulators. They are safe if kept 6 inches or further from these devices (New York University, 2012). Magnets should not be used with pregnant or breastfeeding women. Strong magnets are not recommended for small children.

FUTURE RESEARCH

Claims of positive results from magnet therapies vary greatly, depending on the condition for which they were used. Findings from Western research about the effectiveness of magnets are inconclusive. The variations in the findings may be attributed to the subjective nature of many of the outcome measures used, the inability to control the etiology and severity of the pathological condition, and variation in the types of magnets and treatment parameters. Because anecdotal reports are regarded as being an unreliable source of evidence, many in the scientific and medical communities consider magnet therapy a fraud and quackery. Conducting controlled, scientific experiments on permanent magnet therapy is challenging because participants can notice whether a metal device is magnetized or not. Because there is little evidence that the application of magnets is harmful, it is reasonable to encourage the practice if a patient experiences symptom relief from their use, especially if the use of magnets can reduce the patient's consumption of medications. However, the lack of validated measurement tools and energy markers remain an obstacle to progress in biomagnetic field science and medicine. Continued efforts are needed to enhance our knowledge about the use of magnet therapy. Questions for further knowledge development include:

- What is the scientific evidence for the different effects obtained from the North Pole and the South Pole in magnet therapy?
- What roles do individual (high vs. low vitality) and environmental (northern vs. southern hemisphere) factors play on the effects of magnet therapy?
- What are appropriate methodologies for studying the effects of magnet therapies, particularly the use of sham controls?
- What are the effective measurement tools and their reliability/validity?
- What are the long-term effects of magnet therapy?

REFERENCES

Advanced Magnetic Research Institute. (2005). *Magnetic molecular energizer.* Retrieved from http://www.amri-intl.com/home.html

Arizona Unipole Magnetics. (2008a). *Effects of magnetic energy on living metabolic systems.* Retrieved October 28, 2008, from http://www.azunimags.com/polarity.html

Arizona Unipole Magnetics. (2008b). *Importance of polarity.* Retrieved October 28, 2008, from http://www.azunimags.com/polarity.html

Beattie, A. (2004). *Magnet therapy.* New York, NY: Barnes and Noble.

Bouchlaka, M., Sckisel, G., Wilkins, D., Maverakis, E., Monjazeb, A., Fung, M., . . . Murphy, W. (2012). Mechanical disruption of tumors by iron particles and magnetic field application results in increased anti-tumor immune responses. *PLOS One.* 7(10). Retrieved from http://www.ncbi.nlm.nih.gov/pmc/articles/PMC3485005/

Brockie, S. (2008). Alternative approaches to the menopause. *Practice Nursing, 19*(4), 172–176.

Buetefisch, C. (2007). Magnet for stroke patients. *Massage & Bodywork, 22,* 14. Retrieved from http://connection.ebscohost.com/c/articles/26402537/magnet-therapy-stroke-patients

Chen, Y. (2002). Magnets on ears helped diabetics. *American Journal of Chinese Medicine, 30*(1), 183–185.

Colbert, A., Cleaver, J., Brown, K., Harling, N., Hwang, Y., Schiffke, H., . . . Qin, Y. (2008). Magnets applied to acupuncture points as therapy—A literature review. *Acupuncture in Medicine, 26,* 160–170.

Cope, F. (1980). Magnetoelectric charge states of matter-energy. A second approximation. Part VII. *Physiological Chemistry & Physics, 12*(4), 349–355.

Curtis, P., Gaylord, S., Park, J., Faurot, K, Coble, R., Suchindran, C., . . . Mann, J. (2010). Credibility of low-strength static magnet therapy as an attention control intervention for a randomized controlled study of craniosacral therapy for migraine headaches. *Journal of Alternative and Complementary Medicine, 17*(8), 711–721. doi:10.1089/acm.2010.0277

Eccles, N. K. (2005). A critical review of randomized controlled trials of static magnets for pain relief. *Journal of Alternative & Complementary Medicine, 11*(3), 495–509.

Elahi, B., Elahi, B., & Chen, R. (2008). Effect of transcranial magnetic stimulation on Parkinson motor function-Systematic review of controlled clinical trials. *Movement Disorder, 24,* 357–363. doi:10.1002/mds.22364

Fitzgerald, P. B., Brown, T. L., Marston, N. A., Daskalakis, Z. J., De Catella, A., & Kulkarni, J. (2003). Transcranial magnetic stimulation in the treatment of depression: A double-blind, placebo-controlled trial. *Archives of General Psychiatry, 60*(10) 1002–1008.

Foundation for Alternative and Integrative Medicine. (2012). *Biomagnetic therapy.* Retrieved from http://www.faim.org/newfrontiers/biomagnetictherapy.html

Frankel, R., & Liburdy, R. (1996). Biological effects of static magnetic fields. In C. Polk & E. Postow (Eds.), *Handbook of biological effects of electromagnetic fields* (2nd ed.), 149–183. Boca Raton, FL: CRC.

Fujishiro, T., Enomoto, H., Ugawa, Y., Takahashi, S., Ueno, S., & Kitamura, T. (2000). Magnetic stimulation of the sacral roots for the treatment of stress incontinence: An investigational study and placebo controlled trial. *Journal of Urology, 164,* 1277–1279.

Henry, S., Concannon, M., & Yee, G. (2008). The effect of magnetic fields on wound healing: Experimental study and review of the literature. *Eplasty, 8,* 40.

Kaptchuk, T. J. (1996). Historical context of the concept of vitalism in complementary and alternative medicine. In M. S. Micozzi (Ed.), *Fundamentals of complementary and alternative medicine* (p. 35). New York, NY: Churchill Livingstone.

Kauffmann, C. D., Cheema, M. A., & Miller, B. E. (2004). Slow right prefrontal transcranial magnetic stimulation as a treatment for medication-resistant depression: A double-blind, placebo-controlled study. *Depression and Anxiety, 19,* 59–62.

Macklis, R. (1993). Magnetic healing, quackery, and the debate about the health effects of electromagnetic fields. *Annals of Internal Medicine, 18*(5), 376–382.

Mayo Clinic. (2012). *Transcranial magnetic stimulation.* Retrieved from http://www.mayoclinic.org/transcranial-magnetic-stimulation/

McCarthy, C., Callaghan, M., & Oldham, J. (2006). Pulsed electromagnetic energy treatment offers no clinical benefit in reducing the pain of knee osteoarthritis: A systematic review. *BMC Musculoskeletal Disorders, 7*, 51. doi:10.1186/1471-2474-7-51

Medlearn Matters. (2004). *Electrical stimulation and electromagnetic therapy for the treatment of wounds.* Retrieved from http://www.cms.hhs.gov/medlearn/matters/mmarticles/2004/mm3149.pdf

Meng, Z., Liu, S., Zheng, Y., & Phillips, J. S. (2011). Repetitive transcranial magnetic stimulation for tinnitus. *Cochrane Database Systematic Reviews, 10*, CD007946.

National Center for Complementary and Alternative Medicine. (2012). *Questions and answers about using magnets to treat pain.* Retrieved November 24, 2008, from http://www.nccam.nih.gov/health/magnet/magnet.htm

New York University Langone Medical Center. (2012). *Magnet therapy.* Retrieved from http://www.med.nyu.edu/content?ChunkIID=33778

Nicolakis, P., Kollmitzer, J., Crevenna, R., Bittner, C., Erdogmus, C., & Nicolakis, J. (2002). Pulsed magnetic field therapy for osteoarthritis of the knee—A double blind sham-controlled trial. *Wiener Klinische Wochenschrift, 114*(15–16), 678–684.

Oschman, J. (1997). What is healing energy? Part 2: Measuring the field of life energy. *Journal of Bodywork & Movement Therapies, 1*(2), 117–121.

Oschman, J. (1998). What is healing energy? Part 6: Conclusions: Is energy medicine the medicine of the future? *Journal of Bodywork & Movement Therapies, 2*(1), 46–59.

Pittler, M., Brown, E., & Ernst, E. (2007). Static magnets for reducing pain: Systematic review and meta-analysis of randomized trials. *Canadian Medical Association Journal, 177*(7), 736–742.

Ray, S., Nizamie, S. H., Akhtar, S., Praharaj, S. K., Mishra, B. R., & Zia-ul-Haq, M. (2011). Efficacy of adjunctive high frequency repetitive transcranial magnetic stimulation of left prefrontal cortex in depression: A randomized sham controlled study. *Journal of Affective Disorders, 128*(1/2), 153–159.

Schutter, D. J. (2008). Antidepressant efficacy of high-frequency transcranial magnetic stimulation over the left dorsolateral prefrontal cortex in double-blind sham-controlled designs: A meta-analysis. *Psychological Medicine, 39*, 65–75. doi:10.1017/S0033291708003462

Suen, L., Wong, T., Leung, A., & Ip, W. (2003). The long-term effects of auricular therapy nursing magnetic pearls on elderly with insomnia. *Complementary Therapy Medicine, 11*(2), 85–92.

Sutbeyaz, S., Sezer, N., & Koseoglu, B. (2006). The effect of pulsed electromagnetic fields in the treatment of cervical osteoarthritis: A randomized, double-blind, sham-controlled trial. *Rheumatology International, 26*, 320–324. doi:10.1007/s00296-005-0600-3

Thamsborg, G., Florescu, A., Oturai, P., Fallentin, E., Tritsaris, K., & Dissing, S. (2005). Treatment of knee osteoarthritis with pulsed electromagnetic fields: A randomized, double-blind, placebo-controlled study. *Osteoarthritis Cartilage, 13*(7), 575–581.

Tranulis, C., Sepehry, A. A., Galinowski, A., & Stip, E. (2008). Should we treat auditory hallucinations with repetitive transcranial magnetic stimulation? A metaanalysis. *Canadian Journal of Psychiatry, 53*, 577–586.

Trueman, C. (2000). *History of medicine. Franz Mesmer.* Retrieved from http://www.historylearningsite.co.uk/franz_mesmer.htm

Whitaker, J., & Adderly, B. (1998). *The pain breakthrough: The power of magnet.* Toronto, Ontario: Little, Brown.

Winemiller, M., Billow, R., Laskowski, E., & Harmsen, W. (2005). Effect of magnetic vs. sham-magnetic insoles on nonspecific foot pain in the workplace: A randomized, double-blind, placebo-controlled trial. *Mayo Clinic Proceedings, 80*(9), 1138–1145.

Wolsko, P., Eisenberg, D., Simon, L., Davis, R., Walleczek, J., Mayo-Smith, M. et al. (2004). Double-blind placebo-controlled trial of static magnets for the treatment of OA of the knee. *Alternative Therapies in Health & Medicine, 10*(2), 36–43.

Part VI: Education, Practice, and Research

Consideration of complementary therapies has moved from specific therapies to integrating these procedures into the fabric of practice, education, and research. Nurses have taken the lead in that integration. Although great strides have been made, continuing efforts are necessary if holistic health care is to be available to all people.

Use of complementary therapies in practice settings is increasing, largely because of the public's demand for these treatments. Whether these are well-known therapies such as music, chiropractic care, yoga, and prayer or ones that seem quite foreign to many such as magnets, Alexander technique, and smudging ceremonies, health systems are looking very different from the way they were 50 years ago. As health professions increase content on complementary therapies in curricula, health care systems will continue to reflect holistic care. Within health systems, questions regarding what procedures will be offered, who will pay, and who will provide therapies need to be addressed.

Concerns about the safety and efficacy of many of the complementary therapies continue. Funding for research on complementary therapies by the National Center for Complementary and Alternative Medicine (NCCAM) has increased, thus providing a greater basis for evidence-based practice. Not only is the increase in research important but reviews and meta-analyses of studies on specific procedures provide invaluable assistance to practitioners, educators, and researchers. New methods of inquiry and measurements for outcomes are needed for numerous therapies, particularly those practiced in non-Western and indigenous cultures.

A further help related to safety in the use of complementary therapies are guidelines for the use of complementary treatments that have been developed by professional organizations such as the American Holistic Nurses Association and the Oncology Nurses Association. Additionally, many state boards of nursing have delineated provisions for the use of complementary therapies.

As noted in the education chapter, professional nursing education organizations have specifications for the content on complementary therapies that should be incorporated into the various curricula. If these are to be truly implemented, many more prepared faculty members are needed to provide direction for the inclusion of these procedures in educational programs.

Excitement exists about the integration of complementary therapies into health care. Attention to the use of these therapies in countries across the globe and the therapies used by immigrants is needed. Nurses, as caring, competent professionals, have the opportunity and challenge to be leaders in these efforts.

Chapter 29: Integrating Complementary Therapies Into Education

CARIE A. BRAUN

Nursing curricula are constantly evolving to improve patient care quality and keep pace with the ever-changing health care environment. The challenge to nurse educators is to promote professional nursing education that is attentive to societal and health care changes (Hegarty, Walsh, Condon, & Sweeney, 2009). Such changes include increased globalization, technological advancements, health policy and economics, and increased patient care complexity (Hegarty et al., 2009).

The impact of globalization has heightened the need to seamlessly integrate complementary and alternative therapies into holistic patient care. This is primarily due to the proliferative use of complementary and alternative therapies by the public, safety issues with combining conventional and alternative modalities, cultural competence and the emphasis on patient-centered care, and increasing evidence of the positive impact of integrative health care systems on health care outcomes (Gaylord & Mann, 2007; Institute of Medicine, 2005; Moore, 2010). These influences have permeated the practice of nursing and, as a result, the licensing examination has evolved to emphasize integrative care and holism, which includes a basic knowledge of complementary therapies. The National Council Licensure Examination (NCLEX-RN®), a reflection of actual nursing practice and an important indicator of nursing program quality, has expected knowledge of complementary therapies for entry-level RNs since 2004 (Stratton, Benn, Lie, Zeller, & Nedrow, 2007). The detailed test plan for

NCLEX-RN in 2013 again required the knowledge of health promotion and maintenance, including the safe integration of complementary therapies into the patient's plan of care.

Other documents guiding nursing curricula have been equally influential. The American Association of Colleges of Nursing (AACN) specifically identified baccalaureate generalist practice to include a beginning understanding of complementary and alternative modalities (*Essentials of Baccalaureate Education for Professional Nursing Practice*, 2008). For graduate education, the *AACN Essentials of Master's Education for Advanced Practice Nursing* (2004) and the *AACN Essentials of Master's Education for Nursing* (2011) required master's-level nurses to deliver health care services within integrated care systems. Similarly, the *AACN Essentials of Doctoral Education for Advanced Practice Nursing* (2006) directed Doctor of Nursing Practice (DNP) programs to prepare graduates to synthesize concepts related to clinical prevention and population health, including psychosocial dimensions and cultural diversity. The Institute of Medicine (IOM, 2010) report on the future of nursing affirmed that nurses should practice to the full extent of their education and should achieve higher levels of knowledge to promote quality patient-centered care.

The initial discourse in the 1990s about whether or not complementary therapies *should* be taught in nursing and other health care programs has now been replaced with a pervasive discussion and debate about *what* should be included and *how* to deepen the integration of complementary therapies within a holistic patient-care paradigm (Cutshall et al., 2010).

DEFINING COMPLEMENTARY THERAPY CORE COMPETENCIES

A universally accepted list of complementary therapy core competencies for nursing has yet to be developed. However, the close alignment of nursing with holistic and integrative health care provides solid justification for moving forward. Booth-LaForce and colleagues (2010), Chlan and Halcón (2003), and Kreitzer, Mann, and Lumpkin (2008) have advocated for an integrated curriculum grounded in holistic, patient-centered care beginning at the baccalaureate level. These authors have suggested several core competencies, including:

1. Awareness and assessment of therapies and practices
2. Evaluation of the evidence base underlying therapies and practices
3. Skill development in therapies and practices
4. Self-awareness and self-care, and
5. Awareness of the theoretical basis underlying therapies and practices.

These competencies are evident in the scope and standards for practicing nurses. The American Nurses Association (ANA), in the book *Nursing:*

Scope and Standards of Practice (ANA, 2010), spelled out the practice parameters and responsibilities for all RNs in the United States. The practice standards of assessment, diagnosis, outcome identification, planning, implementation, and evaluation allow for an individualized plan of care that is sensitive to diverse health care practices for all patients. The professional performance standards of quality of practice, practice evaluation, education, collegiality, collaboration, ethics, research, resource utilization, and leadership commit nurses constantly to improve knowledge, skills, and competencies appropriate to the nursing role.

The ANA's *Scope and Standards of Practice* (2010) indicated that nurses must be knowledgeable about and sensitive to a range of health practices so that holistic nursing care can be provided. The document does not identify specific therapies that nurses may or may not incorporate into nursing practice. The *Nursing Interventions Classification* (Bulechek, Butcher, & Dochterman, 2008), however, provides a comprehensive listing of treatments that nurses can perform. This list includes the following complementary therapies, which are within the realm of nursing given the appropriate training or certification: acupressure, animal-assisted therapy, aromatherapy, art therapy, biofeedback, massage, music therapy, self-hypnosis facilitation, and therapeutic touch. Although the knowledge base for many complementary therapies may be part of the educational program, performance proficiency is often not achieved during an undergraduate or even graduate nursing education. Therefore, even though nurses *can* perform these therapies, they *should* perform them only with the appropriate training and certification.

Complementary therapy education expectations are also evident in various Boards of Nursing (BON) documents within the U.S. states and territories that regulate nursing practice to ensure patient safety. Of 53 BONs surveyed in 2001, 47% had statements or positions that included specific complementary therapies or examples of these practices, 13% had them under discussion, and 40% had not formally addressed the topic but did not necessarily discourage these practices (Sparber, 2001). Although this survey has not been repeated, the percentage of BONs with formal position statements is likely to rise. BONs are increasingly aware of and supportive of the integration of complementary therapies into nursing practice, and they are continuously clarifying what is within the scope of nursing practice and identifying basic education and competencies required for nursing practice. Because the interpretation of the nursing scope of practice can vary based on the different state or territorial BONs, nurses must be aware of their own state's position regarding complementary therapies, must have the documented knowledge and competencies to perform the therapy, and must adhere to licensure and credentialing regulations.

Internationally, similar nursing regulatory agencies have articulated the role of the nurse in understanding and practicing complementary therapies. The Nurses Board of Western Australia has published *Guidelines for the Use of Complementary Therapies in Nursing Practice* (2003). The guidelines indicate that "nurses are responsible for acquiring and maintaining their complementary therapy knowledge and competence and for being aware of the limitations of their knowledge and competence in relation to complementary therapies" (p. 1). Selection of the educational program in the specific complementary therapy is the responsibility of the nurse. The Nurses Board of Western Australia cautions that the course must be of adequate quality, be accredited or approved as appropriate, confer the appropriate qualifications and level of practice, and build on the prior learning of the nurse.

Similarly, the College and Association of Registered Nurses of Alberta published the *Alternative and/or Complementary Therapy Standards for Registered Nurses* (2006) to provide "guidance to registered nurses in making decisions about providing care that involves complementary or alternative health-care therapies and natural health products as an adjunct within their nursing practice" (p. 2). These standards require adequate knowledge, skills, and licensure when appropriate to provide the specified alternative/complementary therapy through relevant educational or certificate programs. The provision of such therapies must fall within the current scope of nursing practice for Canadian RNs, if the treatment is being provided under the RN license.

Specialty organizations have also weighed in on the debate about what nurses with specialty certifications can and should perform. The American Holistic Nurses Association (AHNA) and the American Nurses Association (ANA) have jointly developed the *Scope and Standards of Practice for Holistic Nursing* (2007), which includes a core curriculum for integrative health care practice infused with the principles of complementary and alternative therapies and competencies consistent with holistic nursing practice. The certification is not routinely required as part of the nurse's prelicensure or advanced education; however, it offers important insights as to the expectations of holistic nursing practice.

The specialized training required to safely and effectively practice specific complementary therapies is not typically found in general nurse education programs. Increasingly, however, nursing programs are attentive to helping student nurses to better understand the role of complementary therapies in patient health. Multiple authors have suggested specific content applicable to the undergraduate and graduate nursing curriculum (Cuellar, Cahill, Ford, & Aycock, 2003; Gaster, Unterborn, Scott, & Schneeweiss, 2007; Kligler et al., 2004; Lee et al., 2007). The following is a compilation of suggested student learning outcomes that address the necessary dimensions for educating students within general nursing practice:

- Describe the prevalence and patterns of complementary therapy use by the public.
- Compare and contrast the underlying principles and beliefs in Western belief systems and alternative health belief systems.

- Communicate effectively with patients and families about complementary and alternative therapies.
- Critique the scientific evidence available for the most commonly used complementary and alternative therapies.
- Identify reputable sources of information to support continued learning about complementary and alternative therapies.
- Explore the roles, training, and credentialing of complementary and alternative therapy practitioners.
- Reflect on and improve self-care measures and wellness to incorporate complementary therapies for self, where applicable.

CURRENT STATE OF COMPLEMENTARY THERAPIES IN NURSING EDUCATION

Lee and colleagues (2007) recognized that the integration of complementary therapies in nursing education requires little or no shift in philosophical paradigm because issues like wellness, prevention, and holistic health have long been at the core of nursing practice. There is ample evidence to suggest that nursing education programs, albeit inconsistently, are already attending to the knowledge base needed and to understanding the role of complementary therapies in health care. For example, multiple studies have confirmed that nursing faculty and students believe that complementary therapies must be integrated into the nursing curriculum and that nurses must be prepared to advise patients regarding best practices in integrative health care (Al-Rukban et al., 2012; Avino, 2011; Cutshall et al., 2010; Halcón, Chlan, Kreitzer, & Leonard, 2003; Keimig & Braun, 2004; Kim, Erlen, Kim, & Sok, 2006; Kreitzer, Mitten, Harris, & Shandeling, 2002; Kreitzer et al., 2008; Nedrow, Istvan, et al., 2007; Öztekin, Ucuzal, Öztekin, & Issever, 2007; Uzun & Tan, 2004). A few of these studies also determined that nursing students, on graduation, did not feel prepared to integrate complementary therapies and that more education was desired (Keimig & Braun, 2004; Kim et al., 2006; Uzun & Tan, 2004). More recently, Avino (2011) reported students were open to the health benefits of complementary therapies, although they did not want to be overwhelmed with information or trained to personally provide each therapy.

Dutta and colleagues (2003), Fenton and Morris (2003), and Richardson (2003) sampled nursing schools across the United States to determine the extent to which the schools integrated complementary and alternative modalities into their curricula. For all three studies, a large percentage already included complementary therapies in the curriculum (49%–85%) and almost all of the programs were planning to incorporate additional complementary therapies in the future. The same appears to be true for family nurse practitioner programs (Burman, 2003). Very few of the responding schools had a separate required course on complementary therapies (11%–15%); whereas most offered a separate elective course

(37%–84%) and about one third of the schools offered a continuing-education option. The most commonly included therapies were spirituality/prayer/meditation, relaxation, guided imagery, herbals, acupuncture, massage, and therapeutic touch.

Internationally, nursing education programs are also addressing the need to integrate complementary therapies. In 2004, Sok, Erlen, and Kim reported that more than 10 universities in the United Kingdom offered students full-time degree programs in complementary and alternative therapies, such as osteopathy, chiropractic medicine, herbal medicines, acupuncture, and homeopathy. Hon and colleagues (2006) reported that the regulatory body for nursing in Hong Kong now requires that the nursing curriculum contain 20 hours devoted to traditional Chinese medicine (TCM). Similarly, Yeh and Chung (2007) investigated the current and expected levels of competence in TCM that baccalaureate nurses should possess in Taiwan, where Western nursing education is considered mainstream and the expectations that nurses possess skills in TCM have been met with disappointment by consumers. In Korea, one college of nursing science now has a 1-year program that leads to a certificate in complementary and alternative therapies for clinical nurses and researchers (Sok et al., 2004). In contrast, only 13% of nursing colleges in Saudi Arabia introduced complementary therapies briefly within a course. None of the respondents reported having a dedicated complementary therapies course, continuing education related to complementary therapies, or faculty interest/expertise in complementary therapies (Al-Rukban et al., 2012). The authors of this study indicated that the interest in complementary therapies was just beginning and the efforts for further integration were underway.

FACULTY QUALIFICATIONS AND DEVELOPMENT

Although the majority of nursing programs in the United States and throughout the world integrate complementary therapies in some way, the greatest challenges included: finding qualified faculty, an already crowded and changing curriculum, lack of definition for "best practices" in integrative care, and sustainability of complementary therapy content within the curriculum (Avino, 2011; Lee et al., 2007). In one study, the top three therapies for which additional training was desired by faculty included nutritional supplements, herbal medicine, and massage (Avino, 2011). In another survey, greater knowledge was desired in TCM, Qigong, Ayurveda, and energy modulation (Cutshall et al., 2010). Avino (2011) also found that the preferred pedagogy for undergraduate nursing students was direct active learning and the least preferred was through online modules.

Stratton and colleagues (2007) identified essential faculty development needed to facilitate learning in integrative health care. First and foremost, a critical mass of knowledgeable faculty is essential to the successful integration and sustainability of complementary therapies into a nursing curriculum. Viewing complementary therapy information through the lens of evidence-based practice can facilitate acceptance and provide an opportunity for faculty to become more familiar with complementary therapy principles and research (Stratton et al., 2007). Faculty development requires time and resources, access to scholarly writings, reference and research resources, reassigned time, consultations, collaboration, continuing education, and support. Ideally, continuing-education workshops or conferences should be structured using a collaborative approach representing the varying perspectives of complementary and alternative therapy practitioners. Encouraging and supporting faculty research in the area of complementary therapies is another mechanism of generating a team of qualified faculty.

CAM EDUCATION PROJECT

The exploration of best practices in integrative health care education has been an ongoing focus of the National Center for Complementary and Alternative Medicine (NCCAM). The Complementary and Alternative Medicine (CAM) Education Project funded by NCCAM is now completed but the impact continues. The CAM Education Project was designed to incorporate CAM information into the curricula of selected health profession schools (Pearson & Chesney, 2007) and has been highly influential in bringing forward the concept of integrative health care, particularly as it relates to medical education (Nedrow, Istvan, et al., 2007). Integrative medicine combines conventional treatments and complementary/alternative therapies that are proven to be safe and effective (Nedrow, Istvan, et al., 2007). Currently, the 54-member Consortium for Academic Health Centers for Integrative Medicine (www.imconsortium.org) meets regularly to coordinate integrative health systems, including integrative education, research, policy, and patient care. The mission of the consortium is to advance integrative health care within academic institutions. Through this consortium's education subcommittee, core competencies in integrative medicine have been developed and disseminated to U.S. medical schools (Kligler et al., 2004).

A significant example of postbaccalaureate education, stemming from the CAM Education Project, was that described by Amri, Haramati, Sierpina, and Kreitzer (2012). Georgetown University's (Washington, DC) CAM-MS Program in Physiology is a 30-credit-hour graduate degree developed to prepare integrative health care practitioners and scientists and to encourage graduates to pursue future doctoral research in complementary therapies. The curriculum in its current form was initiated in 2009. Nursing education models that have emerged from the CAM Education Project are discussed next.

IMPLEMENTATION MODELS

Integrative Curricula

At least four nursing programs in the CAM Education Project created integrative curricula, inclusive of complementary and alternative health philosophies and practices. For example, the School of Nursing at the University of Minnesota revised curricula to incorporate complementary and alternative therapies into baccalaureate, master's, and doctoral programs (Halcón, Leonard, Snyder, Garwick, & Kreitzer, 2001). The curricular revisions strengthened didactic and experiential learning to encompass complementary therapies theory and research, supported interdisciplinary courses as part of the graduate minor in complementary therapies and healing practices, and incorporated self-care concepts.

At Rush University (Chicago) all students in the undergraduate and graduate (including an entry-level generalist master's and advanced specialty practice) programs were exposed to complementary therapy content through required courses such as pharmacology, health assessment, nutrition, research, and community health nursing. Curricular competencies were outlined for assessment, therapy indications and contraindications, safety, evidence-based practice, and collaboration. Much of the coursework was designed through web-based modules for use in the curriculum and as continuing-education offerings.

The University of Washington School of Nursing (Seattle), in partnership with Bastyr University (Kenmore, WA; San Diego, CA; a leader in the natural health sciences and natural medicine), provided faculty development on complementary therapies through a summer educational program (Booth-LaForce et al., 2010; Fenton & Morris, 2003; Nedrow, Heitkemper, et al., 2007). Faculty used what they learned to support the integration of complementary therapies throughout the nursing curriculum. As a result of this implementation project, about half of faculty incorporated complementary therapy content in class, and more than half indicated their complementary therapy knowledge increased a moderate or great extent. A higher number of students (70%) indicated knowledge of complementary therapies improved with intended self-reported competencies increased throughout the grant period.

Nursing programs throughout the world are implementing integrative educational models to build the complementary therapy knowledge base of generalist nurses. Helms (2006) proposed a sustainable model in which every course included complementary therapy content, with course objectives reflective of complementary and alternative therapy integration in patient care. For example, health care system or policy courses included the history of and philosophical basis for complementary and alternative therapies and health systems. Health assessment courses included history taking inclusive of complementary and alternative therapies. Pharmacology courses were a logical placement for herbal medicines, essential oils, and homeopathic preparations. Nutrition courses added dietary/biologically based therapies. Psychiatric nursing courses emphasized cognitive–behavioral therapy or meditation. And nursing research courses included all aspects of complementary therapy efficacy through the lens of evidence-based practice. In addition, Wetzel, Kaptchuk, Haramati, and Eisenberg (2003) recommended the use of carefully placed case studies as a strategy to integrate complementary therapies throughout the curriculum.

A Course in Complementary Therapies

Another potential approach for learning about complementary and alternative therapies is through specific courses. Groft and Kalischuk (2005) described a 13-week, 3-hour-per-session undergraduate elective course on health and healing. Students explored a range of complementary and alternative therapies commonly used by patients. The course was determined to be highly effective in aiding students' understanding of healing and wholeness. Stephenson, Brown, Handron, and Faser (2007) evaluated a three-semester, 1-hour-per-session elective graduate-level online nursing course designed to: (a) explore the theoretical bases and empirical evidence for various complementary/alternative therapies; (b) explore strategies for integrating evidence-based complementary/alternative therapies; and (c) synthesize advanced knowledge, theory, and research on complementary/alternative therapies into nursing. More recently, van der Reit, Francis, and Levett-Jones (2011) implemented and evaluated an elective course for undergraduate students that included a study tour to Thailand where students learned the techniques of Thai massage and other complementary therapies. The course was positively evaluated and improved global health awareness.

Minor and Major Fields of Study

Similar to the graduate minor in complementary therapies and healing offered at the University of Minnesota, Sofhauser (2002) described the development of a 15-credit, 1-hour-per-session minor in complementary health at the Indiana University, South Bend. Graduate programs with a major in nursing have also been established in integrative health care for advanced practice clinical nurse specialists (Jossens & Ganley, 2006). This program emphasized both Western and CAM practices with two overall goals: (a) to generate nursing leaders with advanced knowledge of, and appreciation for, the diversity of approaches and philosophies concerning health; and (b) to graduate nurses with expertise in the assessment, use, and systematic evaluation of both Western and non-Western practices, contributing to the enhanced health of the community by facilitating the integration of health practices.

Experiential Learning

An experiential component is highly recommended for any students learning about complementary therapies to promote a greater depth of understanding (Wetzel et al., 2003). Chlan, Halcón, Kreitzer, and Leonard (2005) studied the influence of skills lab practice on nursing student confidence levels in performing select complementary therapy skills. Student confidence in the performance of the five therapies (hand massage, imagery, music interventions, reflexology, and breathing/mindfulness) increased after the lab session. The greatest increases in confidence were seen with hand massage, reflexology, and imagery. This study demonstrated the immense value of bringing practical application of CAM into undergraduate nursing education. Similarly, Adler (2009) and Cook and Robinson (2006) implemented an intensive massage therapy experience to promote nursing student competence. The vast majority of student participants indicated that the experience was valuable in their development as nurses by contributing to the nurse–patient relationship and holism in patient care.

Continuing-Education Offerings

For practicing nurses, effective continuing-education opportunities are needed to advance knowledge and skills in complementary therapies. The AHNA has endorsed several continuing-education modules and certification programs that promote holistic nursing practice (www .ahna.org). Nurse practitioners responding to one survey indicated complementary therapy continuing education needed to include information on scientific principles, evidence of efficacy, potential interactions with conventional medicine, and pharmacology. The preferred mechanism for advancing this knowledge was online continuing nursing education (67%), conferences (60%), workshops (60%), and newsletters (51%) (Patterson, Kaczorowski, Arthur, Smith, & Mills, 2003). There are currently a multitude of online (www.healthandhealingny .org/professionals/nurse.asp) and conference opportunities that can assist practicing nurses in improving complementary therapy knowledge and skills.

Also important to note are the ongoing educational models of all forms that continue to evolve. Since the first year of its inception in 2005, the journal *Explore: The Journal of Science and Healing* has featured innovations in integrative health care education. In 2012, columns have focused on interprofessional and exchange programs, student stress reduction, lifelong learning in integrative health, evidence-informed practice, and other innovations in education.

FACILITATING AND EVALUATING STUDENT LEARNING

Creative pedagogies are needed to facilitate student learning and support effective teaching of complementary therapies. According to Lee and colleagues (2007), CAM Education Project schools used a variety of instructional delivery strategies to help students learn about complementary therapies, including classroom-based programs, online modules, and experiential learning. These authors also recognized that personal reflection and self-care are critical components of student learning. At the course level, traditional student learning evaluation methods, such as written papers, examinations, and other projects, were used along with explorative methods, such as through interviews, focus groups, and 1-minute feedback papers, to gain course evaluation information for course improvement (Stratton et al., 2007). Stratton and colleagues (2007) noted:

> In the absence of a single, established set of approved CAM education or competency standards, an array of curricula exist. Consequently, the approaches to evaluating student learning were equally diverse and involved the development and refinement of assessment tools to measure a wide variety of attitudes, beliefs, motivations, knowledge bases, and skills. (p. 959)

WEBSITES

There are an abundance of reputable resources to facilitate effective teaching and student learning in the area of complementary and alternative therapies. Below is a beginning list.

BMJ Clinical Evidence
(www.clinicalevidence.com/x/index.html)

CINAHL: Cumulative Index to Nursing & Allied Health Literature
(www.ebscohost.com/academic/cinahl-plus-with-full-text)

The Cochrane Database
(www.cochrane.org)

MEDLINE Plus: Herbs and Supplements
(www.medlineplus.gov)

MEDLINE: PubMed
(www.ncbi.nlm.nih.gov/entrez/query.fcgi)

Natural Medicine Comprehensive Database
(www.naturaldatabase.com)

NCCAM
(nccam.nih.gov)

CONCLUSIONS

In 2000, Lindeman predicted the future of nursing education would include "greater diversity in clinical experiences to provide contact with people from different cultures, ethnic groups, economic levels, and with alternatives to [W]estern medicine" (p. 11). This certainly has been the case. Avino (2011) affirmed more recently that holistic patient-centered nursing care, including the use of complementary therapies, is a valuable framework to integrate health promotion and wellness in diverse populations. All nursing programs can contribute to the advancement of complementary therapy linkages to health care outcomes through the implementation of clear student learning and program outcomes, rigorous research design, and documentation (Stratton et al., 2007).

The future of nursing education inclusive of complementary therapies requires attention to a set of accepted knowledge and performance core competencies for entry-level and graduate-level nurses (Halcón et al., 2003). Stratton and colleagues (2007), however, recognize that this task represents a moving target, complicated by ever-changing educational and health care environments. Only through thoughtful reflection on the current curricula, adherence to the scope and standards of practice for nurses, and attention to educational and health care influences can we continue to move forward.

Karin Gerber, a nurse educator from South Africa, details the inclusion of complementary therapies within curricula in her country. Content from an interview the author had with Ms. Gerber is found in Sidebar 29.1.

Sidebar 29.1. *Integration of Traditional Healers With Nursing Education in South Africa*

Karin Gerber, Nelson Mandela Metropolitan University (NMMU), Port Elizabeth, South Africa

Throughout the world, nurse educators are responding to the need to integrate complementary and traditional healing into nursing curricula. This sidebar highlights South Africa, the "Rainbow Nation," in which health practices are as diverse as the people. In an interview with two nurse educators from Nelson Mandela Metropolitan University (NMMU), located in Port Elizabeth, South Africa, it was affirmed that traditional African healing practices are presented to the nursing students alongside Western modalities. The nurse educators teach students to be open to various methods of healing but to always seek best practices in their nursing care. The nursing program is science oriented but inclusive of a broad view of therapies based on patient and family

(continued)

Sidebar 29.1. *Integration of Traditional Healers With Nursing Education in South Africa (continued)*

preferences. Of particular note is the collaboration of nursing education with traditional healers within the Nguni and Xhosa societies of South Africa: the diviner (*sangoma* or *amagqirha*) and the herbalist (*inyanga* or *ixwele*).

The diviners and herbalists are highly respected and serve approximately 60% of the people of South Africa. Traditional healers in South Africa greatly outnumber Western-medicine doctors at a rate of 8:1 (Truter, 2007). The distinction between the two types of healers is often blurred; however, in general, the herbalist is concerned with medicines made from plants and animals and the diviner is a spiritualist, using divination for healing purposes. Herbalists make use of more than 3,000 botanical, zoological, and mineral products to bring healing (van Wyk, van Oudtsboorn, & Gericke, 1999). These products are used as a bath water or steaming preparation, ingested (often with a goal to induce vomiting) or inserted as an enema, are placed into incisions in the skin, or inhaled nasally (van Wyk, van Oudtsboorn, & Gericke, 1999). The diviner, through ancestral channeling, prayer, purification, throwing of the bones, use of incense, dream interpretation, or animal sacrifice with a goal of appeasing the spirits, seeks to establish a positive relationship and restitution between the ill person and the spirits causing the illness (Campbell, 1998). The Traditional Health Practitioners Act of 2007 legally recognizes diviners, herbalists, traditional surgeons, and traditional birth attendants as traditional health practitioners. Western-medicine providers continue to study the efficacy of the herbal remedies used, including those for HIV/AIDS, pneumonia, and diarrhea, all major causes of death in South Africa (Campbell, 1998).

Clearly, public acceptance and use of traditional healers has a major influence on the integration of course content at NMMU. The nurse educators interviewed noted that each of the nursing courses has relevant content related to traditional healing, and students often talk about their own personal experiences with the healing modalities. Students are made aware of the risks of the various healing practices because some are known to be toxic, particularly to the kidneys—causing patients to require dialysis. Students are taught how to work together with traditional healers in situations where traditional healing and Western medicine are complementary, such as in the induction of labor. Nurse educators also work with students in the communities to promote optimal health in areas where ritualistic cutting in initiations or as part of traditional healing has led to high rates of infection and mortality. Overall, there is a conscientious effort to help students to understand what is helpful and what can be harmful and how to intervene to promote optimal patient care.

REFERENCES

Adler, P. (2009). Teaching massage to nursing students of geriatrics through active learning. *Journal of Holistic Nursing, 27*, 51–56.

Al-Rukban, M., AlBedah, A., Khalil, M., El-Olemy, A., Khalil, A., & Alrasheid, M. (2012). Status of complementary and alternative medicine in the curricula of health colleges in Saudi Arabia. *Complementary Therapies in Medicine, 20*, 334–339.

American Association of Colleges of Nursing. (2004). *The essentials of master's education for advanced practice nursing.* Retrieved November 27, 2012, from www.aacn.nche.edu

American Association of Colleges of Nursing. (2006). *The essentials of doctoral education for advanced practice nursing.* Retrieved November 27, 2012, from www.aacn.nche.edu

American Association of Colleges of Nursing. (2008). *The essentials of baccalaureate education for professional nursing practice.* Retrieved November 27, 2012, from www.aacn.nche.edu

American Association of Colleges of Nursing. (2011). *The essentials of master's education for nursing.* Retrieved November 27, 2012, from www.aacn.nche.edu

American Holistic Nurses Association & American Nurses Association. (2007). *Holistic nursing: Scope and standards of practice.* Silver Spring, MD: Author.

American Nurses Association. (2010). *Nursing: Scope and standards of practice* (2nd ed.). Washington, DC: American Nurses Association.

Amri, H., Haramati, A., Sierpina, V., & Kreitzer, M. (2012). Georgetown University's graduate program in complementary and alternative medicine: Training future practitioners of integrative healthcare. *Explore: The Journal of Science and Healing, 8*, 258–261.

Avino, K. (2011). Knowledge, attitudes, and practices of nursing faculty and students related to complementary and alternative medicine. *Holistic Nursing Practice, 25*, 280–288.

Booth-LaForce, C., Scott, C., Heitkemper, M., Cornman, J., Lan, M., Bond, E., & Swanson, K. (2010). Complementary and alternative (CAM) attitudes and competencies of nursing students and faculty: Results of integrating CAM into the nursing curriculum. *Journal of Professional Nursing, 26*, 293–300.

Bulechek, G., Butcher, H., & Dochterman, J. (Eds.). (2008). *Nursing interventions classification (NIC)* (5th ed.). St. Louis, MO: Mosby Elsevier.

Burman, M. (2003). Complementary and alternative medicine: Core competencies for family nurse practitioners. *Journal of Nursing Education, 42*, 28–34.

Campbell, S. (1998). *Called to Heal.* Twin Lakes, WI: Lotus Press.

Chlan, L., & Halcón, L. (2003). Developing an integrated baccalaureate nursing education program: Infusing complementary/alternative therapies into critical care curricula. *Critical Care Nursing Clinics of North America, 15*, 373–379.

Chlan, L., Halcón, L., Kreitzer, M., & Leonard, B. (2005). Influence of an experiential education session on nursing students' confidence levels in performing selected complementary therapy skills. *Complementary Health Practice Review, 10*, 189–201.

College & Association of Registered Nurses of Alberta. (2006). *Alternative and/or complementary therapy standards for registered nurses.* Retrieved November 1, 2008, from www.nurses.ab.ca

Cook, N., & Robinson, J. (2006). Effectiveness and value of massage skills training during pre-registration nurse education. *Nurse Education Today, 26*, 555–563.

Cuellar, N., Cahill, B., Ford, J., & Aycock, T. (2003). The development of an educational workshop on complementary and alternative medicine: What every nurse should know. *Journal of Continuing Education in Nursing, 34,* 128–135.

Cutshall, S., Derscheid, D., Miers, A., Ruegg, S., Schroeder, B., Tucker, S., & Wentworth, L. (2010). Knowledge, attitudes, and use of complementary and alternative therapies among clinical nurse specialists in an academic medical center. *Clinical Nurse Specialist, 24,* 125–131.

Dutta, A., Dutta, A., Bwayo, S., Xue, Z., Akiyode, O., Ayuk-Egbe, P., . . . Clarke-Tasker, V. (2003). Complementary and alternative medicine instruction in nursing curricula. *Journal of National Black Nurses Association, 14,* 30–33.

Fenton, M., & Morris, D. (2003). The integration of holistic nursing practices and complementary and alternative modalities into curricula of schools of nursing. *Alternative Therapies, 9,* 62–67.

Gaster, B., Unterborn, J., Scott, R., & Schneeweiss, R. (2007). What should students learn about complementary and alternative medicine? *Academic Medicine, 82,* 934–938.

Gaylord, S., & Mann, D. (2007). Rationales for CAM education in health professions training programs. *Academic Medicine, 82,* 927–933.

Groft, J., & Kalischuk, R. (2005). Nursing students learn about complementary and alternative health care practices. *Complementary Health Practice Review, 10,* 133–146.

Halcón, L., Chlan, L., Kreitzer, M., & Leonard, B. (2003). Complementary therapies and healing practices: Faculty/student beliefs and attitudes and the implications for nursing education. *Journal of Professional Nursing, 19,* 387–397.

Halcón, L., Leonard, B., Snyder, M., Garwick, A., & Kreitzer, M. (2001). Incorporating alternative and complementary health practices within university-based nursing education. *Complementary Health Practice Review, 6,* 127–135.

Hegarty, J., Walsh, E., Condon, C., & Sweeney, J. (2009). The undergraduate education of nurses: Looking to the future. *International Journal of Nursing Education Scholarship, 6*(1), 1–11.

Helms, J. (2006). Complementary and alternative therapies: A new frontier for nursing education? *Journal of Nursing Education, 45,* 117–123.

Hon, K., Twinn, S., Leung, T., Thompson, D., Wong, Y., & Fok, T. (2006). Chinese nursing students' attitudes toward traditional Chinese medicine. *Journal of Nursing Education, 45,* 182–185.

Institute of Medicine. (2005). *Complementary and alternative medicine in the United States.* Washington, DC: National Academy of Sciences.

Institute of Medicine. (2010). *The future of nursing: Leading change, advancing health.* Retrieved December 6, 2012, from http://www.iom.edu

Jossens, M., & Ganley, B. (2006). Integrated health practices: Development of a graduate nursing program. *Journal of Nursing Education, 45,* 16–24.

Keimig, T., & Braun, C. (2004). Student nurses' knowledge and perceptions of alternative and complementary therapies. *Journal of Undergraduate Nursing Scholarship, 6,* 1–9.

Kim, S., Erlen, J., Kim, K., & Sok, S. (2006). Nursing students' and faculty members' knowledge of, experience with, and attitudes towards complementary and alternative therapies. *Journal of Nursing Education, 45,* 375–378.

Kligler, B., Maizes, V., Schachter, S., Park, C., Gaudet, T., Benn, R., . . . Remen, R., Education Working Group, Consortium of Academic Health Centers for Integrative Medicine. (2004). Core competencies in integrative medicine for medical school curricula: A proposal. *Academic Medicine, 79,* 521–531.

Kreitzer, M., Mann, D., & Lumpkin, M. (2008). CAM competencies for the health professions. *Complementary Health Practice Review, 13,* 63–72.

Kreitzer, M., Mitten, D., Harris, I., & Shandeling, J. (2002). Attitudes toward CAM among medical, nursing, and pharmacy faculty and students: A comparative analysis. *Alternative Therapies in Health and Medicine, 8*(6), 44–53.

Lee, M., Benn, R., Wimstatt, L., Cornman, J., Hedgecock, J., Gerick, S., . . . Haramati, A. (2007). Integrating complementary and alternative medicine instruction into health professions education: Organizational and instructional strategies. *Academic Medicine, 82,* 939–945.

Lindeman, C. (2000). The future of nursing education. *Journal of Nursing Education, 39,* 5–12.

Moore, K. (2010). Rationale for complementary and alternative medicine in nursing school curriculum. *Journal of Alternative and Complementary Medicine, 16,* 611–12.

Nedrow, A., Heitkemper, M., Frenkel, M., Mann, D., Wayne, P., & Hughes, E. (2007). Collaborations between allopathic and complementary and alternative medicine health professionals: Four initiatives. *Academic Medicine, 82,* 962–966.

Nedrow, A., Istvan, J., Haas, M., Barrett, R., Salveson, C., Moore, G., . . . Keenan, E. (2007). Implications for education in complementary and alternative medicine: A survey of entry attitudes in students at five health professional schools. *Journal of Alternative and Complementary Medicine, 13,* 381–386.

Nurses Board of Western Australia. (2003). *Guidelines for the use of complementary therapies in nursing practice.* Retrieved November 1, 2008, from www.nbwa.org.au

Öztekin, D., Ucuzal., M., Öztekin, I., & Issever, H. (2007). Nursing students' willingness to use complementary and alternative therapies for cancer patients: Istanbul survey. *Tohoku Journal of Exp Medicine, 211,* 49–61.

Patterson, C., Kaczorowski, J., Arthur, H., Smith, K., & Mills, D.(2003). Complementary therapy practice: Defining the role of advanced nurse practitioners. *Journal of Clinical Nursing, 12,* 816–823.

Pearson, N., & Chesney, M. (2007). The CAM education program of the National Center for Complementary and Alternative Medicine: An overview. *Academic Medicine, 82,* 921–926.

Republic of South Africa, Government Gazette. (2008, January 10). Traditional Healers Act of 2007 (511 No. 42). Retrieved January 31, 2013, from http://www.info.gov.za/view/DownloadFileAction?id=77788

Richardson, S. (2003). Complementary health and healing in nursing education. *Journal of Holistic Nursing, 21,* 20–35.

Sofhauser, C. (2002). Development of a minor in complementary health. *Nurse Educator, 27,* 118–122.

Sok, S., Erlen, J., & Kim, K. (2004). Complementary and alternative therapies in nursing curricula: A new direction for nurse educators. *Journal of Nursing Education, 43,* 401–405.

Sparber, A. (2001). State boards of nursing and scope of practice of registered nurses performing complementary therapies. *Online Journal of Issues in Nursing, 6.* Retrieved from www.nursingworld.org/MainMenuCategories/ANAMarketplace/ANAPeriodicals/OJIN/Tableofcontents/Volume62001/No3Sept01/Article PreviousTopic/complementary TherapiesReport.aspx

Stephenson, N., Brown, S., Handron, D., & Faser, K. (2007). Offering an online course: Complementary and alternative therapies in nursing practice. *Holistic Nursing Practice, 21,* 299–302.

Stratton, T., Benn, R., Lie, D., Zeller, J., & Nedrow, A. (2007). Evaluating CAM education in health professions programs. *Academic Medicine, 82,* 956–961.

Truter, I. (2007). African traditional healers: Cultural and religious beliefs intertwined in a holistic way. *South Africa Pharmaceutical Journal, 74,* 56–60.

Uzun, Ö., & Tan, M. (2004). Nursing students' opinions and knowledge about complementary and alternative medicine therapies. *Complementary Therapies in Nursing & Midwifery, 10*, 239–244.

Van der Reit, P., Francis, L., & Levett-Jones, T. (2011). Complementary therapies in healthcare: Design, implementation, and evaluation of an elective course for undergraduate students. *Nurse Education in Practice, 11*, 146–152.

van Wyk, B., van Oudtshoorn, B., & Gericke, N. (1999). *Medicinal plants of South Africa*. Pretoria, South Africa: Briza.

Wetzel, M., Kaptchuk, T., Haramati, A., & Eisenberg, D. (2003). Complementary and alternative medical therapies: Implications for medical education. *Annals of Internal Medicine, 138*, 191–196.

Yeh, Y., & Chung, U. (2007). An investigation into competence in TCM of BSN graduates from technological universities in Taiwan. *Journal of Nursing Research, 15*, 310–317.

Chapter 30: Integrating Complementary Therapies Into Nursing Practice

Elizabeth L. Pestka and
Susanne M. Cutshall

Complementary therapies are increasingly being offered across the continuum of health care. Nurses are essential for maximizing use of complementary and integrative therapies that support holistic care. The movement toward holism in nursing recognizes the humanistic, caring, healing nature of interventions and often uses many modalities to support the mind–body–spirit on its healing journey (Clark, 2012).

This chapter provides examples of strategies nurses have used to incorporate complementary therapies into their practices. Three health care settings in the Midwest are used to demonstrate the integration of complementary therapies into both inpatient and outpatient hospital nursing practice. The hospitals include one small health campus, Woodwinds Health Campus; one large medical center, Abbott Northwestern Hospital; and one very large health care provider, Mayo Clinic. In addition to traditional nursing roles in hospital settings, examples of nurses incorporating complementary and integrative therapies into community-based care, holistic health and wellness centers, and care provided to military veterans shows the breadth of opportunities for integration into nursing practice.

Health care facilities in the United States are integrating complementary therapies; and this is being done across the world as well. Sidebar 30.1 conveys the use of complementary therapies in Brazil.

Sidebar 30.1. *Use of Complementary Therapies in Brazil*

Milena Flória-Santos, University of São Paulo at Ribeirão Preto College of Nursing, Ribeirão Preto, São Paulo, Brazil

Health care in Brazil includes some traditional medicine that is part of indigenous and popular practices performed by healers and medicine men. Most of these practices provide a search for self-knowledge and focus on the spiritual aspects of culture, religion, and traditions of its users. Brazilian people use these practices because they are easily accessible, have demonstrated relative effectiveness, are congruent with their cultural beliefs, and access to biomedicine is often scarce and expensive in some areas of the country. In western Brazil, traditional practices are undergoing a process of becoming more scientific, specialized, and performed by skilled professionals because they are gradually being disconnected from their traditional cultural context. Use of homeopathy, medicinal plants/phytotherapy, acupuncture, traditional Chinese medicine, anthroposophy medicine, and thermal water therapy are included in the Public Health Unified System.

Spiritist psychiatric hospitals are one example of complementary therapies integrated into care, combining conventional psychiatric treatment and spiritual complementary therapies (Lucchetti et al., 2012). These hospitals include voluntary-based spiritual approaches such as laying-on of hands (fluidotherapy), intercessory prayer, and spirit release therapy (disobsession). Nurses may be trained to provide these therapies. The optional nature of these spiritual complementary therapies seems to increase acceptance by patients and their family members. Outcomes from these interventions have not been scientifically studied.

A recent study found that Brazilian nurses, more so than physicians, are interested in complementary and integrative therapies (Thiago & Tesser, 2011). This is likely due to the belief that nurses use more nonpharmacological interventions to deliver care to patients. For both groups of professionals, acupuncture and homeopathy were the preferred complementary strategies, and acceptance was associated with previous contact with the therapies. Acupuncture was more widely used at public health services where nurses and physical therapists, in addition to physicians, were allowed to use this intervention. The 177 health care professionals who responded to the survey identified the following therapies, which are included in practice: homeopathy, Chinese and Ayurvedic medicine, acupuncture, auriculotherapy, massage, chiropractic and phytotherapy, yoga, biodance, relaxation, meditation, dance, and Tai Chi chuan.

(continued)

Sidebar 30.1. *Use of Complementary Therapies in Brazil (continued)*

Nurses can take elective courses at Brazilian universities and independent courses offered by private organizations to become qualified to use complementary and integrative therapies in their care. More use of complementary and integrative therapies offers growing possibilities for the Brazilian people from individual, health care professional, and health services perspectives.

MEDICAL CENTER SETTINGS

Woodwinds Health Campus

Woodwinds Health Campus located in Woodbury, Minnesota, is an 86-bed not-for-profit facility that opened in 2000. The philosophy of care is based on the creation of an unprecedented healing environment that revolves around the needs of patients and their families, including extensive use of complementary therapies. The vision for the Woodwinds campus of HealthEast Care System was to transform the patient care experience and create compassionate service, holistic care, and a patient-centered care model (Lincoln, 2003). From the spacious main entry to the convenient layout, patients in need of care are easily guided to the area of service they require as quickly and comfortably as possible.

According to Lincoln and Johnson (2009), critical aspects of a healing environment are the relationships and attitudes of health care professionals and administrators in addition to the architectural design elements. The vision of Woodwinds' healing health care model is to be innovative, unique, and a preferred resource for health care. Leadership as well as staff nurses and other employees personally and professionally commit to supporting the principles of holistic care (Lincoln & Johnson, 2009).

Woodwinds Health Campus offers a variety of healing arts therapies designed to complement medical care. These healing arts therapies are also known as integrative therapies or complementary therapies. Integrative treatments are designed to enhance, not replace, traditional therapeutic measures ordered by a primary provider such as medications, exercise, and therapy. A variety of complementary therapies are offered in order to meet the diverse and individualized needs of each patient. Therapies include essential oils, healing touch/energy-based therapies, guided imagery, healing music, acupuncture, acupressure, and massage (Woodwinds Health Campus–HealthEast Care System, 2012a).

In addition to complementary therapies offered by the staff at Woodwinds Health Campus, an outpatient partnership with Northwestern Health Sciences University provides additional care choices such as chiropractic, acupuncture, massage, and naturopathy at the Natural Care Center. This broadens the range of complementary therapies available so that each patient can select options that will help most in the healing process (Woodwinds Health Campus–HealthEast Care System, 2012b).

Nurses play an integral role in providing complementary therapies at Woodwinds. Holistic nursing principles are integrated into the vision for the hospital. Woodwinds Health Campus includes components of holistic nursing in job descriptions and ongoing performance evaluations for nursing staff. The facility continues to attract highly skilled nurses; it maintains a low attrition rate and a high level of staff satisfaction; these factors are associated with the premise that holistic nursing is the foundation for practice. The care environment is collaborative, and individual contributions are honored with nurses providing input on how the holistic care model continues to be implemented (Lincoln, 2003). Woodwinds established a Holistic Practice Council composed of nurses from various patient care units to better understand the needs of staff nurses in providing care and also to strengthen interest and participation in evidence-based practice (Lincoln & Johnson, 2009).

Education for all nurses at Woodwinds includes holistic nursing-related courses: one focusing on healing touch and the second including training in other complementary/alternative modalities such as music therapy, guided imagery, and use of essential oils. In addition, nurses are required to complete at least three educational contact hours annually in holistic nursing. Nurses are expected to include what they have learned in these courses in the care provided to each patient (Lincoln, 2003). The "Woodwinds way" requires nurses to take personal and professional steps to practice from a place of healing, compassion, and love, while also performing with high clinical competence (Lincoln & Johnson, 2009).

Nurses are encouraged to use complementary therapies themselves. They are able to use the many healing spaces in the integrative services area at Woodwinds to enhance their own well-being. They can take "spirit breaks" to rejuvenate themselves during their work shifts. For nurses employed at Woodwinds, using integrative therapies becomes an aspect of their own lives (Lincoln, 2003).

Woodwinds' impact goes beyond its own campus and into the surrounding community. The facility has formed wellness initiatives with local corporations such as 3M and Medtronic. Medtronic has created an Integrative Health Council and invited staff from Woodwinds to conduct a healing harp seminar on their premises (Olson, 2010).

Abbott Northwestern Hospital

Abbott Northwestern Hospital, a part of the Allina Health System, is a 627-bed, tertiary care, not-for-profit hospital in Minneapolis, Minnesota. The nursing department's philosophy at Abbott Northwestern is supported by a patient-centered, holistic framework for practice. In 1999, a complementary and alternative medicine program for cardiovascular inpatients was initiated and has grown into a nationally recognized model for providing integrative care (Sendelbach, Carole, Lapensky, & Kshettry, 2003).

Abbott Northwestern Hospital, in collaboration with the Minneapolis Heart Institute, identified a mission to provide an exceptional health care experience for patients with cardiovascular disorders, and to support this they established a holistic nursing framework for practice. The prevalence of the public's use of complementary/alternative therapies identified in the literature, along with an increasing number of patient and family requests for these interventions, motivated Abbott Northwestern Hospital to initiate its original innovative program, which was called "Healing the Hearts" and which include therapeutic interventions such as music and massage (Sendelbach et al., 2003).

Nursing involvement has been critical to the ongoing success of integrative therapies. An Integrative Practice Advisory Board was established in 2001, and one of the three key areas identified for growth was to further develop holistic nursing to complement the interventions received by patients. The interventions were assessed to be congruent with the nursing department's philosophy and the cornerstones of the patient care model. Work was also focused on enhancing a total healing environment that includes developing positive and collaborative relationships between nurses and physicians because this has been shown to influence patient outcomes (Sendelbach et al., 2003).

With initial success and institutional support, along with continuing education for providers, the inpatient cardiovascular integrative therapy program developed into a national model for not only inpatient care but also for outpatient care, research, and education. The Penny George Institute for Health and Healing is the largest hospital-based program of its kind in the United States and is a role model for enhancing health through an integrative approach. The mission of this innovative program is to transform health care locally by providing outstanding integrative care and to transform health care nationally through development and dissemination of integrative practices that enhance quality, ensure safety, and reduce costs (Allina Health, 2012a).

The Penny George Institute for Health and Healing offers inpatient services that include: acupressure/acupuncture; aromatherapy; energy healing, including Reiki and healing touch; healing arts; Korean hand therapy; mind/body therapies, including relaxation response, guided imagery, and biofeedback; music therapy; reflexology; and therapeutic massage (Allina Health, 2012a). Outpatient services include: Oriental medicine/acupuncture; Ayurveda; energy healing; healing coaching; herbal consultations; integrative medicine physician consultations; integrative nutrition counseling; mind/body therapies, including biofeedback, spiritual coaching, massage therapy, therapeutic yoga, classes and workshops on aromatherapy, drum circle, and healing through the arts. Integrative therapy practitioners have provided more than 900 interventions to patients in the inpatient setting, as well as 700 appointments including complementary therapies in the outpatient clinic per month. More than 60,000 inpatients have benefited from these services since the beginning of the program in 2003 (Allina Health, 2012b).

The holistic nurse clinicians and other members of the integrative therapy team provide ongoing education to the staff. Together with the Bravewell Collaborative, Abbott Northwestern Hospital sponsors physician and nurse practitioner training in integrative medicine and advocates for integrative health in health care reform. Education programs are focused on integrative therapies, promoting self-managed health and wellness, community education classes, nurse training programs, and local health care conferences. Ongoing classes and programs for the community on topics including yoga, stress reduction, nutrition, and fitness provide up-to-date information to more than 800 participants a year (Allina Health, 2012b).

Research to measure patient outcomes and identify best practices is also a key to expanding this innovative model. Nurses are involved with ongoing clinical trials using integrative therapies and data analysis to provide evidence for integrating complementary/alternative therapies into clinical practice. The impact of integrative therapies has been documented to provide immediate and beneficial effects on pain among hospitalized patients. Following integrative therapy interventions, the average pain reduction was over 55% (Dusek, Finch, Plotnikoff, & Knutson, 2010).

Mayo Clinic

Mayo Clinic, located in Rochester, Minnesota, is a large tertiary medical center with almost 2,000 hospital beds, as well as affiliated facilities around the nation. Mayo Clinic defines quality as a comprehensive look at all aspects of a patient's experience (Mayo Clinic: Quality and Mayo Clinic, 2012b). Comprehensive individualized care addresses the mind, body, and spirit to promote healing and wellness with complementary therapies integrated into practice.

The Mayo Nursing Care Model is based on the nursing theory of human caring proposed by Dr. Jean Watson, which honors every patient as a unique person with potential to heal holistically, and is nurtured by the intentional presence of a nurse who connects with the patient in the moment, expressing care through words, actions, and empathy (Mayo Clinic: Department of Nursing, 2012). Nurses across the continuum of care include complementary therapies as part of the holistic healing process.

All nurses, both inpatient and outpatient, are encouraged to include complementary therapies as part of ongoing pain management. One of the policy statements in the institution's procedure guideline on pain management states that complementary interventions such as relaxation techniques, imagery, and music therapy are incorporated in the pain management plan when appropriate (Mayo Clinic: Procedural Guideline, 2012a). A pain action plan also is available that lists several ideas for patients to consider for including complementary interventions in ongoing treatment. Identification of resources to support use of complementary therapies for pain management has been included in departmental orientation for nurses new to the organization and in ongoing staff development sessions. A class in complementary therapies for pain management is offered for nurses to learn more about specific evidence-based practices. The course reviews mind–body modalities, energy-based therapies, biologically based approaches, and manipulative-based methods.

As part of patient education, a brochure nurses provide to patients in many specialties is titled *Introduction to Relaxation Skills* (Mayo Foundation for Medical Education and Research, 2008). This handout focuses on the importance of relaxation to eliminate tension in the body and mind. It describes the complementary therapies of relaxed breathing; progressive muscle relaxation; autogenic relaxation; imagery; and other activities such as Tai Chi, self-hypnosis, yoga, and meditation. The nurse uses this resource to introduce complementary therapies to assist a patient with holistic healing and to emphasize that learning relaxation skills may improve overall health and quality of life.

Other strategies nurses use to integrate complementary therapies into a patient's care include a television channel with continuous relaxing music in each patient's room; compact disc (CD) players and CDs available for patient use on each unit for music therapy; CDs with audio-guided imagery that a patient can use in the hospital and take home at discharge; journals available for patients to write in; a chaplain service that can be requested to provide spirituality support; and the ongoing basics of nursing presence, touch, and humor.

Healing Enhancement Program

The Healing Enhancement Program was initiated in the inpatient setting based on patient feedback and review of the patient experience for cardiovascular surgery patients. A team including nurses was formed to address the needs of patients that often occur with and after cardiac surgery: managing pain, anxiety, tension, stress, sleeplessness, and nausea. When the team realized that initial orders focused on pain medications were not enough, a trial of massage and music therapies targeted at reducing patients' complaints of musculoskeletal pain and decreasing anxiety and tension after surgery was initiated. Studies confirmed positive findings (Cutshall et al., 2007).

Nurses educate patients and their family members about complementary/alternative resources and coordinate the delivery of services. Nurses promote patient use of a wide array of opportunities. A massage therapist is available to provide treatment for back, neck, and shoulder pain. CD players are available in each of the cardiac surgical rooms for music therapy with a small CD library available on each unit and additional CDs in the patient library. The Patient Education Section made guided-imagery CDs specific to "Successful Surgery" and "Healthful Sleep" available on each patient's television, as well as other CD resources for passive muscle relaxation, stress management, and additional imageries. Patient education classes on stress and wellness and healing movement are offered on an ongoing basis. Live, soothing music is sometimes available in clinical areas; patients are able to select art pieces for their hospital room; and some hospital volunteers are trained to offer hand massage to patients, family members, and staff (Cutshall et al., 2007).

The success of the Healing Enhancement Program has led to replication in other surgical areas at Mayo Clinic, including the colorectal surgery and transplant surgery specialties. Recognizing the benefits to patients, nurses continue to collaborate with other health care providers and the outpatient Complementary and Integrative Medicine Program to expand resources and opportunities for additional services and patient populations. An advanced practice nurse/integrative health specialist is available to assist patients regarding incorporating integrative therapies into their plan for preparing for and recovering from surgery. There is also an inpatient consult service for integrative therapies that includes massage therapy, acupuncture, animal-assisted therapy, integrative health specialist nurse and integrative medicine physician consults.

Pain Rehabilitation Center

The Mayo Clinic Pain Rehabilitation Center (PRC) is an exemplary outpatient model of nurses integrating complementary/alternative therapies into their practice. It was among the first pain rehabilitation programs in the United States, established in 1974, and is now one of the largest interdisciplinary pain rehabilitation programs. The PRC focuses on functional restoration with a cognitive–behavioral basis and extensive use of complementary therapies (Mayo Foundation for Medical Education and Research, 2006).

A team of health care professionals, with nurses being integral members of the group, deliver care to patients in the program. Patients are provided education on medication management, cognitive–behavioral therapy, complementary therapies, stress and emotional management, physical therapy, occupational therapy, biofeedback, sleep hygiene, and lifestyle management. Complementary therapies included have been carefully researched and proven to be helpful, including biofeedback, deep diaphragmatic breathing, guided imagery, yoga, Tai Chi, music, art, exercise, and humor.

The PRC always tapers patients off opioid medications because there is evidence that these individuals can experience significant and sustained improvement in pain severity and functioning following participation in a comprehensive pain rehabilitation program without these substances (Townsend et al., 2008). Many people who have lived with chronic pain for much of their lives inform the nurses that they are skeptical that if large dosages of medication have not helped their pain, nonpharmacological methods such as complementary therapies are unlikely to be effective. Program outcomes data support not only overwhelming patient satisfaction with the program (94%), but also a reduction in depressive symptoms (79%), a gain in activity level (75%), and a reduction in pain severity in 73% of the patients (Mayo Foundation for Medical Education and Research, 2006). Program participants credit complementary therapies as one of the most effective elements of their pain rehabilitation program and improved quality of life.

Research Related to the Use of Integrative Therapies

Research to provide evidence for integrative therapies is supported at Mayo Clinic. Investigators have conducted more than 30 clinical trials of various complementary therapies for treating cancer and controlling symptoms. For example, using oral cryotherapy (having patients suck on ice chips for 30 minutes) before and during administration of the chemotherapy agent 5-FU decreases the incidence of mouth sores by 50% (Sencer, 2010). The Mayo Clinic Cancer Education Program supports a model of nurses providing leadership and education on complementary/integrative therapies. A nurse coordinates a program that provides patients, visitors, and staff with an opportunity to explore integrative/complementary medicine approaches and creative expression. Several nurses also teach classes to oncology patients on aromatherapy, mindfulness, and yoga. Other integrative medicine practitioners and community-based practitioners also present on topics such as acupuncture, mandalas, and music therapy. These free educational programs enhance self-care and support the experience of holistic healing.

Healthy Living Center

The Dan Abraham Healthy Living Center at Mayo Clinic provides access to complementary and integrative health and wellness programs for staff. These include cooking demonstrations, group fitness classes, individual wellness evaluations, massage therapy, wellness coaching, small-group training, stress management programs, massage therapy, Reiki, acupressure, yoga, Tai Chi, Alexander technique, and weight-loss programs. The

Healthy Living Center has initiated a Wellness Champions Program to promote health and wellness activities in local areas. Several nurses have volunteered to participate in this program and serve as leaders in their work locations. The department of nursing has a Wellness Champions Steering Group to help support nurse engagement in wellness offerings (Mayo Clinic: Dan Abraham Healthy Living Center, 2012).

COMMUNITY-BASED HEALTH CARE SETTINGS

Holy Redeemer Hospice

Many hospice programs include complementary therapies as part of their care. One program, Holy Redeemer Hospice in southeastern Pennsylvania, provides an innovative model with a team of nurses certified in complementary therapy modalities (Hansen, 2012). This approach enables experienced hospice nurses who really know hospice care to have another set of tools in their toolbox. Hospice care does not end when the patient who is being cared for dies because nurses continue to provide support to family members following the loss. Complementary therapies can help family members relax and address their stress level and cope more effectively.

Pillsbury House Integrated Health Clinic

The Pillsbury House Integrated Health Clinic uses student practitioners and serves patients living in south Minneapolis, Minnesota, and the surrounding communities. All services are free and open by appointment to the public. Patients receive integrative care from student interns who are supervised by licensed faculty. The care is planned and delivered by a team of students and providers from several disciplines, including chiropractic care, acupuncture, massage therapy, and health coaching. Nursing students from the University of Minnesota and the Center for Spirituality and Healing are involved in providing information at the Pillsbury House. Nurses may be involved in collaborative planning for patients, and nurses who are health-coaching students may also be offering services (Pillsbury United Communities, 2012).

Mayo Clinic Affiliated Practices

Community services are sometimes part of larger health care networks. Nurses who work at Mayo Clinic Affiliated Practices are integrating complementary therapies into practice in local communities. Mayo Clinic Health System in Red Wing, Minnesota, formerly part of another health care group, has initiated a Healing Arts Program. The program offers guided imagery, essential oils, healing music, antinausea acupressure bands, healing touch, massage therapy, reflexology, and yoga in the community. Several nurses are trained in these healing arts practices and discuss the programs with patients (Carstensen, 2012).

Another extension of the Mayo Clinic system to a community-based setting is The Center for Health and Healing Healthcare in Onalaska, Wisconsin. Patients and other interested persons in the community are offered access to integrative therapies. The services provided in this center include acupuncture, healing oils, osteopathic medicine, Qigong, spiritual direction, healing touch, massage therapy, Reiki, yoga, guided imagery, life coaching, meditation, and Shen. Nurses are actively involved in leadership of the center and serve as practitioners for some of the offerings. Nurses are also leaders in providing education within the health care setting on the complementary and integrative therapies and providing guidance for nursing practice (Mayo Clinic: Health System, 2012).

HOLISTIC HEALTH AND WELLNESS CENTERS

Hermitage Farm Center for Healing

Nurses may work as instructors and practitioners in community-based holistic health and wellness centers. An example of such a community-based program initiated by nurses is the Hermitage Farm Center for Healing in Rochester, Minnesota. This center was founded by an advanced practice nurse and several of the practitioners affiliated with the center are nurses with advanced skills in complementary and integrative therapies. These nurses interact and collaborate with other complementary and integrative health practitioners to provide a variety of services. The classes offered are related to energy healing, stress management, and mindfulness-based stress reduction. Practitioners also provide therapies such as Reiki, energy healing, and massage therapy (Hermitage Farm Center for Healing, 2012). The Southeast Minnesota chapter of the Holistic Nurses Association meets at this location.

Pathways

Pathways, in Minneapolis, Minnesota, is another example of a community-based holistic wellness center that provides classes focused on the mind, body, and spirit. Volunteers provide therapies free of charge. Nurses are active in providing therapies and also teach classes. The Minnesota chapter of the Holistic Nurses Association meets at this location and these meetings serve as an opportunity for networking and sharing resources for practice and self-care (Pathways, 2012).

Well Within

Another example of a nonprofit holistic wellness community center, Well Within, in Minneapolis, is a resource that offers innovative programs, support, and services to those seeking well-being and healing of body, mind, and spirit. The center provides services to individuals, groups, and as outreach to the community. The services offered at the community center include: health and wellness coaching, integrative psychotherapy, energy healing, mind–body practice groups, and integrative healing programs. Nurses are involved in this center as a part of the board of directors, practitioners, and educators (Well Within, 2012).

VETERANS ADMINISTRATION

Complementary therapies are increasingly becoming part of care provided to military veterans. Results of a 2011 survey were presented at a meeting discussing complementary practice in the Department of Veterans Affairs. According to this survey, 89% of Veterans Administration (VA) facilities offered complementary therapies compared to 84% in 2002. The five most common therapies provided are meditation (72% of hospitals), stress management/relaxation therapy (66% of hospitals), guided imagery (58% of hospitals), progressive muscle relaxation (53% of hospitals), and biofeedback at 50% of hospitals (U.S. Department of Veterans Affairs, 2011).

There is much interest in using complementary therapies to treat chronic pain and posttraumatic stress disorder (PTSD) because these are growing concerns in the VA. A July 2012 report from the Institute of Medicine states that an estimated 13% to 20% of the more than 2.6 million U.S. service members deployed to Iraq or Afghanistan since 2001 develop PTSD (Kennedy, 2012). Review of research evidence showed the highest quality evidence supported the use of acupuncture; however, strong conclusions cannot be drawn without further evidence. Findings in studies using forms of breathing and muscle relaxation were positive overall but also need more studies (U.S. Department of Veterans Affairs, 2011).

The VA is committed to maximizing roles that nurses can play in comprehensive holistic care for veterans. The Office of Nursing developed the Clinical Practice Program to support nursing clinical practice. Seven specialty advisory committees consisting of a clinical nurse advisor and nurses actively involved in clinical practice focus on identifying and developing recommendations for best practice, practice guidelines, patient care standards, and policy guidance (U.S. Department of Veterans Affairs, 2012). Each of these specialty committees is examining evidence for integrating complementary therapies into comprehensive recommendations.

For example, many veterans return from active duty with symptoms of insomnia that are disruptive to their lives. A study by Epstein, Babcock-Parziale, Hayes, and Herb (2012) examined treatment acceptability and preferences of male Iraq and Afghanistan combat veterans. Veterans considered pharmacotherapy as an option but recognized it might be a quick fix that could lead to problems with dependence. Relaxation therapies such as mindfulness and guided imagery were considered acceptable and could be used to not only treat symptoms of insomnia but also symptoms of anxiety and stress. Persons with insomnia can use the relaxation skills to fall asleep more easily and can incorporate them into their everyday lives to cope with stressful situations. The veterans participating in this study emphasized the need for interventions that could be given in an individual treatment delivery method and obtained with a minimum of appointments. Use of electronic resources such as digital video discs (DVDs) to augment initial education was supported by both veterans and providers.

NURSES USING COMPLEMENTARY THERAPIES

Nurses are in a key position to help integrate complementary and alternative therapies into clinical practice. They are in a position to guide and impact the growth and use of complementary therapies in the continuum of health care environments. Nurses have a background and educational curriculum that focuses on holistic mind, body, and spiritual care. The nursing profession has long been a strong advocate of integrated care (Clark, 2012; O'Connell & Russel, 2003).

A national survey of critical care nurses was conducted by Tracy and colleagues (2005) to determine attitudes, knowledge, perspectives, and use of complementary and alternative therapies. The study used a random sample of members of the American Association of Critical Care Nurses with 726 respondents. Most of the 726 respondents were using one or more complementary and alternative therapies in practice. The most common therapies mentioned were diet, exercise, relaxation techniques, and prayer. A majority of the nurses had some knowledge of more than half of the 28 therapies listed on the survey, and a majority desired additional training for 25 therapies. The participants generally required more evidence before using or recommending conventional therapy than before using or recommending complementary and alternative therapies. Overall the respondents viewed complementary and alternative therapies positively and were open to use of the therapies and perceived them as legitimate and beneficial to patients for a variety of symptoms.

A majority of the respondents desired an increase in the availability of therapies for patients, families, and nursing staff. Respondents' professional use of the therapies was related to having more knowledge about them, perceiving benefits from them, total number of therapies they rec-ommended to patients, personal use, and affiliation with a mainstream religion. This study concluded that there would be benefit to having edu-cational programs that provide information about complementary and alternative therapies, and evidence for use of therapies would increase the appropriate use of these therapies (Tracy et al., 2005).

Nursing as a profession is well rooted in understanding the support-ive needs of patients to reduce stress to allow for healing from illness or disease. Nurses are exposed to stress in their own lives and in the work environment. Nurses can personally benefit from stress-reducing comple-mentary and integrative medicine therapies for their own self-care and to prevent professional burnout. There is especially a great potential for turmoil, stress, and burnout among new nurses (Boychuk, Duchscher, & Cowin, 2006). In a recent study of new nurses with less than 2 years' tenure, 66% were found to have symptoms of burnout, mental exhaustion, and depression (Cho, Laschinger, & Wong, 2006). Complementary thera-pies aimed at stress reduction and relaxation may be helpful in allowing new nurses, and nurses currently working in the profession, to manage ongoing stressful activities and events.

A recent study by Tucker, Weymiller, Cutshall, Rhudy, and Lohse (2012) on stress ratings and health-promotion practices among registered nurses that included more than 2,200 nurses highlighted the importance of continued focus on the health of nurses and recognized a huge oppor-tunity for incorporating complementary therapies into nursing self-care. Study results indicated that although overall stress levels of nurses who participated were similar to the national average, the stress levels were inversely correlated with overall health-promotion behavior scores. Nurses with caregiver responsibilities outside of their nursing roles were associ-ated with higher stress and lower health-promoting behavior scores. In a multivariate analysis, health responsibility, spiritual growth, and stress management accounted for most of the variance in perceived stress scores. The findings support work-site interventions that promote nurses' health and wellness and a focus on reducing work and home stress using comple-mentary relaxation and exercise strategies.

Another study examined the effects of a brief stress management inter-vention for nurse leaders. Nurse leaders were assigned to a randomized controlled trial of a brief mindfulness meditation course or a leadership course. Results supported preliminary effectiveness of a 4-week mindful-ness meditation course in reducing self-reported stress symptoms among nurse leaders, demonstrating positive results for this complementary therapy intervention (Pipe et al., 2009).

A related study evaluated results of HeartMath™, an approach incor-porating complementary therapies into an educational intervention, on the stress of health team members. The compelling imperative for the project was to find a positive and effective way to address the documented stress levels of health care workers. A pilot study of primarily nurses includ-ing oncology staff (n = 29) and health care leaders (n = 15) explored the impact of a positive coping approach on Personal and Organizational Quality Assessment-Revised (POQA-R) (Institute of HeartMath and Caring Management Consulting, 1999–2002) scores at baseline and at 7 months using paired t-tests. Baseline measures of distress demonstrated that stress and its symptoms are problematic issues for hospital and ambulatory clinic staff nurses. This workplace intervention including complementary thera-pies was feasible and effective in promoting positive strategies for coping and enhancing well-being, personally and organizationally (Pipe et al., 2011).

By gaining a greater appreciation of the value of complementary ther-apies for their own well-being, nurses can be very instrumental in further integration of these modalities into comprehensive holistic care. Nurses can continue serving as strong advocates for patients, families, and com-municate with interdisciplinary team members promoting use of comple-mentary therapies. Motivated nurses can have an influence on standards and guidelines for clinical nursing and complementary/alternative thera-pies polices. Nurses can also develop frameworks and practice models for hospital-based complementary alternative services.

REFERENCES

Allina Health–Penny George Institute for Health and Healing. (2012a). Retrieved from http://www.allinahealth.org/ahs/anw.nsf/page/ihh_home

Allina Health–Penny George Institute for Health and Healing. (2012b). *Overview and outcomes report 2010*. Retrieved from http://www.allinahealth.org/ahs/anw.nsf/page/ihh_home

Boychuk Duchscher, J. E., & Cowin, L. S. (2006). The new graduates' professional inheritance. *Nursing Outlook, 54*(3), 152–158.

Carstensen, R. (2012). Fairview will soon offer "healing touch." *Red Wing Republican Eagle*. Retrieved from http://www.republican-eagle.com/event/article/id/80063/publisher_ID/16/

Clark, C. S. (2012). Beyond holism: Incorporating an integral approach to support caring-healing-sustainable nursing practices. *Holistic Nursing Practice, 26*(2), 92–102.

Cho, J., Laschinger, H .K. S., & Wong, C. (2006). Workplace empowerment, work engagement and organizational commitment of new graduate nurses. *Canadian Journal of Nursing Leadership, 19*(3), 43–60.

Cutshall, S., Fenske, L., Kelly, R., Phillips, B., Sundt, T., & Bauer, B. (2007). Creation of a healing enhancement program at an academic medical center. *Complementary Therapies in Clinical Practice, 13*, 217–223.

Dusek, J. A., Finch, M., Plotnifkoff, G., & Knutson, L. (2010). The impact of integra-tive medicine on pain management in a tertiary hospital. *Journal of Patient Safety, 6*(1), 48–51.

Epstein, D. R., Babcock-Parziale, J. L., Hayes, P. L., & Herb, C. A. (2012). Insomnia treatment acceptability and preferences of male Iraq and Afghanistan com-bat veterans and their healthcare providers. *Journal of Rehabilitative Research & Development, 49*(6), 867–878.

Hansen, S. (2012). Complementary therapy program at hospice puts nurses in unique role. Retrieved from http://news.nurse.com/article/20120827/PA01/108270027

Hermitage Farm Center for Healing. (2012). Retrieved from http://www.hermitagefarm.org/about.html

Institute of HeartMath and Caring Management Consulting. (1999–2002). *POQA-R Personal and Organizational Quality Assessment-Revised.* Boulder Creek, CA: Author.

Kennedy, M. S. (2012). The hidden wounds of war. *American Journal of Nursing, 112*(11), 7.

Lincoln, V. (2003) Creating an integrated hospital: Woodwinds Health Campus. *Integrative Nursing, 2*(1), 12–13.

Lincoln, V., & Johnson, M. (2009). Staff nurse perceptions of a healing environment. *Holistic Nursing Practice, 23*(3), 183–190.

Lucchetti, G., Aguiar, P. R., Braghetta, C. C., Vallada, C. P., Moreira-Almeida, A., & Vallada, H. (2012). Spiritist psychiatric hospitals in Brazil: Integration of conventional psychiatric treatment and spiritual complementary therapy. *Culture, Medicine and Psychiatry, 36*(1), 124–135.

Mayo Clinic. (2012a). *Procedural Guideline: Pain Management.* Retrieved from http://mayocontent.mayo.edu/mcnursing/DOCMAN-0000053838

Mayo Clinic. (2012b). *Quality and Mayo Clinic.* Retrieved from http://www.mayoclinic.org/quality

Mayo Clinic: Dan Abraham Healthy Living Center. (2012). *About DAHLC.* Retrieved from http://mayoweb.mayo.edu/dahlc

Mayo Clinic: Department of Nursing–Relationship-Based Caring. (2012). Retrieved from http://nursing.mayo.edu/nursing-care-model/

Mayo Clinic: Health System. (2012). Retrieved from http://mayoclinichealthsystem.org/locations/onalaska/medical-services/complementary-medicine/center-for-health-and-healing

Mayo Foundation for Medical Education and Research. (2006). *Comprehensive pain rehabilitation center: Program guide* (Brochure). Rochester, MN.

Mayo Foundation for Medical Education and Research. (2008). *Introduction to relaxation skills* (Brochure). Rochester, MN.

O'Connell, E., & Russel, G., (2003). Federal CAM policy: Politics and practice. *Critical Care Nursing Clinics of North America, 15,* 381–386.

Olson, P. (2010). Woodwinds Health Campus supports integrative care. *Edge magazine.net.* Retrieved from http://edgemagazine.net/2010/05/woodwinds-health-campus-supports-integrative-care/

Pathways. (2012). *About us.* Retrieved from http://www.pathwaysminneapolis.org/

Pillsbury United Communities. (2012). *Pillsbury House integrated health clinic.* Retrieved from http://puc-mn.org/NeighborhoodCenters/PillsburyHouse/IntegratedHealthClinic/tabid/518/Default.aspx

Pipe, T., Bortz, J., Dueck, A., Pendergast, D., Buchda, V., & Summers, J. (2009). Nurse leader mindfulness meditation program for stress management: A randomized controlled trial. *Journal of Nursing Administration, 39*(3), 130–137.

Pipe, T., Buchada, V., Launder, S., Hudak, B., Hulvey, L., Karns, K., & Pendergast, D. (2011). Building personal and professional resources of resilience and agility in the healthcare workplace. *Stress Health.* Published online in Wiley Online Library (wileyonlinelibrary.com). doi:10.1002/smi.1396

Sencer, S. (2010, October). The best of both worlds. *Minnesota Medicine.* Retrieved from: http://www.minnesotamedicine.com/Default.aspx?tabid+3575

Sendelbach, S., Carole, L., Lapensky, J., & Kshettry, V. (2003). Developing an integrative therapies program in a tertiary care cardiovascular hospital. *Critical Care Nursing Clinic of North America, 15,* 363–372.

Thiago, S. C. S., & Tesser, C. D. (2011). Family health strategy doctors and nurses' perceptions of complementary therapies. *Rev Saude Publica*, *45*(2), 1–8. Retrieved from www.scielo.br/rsp

Townsend, C. O., Kerkvliet, J. L., Bruce, B. K., Rome, J. D., Hooten, W. M., Luedtke, C. A., & Hodgson, J. E. (2008). A longitudinal study of the efficacy of a comprehensive pain rehabilitation program with opioid withdrawal: Comparison of treatment outcomes based on opioid status at admission. *Pain*, *140*, 177–189.

Tracy, M. F., Lindquist, R., Savik, K., Watanuki, S., Sendelbach, S., Kreitzer, M. M., & Berman, B. (2005). Use of complementary and alternative therapies: A national survey of critical care nurses. *American Journal of Critical Care*, *14*(5), 404–414.

Tucker, S. J., Weymiller, A. J., Cutshall, S. M., Rhudy, L. M., & Lohse, C. M. (2012). Stress ratings and health promotion practice among RN's at Mayo Rochester: A case for action. *Journal of Nursing Administration*, *42*(5), 282–292.

U.S. Department of Veterans Affairs. (2011). *PTSD and complementary alternative medicine–Research opportunities*. Retrieved from http://www.research.va.gov/news/research_highlights/ptsd-cam-051711.cfm

U.S. Department of Veterans Affairs. (2012). Office of Nursing Services. *The clinical practice program*. Retrieved from http://www.va.gov/NURSING/featured_initiatives.asp

Well Within. (2012). *About us*. Retrieved from http://wellwithin.org/about.us/

Woodwinds Health Campus–HealthEast Care System. (2012a). *About us*. Retrieved from http://www.healtheast.org/woodwinds/about.html

Woodwinds Health Campus–HealthEast Care System (2012b). *Healing arts at Woodwinds*. Retrieved from http://www.healtheast.org/woodwinds/healing-arts.html

Chapter 31: Perspectives on Future Research

RUTH LINDQUIST, YEOUNGSUK SONG,
AND MARIAH SNYDER

Nursing's commitment to the generation of high-quality, cost-effective patient outcomes requires that a sound scientific basis for practice be established. Previous chapters have identified existing research related to the therapies reviewed; however, most chapters end with statements that more research is needed. The need for more evidence related to the safety, efficacy, timing, "dose," and specific indications for most therapies is clearly evident. As previously noted, there is a considerable and growing interest in and use of complementary therapies by the public. In a large and comprehensive examination of the use of complementary and alternative therapies, the number of annual visits to providers of complementary and alternative therapies was found to outnumber visits to primary care physicians (Institute of Medicine [IOM], 2002). Subsequently, the 2007 annual National Health Survey, a comprehensive in-person survey of Americans regarding their health, found that 38.8% of adults and 11.8% of children surveyed in the United States reported use of a form of complementary and alternative medicine in the preceding 12 months (Barnes, Bloom, & Nahin, 2008; NCCAM, 2008). More recently, a 2010 phone survey of more than 1,000 persons 50 years of age and older reported that more than one half of the respondents used some form of complementary and alternative medicine; however, only a little more than one half of those who reported use said that they had ever discussed their use with their health care providers (NCCAM, 2012a).

Interest in complementary therapies is encountered in a broad range of health care practice settings. Along with public and patient interest, there is a concomitant interest on the part of providers who not only want to deliver these therapies to patients but also have an interest in the same therapies for their own personal use (Lindquist, Tracy, & Savik, 2003). However, despite provider interest, it has been noted that the complementary and alternative therapies most often used by patients are not those that providers are familiar with or which are most understood (Zhang, Peck, Spalding, Jones, & Cook, 2012). In addition to the significant demand, common use, and lack of understanding of even commonly used complementary and alternative therapies, there is an urgency to increase knowledge among providers, and to expand the evidence base that supports their safety and efficacy, and which guides their use.

The world is shrinking. New therapies and new uses for old therapies are shared across continents. Health providers and researchers are challenged to create and employ a solid evidence base to undergird the broad range of complementary therapies used by substantial segments of the U.S. population and persons throughout the world. There is an acute need to know and understand benefits of therapies and whether they work according to the purpose for which they are used; there is also a need to ensure the safety and efficacy of complementary therapies and to understand their effects and interactions when used in combination with other complementary and allopathic therapies. In this chapter, the need for more evidence to support the expanding use of complementary therapies in practice is presented, research designs appropriate for the study of complementary therapies are explored, the overall state of research on complementary therapies is described, and implications that the state of evidence and expanded use of complementary therapies have for future nursing research are identified.

NEED TO EXPAND THE EVIDENCE BASE

The documented growing interest in and use of alternative and complementary therapies and alternative systems of care have caused health care providers to consider the appeal of these therapies to consumers as well as the consideration of their safety and efficacy. Concomitantly, questions regarding costs and cost-effectiveness for third-party payment and for individuals paying out-of-pocket need to be answered. Questions need to be answered through research related to which therapies and how many treatment sessions should be covered, and what results from the treatment can be expected and for what conditions. The optimal mix and relative cost of the complementary or alternative therapies versus traditional Western treatments must be determined.

With the widespread use of complementary and alternative therapies, there is reason for concern regarding the safety of their use and about their potential interactions with Western medicine (Bent, 2008). An example is the interaction of herbal remedies such as St. John's wort with prescribed pharmacotherapy, including psychotropic agents, in the family of selective serotonin reuptake inhibitors. Contributing to the difficulty is the lack of regulation of complementary and alternative therapies such as herbal products (Bent, 2008), although increasing attention is being paid to this in an effort to provide guidance for use. The creation of the World Health Organization's policy on herbal medicine recognizes the value of herbal medicine, but calls for systematic inventory and assessment, and regulatory measures to ensure quality control, and calls for international cooperation and coordination to conserve medicinal plants for future generations (World Health Organization, 1998). Indeed, scientific data in this area are needed by providers to inform their practice. Accurate and reliable knowledge is also needed by consumers who wish to make informed decisions regarding their own health practices.

There is a rising interest in and indeed a mandate for evidence-based practice. Evidence-based practice (EBP) has been defined simply as, "applying the best available research results (evidence) when making decisions about health care" (AHRQ, 2013). Further, "health care professionals who perform evidence-based practice use research evidence along with clinical expertise and patient preferences" (AHRQ, 2013). Indeed, nurses and other providers practicing in the context of conventional allopathic care rely on an evidence base. So, too, nurses and other health professionals are relying on or requiring similar evidence in their use of complementary therapies. However, in a national survey, critical care nurses generally reported that they required more evidence for conventional allopathic remedies than they did for complementary and alternative therapies (Tracy et al., 2005).

It is important that resources to access knowledge about complementary and alternative therapies be identified, made available, and used by providers. Research findings regarding the safety and efficacy of therapies must be disseminated broadly to practitioners, who need to be informed so that the safety of patients can be protected and the potential benefits of therapies realized. A number of personal data assistants (PDA)–based resources provide access to authoritative information as a resource to professional practice. Databases of research findings (e.g., the Cochrane Database of Systematic Reviews) are good resources for synthesized research findings (www.cochrane.org/re-views). As of 2013, a simple search of "complementary and alternative therapies" on this online source produced 204 hits, including, but not limited to, reviews related to healing therapies such as healing touch, dietary products, acupuncture, reflexology, meditation, relaxation techniques, herbal medicine, manual therapies, mind–body therapies, hypnosis, aromatherapy, and homeopathy. These reviews are an excellent source of well-integrated research-based knowledge about what is known regarding the use of therapies for specific conditions. Additionally, websites of government agencies, such as the National Institutes of Health's (NIH) National Center for Complementary and Alternative Medicine (NCCAM) (nccam .nih.gov/health/bytreatment.htm) or the Office of Cancer Complementary and Alternative Medicine (OCCAM), provide other sources of information on a wide range of complementary and alternative therapies. The Natural Standard Database provides high-quality information, graded to reflect the level of scientific evidence available on a scale ranging from A to F, regarding herbs, dietary supplements, natural products, and other complementary therapies used for specific health conditions (Natural Standard, 2013) (www.naturalstandard.com).

NCCAM supports investigator-initiated research and interdisciplinary research training initiatives (NCCAM, 2013). With a special encouragement of research that focuses on complementary and alternative therapies that are commonly used by the American public, NCCAM has begun building a solid foundation from which therapies can be selected and delivered with growing confidence as to their safety and efficacy. However, there is much work to be done. The ideal evidence base for complementary therapies would support decision making in a broad range of complex patient situations. It would differentiate effects on and appropriateness for persons with diverse characteristics (e.g., age, gender, body mass), from various cultures (accounting for dietary practices, social acceptability, and cultural traditions, and so forth), and genetic make-up, and would outline the potential differing effects and indications for persons suffering the full range of pathologies and comorbidities.

There are legitimate safety concerns related to therapy selection, quality of the product (the purity or technique of delivery), dose, timing, duration, and other considerations related to specific therapies such as herbal therapies, nutraceuticals, and supplements. For example, more research is needed to identify potentially adverse drug–herb interactions, to answer questions related to whether particular drugs and herbs can be ingested simultaneously; if not, the half-life of herbs in the body, or their "washout" times, need to be determined. Research is also needed to provide data to document the relative risks and benefits of therapies such as the use of diet therapy for hypertension (as opposed to standard allopathic pharmacological therapies), or to consider the potential reduction of the side effects of an allopathic agent if used at a reduced dose in combination with a complementary therapy.

The growing evidence base provides much needed information for the consumer and provider. However, additional research is needed to determine the potential beneficial outcomes of complementary therapies. Likewise, studies are necessary to generate findings that protect the public from harm or from needless, costly therapies that have no evidence to support them, or when evidence clearly shows no benefit. For example, therapies such as the use of laetrile to combat cancer caused concern among allopathic providers who feared that the false hope of cure would dissuade patients from seeking legitimate forms of cancer therapy while bleeding fortunes from desperate families, despite the fact that there was no basis for its claims of beneficial effects (National Cancer Institute, 2012; Pinn, 2001). Extramural funding opportunities and the peer review system of NIH ensure the continued accumulation of high-quality evidence and encourage investigators who have the ideas, curiosity, and scientific expertise to explore potential therapies for human use.

RESEARCH DESIGNS FOR COMPLEMENTARY THERAPIES

Most scientists would agree that the most rigorous design to test complementary and alternative therapies is the randomized, placebo-controlled, double-blind design that has long been the standard for testing therapies and advancing fields of inquiry (Duley & Farrell, 2002; Misra, 2012). However, this design is not the only one that provides useful information, and data that are generated from quantitative studies are not the only available evidence base for practice. Other designs and sources of evidence are also important and contribute to our knowledge and understanding of patients' responses to therapies, both allopathic and nonallopathic.

Consumers may be increasingly reluctant to enroll in clinical trials; hence, alternative study designs and strategies for the conduct of clinical research to advance the field have been called for (Gross & Fogg, 2001). The Committee on the Use of Complementary and Alternative Medicine by the American Public was commissioned by the Institute of Medicine, the AHCRQ, NCCAM, and 15 other agencies and institutes of NIH to study and provide specific recommendations regarding complementary and alternative therapies. As part of their report (IOM, 2002), innovative alternative designs to provide information about the effectiveness of therapies were identified, including:

- **Preference randomized controlled trials** (RCTs)—trials that include randomized and nonrandomized arms, which then permit comparisons between patients who chose a particular treatment and those who were randomly assigned to it
- **Observational and cohort studies**—studies that involve the identification of patients who are eligible for study and who may receive a specified treatment as part of the study
- **Case-control studies**—studies that involve identifying patients who have good or bad outcomes, then "working back" to find aspects of treatment associated with those differing outcomes

■ **Studies of bundles of therapies**—analyses of the effectiveness, as a whole, of particular packages of treatments

■ **Studies that specifically incorporate, measure, or account for placebo or expectation effects**—patients' hopes, emotional states, energies, and other self-healing processes are not considered extraneous, but are included as part of the therapy's main "mechanism of action"

■ **Attribute-treatment interaction analyses**—a way of accounting for differences in effectiveness outcomes among patients within a study and among different studies of varying design (p. 3)

In an effort to identify major issues in research design in funding proposals submitted to a specific funding program for clinical trials of complementary and alternative medicine for cancer symptom management, a number of problems with scientific methodology were found (Buchanan et al., 2005). Common issues included "unwarranted assumptions about the consistency and standardization of CAM interventions, the need for data-based justifications for the study hypothesis, and the need to implement appropriate quality control and monitoring procedures during the course of the trial" (Buchanan et al., p. 6682). Such problems need to be addressed and resolved, to ensure the rigor and merit of studies of therapies for cancer symptom management as well as the study of a broader array of therapies.

Another important and challenging area for investigators involves the placebo effect and placebo/attention control groups (Gross, 2005). The placebo effect has been studied with respect to pain and analgesia, neuroimmunology, fear, anxiety, and pharmacotherapy and may have the capacity to stimulate dramatic healing (Harrington, 1997). The power of the placebo effect, and cautions that it should not be underestimated, have long been appreciated (Turner, Deyo, Loesser, Von Korff, & Fordyce, 1994). Placebo effects may lead to improvements in well over 50% of subjects in trials of medical therapies. There is evidence that the placebo effect in clinical trials of CAM is similar to the placebo effect observed in clinical trials of conventional medicine (Dorn et al., 2007). Methods to manage placebo effects must be carefully considered in research on complementary therapies. In addition, when assessing the overall effects of a therapy, the potential added impact of the healer and the therapeutic relationship on the outcome must be considered (Quinn, Smith, Ritenbaugh, Swanson, & Watson, 2003). New methods for exploring some therapies are needed, as it is difficult to use sham therapy for some therapies or to identify a suitable control group for others. For example, in the case of the study of aromatherapy to enhance sleep, will subjects remain blinded to condition or will they detect the aroma? If a "sham" aroma is administered to the control group, may it also have undocumented effects beyond a placebo effect?

Complementary therapies are often administered in the context of other therapies. This makes it challenging to differentiate the effects of the complementary therapies from those of other therapies given simultaneously while dissecting out effects of other concomitant disease processes and their treatments. Therapies may have both direct and indirect effects as well as salutary and adverse effects. These must be determined through systematic observation and research. The mechanism of action of many therapies remains elusive. It is hard to understand the effects without framing the therapy within the culture or practice of the healing tradition. Also the terms and measures of outcomes across cultures may not be the same, resulting in barriers for transglobal communication and learning from a commonly held and supported evidence base.

Simply knowing that a therapy may be beneficial is not enough. Questions need to be answered; for example: What are the conditions under which it is effective? What is the dose needed? What dose is too much? How often must a therapy be delivered to achieve a benefit? How long does the effect last? How much therapy should insurers cover? There is a need for studies on the cost-effectiveness of complementary therapies and for research that compares and contrasts complementary therapies with other conventional therapies. There is also a need to examine safety and effectiveness of complementary therapies when used in combination with or as adjuncts to other allopathic pharmacological or nonpharmacological interventions.

Cultural Considerations

Studies of therapies relevant to aging populations, populations at varied ages/developmental stages, and those having varied cultural backgrounds are also needed. These populations present challenges for the design, recruitment, and implementation of studies. Older subjects often have multiple comorbidities and may be taking multiple medications. Language and lack of cultural understanding may pose barriers to the inclusion of new immigrants. Access to young children, adolescents, vulnerable adults, and the unique ethical issues surrounding their recruitment and participation may also be perceived as barriers to the inclusion of these groups.

Research methods and findings from one country can inform the design and implementation of studies in other countries. Findings may be relevant across the globe or interesting nuances or differences can be identified. It is appropriate that native scholars build a culturally relevant evidence base of complementary and alternative therapies for use. The work of nurse scholars in South Korea described in Sidebar 31.1 illustrates this point.

There are other outcomes sought by health care consumers. That a therapy is shown to have beneficial health effects is not the only legitimate reason for its use. Immigrants tend to use complementary and alternative therapies first and then seek conventional medical help if these are not effective (Garcés, Scarinici, & Harrison, 2006). Such patterns and the use of

Sidebar 31.1. *Complementary and Alternative Therapy Implemented by Nurses in Korea*

Sohye Lee, South Korea

In South Korea, complementary and alternative therapies (CATs) based on Chinese medicine and folk remedies have been used since ancient times. Certain types of therapy have known side effects when administered to patients, whereas other types of therapy have been experimentally demonstrated to be effective as used in the treatment of selected health conditions. Many patients who have chronic conditions, such as cancer, stroke, arthritis, cardiovascular disease, diabetes, and obesity, tend to seek CATs to reduce their pain and alleviate anxiety. Today, these therapies have also become very popular for healthy people to improve their health and well-being.

Complementary therapies are practiced by South Korean nurses in the provision of care in many clinical specialty areas. Back, hand, and foot massage, as well as patient position changing, are techniques used by nurses to help patients' body circulation, and to prevent patient pressure ulcers in many intensive care units. Nurse midwifery and obstetric and gynecology nurses use imagery therapy, aromatherapy, reflexology, or hand therapy to reduce patients' pain and anxiety. Anesthesia nurses offer music therapy, aromatherapy, or foot massage to relieve patients' pain and anxiety during and after surgery. Oncology nurses recommend mind therapy (meditation) to their cancer patients for alleviating symptoms and maintaining mental stability.

Hand therapy is one of the CATs performed by nurses in Korea. Many studies support the effectiveness of hand therapy. Park (2011) studied effects of hand therapy on bowel symptoms and stress of college women with irritable bowel syndrome, and she concluded that 3 weeks of hand therapy helped to reduce the bowel symptoms and stress. Ko and her colleagues (2011) investigated the effects of hand therapy on an older woman with knee pain and depression, and the investigators concluded that hand therapy relieved knee pain and depression in the older woman. Research has shown that many nurses are interested in studying hand therapy and they want to develop it as a nursing intervention.

According to the Korean Nurses Association for Complementary and Alternative Therapy, there are many areas being developed: hand therapy, aromatherapy, foot therapy, alternative dietary therapy, hortitherapy, and hypogastric breathing. Even though there still remain the difficulties of applying the CATs to patients without strong scientific foundations, nurse researchers are trying to develop and test these

(continued)

> ## Sidebar 31.1. *Complementary and Alternative Therapy Implemented by Nurses in Korea* *(continued)*
>
> CATs within nursing's holistic view. They also want to develop these CATs as nursing interventions to help their patients in many areas.
>
> ### References
>
> Park, S. H. (2011). *Koryo hand therapy on bowel syndromes and stress of college women with irritable bowel syndrome* (Unpublished master's thesis). Chungang University, Seoul, Korea.
> Ko, H. J., Jung, M. K., & Kwan, Y. H. (2011). Effects of Koryo hand therapy on woman elder's knee pain. *Korea Academia-Industrial Cooperation Society, 12*(9), 4022–4029.

complementary therapies as an alternative to conventional care may also be attributable in part to barriers to conventional care or lack of insurance (Zhang, 2011). Certain therapies may also have cultural significance or be intricately tied with healing traditions; therapies may lead to patients' peace of mind; they may meet patient and family expectations, or lead to their increased satisfaction. If they have come to the United States from other countries, the cultural belief in alternative or complementary medicine is not changed. In considering the use of complementary therapies, the costs, risks, and value to recipients must be carefully weighed.

Longitudinal Studies

Many studies have employed small samples and examined the short-term effects of therapies. If we want to know the real risks and benefits of complementary and alternative therapies, we need longitudinal studies because, with some complementary and alternative therapies, we can determine the severity and occurrence of adverse events only when they are applied on a long-term basis. Although similar longitudinal studies using the same design are performed, different results may be obtained from persons from different cultures. Therefore, it is important that we study complementary and alternative therapy using the same or similar design in other countries and different cultures.

NCCAM's strategic plan created two interrelated offices to address ethnic and cultural issues: The Office of Special Populations (to eliminate racial and ethnic disparities), and the Office of International Health Research (to identify promising international CAM practices, foster rigorous scientific study, and develop effective CAM applications through productive international scientific collaborations while embracing the heritage and practices of indigenous peoples; NCCAM, 2002). NCCAM program initiatives are further described in the next section.

CURRENT STATE OF RESEARCH ON COMPLEMENTARY THERAPIES

As previously noted, chapter authors have included the most recent research and have identified where more research is needed to provide knowledge to guide practice. Specific research challenges include the need for data-based decision support resources for the combination of therapies. Such resources would include data related to potential adverse interactions or the potentiating effects of therapies when given in combination. There is a need for research to be conducted with special populations, including children, frail older adults, and the critically ill. Research is needed to study the effects of complementary therapies in specific health conditions or disease states. Clearly, research lags behind the public's appetite for complementary therapies; knowledge of the putative mechanisms of action, the qualities of therapies, and the predictability of outcomes is uneven across therapies. Historically, the Institute of Medicine report, *Complementary and Alternative Therapies in the United States* (IOM, 2004), provides perhaps the most comprehensive, authoritative summary of the research and knowledge base in the field. The report provides an assessment of what is known about complementary and alternative therapies and their use; it also proposes research methods and priorities for research and product evaluation.

Insistence on the use of standard conventions of scientific inquiry has been helpful in increasing the amount of evidence that has been systematically obtained to provide information for decision making in complementary therapies. However, information is lacking on the appropriate dose and timing of interventions and on those for whom the interventions may have the most beneficial effects. A solid evidence base for complementary therapies would support decision making in broad and complex patient situations. Complementary therapies may have different effects on people of diverse ethnic backgrounds and demographic characteristics. So, too, they may have potentially different indications and effects in persons suffering from differing pathologies or medical conditions. The lack of such information is limiting to practitioners who rely on a more fully developed evidence base, and this may hinder the full integration of the use of complementary therapies in practice.

Often, studies have been done that have relatively small sample sizes; meta-analyses can be conducted on such studies to synthesize findings to estimate "effect size" of therapies when examined across studies. Also, large, multicenter studies may facilitate the recruitment of participants so that studies have overall larger sample sizes to enable testing of hypotheses; such studies are important to scientifically test the effects of alternative and complementary therapies (Singendonk et al., 2013). Synthesis and review articles would also contribute to the availability of well-organized, available information.

The NCCAM, established by Congress in 1999, has as its mission "to define, through rigorous scientific investigation, the usefulness and safety of complementary and alternative medicine interventions and their roles in improving health and health care. The Center's vision is that scientific evidence informs decision making by the public, by health care professionals, and by health policymakers regarding use and integration of these approaches" (National Institutes of Health [NIH], 2013). As previously mentioned, the NCCAM website (nccam.nih.gov) provides updated online information about the research conducted in the area of these therapies. It also provides a listing of clinical trials that are alphabetized by the name of the therapies and further organized by the domains of complementary and alternative therapies (the same domains used to organize chapters in the intervention sections of this book). NCCAM has played a vital role in promoting the generation, organization, and dissemination of data for practice and research. It has fostered a standard language and is a source for arguably the most definitive information, and for funding. The work of this NIH center promises to increase the scientific evidence base and improve the context and delivery of therapies in years to come.

As part of its efforts to achieve its mission, NCCAM has created and funded research centers to foster more rapid development of the scientific knowledge base for the use of complementary and alternative therapies. These centers, their structure, functioning, and productivity have received intensive review, resulting in changes in focus and mechanisms of funding over time (NCCAM, 2012b).

IMPLICATIONS FOR NURSING RESEARCH

There is a great need for nurses and scientists in other disciplines to develop ongoing programs of research related to specific complementary therapies. As primary care providers, nurses are in an excellent position to address patients' need for complementary therapies. Nurses have a vested interest in generating information that can be used to build the knowledge database underlying the use of specific therapies that may benefit patients. They may also generate data that refute the use of therapies or reveal adverse risk/benefit ratios. Nurses have conducted research on a number of complementary therapies. Most nurse scientists are educated in both qualitative and quantitative designs. This gives them an understanding of multiple ways to construct research studies to determine effects of complementary therapies. The need for the expansion and dissemination of evidence and access to it has particular significance for the discipline of nursing and underlies recommendations for future directions in nursing research.

The need to generate information that can be used to build the evidence base for complementary therapies is compelling for nurse scientists.

Specialized clinical expertise of nurse researchers can be used to select therapies to test and to target outcomes of importance to their patient populations. Specialized clinical knowledge has the potential to enhance the identification of instruments that are sensitive enough to assess potential effects of therapies (subjective, objective, or behavioral). Nurses play important roles in generating, disseminating, and using the evidence base for practice.

The *Research Teams of the Future* program of the NIH was initiated to harness and extend advances in science through interdisciplinary research (NIH, 2004). Interdisciplinary collaborations between nurse investigators and investigators from other disciplines who bring complementary strengths from basic science, genetics, complementary therapies, or clinical practice may lead to growth of the knowledge base and its breadth, depth, and relevance, which should ultimately improve the quality of care for patients. Collaborations between scientists who are capable of conducting research across disciplines may lead to new breakthroughs in regard to CAM therapies.

Broadening frames of reference of nurse scientists to include global perspectives, genetic breakthroughs, new technologies, and information from around the world will ensure an appropriate and comprehensive view of the field. The World Health Organization launched a global strategic initiative in 2002 to assist countries in blending complementary therapies with the respective countries' established system(s) of health care (World Health Organization, 2002).

Such global initiatives should serve as catalysts in making information available to practitioners worldwide and should advance the field of complementary/alternative medicine. Electronic means of posting new knowledge, warnings, or updated information on clinical trials speeds the availability of information and literally has the potential to bring a world of information to bear on practice—but only if used. Electronic publishing speeds the transfer of research findings to practice settings. The mandate set forth by prominent medical publishers that requires investigators to enroll their studies in a registry of clinical trials in order for their results to be published in highly distinguished medical journals was a step in the right direction (DeAngelis et al., 2004).

Clinical research is costly. Advanced research training may help to hone nurse-investigators' grant-writing skills to pursue needed funds for investigative work to generate new knowledge in the field. Design skills that permit nurse investigators to rigorously test interventions and advance clinical knowledge about the use of complementary therapies are critical. However, studies conducted in nonclinical settings, including surveys of public use of complementary therapies, are also important. Nursing research is also needed to focus on the costs, relative cost-versus-benefits ratio, and ethical issues surrounding access to and delivery of therapies.

Nurses and other providers have responsibilities to provide the public with guidance in the use of complementary therapies, to interpret and share scientific information, and to contribute to the development of the knowledge base through investigation and research dissemination. Guidelines that are founded in the evidence are clearly needed to set standards for appropriate use of complementary therapies.

Making optimal use of available knowledge and methods to disseminate research electronically and making information available at the point of care are important. However, as noted in the concluding sections of the intervention chapters of this book, many questions remain to be answered for the application of therapies in general and also for gender, culture, age, and comorbidities. More research is needed and it is increasingly recognized that interdisciplinary, multicultural, and transglobal partnerships may be the most fruitful in answering these questions.

Imagine the future with a new culture of care: one that is open and that offers patient-centered care grounded in a well-established evidence base; a future world in which care is viewed through the lens of the patient experience and integrates the best of Western medicine with the best of available nonallopathic remedies. The exploration of therapeutic options includes the consideration of allopathic and nonallopathic remedies by patients and their providers, followed by the evaluation of the outcomes of the therapies selected. With the exploding increase in the use of complementary therapies, there will be new and interesting therapies explored and adopted based on evidence that supports their efficacy. Imagination aside, new information regarding the health practices of immigrant groups, increased global sharing of healing practices, and the public's appetite for new ways to achieve better health, to effect cures, or to forestall aging, all guarantee that the future of the use of complementary therapies by nurses, health care providers, and the public will always be fresh and interesting.

REFERENCES

Agency for Healthcare Research and Quality (AHRQ). (2013). *Effective Health Care Program. Glossary of terms. Evidence-based practice.* Retrieved from http://effectivehealthcare .ahrq.gov/index.cfm/glossary-of-terms/?pageaction=showterm&termid=24

Barnes, P. M., Bloom, B., & Nahin, R. L. (2008, December). Complementary and alternative medicine use among adults and children: United States, 2007. *National health statistics reports; no.12.* Hyattsville, MD: National Center for Health Statistics.

Bent, S. (2008). Herbal medicine in the United States: Review of efficacy, safety and regulation. *Journal of General Internal Medicine, 23*(6), 854–859.

Buchanan, D. R., White, J. D., O'Mara, A. M., Kelaghan, J. W., Smith, W. B., & Minasian, L. M. (2005). Research-design issues in cancer-symptom-management trials using complementary and alternative medicine: Lessons from the National Cancer Institute Community Clinical Oncology Program experience. *Journal of Clinical Oncology, 23*(27), 6682–6689.

DeAngelis, C. D., Drazen, J. M., Frizelle, F. A., Haug, C., Hoey, J., Horton, R., . . . Van Der Weyden, M. B. (2004). Clinical trial registration: A statement from the International Committee of Medical Journal Editors. *Journal of the American Medical Association, 292*(11), 1363–1364.

Dorn, S. D., Kaptchuk, T. J., Park, J. B., Nguyen, L. T., Canenguez, K., Nam, B. H., Lembo, A. J. (2007). A meta-analysis of the placebo response in complementary and alternative medicine trials of irritable bowel syndrome. *Neurogastroenterology & Motility, 19*(8), 630–637.

Duley, L., & Farrell, B. (Eds.). (2002). *Clinical trials.* London, UK: BMJ Books.

Garcés, I. C., Scarinici, I. C., & Harrison, L. (2006). An examination of sociocultural factors associated with health and health care seeking among Latina immigrants. *Journal of Immigrant Health, 8,* 377–385.

Gross, D. (2005). On the merits of attention-control groups. *Research in Nursing & Health, 28,* 93–94.

Gross, D., & Fogg, L. (2001). Clinical trials in the 21st century: The case for participant-centered research. *Research in Nursing & Health, 24,* 530–539.

Harrington, A. (1997). Introduction. In A. Harrington (Ed.), *The placebo effect: An interdisciplinary exploration* (pp. 1–11). Cambridge, MA: Harvard University Press.

Institute of Medicine. (2004). *Complementary and alternative medicine (CAM) in the United States* (Executive Summary, pp. 1–11). Washington, DC: National Academies Press.

Institute of Medicine, Committee on the Use of Complementary and Alternative Medicine by the American Public. (2002). *Executive summary: Complementary and alternative medicine in the United States.* Washington, DC: National Academies Press. Retrieved August 5, 2009, from http://books.nap.edu/catalog/11182.html

Lindquist, R., Tracy, M. F., & Savik, K. (2003). Personal use of complementary and alternative therapies by critical care nurses. *Critical Care Nursing Clinics of North America, 15*(3), 393–399.

Misra, S. (2012). Randomized double blind placebo control studies, the "Gold Standard" in intervention based studies. *Indian Journal of Sexually Transmitted Diseases, 33*(2), 131–134.

National Cancer Institute. (2012). *Summary of the evidence for Laetrile/amygdalin.* Retrieved from http://www.cancer.gov/cancertopics/pdq/cam/laetrile/Health Professional/page7

National Center for Complementary and Alternative Medicine. (2002, June). *Office of International Health Research expanding global horizons of health care 5-year strategic plan.* Retrieved April 26, 2009, from http://nccam.nih.gov/about/plans/oihr/#jump3

National Center for Complementary and Alternative Medicine. (2008, December). *The use of complementary and alternative medicine in the United States.* Retrieved April 27, 2009, from http://nccam.nih.gov/news/camstats/2007/camsurvey_fs1.htm#use

National Center for Complementary and Alternative Medicine. (2012a). *Complementary and alternative medicine: What people aged 50 and older discuss with their health care providers. AARP & NCCAM Survey Report (2010).* Retrieved from http://nccam.nih.gov/news/camstats/2010

National Center for Complementary and Alternative Medicine. (2012b). *NCCAM Research Centers Program expert panel review.* Retrieved from http://nccam.nih.gov/about/plans/centers/expertreview.htm

National Center for Complementary and Alternative Medicine. (2013). *Grants and funding.* Retrieved from http://nccam.nih.gov/grants

National Institutes of Health (2013). The NIH Almanac: National Center for Complementary and Alternative Medicine. Retrieved from http://www.nih.gov/about/almanac/organization/NCCAM.htm

National Institutes of Health. (2004, February). *NIH roadmap for medical research: A briefing by the NIH director and senior staff, February 27, 2004.* Retrieved May 29, 2005, from http://nihroadmap.nih.gov/briefing/executive summary.asp

Natural Standard. (2013). *Natural Standard. The authority on integrative medicine.* Retrieved from www.naturalstandard.com

Pinn, G. (2001). Herbal medicine in oncology. *Australian Family Physician, 30*(6), 575–580.

Quinn, J. F., Smith, M., Ritenbaugh, C., Swanson, K., & Watson, M. J. (2003). Research guidelines for assessing the impact of the healing relationship in clinical nursing. *Alternative Therapies in Health and Medicine, 9*(3), Suppl. A, 65–79.

Singendonk, M., Kaspers, G.-J., Naafs-Wilstra, M., Schouten-van Meeteren, A., Loeffen, J., & Vlieger, A. (2013). High prevalence of complementary and alternative medicine use in the Dutch pediatric oncology population: A multicenter survey. *European Journal of Pediatrics, 172*(1), 31–37.

Tracy, M. F., Lindquist, R., Savik, K., Watanuki, S., Sendelbach, S., Kreitzer, M. J., & Berman, B. (2005). Use of complementary and alternative therapies: A national survey of critical care nurses. *American Journal of Critical Care, 14*(5), 404–414.

Turner, J., Deyo, R., Loesser, J., Von Korff, J., & Fordyce, W. E. (1994). The importance of placebo effects in pain treatment and research. *Journal of the American Medical Association, 271*(10), 1609–1614.

World Health Organization. (1998). *Guidelines for the appropriate use of herbal medicines. WHO's policy on herbal medicines.* Retrieved from http://apps.who.int/medicinedocs/en/d/Jh2945e/2.2.html

World Health Organization. (2002). *WHO traditional medicine strategy: 2002–2005.* Geneva, Switzerland: World Health Organization. Retrieved from http://whqlibdoc.who.int/hq/2002/who_edm_trm_2002.1.pdf

Zhang, L. (2011). *Use of complementary and alternative medicine (CAM) in racial, ethnic and immigrant (REI) populations: Assessing the influence of cultural heritage and access to medical care [dissertation].* Retrieved from http://conservancy.umn.edu/bitstream/104632/1/Zhang_umn_0130E_11782.pdf

Zhang, Y., Peck, K., Spalding, M., Jones, B. G., & Cook, R. L. (2012). Discrepancy between patients' use of and health providers' familiarity with CAM. *Patient Education and Counseling, 89*(3), 399–404.

Index

nursing curricula (*continued*)
governance (*see* Boards of
Nursing)
learning outcomes, 495–496
facilitation, 501
NCLEX-RN certification
(*see* National Council
Licensure Examination)
Nursing Interventions Classification
(Bulechek, Butcher, &
Dochterman), 493
*Nursing: Scope and Standards of
Practice* (ANA), 492–493
nutraceuticals
Coenzyme Q10, 369–370
cultural considerations, 375–376
definition, 366
future research, 376
glucosamine and chondroitin
sulfate, 368–369
outcome measures, 372–373
patient use assessment, 371
probiotics, 370
safety mechanisms, 373
use, 373–375
web resources, 372
See also functional foods
Nutrition Labeling and Health Act
(1989), 347

observational studies, 531
Office of Alternative Medicine.
See National Center for
Complementary and
Alternative Medicine
(NCCAM)
ointments, 325
older adults
exercise interventions, 309–310,
313 (*see also* Tai Chi; yoga)
light therapy, 389–390
massage therapy concerns, 264
music intervention concerns,
106–107
storytelling practices, 222–223
therapeutic humor, 132–133
optimal healing environment
case study applications, 62–65

cultural applications, 65
elements, 56–57
in home space, 66
physical structure
design strategies, 58–60
biophilic design, 59–61
case studies, 62–65
chronotherapeutics, 61–62
cultural considerations, 65–68
orality, 215–216
osteoarthritis
glucosamine and chondroitin
sulfate use, 368–369
imagery interventions, 84
magnet therapy, 482

pain management
acupressure treatment, 451–452
animal-assisted therapy, 234–235
imagery techniques, 82–86
magnet therapy, 481, 482
massage therapy, 258, 266
reflexology, 466–467
Reiki practice, 426–427
relaxation techniques, 292
Pain Rehabilitation Center at Mayo
Clinic, 516–517
Palestine, complementary therapies
in, 11–12
palliative care, 21–22
Parkinson's disease, 483
Passy-Muir tracheal valves, 47
Pathways (Minnesota), 519
Patient Protection and Affordable
Care Act, 9
patient space in health care facilities,
62, 63, 64–65
Paws 4 Therapy organization, 246
percussion strokes, 260
peripheral artery disease, 311
permanent magnets, 477–478
efficacy, 481, 482
Perú
Healing Touch (HT) practice,
409–410
journaling use, 212–213
Pet Partners (Delta Foundation
[Society]), 230, 246